T0251393

Edited by
Ingrid Kohlstadt, MD, MPH
Kenneth Cintron, MD, MBA

Metabolic Therapies in Orthopedics

Second Edition

Edited by
Ingrid Kohlstadt, MD, MPH
Kenneth Cintron, MD, MBA

Metabolic Therapies in Orthopedics

Second Edition

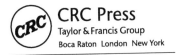

CRC Press
Taylor & Francis Group
Boca Raton   London   New York

CRC Press is an imprint of the
Taylor & Francis Group, an **informa** business

CRC Press
Taylor & Francis Group
6000 Broken Sound Parkway NW, Suite 300
Boca Raton, FL 33487-2742

First issued in paperback 2021

© 2019 by Taylor & Francis Group, LLC
CRC Press is an imprint of Taylor & Francis Group, an Informa business

No claim to original U.S. Government works

Printed on acid-free paper

ISBN-13: 978-1-138-03921-6 (hbk)
ISBN-13: 978-1-03-209485-4 (pbk)

Visit the Taylor & Francis Web site at
http://www.taylorandfrancis.com

and the CRC Press Web site at
http://www.crcpress.com

Contents

Preface...ix
Acknowledgments...xi
Editors..xiii
Contributors..xv

SECTION I Cross-Cutting Technologies

Chapter 1 Regenerative Orthopedics Enabled by Cross-Cutting Technologies 3

   Kenneth Cintron, MD, MBA

Chapter 2 Orthogenomics: Genome-Directed Therapies in Orthopedics 21

   Joseph R. Veltmann, PhD, DCCN and Roberta L. Kline, MD

Chapter 3 Predictive Biomarkers in Personalized Laboratory Diagnoses and Best Practices Outcome Monitoring for Musculoskeletal Health.......................................39

   Russell Jaffe MD, PhD, CCN and Jayashree Mani, MS, CCN

Chapter 4 Veterinary Medicine's Advances in Regenerative Orthopedics.................................59

   Sophie H. Bogers, BVSc, MVSc, PhD and Jennifer G. Barrett, DVM, PhD

Chapter 5 Biotensegrity: How Ultrasound Diagnostics Guide Regenerative Orthopedic Therapies to Restore Biomechanical Function..93

   Bradley D. Fullerton, MD

Chapter 6 Photobiomodulation Therapy in Orthopedics: Metabolic Effects 113

   Michael R. Hamblin, PhD

SECTION II Clinical Approaches to Preventing and Treating Metabolic Dysfunction

Chapter 7 Safeguarding Musculoskeletal Structures from Food Technology's Untoward Metabolic Effects 141

   Ingrid Kohlstadt, MD, MPH

Chapter 8 Inflammatory Responses Acquired Following Environmental Exposures Are Involved in Pathogenesis of Musculoskeletal Pain..159

   Ritchie C. Shoemaker, MD and James C. Ryan, PhD

Chapter 9 Periodontal Disease: Treatable, Nutrition-Related, and with Systemic Repercussions 185

David Kennedy, DDS

Chapter 10 Reduction in Orthopedic Conditions through Teledontic Treatment of Pharyngorofacial Disorders 193

Joseph Yousefian, DMD, MS and Michael N. Brown, DC, MD

Chapter 11 Drug-Related Muscular Pain 215

Sahar Swidan, PharmD

Chapter 12 Metabolic Interventions for Sarcopenic Obesity 223

Gabrielle Lyon, DO and Jamie I. Baum, PhD

Chapter 13 Drug-Related Sarcopenia 239

Sahar Swidan, PharmD

Chapter 14 Sex Hormones and Their Impact on Sarcopenia and Osteoporosis 251

Pamela W. Smith, MD, MPH, MS

Chapter 15 Treating the Dysmetabolism Underlying Osteoporosis 263

Xaviour Walker, MD, MPH, DTMH and Joseph Lamb, MD

Chapter 16 Nutritional Status and Interventions for Reducing Stress Fracture Risk among Military Personnel 283

James McClung, PhD

SECTION III   Metabolic Therapies for Specific Orthopedic Conditions

Chapter 17 Perioperative Metabolic Therapies in Orthopedics 293

Frederick T. Sutter MD, MBA

Chapter 18 Metabolic Therapies for Muscle Injury 319

Ana V. Cintrón, MD and Kenneth Cintron, MD, MBA

Chapter 19 Tendinopathy: Addressing the Chronic Pain and Pathophysiology 339

David Musnick, MD

Chapter 20 Metabolic Therapies in the Management of Heel Pain...................................349

Emily M. Splichal, DPM, MS

Chapter 21 Fascial Syndromes: Emerging, Treatable Contributors to Musculoskeletal Pain 357

David Lesondak, BCSI, ATSI, FST, FFT

Chapter 22 Metabolic Approaches to the Treatment of Back Pain..369

Carrie Diulus, MD and Patrick Hanaway, MD

Chapter 23 Optimizing Metabolism to Treat Fractures and Prevent Nonunion........................389

Jacob Wilson, MD, Scott Boden, MD, Kenneth Cintron, MD, MBA and
Mara Schenker, MD

Chapter 24 Treating the Underlying Causes of Synovitis, Degenerative Joint Disease and
Osteoarthritis in Primary Care 403

John C. Cline, MD, BSc

Chapter 25 Osteoarthritis: Comprehensive Treatment 419

David Musnick, MD and Richard D. Batson, ND

Chapter 26 Integrative Approaches to Autoimmune Arthritis 449

George E. Muñoz, MD

Index...465

Preface

ENABLING A PERSONALIZED APPROACH

Medicine is personalized. The best of clinical medicine draws from all available resources to tailor a treatment for each patient. The gold standard of medical care is and should be an "n" of 1, epidemiologically speaking. This textbook explores what it means to deliver n of 1 care to patients with musculoskeletal conditions.

One characteristic of personalized medicine is that assessment reaches beyond population averages. Selection and dosing of prescription medications involves individual patient data such as genetics, environmental exposures, lifestyle and metabolomics. The timing of and the need for palliative surgery considers emerging therapies such as photobiomodulation, biotensegrity, teledontics and molecular regenerative approaches. Additionally, pain control for often chronic musculoskeletal conditions is opioid-sparing because treatment can be more precise by modifying the patient's specific metabolic pathways.

WHY PROACTIVE ORTHOPEDICS WORKS

Personalized medicine enables prevention. It allows patients to participate more fully in their care, effectively replacing reactive approaches to orthopedics.

Proactive orthopedics works with the body's innate healing mechanisms. We know that ancient physicians of both East and West marveled at the powerful healing from within elicited by diet, lifestyle and simple metabolic approaches. Today we see emerging technologies buttressing Antiquity's practice of observing, describing and quantifying the human body's regenerative potential. 21st Century therapies accelerate the human body's self-healing mechanisms.

The musculoskeletal system is especially responsive to the innate healing mechanisms. The explanation for the suppleness of muscle, bone and connective tissue is rooted in the fundamentals of metabolism. Look at it like this: Musculoskeletal structures are like nutrient warehouses. When pH drops, bone is metabolized for buffering. When fat metabolism is impaired muscle protein is catabolized for energy. Also, system-wide inflammation inhibits optimal repair of soft tissues. Further, the study of scaling and proportions called allometry demonstrates how sarcopenic obesity contributes to dehydration, detoxification and utilization of fat-soluble nutrients. Correcting metabolism in each of these examples confers a healing advantage to a beleaguered musculoskeletal system.

CREDIBILITY FOR THE INFORMATION AGE

Emerging therapies and the comprehensive evidence behind them are not enough to justify the compilation of chapter authors for this book. Our combined vision for how this book can serve health care professionals and their patients reach even further. It harmonizes the expert opinions of 35 thought leaders in diverse specialties across the practice of medicine. Their consensus of opinion provides readers with a resource greater than the sum of its chapters.

Both authoritative and patient-focused, *Metabolic Therapies in Orthopedics, 2nd Edition* gives health care practitioner's a solid hook on which to confidently hang their stethoscope, figuratively speaking. It's practical, written by clinicians for clinicians. These clinicians "walk the talk," providing empowerment by teaching effective, safe and valuable practice guidelines. Their work serves the interest of important constituencies of the healthcare system, patients, families, providers, and the community. It's a practical tool, one can translate its contents into a realistic medical practice.

Designed to be used efficiently, the chapters are intended to save readers time by synthesizing a broad and fast-moving field of medicine. The authors' collective knowledge is an unprecedented synthesis of orthopedic medicine, which draws from informatics, genomics, microbiology, ecology, biophysics, agriculture, pharmacology, and veterinary medicine.

The Information Age can't diminish the value of textbooks that are created with the forethought utilized for creating this reference book. If anything, the internet increases the book's value, because of health care practitioners' growing need for discernment. The internet promulgates valuable information, unsubstantiated and unripe therapies, sometimes marketed directly to our proactive patients. If we are savvy we concurrently reach for emerging evidence-based therapies and help patients navigate around modern iterations of P.T. Barnum-style hoaxes, and "fake news," call them what you want. This book empowers health care providers to readily distinguish hope from hype, and engenders forward-thinking healers and adherers to "first-do-no-harm."

CONTINUING THE CALL FROM ONE DECADE TO THE NEXT

Metabolic Therapies in Orthopedics, 2nd Edition stands on the sturdy shoulders of its first edition published in 2006 under the title *Scientific Evidence for Musculoskeletal, Bariatric and Sports Nutrition*. Still in print, the book was the first to be written by doctors for doctors as a synthesis of the scientific evidence supporting metabolic therapies for musculoskeletal conditions. The team of experts include new luminaries and returning authors who present the next decade of breakthroughs:

- New opioid-sparing pain management strategies
- How orthopedic surgeons use metabolic therapies to prevent delayed union of bone
- Metabolic therapies that restructure the pharmacocentric medical framework
- Metabolic strategies for improving surgical outcomes
- Orthogenomics
- Photobiomodulation
- Regenerative orthopedic therapies including those used in veterinary medicine with anticipated human uses in the near future
- Improving oxygenation
- Treating fascia, the body's ancient and overlooked metabolic roads

Please join the conversation at *www.BetterOrthopedics.com*, the book's dedicated website. And on behalf of the entire Metabolic Therapies in Orthopedics, 2nd Edition team, thank you for using this book to put "personalized" back into clinical medicine.

ABOUT HELPING TODAY'S PATIENTS

This book is written by doctors for doctors. For medical legal purposes it is important to note that this book does not claim to represent guidelines, recommendations, or the current standard of medical care. On behalf of the authors and editorial staff, I thank you for caring and going the extra step in finding healing answers for your patients.

Acknowledgments

Our textbook has a unique feature, its own website. The website www.BetterOthopedics.com is a forum to bring together clinicians and researchers from all fields of medicine. The website is possible because of the vision and generosity of many people.

We would like to acknowledge the support of Home Orthopedics and its president Mr. Jesus Rodriguez for his unconditional help regarding www.BetterOrthopedics.com. Mr. Nelson Rodriguez, president of RMC and Arthrex of Puerto Rico has been a great supporter since the early days of the project.

They stand out and are strong believers of innovation, perseverance and hard work. They believe in our vision and goals of improving results and the quality of life of our orthopedic patients – our gratitude to both.

Editors

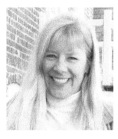

Dr. Ingrid Kohlstadt, M.D., M.P.H. is a 1993 physician graduate of Johns Hopkins School of Medicine and is currently a faculty associate at Johns Hopkins Bloomberg School of Public Health, Center for Human Nutrition. Dr. Kohlstadt earned a Master's Degree in Public Health to add epidemiology and tropical medicine to her skills in diagnosing and treating metabolic conditions. She is a Fellow of the American College of Nutrition and a Fellow of the American College of Preventive Medicine.

Dr. Kohlstadt specializes in optimizing the body's metabolism for vibrant health and longevity. On this topic she conducts research and lectures at Johns Hopkins University; consults for Gerson Lehrman Group; contributes to TIME and Townsend Letter; and unites thought leaders from around the world by editing two prominent medical references Advancing Medicine with Food and Nutrients commencing its 3rd edition and Metabolic Therapies in Orthopedics, now in its 2nd edition.

Dr. Kohlstadt has set out to repair the metabolism of her patients in the Indian Health Service, for the Florida Orthopaedic Institute, with the Johns Hopkins Weight Management Center, and on every continent including as station doctor in Antarctica.

Augmenting her clinical efforts Dr. Kohlstadt has taken a public health approach to optimizing metabolism. She was an inaugural U.S. Food and Drug Administration Commissioner's Fellow in the Office of Pediatric Therapeutics; directed a state capitol's health department; assists hospitals with interpreting medical records through FairCode Associates; and served at the CDC and the USDA.

Because longevity starts with youth, Dr. Kohlstadt has developed and researched an intervention for medically at-risk youth. Her research findings compelled her into social entrepreneurship. She founded NutriBee National Nutrition Competition and serves as its executive director. Dr. Kohlstadt newly brings her longstanding professional passion - innovating metabolic shortcuts to longevity - to Carolina Longevity Institute.

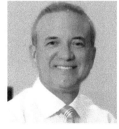

Dr. Kenneth Cintron, M.D, M.B.A. was born and raised in Ponce, Puerto Rico. During his youth days he was an elite baseball player and an outstanding student. He completed his bachelor and medical degree from the University of Puerto Rico with honors. Moved for his interest in sports, he became an orthopedic surgeon and then completed a Foot and Ankle surgery fellowship from Emory University during the Olympic year of 1996. Recently, he obtained an MBA degree from the Physician Executive program of the University of Tennessee in Knoxville.

Dr. Cintron is board certified by the American Academy of Orthopedic Surgeons and has more than 20 years of clinical experience. He is currently the Chief of Orthopedics at the Veterans Administration Hospital in San Juan and holds an Ad honorem appointment from the Department of Orthopedic Surgery of the University of Puerto Rico. Has served as a team physician in Puerto Rico and in the USA for multiple professional, college and national athletic teams. He has also served in several national and international athletic competitions like Central-American, Pan-American and Olympic Games. He is past-president of the Society of Orthopedic and Traumatology Surgeons of Puerto Rico and current President of the Caribbean, Mexico and Central-American Region for the Latino-American Society of Orthopedic and Traumatology Surgeons.

He has a kind interest and special training in wellness, nutrition and non-toxic therapies. His passion for the emerging field of Functional Medicine started nine years ago when her older daughter was diagnosed with type 1 diabetes at 14 years of age. He decided then to join the American Academy of Anti-Aging Medicine and completed a two year fellowship in Functional, Integrative and Regenerative Medicine. He was president and owner of BodylogicMD of San Juan, a national network of highly trained physicians specializing in natural bio-identical hormone replacement therapy. His training has helped tremendously his daughter and family to enjoy and optimize their health and lifestyle. He has published and collaborate in multiple scientific articles, studies and international congresses. Dr. Cintron has a double board certification in both Orthopedic Surgery (AAOS) and Integrative Medicine (ABOIM).

The medical community has welcomed his visionary concept of applying preventative and nutritional medicine to the field of orthopedics and regenerative medicine. His experience in Sports medicine and his passion for this new field has transformed the way he practices the art of medicine. Dr. Cintron has successfully incorporated into his practice the important concepts of age management including cellular physiology, epigenetics, nutrigenomics, regenerative medicine, hormone balance and metabolic optimization to improve the quality of life and the athletic performance of his patients.

Contributors

Jennifer G. Barrett, DVM, PhD, Diplomate ACVS, Diplomate ACVSMR
Professor of Equine Surgery at the Marion duPont Scott Equine Medical Center
Virginia Tech
Leesburg, VA
and
Founding director of the North American Veterinary Regenerative Medicine Association
and
Chief Editor of the Veterinary Regenerative Medicine specialty section in the *Frontiers in Veterinary Science* journal.
and
Member of the American Veterinary Medical Association.

Richard D. Batson, ND, ABAAHP
Co-founder and Medical Director of Neurevolution Medicine, LLC
Bellevue, WA
and
Naturopathic physician,
WA

Jamie I. Baum, PhD
Associate Professor
Director, Center for Human Nutrition
Department of Food Science
University of Arkansas
Fayetteville, AR

Scott Boden, MD
Chief Medical Officer/Chief Quality Officer at Emory University Orthopedics and Spine Hospital
Atlanta, GA
and
Professor of Orthopaedic Surgery at the Emory University School of Medicine
and
Vice-Chairman of the Department of Orthopaedics
and
Director of Emory Orthopaedics & Spine Center

Sophie H. Bogers BVSc, MVSc, PhD
College of Biomedical and Veterinary Sciences
Virginia Tech
Blacksburg, VA
and
Diplomate of the American College of Veterinary Surgeons (Large Animal)

Michael N. Brown, DC, MD
Interventional Regenerative Orthopedic Medicine Institute (IROM)
Belleveue, WA

Ana V. Cintrón, MD, FAAPMR
Diplomate of the American Board of Physical Medicine & Rehabilitation
Assistant Professor - Department of Physical Medicine & Rehabilitation of the University of Puerto Rico of School of Medicine
and
Attending physician at the VA Caribbean Healthcare System,
Department of Physical Medicine & Rehabilitation
and
Medical Director of the VA Polytrauma Amputation Network System
and
Member of the Executive Board of the Puerto Rico Sports Medicine Federation

Kenneth Cintron, MD, MBA, FAAOS
University of Puerto Rico School of Medicine
San Juan, Puerto Rico

John Cline, MD, BSc., IFMCP
Cline Medical Center
Nanaimo, British Columbia, Canada

Carrie Diulus, MD
Crystal Clinic Orthopaedic Center
Akron, OH

Bradley D. Fullerton, MD, FAAPMR
Diplomate of the American Board of Physical
Medicine & Rehabilitation
and
Clinical Assistant Professor, Department of
Internal Medicine, Texas A&M College of
Medicine
and
Past President, American Association of
Orthopaedic Medicine (AAOM)
and
Private practice at ProloAustin
Austin, TX

Michael R Hamblin, PhD
Department of Dermatology
Harvard Medical School
Boston, MA
and
Wellman Center for Photomedicine
Massachusetts General Hospital
Boston, MA
and
Harvard-MIT Division of Health Sciences and
Technology
Cambridge, MA

Patrick Hanaway, MD
Cleveland Clinic Center for Functional
Medicine
Cleveland, OH

Russell Jaffe, MD, PhD, CCN
FASCP, FACN, FACAAI, FRCM
Fellow, Health Studies Collegium
Adjunct Faculty, George Washington Medical
School
Chairman and CEO, PERQUE® Integrative
Health/Health Studies Collegium
Ashburn, VA
and
Chairman and CEO, ELISA/ACT®
Biotechnologies
Sterling, VA
and
Chairman and CEO, MAGique
BioTherapeutics™
Vienna, VA

Roberta L. Kline, MD, FACOG
Co-Founder, CEO
Genoma International
Santa Fe, NM

David Kennedy, DDS
International Academy of Oral Medicine and
Toxicology
San Diego, CA

Ingrid Kohlstadt MD, MPH, FACN, FACPM
Fellow of the American College of Nutrition
Fellow of the American College of Preventive
Medicine
Associate, Johns Hopkins University
Center for Human Nutrition
Baltimore, MD
and
Founding Director, NutriBee National
Nutrition Competition, Inc.
Annapolis, MD

Joseph Lamb, MD
St. Thomas Medical Group
Hypertension Institute of Nashville
Nashville, TN
and
Medical Director
The Hughes Center for Research and
Innovation
Nature's Sunshine Products
Lehi, UT

**David Lesondak, BCSI, ATSI, FFT,
FST, VMT**
University of Pittsburgh Medical Center
Center for Integrative Medicine
Pittsburgh, PA

Gabrielle Lyon, DO
The Ash Center for Comprehensive Medicine
New York, NY

Jayashree Mani, MS, CCN
Nutrition Specialist and Clinical Coordinator
PERQUE Integrative Health
ELISA/ACT Biotechnologies
Ashburn, VA

James P. McClung, MS, PhD
Chief, Military Nutrition Division
US Army Research Institute of Environmental
Medicine
Natick, MA

George E. Muñoz, MD
Chief, Integrative Rheumatology AARA
(American Arthritis & Rheumatology
Associates)
and
Chief Medical Officer
The Oasis Institute
Miami, FL

David Musnick, MD
Board Certified in Sports Medicine, Functional
Medicine and Internal Medicine practice
Peak Medicine Center
Bellevue, WA
and
Clinical Instructor in Sport Medicine
University of Washington
Seattle, WA

James C. Ryan, PhD
Co-Founder
Progene Dx, LLC
Deerfield Beach, FL

Mara L. Schenker, MD
Emory University Orthopaedic Surgery
Grady Memorial Hospital
Atlanta, GA

Ritchie C. Shoemaker, MD
Center for Research on Biotoxin Associated
Illnesses
Pocomoke, MD

Pamela W. Smith, MD, MPH, MS
Center for Personalized Medicine
Co-Director, Masters Program in Medical
Sciences with a concentration in Metabolic and
Nutritional Medicine
Morsani College of Medicine
University of South Florida
Tampa, FL

Emily M. Splichal, DPM, MS
Center for Functional and Regenerative
Podiatric Medicine
Fellow of the American Academy of Antiaging
Medicine
New York, NY

Frederick Sutter, MD, MBA
Center for Wellness Medicine
Annapolis, MD

**Sahar Swidan, Pharm.D., BCPS, ABAAHP,
FAARM, FACA**
President and Chief Executive Officer
Pharmacy Solutions
Ann Arbor, MI
and
Executive Director
Slyngshot Health
Chicago, IL
and
Adjunct Associate Professor
George Washington University
School of Medicine
Washington, D.C.

Joseph R. Veltmann, PHD, FAAIM, DCCN
Co-Founder and Chief Science Officer
Genoma International
Santa Fe, NM

Xaviour Walker, MD, MPH, DTMH
Geriatrician, Hospitalist, Public Health and
Preventive Medicine Physician
Kaiser Permanente
Orange, CA
and
University of California
Irvine, CA

Jacob Wilson, MD
Emory University Orthopedics
Atlanta, GA

Joseph Z. Yousefian, DMD, MS, MA
Diplomate, American Board of Orthodontics
Diplomate, American Board of Dental Sleep
Medicine
Bellevue, WA

Section I

Cross-Cutting Technologies

1 Regenerative Orthopedics Enabled by Cross-Cutting Technologies

Kenneth Cintron, MD, MBA, FAAOS, ABOIM

INTRODUCTION

Biologic therapies for tissue repair and regeneration has been a topic of intense interest during the last 20 years. As we recognize the innate healing potential of the human body, the goal is to repair or replace damaged or diseased tissue with healthy and functional tissue that replicates the pre-injury state. The use of orthobiologics by trained providers has been the core of treatments and successful outcomes for many musculoskeletal conditions in patients. Continued research and technologic advances are making platelet-rich plasma (PRP) and stem cells increasingly effective and safe options for the clinical practice of regenerative orthopedics. In this chapter, we present current and potential future regenerative therapies for common musculoskeletal issues.

ORTHOBIOLOGICS

PRP

PRP was first utilized by Ferrari et al. in 1987 to stop blood loss in open heart surgery [1]. Since then, PRP has been used extensively in dentistry, orthopedics, ophthalmology, neurosurgery, maxillofacial surgery, and cosmetic surgery for over 30 years. PRP therapy appears to augment the body's own healing process by reducing pain and improving function. Multiple studies have demonstrated these outcomes in a variety of treatments for tendinopathies, cartilage degenerative diseases, muscle injuries, and arthroscopic repair. PRP is thought to work via growth factors, anti-inflammatory cytokines, and chemokines that help inhibit the destruction or even promote the regeneration of connective tissue [2].

How Does PRP Work?

A basic definition of PRP can be described as "a volume of plasma that has a platelet count above baseline [of whole blood]." However, in the clinical setting this concentration can be over 200% [3]. Platelets are a crucial component not only of hemostasis, but also of tissue repair [4]. They contain over 1100 proteins that act as growth factors, cytokines, chemokines, or enzymes involved in the reparative process [5]. Most of these growth factors and cytokines are thought to be contained in organelles called *α-granules*. When platelets are activated, usually by either *in vivo* exposure of endothelial collagen, shear forces, the von Willebrand factor, or thrombin, they release the contents of these granules [4].

The most studied growth factors (GF) are platelet-derived growth factor (PDGF), transforming growth factor (TGF-β), platelet derived angiogenesis factor (PDAF), vascular endothelial growth factor (VEGF), epidermal growth factor (EGF), platelet-derived endothelial growth factor (PDEGF), epithelial cell growth factor (ECGF), and insulin-like growth factor (IGF-I) [3, 4, 6]. Studies have shown that these factors may promote migration of reparative cells, differentiation of mesenchymal stem cells into connective tissue, angiogenesis, cellular proliferation, and matrix synthesis [7, 8].

PRP Preparation

The fundamental process of creating PRP usually begins with the collection of whole blood through venipuncture in the presence of an anticoagulant to prevent premature activation of platelets through the clotting cascade. In most cases, PRP is prepared using the patient's own platelets, which is advantageous because of the unlikely probability of provoking an immune response (Figure 1.1) [4]. There are three different methods of PRP preparation: (a) blood filtration and plateletpheresis, which allows the production of PRP products with high concentrations of human platelets, growth factors, and low numbers of contaminating leucocyte; (b) centrifugation by a "single-spinning" technique that allows for a concentration of platelets up to three times higher than baseline level, while also avoiding the presence of leukocytes; (c) centrifugation by a "double-spinning" technique, from which a higher concentration of platelets, up to eight times higher than baseline level, may be produced, while also containing a high content of leukocytes [3].

A basic understanding of these techniques is important to understand the scientific background behind the clinical process.

There are four different preparations of PRP as suggested by Dohan Ehrenfast [9]: P-PRP (pure platelet-rich plasma, which contains low levels of leukocytes), L-PRP (leukocyte-rich PRP), P-PRF (platelet-rich fibrin matrix with low levels of leukocytes), and L-PRF (leukocyte-rich and platelet-rich fibrin matrix) [3, 8]. Essentially, these products can vary in (a) the volume of whole blood harvested, which correlates with platelet concentration; (b) the inclusion or exclusion of leukocytes; (c) the exogenous activation of platelets, through either $CaCl2$, thrombin, or ultraviolet radiation creating an upregulation of leukocyte anti-inflammatory cytokines and downregulation of pro-inflammatory cytokines; and (d) the formation of a fibrin matrix [9].

Platelet-rich fibrin matrices have a higher concentration of platelets than other PRP formulations and the shape of a moldable tri-dimensional gel [10]. This gel can be readily applied to sutures or bone or cartilage defect sites. In addition, the fibrin-rich matrix has been shown to delay the release of growth factors for up to 7 days, whereas normally platelets release all their GFs in about an hour in the absence of a fibrin matrix or other type of scaffold [5, 11]. These fibrin matrices, especially the L-PRF formulation, have been successfully used in rotator cuff repair procedures and in maxillofacial surgery [12].

The inclusion of leukocytes in PRP is a topic of debate in literature. L-PRP has demonstrated to have antimicrobial effects and a greater presence of catabolic cytokines such as matrix metalloproteinase-9 (MMP-9) and interleukin-1 β (IL-1β), as well as a greater number of platelets [13].

PROCESS OF **PRP THERAPY**

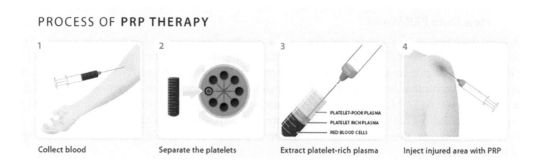

| Collect blood | Separate the platelets | Extract platelet-rich plasma | Inject injured area with PRP |

FIGURE 1.1 Process of PRP therapy. Step 1. 30–60 ml of blood is drawn from the patient's arm. Step 2. The blood is then placed in a centrifuge. The centrifuge spins and separates the platelets from the rest of the blood components. Step 3. 3–6 ml of platelet-rich plasma is extracted. Step 4. Using the concentrated platelets, the growth factors are increased many times, which promotes relief and stops inflammation.

However, in a recent preclinical study, L-PRP seems to have caused greater inflammatory reactions and adverse effects than P-PRP following the injection at the lesion site [14]. Moreover, a study by Filardo et al. compared the efficacy and safety of a single-spinning prepared PRP and a double-spinning prepared PRP in osteoarthritic (OA) knees, which resulted in significantly more adverse events (pain and swelling) detected in the group treated with the PRP developed by the double-spinning approach [15]. However, it should be noted that both groups resulted in statistically significant beneficial outcomes in the treatment of knee OA. Currently, more studies are conducted to ensure the efficacy, advantages, and safety of leukocyte-rich PRP formulations.

Clinical Applications of PRP

The general indication for offering PRP seems to be in patients with specific isolated injuries where other standard-of-care treatments such as corticosteroid therapy may pose a greater systemic risk. It may become a therapy for patients that have utilized other standard-of-care treatments with minimal benefit and patients interested in nonsurgical procedures [4]. It has been observed that younger patients with less severe forms of OA respond more favorably to PRP [16, 3].

The overwhelming recent literature for the use of PRP in orthopedics and sports medicine has increased the preclinical and clinical evidence supporting its use as a treatment option [17]. Here, we describe some of the most current clinical studies on the treatment of tendinopathies, osteoarthritis, and orthopedic reconstructive surgery.

Tendinopathies

PRP has been utilized in the treatment of lateral epicondylitis (LE) with significant beneficial results [18, 4]. In a randomized control trial (RCT), the authors were trying to determine the effectiveness of PRP compared with corticosteroid injections in patients with chronic LE with a 2-year follow-up. One hundred patients with chronic lateral epicondylitis were randomly assigned to a L-PRP injection or the corticosteroid injection using a peppering technique with no activating agents into the common extensor tendon. The study showed statically significant reduced pain (VAS scores) and increased functionality (DASH) in the group treated with L-PRP and no serious complications after a 2-year follow-up.

Recently, in a prospective multicenter cohort study, PRP was found to be an effective treatment modality for distal biceps tendonitis. Twelve patients were recruited and were injected with L-PRP under ultrasound guidance into the distal biceps tendon. After a median follow-up time of 47 months, all patients showed significant improvement in pain and functional outcome. Median resting VAS score improved from 6 to 0.5, and the activity VAS score improved from 8 to 2.5. In addition, elbow functional assessment scores improved from 63 to 90 [19].

According to the literature, the use of PRP in Achilles tendinopathy has mixed results. One RCT found no significant difference in complete Achilles tendon tears between PRP and placebo [20]. Others have noted better results utilizing PRP in partial Achilles tendon tears [4]. In this radiological study, 30 patients suffering from chronic pain and degeneration of the Achilles tendon were treated with PRP. Six months after treatment, a magnetic resonance imaging (MRI) of the tendon showed that most lesions had healed (27 out of 29 MRIs) [21]. Even though there is good evidence showing the effectiveness of PRP on Achilles tendinopathies, further studies need to be performed.

Osteoarthritis

The orthopedic literature has overwhelming studies showing the effectiveness and safety of PRP for OA (Figure 1.2). In a recent meta-analysis of 14 RCTs, PRP was found to be more effective at reducing pain and increasing functional outcomes in OA knees when compared to hyaluronic acid (HA), corticosteroid, ozone, and saline-placebo intra-articular injections [7, 16, 22]. Data analysis consistently showed that intra-articular PRP injections worked better to significantly reduce knee pain and improve physical function and total WOMAC scores than control or other standard intra-articular injections. Such superiority was observed at 3, 6, and 12 months after treatment [16].

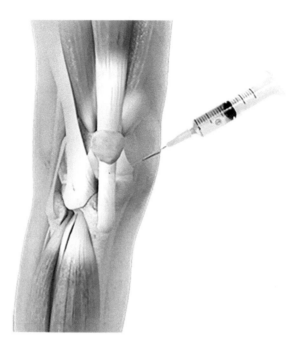

FIGURE 1.2   Meta-analyses have concluded that PRP is an effective and safe treatment for knee osteoarthritis.

This temporal effect has varied slightly throughout studies. One study by Filardo et al. reported that 90 patients affected by chronic degenerative joint of the knee and treated with PRP intra-artic-ular injections yielded a sustained good clinical outcome at 6-month follow-up. It is hypothesized that this temporal effect of PRP consists in reducing synovial membrane hyperplasia and modu-lating the cytokine level in the arthritic joint, rather than a long-lasting chondro-regenerative and chondro-protective effect [15]. A review article by Marmotti et al. proposed some suggestions for yielding best results with PRP treatment. According to this article, PRP works best (a) on younger patients, (b) on those with a lower degree of cartilage degeneration, (c) on those of male gender, (d) on those with a low BMI, and (e) after short-term follow-up, 9 months being the median duration of the efficacy of PRP injections [3].

The amount of PRP injections and timing between injections have been a matter of debate. Whereas some cases have shown positive effects with only one injection, other RCTs have found increased pain relief and functional outcomes compared to HA utilizing three or more weekly injections [7]. In terms of OA of the hip, ankle, and shoulder, there are only a few high-level stud-ies available with varying and promising results. Multiple RCTs, comparative studies, reviews, and meta-analyses have concluded that PRP is an effective and safe treatment for knee OA [2, 3, 9, 16].

Rotator Cuff Injuries

Research has shown positive results in the use of PRP for rotator cuff tear treatment, specifically grade 1 and 2 partial tears (Figure 1.3). In a sub-group of a 2-year follow up prospective RCT, they found increased strength upon external rotation (SER) and good shoulder constant scores in patients treated with injections of activated double-spin PRP. For patients with complete rotator cuff tears, there was reduction in pain only during the first month of recovery when compared to the control group. The authors found PRP to decrease post-operative pain at early follow-ups and to improve the early healing process after rotator cuff repair [22]. Various authors also agreed a preferential use of PRP injections for the treatment of partial tears [4]. In terms of PRP's use in surgical repair, a study by Chahal et al. did not find any change in the incidence of re-lesions [23].

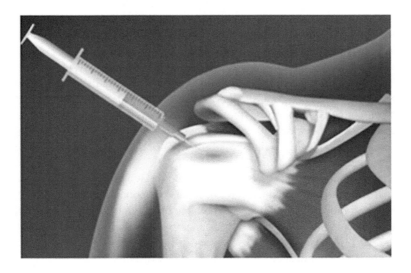

FIGURE 1.3 Studies have shown that PRP improves postoperative pain and the early healing process after rotator cuff repair.

ACL Reconstruction

According to the literature, PRP use in ACL reconstruction is still being discussed. Pre-clinical studies have shown improvements in ACL healing; however, few human studies have resulted in significant beneficial outcomes in pain management. There have been some studies that have shown normalization of grafted tissue through MRI studies after PRP with patellar tendon grafts and second-look arthroscopies [24, 25]. Bio-enhanced repair augments classic ACL repair with a collagen–platelet composite scaffold that enhances cell migration, proliferation, and collagen synthesis *in vitro* [26, 27]. Even though some studies have shown increased tissue normalization, one RCT found no significant clinical difference between ACL reconstructions that utilized PRP and those that did not after 2 years of follow-up [28].

LIMITATIONS OF PRP

The success or failure of a specific PRP product is not necessarily predictive of all PRP preparations due to the many variables involved in the process, like blood volume collected, inter-individual differences in platelet counts, inclusion or exclusion of leukocytes, and activation methods [3]. Thus, this inconsistency makes it difficult to draw generalizable conclusions for the efficacy and use of PRP. Well-designed, prospective, randomized, level 1 clinical studies are needed to carefully and comprehensively investigate the role of different PRP preparations in augmenting connective tissue healing as an opportunity to customize the concentrate to the patient's needs for a specific lesion, anatomic site, tissue type, and medical and nutritional status.

STEM CELLS

Stem cells (SC) are a very useful tool and are of interest in the field of regenerative orthopedic medicine. They possess many unique characteristics that set them apart from other cell types [29]. A difference must be made between different stem-cell types, embryonic stem cells (ESC) and adult multipotent stem cells [30], because of how they are used clinically. The practical and clinical use of these unique cells, as well as their limitations, remain to be determined [31]. The use of human stem cells is currently an intensively researched field and may be controversial from an ethical and legal standpoint [31, 32].

Among the different varieties of stem cells, mesenchymal stem cells (MSCs) hold significance for the field of regenerative orthopedics [33]. Initially identified in bone marrow aspirates, MSCs have since been isolated from almost every tissue and organ in the body and remain the cell of choice for many investigators. MSCs can be harvested from various sources, such as the periosteum, umbilical cord, bone marrow, muscle, and adipocyte. Interestingly, the source tissue used to isolate MSCs can affect differentiation capabilities, colony size, and growth rate. Sub-dermal fat is a readily accessible source of MSCs. Additionally, lipoaspirates provide, in addition to MSCs, endothelial precursor cells, monocytes, smooth muscle cells, macrophages, and T and B lymphocytes, among others [34]. Because populations generated from bone marrow contain cells with the ability to differentiate along various lineages of importance to the skeletal system, they are of wide significance to regenerative orthopedics.

Another popular source for stem cells is umbilical cord (UC) tissue, and that is why UC banking and commercial "off the shelf" products have become very popular in the United States and many other countries. Theoretically, it is potentially possible for patients to reserve their future personalized medicine in a bank. UC derived SC have been proven clinically useful for numerous diseases, as have been MSCs [31]. It is possible to use successfully allograft MSCs, which raises the possibility of facilitating clinical application with universal donor lines [35, 36].

Additionally, MSCs have anti-inflammatory properties, which confers potential benefits when regeneration should occur in an inflammatory environment. The ideal source material for MSCs will depend in part on the treatment goals and the procedure in which they will be applied; examples of their possible uses will be given in this section.

CELLULAR THERAPY FOR TISSUE REPAIR

Tendon Regeneration

Tendon injuries confer additional complexity in their treatment, as they tend to heal slowly, and even then, structural integrity cannot always be fully restored despite surgery. To regenerate the tendon and ligaments, mesenchymal stem cells (MSC) – which are a lineage of adult multipotent stem cells that lead to cell types such as chondrocytes (cartilage cells), osteoblasts (bone cells), myocytes (muscle cells) and adipocytes (fat cells) – are being used as therapeutic options among other breakthrough therapies. One such cellular therapy has shown that injection of autologous adipose derived stem cells (ADSC) in sufficient numbers are able to heal or regenerate damaged tendons. Dosage effects on cellular responses and cytokine have been reported [37]. Interestingly, some studies show that a lower dose of cells proved to be more effective in improving functional properties; further studies are required to determine the optimal number of cells needed for maximum healing [31].

Skeletal muscle cells and bone marrow–derived stromal cells have also been used to compare the differentiation capabilities in the tendon with promising results. Alternatively, many approaches attempt to mimic the chemical and mechanical micro-environment that may be necessary to provide MSCs or tendon-derived cells with the cues to develop into tendocytes and ligamentocytes. Mechanical forces are important in the formation and maturation of ligament and tendon; tensile stress, for instance, is known to upregulate the expression of scleraxis by MSCs, an important transcription factor in the development of tendon tissue and muscle attachment [38]. For example, tendon-derived MSC fabricated in a mechanically loaded, linear collagen gel construction assumes a phenotype that is similar to that of a native tendon in terms of appearance and expression.

Another approach to this problem is to use scaffolds containing multiple cells types. In one study, a scaffold was seeded with ligament cells at one end, osteoblasts at the other, and chondrocytes in between [39]. As study in this field progresses, a more practical approach to ligament attachment may be to use a single stem-cell type and induce zone-specific differentiation by spatial differences in the matrix. However, a variety of devitalized extracellular matrix scaffolds are used clinically to augment repair [35].

Practical application of these regenerative techniques and studies can be employed to accelerate healing and rehabilitation in Achilles repair in humans. In the assessment of stem-cell use for this purpose with humans, a study was conducted that reviewed 28 sports-related Achilles tendon ruptures in 27 patients treated with open repair and bone marrow aspirate concentration (BMAC) injection. On follow-up, there were no reported re-ruptures, with 92% reporting a return to sport at 5.9 months and excellent clinical outcomes. This small cohort study found no adverse outcomes related to the BMAC addition and thus proposed further study of the efficacy of stem-cell treatment for Achilles tendon repair [40].

Bone Regeneration

Bone is proving to be particularly challenging to regenerate, even though it is known to be an organ that often heals itself. Utilizing stem cells and other cell-based approaches to regenerating bone are becoming popular and have a substantial role in the current field of research [33]. Most of the current research in bone regeneration is focused in four areas: fractures that fail to heal (nonunions), critical size defects in long bones, spine fusion, and calvarial defects [35]. Perhaps the most remarkable example of successful bone regeneration concerns the regeneration of the entire distal phalanx of the human thumb by Vacanti CA et al. This was achieved by implanting autologous, expanded OSC from the patient's periosteum loaded onto a porous hydroxyapatite scaffold. No transcription factors or other developmental cues were required [41].

Osteonecrosis has been also treated in a clinical setting with marrow-derived MSCs. When MSCs were administered before collapse of the femoral head, only 6.2% of hips went on to require total arthroplasty. In contrast, 56.8% of hips required arthroplasty when cells were administered post collapse. Better outcomes were associated with the administration of larger numbers of MSC, this in contrast to tendon tissue, where lower numbers achieved better results.

The current challenge in bone regeneration is to develop robust technologies that can perform in demanding models such as large animals, justifying human trials. Many opportunities exist to translate MSC technologies into clinical treatments for bone regeneration, as is the case with tendon tissue, even though implementation challenges remain [35]. To overcome some of these challenges, identifying a sustainable source of MSCs that can be manufactured in sufficient quantities is important for clinical success.

Cartilage Regeneration

By far, the most advanced in terms of clinical trials is the treatment of cartilage lesions by means of cellular therapy. Articular cartilage has almost no intrinsic ability to regenerate, unlike bone, which has inherent capacity to repair itself. The lack of a repair process is usually attributed to the lack of blood flow, low cellularity of the tissue, and absence of lymph and innervation [42]. Damaged cartilage can predispose to OA, which is a rising global burden among musculoskeletal diseases and often leads to joint pain.

There is a need for optional treatments in moderate and severe OA, as there are currently no disease-modifying treatments for OA. This treatment gap paves the way for cellular therapy. Autologous chondrocyte implantation was the first cellular treatment to regenerate cartilage. One such therapy involved arthroscopic injection of MSCs by the way of a single-stage arthroscopic cartilage repair procedures, which was evaluated in 30 patients. The surgical procedure involved debridement of the lesion, microfracture, and application of concentrated bone marrow aspirate concentric cells with hyaluronic acid and fibrin gel under CO_2 insufflation. Clinical outcome showed significant benefit, but the effect of only the cells on the healing process should be evaluated [43]. The efficacy of cellular therapy can be augmented by combining it with minor surgery, multiple injections, arthroscopic injection, and biomimetic composites [31].

Composites such as biomaterial scaffolds, nanofibrous scaffolds, and hydrogels are an interesting area of research, as they are known to promote cartilage regeneration [31]. Because cartilage is a highly hydrated tissue, most of the scaffolds being developed are hydrogels. Materials utilized in these scaffolds include fibrin, hyaluronic acid, collagen, chitosan, silk, alginate, and synthetic polymers such as polylactic acid (PLA) and polyglycolic acid (PGA). Newer hydrogels are based on self-assembling peptides, polyethylene glycol (PEG), and electrospun nanofibers. Electrospinning allows the formation of nanofibers that can provide complex, anisotropic, biomimetic structures [35]. Advanced imaging and fabrication techniques allow designed scaffolds to be anatomically shaped to individual patients. MSCs differentiate in response to varied surface nanotopography, highlighting the importance of incorporating topographical design in scaffolds for cartilage tissue engineering [44].

Recent treatment modalities in cartilage repair consist of inducing regeneration in a cartilaginous lesion by way of gene introduction. Gene delivery provides an alternative route of gene introduction in the form of cDNA. This molecule encodes protein and will ultimately result in synthesis of an endogenous product that can be regulated and work intra-cellularly. Additionally, scaffolds may also be associated with gene delivery vectors to form gene-activated matrices (GAMs) that both provide both support and deliver cDNA molecules. Furthermore, gene therapy could also be used in conjunction with MSCs from various tissue sources [34].

In addition to their regenerative potential, MSCs demonstrate potent anti-inflammatory properties, increasing their usefulness in the setting of OA [45, 46]. Multiple human trials have been published that demonstrate the efficacy of MSC injections into patients with OA [47, 48]. For example, a recent randomized control trial of patients with knee OA reported improved cartilage and quality of life outcomes at 1 year following MSC injection compared to a control group receiving a hyaluronic acid injection [48]. Another study evaluating a MSC injection into elderly patients (age > 65 years) with knee OA found that 88% demonstrated improved cartilage status at 2-year follow-up, while no patient underwent a total knee arthroplasty during this time period [49]. Interestingly, a study investigating patients with unicompartmental knee OA with varus alignment undergoing high tibial osteotomy and microfracture showed better patient-reported, clinical, and MRI-based outcomes in a group receiving a pre-operative MSC injection compared to a control group. In addition to knee OA, studies have also reported improvement in ankle OA following MSC injection [50]. While promising, additional large-scale randomized studies are required in hopes of validating these preliminary findings concerning MSC therapies in the treatment of OA [48].

STEM CELLS CONTRAINDICATIONS

Most of the contraindications that have been discussed in the literature were established by the International Cellular Medicine Society (ICMS). The ICMS published guidelines on the use of orthobiologics therapy and lists the following conditions as absolute contraindications to its use: platelet dysfunction syndrome, critical thrombocytopenia, hemodynamic instability, septicemia, local infection at the procedure site, and patient unwillingness to accept risks. Patients with a history of bone marrow–derived cancer, metastatic disease, anemia, or other blood dyscrasias should not have BMAC procedure [17]. In addition, relative contraindications include use of NSAIDs within 48 hours of the procedure, corticosteroid injection at the treatment site within 1 month, systemic use of corticosteroids within 2 weeks, tobacco use, recent fever or illness, hemoglobin < 10 g/dL, or a platelet count <105/μL [51].

The presence of co-morbidities has not been fully studied enough to be considered as a contraindication since these patient populations are regularly excluded from RCTs in most clinical studies [16, 2].

FUTURE TRENDS

The use of ultrasound guided injection has become the gold standard for the application of orthobiologics. Fortunately, a desire to improve image quality is pushing ultrasound manufacturers beyond the capabilities of traditional 2-D imaging and increasing the roll-out of 3-D and even 4-D ultrasound systems. The b-mode technology has improved enormously in terms of transducer sensitivity, the beam former, image processing speed, and the quality of the final data display. Volumetric ultrasound has also continued to improve. Transducers now allow for the acquisition of real-time volumes of tissue allowing us to image in multiple planes – for example, the transverse and sagittal dimensions – simultaneously. Sonoelastography measures the mechanical characteristics of tissues and then displays those mechanical characteristics overlaid on the conventional b-mode ultrasound image, giving physicians the ability to see stiffer and softer areas inside the tissue. As this technology continues to improve, it will enhance the accuracy, effectiveness, and outcomes of the application of these orthobiologic treatments.

Orthobiologics are being incorporated as a standard of care to improve PRP and stem-cell application protocols; platelet and stem-cell activation procedures with L-PRP; nutritional, hormonal and inflammation optimization; and other novel approaches to modulating specific features of orthobiologics [52–54]. In a recent study, it was found that the activity of PRP may be enhanced in presence of specific biphasic tridimensional porous scaffolds made of collagen type I and glycosaminoglycan. It was proposed that the combination of collagen and glycosaminoglycan led to a spontaneous activation of PRP without the need for thrombin or any other activation factors and a sustained release of platelet growth factors such as PDGF, FGF-2, and TFG-beta [55].

The interaction and convergence of advanced biologic therapies and technological progresses are dictating the future of the regenerative orthopedic field. High-level research and clinical studies are in progress and many more are on the way in the years to come due to the excellent outcomes obtained and the interest this exciting field has aroused among the public and in the medical industry.

ORTHOBIOLOGICS CLINICAL TIPS

As a general rule, PRP should be used in tendons, ligaments, and other soft-tissue conditions, and in combination with a fat graft, ADSC, or BMAC to add the growth factors that stem cells need to do their work. However, excellent results have been obtained for knee OA as well. PRP, leukocyte rich or not, is a more controversial decision and is subject to clinical experience, equipment availability, and preference.

Stem cells of some type should be used for joints issues. ADSC are the richest source of stem cells in the body, providing 500–2500 times more MSC than BMAC. Its abundance and the ability to safely collect large amounts of adipose tissue via liposuction eliminates the need for tissue culturing. The liposuction technique is simple, safe, and cost effective and requires minimal learning and time investment. Adipose tissue contains a number of cytokines that are key for tissue regeneration: vascular endothelial growth factor, placental growth factor, and transforming growth factor-beta, among others. BMAC is obtained, preferably from the posterior iliac crest, under local anesthesia, with a simple aspiration technique. The procedure is usually performed under ultrasound or c-arm imaging guidance, and approximately 60cc of aspirate is removed and used for centrifugation. This will produce a concentrate of 7–10 ml for injection, but this concentrate also contains PRP. BMAC contains IGF-1 growth factor and others that remain to be discovered.

Orthobiologics will work better if the metabolic microenvironment where they are injected has previously been optimized. Vitamins and mineral deficiencies should be corrected, and hormonal balance and inflammation control therapies must be implemented. The use of the appropriate supplements and nutritional interventions for metabolic correction and optimization are therefore warranted.

The goals of orthobiologic therapies are to reduce pain, increase mobility, improve function, allow the patient to return to activities at least at the pre-injury level, and, most importantly, to prevent a recurrent ipsilateral or contralateral injury.

REGENERATIVE IMMUNOLOGY

The immune system has a very important role in orthopedics. Regenerative therapies that use allogeneic cells are likely to encounter immunological barriers like those that occur with transplantation of solid organs and allogeneic hematopoietic stem cells. Orthopedic implants are very sensitive to immune system responses.

Immunologic responses (e.g. cell-mediated hypersensitivity) associated with metal components used in some total joint arthroplasties (TJA) are well documented in the orthopedic literature. Both soluble and particulate debris derived from cobalt alloy implants can induce monocyte/macrophage activation and secretion of proinflammatory IL-1b, TNF-a, IL-6, and IL-8; and can upregulate transcription factor NFkB-b and downstream proinflammatory cytokines [56, 57]. Debris-induced immune reactivity, aseptic inflammation, and subsequent early failure has been reported to be as high as 4%–5% at 6–7 years for particular orthopedic implants [58–60].

The incidence of metal sensitivity among the general population is approximately 10% and among patients with well-functioning and poorly functioning implants is approximately 25% and 60%, respectively, in reported compiled analyses of numerous investigations. The most common orthopedic soluble metal (ions) sensitizers include nickel (Ni), cobalt (Co), and chromium (Cr), while occasional responses have been reported to tantalum (Ta), titanium (Ti), and vanadium (V) [61–63].

Certainly, the immune system has been a topic of great clinical interest and research for the orthopedic community in the past and present. For the regenerative field, the immune system is clearly influencing and conducting the future. The term *regenerative immunology* was coined by Dr. Jennifer Elisseeff, a biomedical investigator, Jules Stein Chair in Ophthalmology and Director of the Translational Tissue Engineering Center at Johns Hopkins University, characterizing the emergence of immunology in regenerative medicine as a paradigm shift.

"We've seen stem cells get injected and they just disappear. With immunology, we're looking earlier in the healing process to create that better environment to enhance stem cell survival after migration or implantation," Elisseeff says. In a recent study, they presented a flow cytometric analysis of cellular recruitment to tissue-derived extracellular matrix scaffolds, where they quantitatively described the infiltration and polarization of several immune subtypes, including macrophages, dendritic cells, neutrophils, monocytes, T cells, and B cells [64].

Studies have shown the ability of acellular biologic scaffold materials to modulate the host immune response and promote a functional tissue replacement outcome, and strategies have been created within the fields of tissue engineering and biomaterials to develop immune-responsive and immunoregulatory biomaterials [65]. Different types of nanofibrous scaffolds have been described to enhance the osteogenic differentiation and the regulation of adhesion, proliferation, cytoprotection, and stemness preservation of adipose-derived mesenchymal stem cells, representing a hopeful approach for use in stem cell–based regenerative medicine [66, 67].

Novel scientific concepts and advanced biological treatment techniques that apply modern tissue engineering promise further enhancement in the outcomes of orthopedic patients.

NANOTECHNOLOGY

Nanotechnology is the "science, engineering and technology conducted at the nanoscale, which is about 1 to 100 nanometers." Nanoscience and nanotechnology involve the ability to see and manipulate individual atoms and molecules [68]. Nanotech has affected many different aspects of life, such as the industrial and medical fields. Manufacturers have used nanotech to improve products such as cosmetics and electronics [69, 70].

Nanomedicine, the application of nanotechnology to medicine, can be applied in almost every branch of medicine but has had a particular impact on orthopedic surgery. Certain nanomaterials including gelatin, bioactive ceramics, biodegradable polymers, and polysaccharides such as agarose have physical characteristics that work well within the human body and promote cell growth and tissue regeneration [71]. The addition of nanomaterials to implants can improve biocompatibility and osteointegration to promote a healthier bone stimulation than in conventional implants [72]. It has dissipated some of the complications that come with bone allografts and autografts, which compose 80% of surgeries related to bone defects. They include risks of complications by infections, immune rejection, long recovery times, and low bone availability [71]. The additional surface area created by nanomaterial also aids in tissue regeneration and reduction of infection rates. Implants can be made up of nanomaterial, or the implants can be coated with it to provide for scaffolding [73]. This has been shown to promote bone formation and fusion and a better surface of adhesion for interaction with surface protein, compared to conventional implant surfaces [71]. In addition to lowering infection risk, another of the many positive clinical outcomes of nanotech in implants is the improvement of scar appearance [74, 75]. Scaffolds from nanomaterials are not limited to bone defects. Peripheral nerve injuries have shown an increase in nerve regeneration when scaffolds with nanotechnology were used compared to standard collagen scaffolds [76].

Nanomaterials have become fundamental in total joint replacement (TJR). Over 600,000 joint replacements are performed annually in the United States alone. This number increases each year, and TJR is estimated to cost more than 3 billion dollars worldwide. Aseptic loosening or the failure of the bond between an implant and the bone in absence of an infection occurs in up to 10% of patients with TJRs by 10–15 years post implantation and is a major cause of failure and increasing costs in TJRs [77]. By improving osteoblast adhesion and osteointegration, nanomaterial reduces the risk of aseptic loosening [73].

Nanotech has also been applied in methods of detection and diagnosis. Detection devices have been developed that can diagnose bone diseases such as Paget's disease, renal osteodystrophy, and osteoporosis [72, 78]. For example, a chip has been developed in which gold nanoparticles are used in sensors to accurately assess the condition of the bone and diagnose osteoporosis. [127] Unprecedented methods such as this provide precise data in a noninvasive, affordable, and timely manner [73].

Upcoming sensors created with nanotechnology can also be coupled to drug delivery. They can sense new bone formation, and if it is not happening, drugs that promote bone growth can be released as needed [72]. Even without being combined with sensors, nanotechnology provides greater precision in drug delivery [73]. For example, gold nanoparticles have been shown to improve the efficacy of anti-inflammatory agents in rats and successfully delivered iontophoresis, treating tendonitis in other preclinical animal studies [79, 80].

Nanotech drug delivery can potentially be applied to TJR by targeting release of an antibiotic right after implantation, where and when it is needed, while promoting bone growth and decreasing the risk of infection [79, 81]. Nanomaterials have also been shown to be effective in identifying cancerous bones and delivering drug therapies accordingly [82].

Even though nanotech has revolutionized the medical industry, specifically orthopedics, more research must be done before it is widely accepted in medicine [73]. Since nanotech is relatively new, further investigation is warranted until long-term safety and toxicity risks have been evaluated. Risks of cytotoxicity and inflammation of internal organs have been suggested by early research [79, 83]. In addition to the biological research needed to improve the function and viability of nanotechnology, other issues such as accessibility and cost need to be addressed if it is to reach its full potential.

MITOCHONDRIAL MEDICINE

Mitochondria are double-membrane organelles that are well known for being responsible for the production of adenosine triphosphate (ATP), the energy that mediates the cellular metabolic reaction. These organelles produce over 90% of this cellular energy via oxidative phosphorylation, a process that couples glucose oxidation to an electron transport chain and to the flow of protons down a gradient, which results in ATP synthesis via a rotary engine of the cell called *ATP synthetase* [84].

Besides ATP production, new perspectives on mitochondrial functions include responsiveness to microbial infections, promoting or resisting cell death via apoptosis or necrosis, and the ability to trigger sustained inflammation via NFkB activation.

Because most of the mitochondrial genome is scattered throughout chromosomal DNA, the mitochondria is considered a semiautonomous organelle. Its communication relies on the nucleus for expression of all its enzyme complexes and molecular constituents [85].

Mitochondria are inherited in maternal fashion, and unlike nuclear DNA, mitochondrial DNA lacks protective histones and hence is particularly susceptible to DNA damage from free radicals. For this reason, many factors can negatively influence mitochondrial function, and once initiated, it becomes a progressive vicious cycle of sustained inflammation. Pharmaceutical drugs and toxic environmental chemicals like herbicides and pesticides, metabolic toxins produced by endogenous bacteria within the gastrointestinal tract, cyanide found in tobacco smoke, and vitamin and mineral deficiencies clearly and commonly cause mitochondrial dysfunction.

Recent studies have shown that mitochondrial dysfunction may affect several of the specific pathways involved in osteoarthritis (OA) pathology, including oxidative stress, chondrocyte apoptosis, cytokine-induced chondrocyte inflammation, and matrix cartilage catabolism and calcification. OA chondrocyte mitochondrial dysfunction may originate from somatic mutations in the mitochondrial DNA or from the direct effects of proinflammatory cytokines, prostaglandins, reactive oxygen species, and nitric oxide on the mitochondrial respiratory chain and ATP synthesis [86].

As mitochondrial dysfunction explains several of the events occurring during the pathogenesis of OA, improving mitochondrial activity may prove to be a therapeutic alternative for patients with this disease. New strategies for discovering and verifying OA biomarkers have emerged, among which are genomic, proteomic, and metabolomic technologies. Mitochondrial DNA haplogroups may serve as useful biomarkers for the diagnosis or prognosis of OA and might define distinct, specific OA phenotypes with different levels of serum OA biomarkers [86].

Promising epigenetic and pharmacological therapies for OA include those that target mitochondrial regulatory proteins and the basic mitochondrial processes, particularly energy metabolism and free-radical generation.

ORTHOGENOMICS

In 2003, after more than a decade of research, the Human Genome Project was completed by the US Department of Energy and the National Institutes of Health. The genome consists of an organism's total DNA, including its genes. It is the blueprint for each person's body, influencing how we look, our genetic predispositions for certain medical conditions, how well our bodies fight disease or metabolize food, and which therapies our bodies do and do not respond to.

Single nucleotide polymorphisms, frequently called *SNPs* (pronounced "snips"), are the most common type of genetic variation among people. Each SNP represents a difference in a single DNA building block, called a *nucleotide*. SNPs occur normally throughout a person's DNA. They occur once in every 300 nucleotides on average, which means there are roughly 10 million SNPs in the human genome. Most commonly, these variations are found in the DNA between genes. They can act as biological markers, helping scientists locate genes that are associated with disease. When SNPs occur within a gene or in a regulatory region near a gene, they may play a more direct role in disease by affecting the gene's function. Some of these genetic differences, however, have proven to be very important in the study of human health. Researchers have found SNPs that may help predict an individual's response to certain drugs, susceptibility to environmental factors such as toxins, and risk of developing diseases [87].

The field of *orthogenomics*, defined here as the application of genomic principles to orthopedic pathology, has produced findings that could affect the practice of orthopedics. Currently, orthopedic oncology may be the best-studied orthogenomic discipline, focusing on pathologic identification and chemotherapeutic management rather than on surgical management [88]. With SNP analysis, new areas of the genome have been associated with disease, as with osteoporosis and genes in the major histocompatibility complex. Bone marrow density has been estimated to have a heritability of more than 70% [89]. The contribution of genetics to OA has been estimated to be 65% for the knee, 60% for the hip, and 39% for the hand [90].

Adolescent idiopathic scoliosis is an example of orthogenomics. It is now possible to analyze a combination of 53 genetic markers together with the presenting Cobb angle to stratify patients based on predicted risk of progression [91]. Orthopedic trauma patients who are at risk of multiple complications and genetic associations have been identified for conditions like acute respiratory distress syndrome, trauma-associated complicated sepsis, and deep vein thrombosis (DVT) [92–94].

Although the application of genomics in orthopedic practice remains limited, the framework for identifying practical interventions has begun to be constructed. In adult reconstructive surgery, there is a high degree of variability in patient outcomes, complications, and overall satisfaction. The key to understanding the cause of such varied outcomes may well lie in our understanding of the genetic basis of degenerative joint diseases and the genetic response to treatment. A number of conditions that occur in patients undergoing adult reconstructive orthopedic surgery may be modifiable through the use of genomics, and the use of biomarkers and genetic testing may aid in preventing postoperative complications. In a near future, orthogenomics may allow orthopedic surgeons to preoperatively stratify patients according to risk on the basis of their genetic profile and establish patient-specific strategies that will optimize results after surgery [95].

Orthogenomics is the foundation for a personalized orthopedics practice. It will improve the ability to make better informed medical decisions, result in a reduced probability of negative side effects, benefit the patient by suggesting preventive lifestyle choices that will help counteract the biological risk, and reduce healthcare costs.

CONCLUSION

Orthobiologics is a relatively new science that involves the application of naturally found materials from biological sources (cell-based therapies) and offers exciting new possibilities for the promotion and acceleration of bone and soft tissue healing. Personalizing orthopedic care bring opportunities to optimize the metabolism of orthopedics patients. As part of this therapeutic evolution, we should integrate metabolic medicine into orthopedic practice as a consequence of this integrative and functional model.

Although much progress has been made in the last 5 years, medically based studies to integrate and systematically determine the safety and cost effectiveness of these new therapeutic technologies are currently ongoing.

Emerging technologies and therapeutic concepts are having a direct impact on musculoskeletal health and treatment options; the remaining chapters of this book will guide you in how to provide them in a safe and effective way for your patients.

ACKNOWLEDGMENT

The author would like to express his appreciation to Dr. Ricardo Abreu, Mr. Frank Soto, and Miss Amanda Cintron for their kind interest and important collaboration in this manuscript.

REFERENCES

1. Ferrari M, Zia S, Valbonesi M, et al. A new technique for hemodilution, preparation of autologous platelet rich plasma and intraoperative blood salvage in cardiac surgery. *Int J Artif Organs.* 1987;10(1):47–50.
2. Tietze DC, Geissler K, Borchers J. The effects of platelet-rich plasma in the treatment of large-joint osteoarthritis: A systematic review. *Phys Sportsmed.* 2014;42(2):27–37.
3. Marmotti A, Rossi R, Castoldi F, Roveda E, Michielon G, Peretti G. PRP and articular cartilage: A clinical update. *Biomed Res Int.* 2014;2015(Article ID 542502):19 pages.

4. Lana J, Helena M, Belangero W, Cristina A. *Platelet-Rich Plasma Regenerative Medicine: Sports Medicine, Orthopedic, and Recovery of Musculoskeletal Injuries*. Berlin: Springer; 2016.

5. Arnoczky SP, Delos D, Rodeo SA. What is platelet-rich plasma? *Oper Tech Sports Med*. 2011;19:142–148.

6. Civinini R, Nistri L, Martini C, Redl B, Ristori G, Innocenti M. Growth factors in the treatment of early osteoarthritis. *Clin Cases Miner Bone Metab*. 2013;10(1):26–29.

7. Sánchez M, et al. Randomized clinical trial evaluating plasma rich in growth factors (PRGF-Endoret) versus hyaluronic acid in the short-term treatment of symptomatic knee osteoarthritis. *Arthroscopy*. 2012;28(8):1070–1078.

8. Dohan Ehrenfest DM, Andia I, Zumstein MA, Zhang C-Q, Pinto NR, Bielecki T. Classification of platelet concentrates (platelet-rich plasma – PRP, platelet-rich fibrin – PRF) for topical and infiltrative use in orthopedic and sports Research International medicine: Current consensus, clinical implications and perspectives. *Muscles Ligaments Tendons J*. 2014;4(1):3–9.

9. Paterson K, Nicholls M, Bennell K, Bates D. Intra-articular injection of photo-activated platelet-rich plasma in patients with knee osteoarthritis: A double-blind, randomized controlled pilot study. *BMC Musculoskelet Disord*. 2016;17:67.

10. Mazzucco L, Balbo V, Cattana E, Guaschino R, Borzini P. Not every PRP-gel is born equal. Evaluation of growth factor availability for tissues through four PRP-gel preparations: Fibrinet, RegenPRP-Kit, Plateltex and one manual procedure. *Vox Sanguinis*. 2009;97(2):110–118.

11. Anitua E, Zalduendo MM, Alkhraisat MH, Orive G. Release kinetics of platelet-derived and plasma-derived growth factors from autologous plasma rich in growth factors. *Ann Anat*. 2013;195(5):461–466.

12. Zumstein MA, Berger S, Schober M, et al. Leukocyte- and platelet-rich fibrin (L-PRF) for long-term delivery of growth factor in rotator cuff repair: Review, preliminary results and future directions. *Curr Pharm Biotechnol*. 2012;13(7):1196–1206.

13. Braun HJ, Kim HJ, Chu CR, Dragoo JL. The effect of platelet-rich plasma formulations and blood products on human synoviocytes: Implications for intra-articular injury and therapy. *Am J Sports Med*. 2014;42(5):1204–1210.

14. Dragoo JL, Braun HJ, Durhamet JL, et al. Comparison of the acute inflammatory response of two commercial platelet-rich plasma systems in healthy rabbit tendons. *Am J Sports Med*. 2012;40(6):1274–1281.

15. Filardo G, Kon E, Buda R, et al. Platelet-rich plasma intraarticular knee injections for the treatment of degenerative cartilage lesions and osteoarthritis. *Knee Surg Sports Traumatol Arthrosc*. 2011;19:528–535.

16. Shen L, Yuan T, Chen S, Xie X, Zhang C. The temporal effect of platelet-rich plasma on pain and physical function in the treatment of knee osteoarthritis: Systematic review and meta-analysis of randomized controlled trials. *J Orthop Surg Res*. 2017;12:16.

17. Jang S, Kim J, Cha S. Platelet-rich plasma (PRP) injections as an effective treatment for early osteoarthritis. *Eur J Orthop Surg Traumatol*. 2013;23:573–580.

18. Gosens T, Peerbooms J, Laar W, Oudsten B. Ongoing positive effect of platelet-rich plasma versus corticosteroid injection in lateral epicondylitis: A double-blind randomized controlled trial with 2-year follow-up. *Am J Sports Med*. 2011;39(6):1200–1208.

19. Sanli I, Morgan B, Tilborg F, Funk L, Gosens T. Single injection of platelet-rich plasma (PRP) for the treatment of refractory distal biceps tendonitis: Long-term results of a prospective multicenter cohort study. *Knee Surg Sports Traumatol Arthrosc*. 2016;24:2308–2312.

20. De Vos R, Weir A, van Schie H, Bierma-Zeinstra S, Verhaar J, Weinan H, Tol J. Platelet-rich plasma injection for chronic Achilles tendinopathy: A randomized controlled trial. *JAMA*. 2010;303(2):144–149.

21. Monto R. Platelet rich plasma treatment for chronic Achilles tendinosis. *Foot Ankle Int*. 2012;33(5):379–385.

22. Randelli P, Arrigoni P, Ragone V, Enga M, Aliprandi A, Cabitza P. Platelet rich plasma in arthroscopic rotator cuff repair: A prospective RCT study, 2-year follow-up. *J Shoulder Elbow Surg*. 2011; 20: 518–528.

23. Chahal G, Mall N. The role of platelet-rich plasma in arthroscopic rotator cuff repair: A systematic review with quantitative synthesis. *Arthroscopy*. 2013 [In press].

24. Radice F, Yanez R, Gutierrez V, Rosales J, Pinedo M, Coda S. Comparison of magnetic resonance imaging findings in anterior cruciate ligament grafts with and without autologous platelet-derived growth factors. *Arthroscopy: J Arthroscopic Relat Surg*. 2010;26(1):50–57.

25. Sanchez M, Anitua E, Azofra J, Prado R, Muruzabal F, Andia I. Ligamentization of tendon grafts treated with endogenous preparation rich in growth factors: Gross morphology and histology. *Arthroscopy*. 2010;26(4):470–480.

26. Nin J, Gasque G, Azcarate A, Beola J, Gonzalez M. Has platelet-rich plasma any role in anterior cruciate ligament allograft healing? *Arthroscopy*. 2009;25(11):1206–1213.
27. Murray M, Spindler K, Abreu E, Muller J, Nedder A, Kelly M. Collagen-platelet rich plasma hydrogel enhances primary repair of the porcine anterior cruciate ligament. *J Orthop Res*. 2007;25(1):81–91.
28. Joshi S, Mastrangelo A, Murray M. Collagen-platelet composite enhances histologic healing of the ACL. *55th ORS*, Las Vegas, 22–25 Feb. 2009.
29. Schmitt A, van Griensven M, Imhoff AB, Buchmann S. Application of stem cells in orthopedics. *Stem Cells Int*. 2012;2012:394962.
30. Hernigou P. Bone transplantation and tissue engineering, part IV. Mesenchymal stem cells: History in orthopedic surgery from Cohnheim and Goujon to the Nobel Prize of Yamanaka. *Int Orthop*. 2015;39(4):807–817.
31. Noh MJ, Lee KH. Orthopedic cellular therapy: An overview with focus on clinical trials. *World J Orthop*. 2015;6(10):754–761.
32. Oh JH, Chung SW, Kim SH, Chung JY, Kim JY. 2013 Neer Award: Effect of the adipose-derived stem cell for the improvement of fatty degeneration and rotator cuff healing in rabbit model. *J Shoulder Elb Surg*. 2014;23(4):445–455.
33. Akpancar S, Tatar O, Turgut H, Akyildiz F, Ekinci S. The current perspectives of stem cell therapy in orthopedic surgery. *Arch Trauma Res*. 2016;5(4):e37976.
34. Menssen A, Häupl T, Sittinger M, Delorme B, Charbord P, Ringe J. Differential gene expression profiling of human bone marrow–derived mesenchymal stem cells during adipogenic development. *BMC Genomics*. 2011;12:461.
35. Evans CH. Advances in regenerative orthopedics. *Mayo Clin Proc*. 2013;88(11):1323–1339.
36. Yang YJ, Li XL, Xue Y, et al. Bone marrow cells differentiation into organ cells using stem cell therapy. *Eur Rev Med Pharmacol Sci*. 2016;20(13):2899–2907.
37. Saether EE, Chamberlain CS, Leiferman EM, Kondratko-Mittnacht JR, Li WJ, Brickson SL, Vanderby R. Enhanced medial collateral ligament healing using mesenchymal stem cells: Dosage effects on cellular response and cytokine profile. *Stem Cell Rev*. 2014;10:86–96 [PMID: 24174129 DOI:10.1007/s12015-013-9479-7].
38. Kuo CK, Tuan RS. Mechanoactive tenogenic differentiation of human mesenchymal stem cells. *Tissue Eng Part A*. 2008;14:1615–1627. [PubMed: 18759661].
39. Spalazzi JP, Dagher E, Doty SB, Guo XE, Rodeo SA, Lu HH. In vivo evaluation of a multiphased scaffold designed for orthopaedic interface tissue engineering and soft tissue-to-bone integration. *J Biomed Mater Res A*. 2008;86:1–12. [PubMed: 18442111].
40. Stein BE, Stroh DA, Schon LC. Outcomes of acute Achilles tendon rupture repair with bone marrow aspirate concentrate augmentation. *Int Orthop*. 2015;39(5):901–905.
41. Vacanti CA, Bonassar LJ, Vacanti MP, Shufflebarger J. Replacement of an avulsed phalanx with tissue-engineered bone. *N Engl J Med*. 2001;344:1511–1514. [PubMed: 11357154].
42. Latief N, Raza FA, Bhatti FU, Tarar MN, Khan SN, Riazuddin S. Adipose stem cells differentiated chondrocytes regenerate damaged cartilage in rat model of osteoarthritis. *Cell Biol Int*. 2016;40(5):579–588.
43. Shetty AA, Kim SJ, Bilagi P, Stelzeneder D. Autologous collagen-induced chondrogenesis: Single-stage arthroscopic cartilage repair technique. *Orthopedics*. 2013;36:e648–e652. [PMID: 23672920 DOI:10.1007/s13770-014-0061-4].
44. Wu YN, Law JB, He AY, Low HY, Hui JH, Lim CT, Yang Z, Lee EH. Substrate topography determines the fate of chondrogenesis from human mesenchymal stem cells resulting in specific cartilage phenotype formation. *Nanomedicine*. 2014;10:1507–1516. [PMID: 24768908 DOI:10.1016/j.nano.2014.04.002].
45. Koh YG, Choi YJ. Infrapatellar fat pad–derived mesenchymal stem cell therapy for knee osteoarthritis. *Knee*. 2012;19(6):902–907.
46. Filardo G, Madry H, Jelic M, Rof A, Cucchiarini M, Kon E. Mesenchymal stem cells for the treatment of cartilage lesions: From preclinical findings to clinical application in orthopaedics. *Knee Surg Sports Traumatol Arthrosc*. 2013;21(8):1717–1729.
47. Wyles CC, Houdek MT, Behfar A, Sierra RJ. Mesenchymal stem cell therapy for osteoarthritis: Current perspectives. *Stem Cells Cloning*. 2015;8:117–124.
48. Vega A, Martín-Ferrero MA, Del Canto F, et al. Treatment of knee osteoarthritis with allogeneic bone marrow mesenchymal stem cells: A randomized controlled trial. *Transplantation*. 2015;99(8):1681–1690.
49. Koh YG, Choi YJ, Kwon SK, Kim YS, Yeo JE. Clinical results and second-look arthroscopic findings after treatment with adipose-derived stem cells for knee osteoarthritis. *Knee Surg Sports Traumatol Arthrosc*. 2015;23(5):1308–1316.

50. Kim YS, Lee M, Koh YG. Additional mesenchymal stem cell injection improves the outcomes of marrow stimulation combined with supramalleolar osteotomy in varus ankle osteoarthritis: Short-term clinical results with second-look arthroscopic evaluation. *J Exp Orthop.* 2016;3(11):12.

51. International Cellular Medicine Society. Guidelines for the use of platelet rich plasma (adopted 2011). Available at: http://www.cellmedicinesociety.org/attachments/206_ICMS%20-%20Guidelines%20for%20the%20use%20of%20Platelet%20Rich%20Plasma%20-%20Draft.pdf. Accessed July 25, 2017.

52. Mifune Y, Matsumoto T, Takayama K, et al. The effect of platelet-rich plasma on the regenerative therapy of muscle derived stem cells for articular cartilage repair. *Osteoarthritis Cartilage.* 2013;21(1):175–185.

53. Zhu Y, Yuan M, Meng HY, et al. Basic science and clinical application of platelet-rich plasma for cartilage defects and osteoarthritis: A review. *Osteoarthritis Cartilage.* 2013;21(11):1627–1637.

54. Turajane T, Thitiset T, Honsawek S, Chaveewanakorn U, Aojanepong J, Papadopoulos KI. Assessment of chondrogenic differentiation potential of autologous activated peripheral blood stem cells on human early osteoarthritic cancellous tibial bone scaffold. *Musculoskelet Surg.* 2014;98(1):35–43.

55. Getgood A, Henson R, Brooks F, Fortier LA, Rushton N. Platelet-rich plasma activation in combination with biphasic osteochondral scaffolds-conditions for maximal growth factor production. *Knee Surg Sports Traumatol Arthrosc.* 2011;19(11):1942–1947.

56. Sethi RK, Neavyn MJ, Rubash HE, et al. Macrophage response to cross-linked and conventional UHMWPE. *Biomaterials.* 2003;24:2561–2573.

57. Catelas I, Petit A, Zukor DJ, et al. TNF-alpha secretion and macrophage mortality induced by cobalt and chromium ions in vitro-qualitative analysis of apoptosis. *Biomaterials.* 2003; 24:383–391.

58. Jacobs JJ, Hallab NJ. Loosening and osteolysis associated with metal-on-metal bearings: A local effect of metal hypersensitivity? *J Bone Joint Surg Am.* 2006; 88:1171–1172.

59. Korovessis P, Petsinis G, Repanti M, et al. Metallosis after contemporary metal-on-metal total hip arthroplasty. Five to nine-year follow-up. *J Bone Joint Surg Am.* 2006;88:1183–1191.

60. Milosev I, Trebse R, Kovac S, et al. Survivorship and retrieval analysis of Sikomet metal-on-metal total hip replacements at a mean of seven years. *J Bone Joint Surg Am* 2006; 88:1173–1182.

61. Catelas I, Petit A, Marchand R, et al. Cytotoxicity and macrophage cytokine release induced by ceramic and polyethylene particles in vitro. *J Bone Joint Surg Br.* 1999; 81:516–521.

62. Liden C, Wahlberg JE, Maibach HI. *Skin.* New York: Academic Press; 1995. pp. 47–64.

63. Lalor PA, Revell PA, Gray AB, Wright S, Railton GT, Freeman MA. Sensitivity to titanium. A cause of implant failure. *J Bone Joint Surg.* 1991;73-B:25–28.

64. Sadtler K, Allen BW, Estrellas K, Housseau F, Pardoll DM, Elisseeff JH. The scaffold immune microenvironment: Biomaterial-mediated immune polarization in traumatic and nontraumatic applications. *Tissue Eng Part A.* 2017;23(2019–20):1044–1053.

65. Dziki JL, Huleihel L, Scarritt ME, Badylak SF. Extracellular matrix bioscaffolds as immunomodulatory biomaterials. *Tissue Eng Part A.* 2017;23(2019–20):1152–1159.

66. Tavangar B, Arasteh S, Edalatkhah H, Salimi A, Doostmohammadi A, and Seyedjafari E. Hardystonite-coated poly(l-lactide) nanofibrous scaffold and efficient osteogenic differentiation of adipose-derived mesenchymal stem cells. *Artif Organs.* 27 June, 2017.

67. Dadashpour M, Pilehvar-soltanahmadi Y, Mohammadi SA, et al. Watercress-based electrospun nanofibrous scaffolds enhance proliferation and stemness preservation of human adipose-derived stem cells. *Artif Cells Nanomed Biotechnol.* 46(4), 819–830. doi:10.1080/21691401.2017.1345925

68. Available at: https://www.nano.gov/nanotech-101/what/definition Accessed July 19, 2017.

69. Available at: https://www.nano.gov//timeline. Accessed July 19, 2017.

70. Available at: http://www.nanotechproject.org/inventories/medicine/. Accessed July 19, 2017.

71. Parchi PD, Vittorio O, Andreani L, Piolanti N, Cirillo G, et al. How nanotechnology can really improve the future of orthopedic implants and scaffolds for bone and cartilage defects. *J Nanomedine Biotherapeutic Discov.* 2013;3:114.

72. Mazaheri M, Eslahi N, Ordikhani F, Tamjid E, Simchi A. Nanomedicine applications in orthopedic medicine: State of the art. *Int J Nanomedicine.* 2015;10:6039–6053.

73. Garimella R, Eltorai A. Nanotechnology in orthopedics. *J Orthopaedics.* 2017;14:30–33. 10.1016/j.jor.2016.10.026.

74. Webster TJ, Ergun C, Doremus RH, Siegel RW, Bizios R. Enhanced functions of osteoblasts on nanophase ceramics. *Biomaterials.* 2000;21:1803–1810.

75. Shirwaiker RA, Samberg ME, Cohen PH, Wysk RA, Monteiro-Riviere NA. Nanomaterials and synergistic low-intensity direct current (LIDC) stimulation technology for orthopedic implantable medical devices. *Wiley Interdiscip Rev Nonacid Nanobiotechnol.* 2013;5:191–204.

76. Ding T, Luo ZJ, Zheng Y, Hu XY, Ye ZX. Rapid repair and regeneration of damaged rabbit sciatic nerves by tissue-engineered scaffold made from nano-silver and collagen type I. *Injury*. 2010;41:522–527.

77. Christenson EM, Anseth KS, van den Beucken JJ, Chan CK, Ercan B, et al. Nanobiomaterial applications in orthopedics. *J Orthop Res*. 2007;25:11–22.

78. Yun YH, Eteshola E, Bhattacharya A, Dong Z, Shim JS, Conforti L, Kim D, Schulz MJ, Ahn CH, Watts N. Tiny medicine: Nanomaterial-based biosensors. *Sensors (Basel)*. 2009;9(11):9275–9299.

79. Sullivan MP, McHale KJ, Parvizi J, Mehta S. Nanotechnology: Current concepts in orthopaedic surgery and future directions. *Bone Joint J*. 2014;96-B(5):569–573.

80. Dohnert MB, Venâncio M, Possato JC, et al. Gold nanoparticles and diclofenac diethylammonium administered by iontophoresis reduce inflammatory cytokines expression in Achilles tendinitis. *Int J Nanomedicine*. 2012;7:1651–1657.

81. Li H, Ogle H, Jiang B, Hagar M, Li B. Cefazolin embedded biodegradable polypeptide nanofilms promising for infection prevention: A preliminary study on cell responses. *J Orthop Res*. 2010;28(8):992–999.

82. Mohamed M, Borchard G, Jordan O. In situ forming implants for local chemotherapy and hyperthermia of bone tumors. *J Drug Deliv Sci Technol*. 2012;22:393–408.

83. Polyzois I, Nikolopoulos D, Michos I, Patsouris E, Theocharis S. Local and systemic toxicity of nanoscale debris particles in total hip arthroplasty. *J Appl Toxicol*. 2012;32(4):255–269.

84. Zeviar DD, et al. The role of mitochondria in cancer and other chronic diseases. *J Orthomolecular Med*. 2014;29(4):157–166.

85. Wallace DC. A mitochondrial paradigm of metabolic and degenerative diseases, aging, and cancer: A dawn for evolutionary medicine. *Annu Rev Genet*. 2005;39:359–407.

86. Blanco FJ, Rego I, Ruiz-Romero C. The role of mitochondria in osteoarthritis. *Nat Rev Rheumatol*. 2011;7(3):161–169.

87. Genetics Home Reference. Available at: https://ghr.nlm.nih.gov/. [Accessed July 22, 2017].

88. Bond M, Bernstein ML, Pappo A, et al. A phase II study of imatinib mesylate in children with refractory or relapsed solid tumors: A Children's Oncology Group study. *Pediatr Blood Cancer*. 2008;50(2):254–258.

89. Arden NK, Baker J, Hogg C, Baan K, Spector TD. The heritability of bone mineral density, ultrasound of the calcaneus and hip axis length: A study of postmenopausal twins. *J Bone Miner Res*. 1996;11(4):530–534.

90. Spector TD, MacGregor AJ. Risk factors for osteoarthritis: Genetics. *Osteoarthritis Cartilage*. 2004;12 suppl A:S39–S44.

91. Ward K, Ogilvie JW, Singleton MV, Chettier R, Engler G, Nelson LM. Validation of DNA-based prognostic testing to predict spinal curve progression in adolescent idiopathic scoliosis. *Spine (Phila Pa 1976)*. 2010;35(25):E1455–E1464.

92. Zhai R, Gong MN, Zhou W, et al. Genotypes and haplotypes of the VEGF gene are associated with higher mortality and lower VEGF plasma levels in patients with ARDS. *Thorax*. 2007;62(8):718–722.

93. O'Keefe GE, Hybki DL, Munford RS. The GA single nucleotide polymorphism at the -308 position in the tumor necrosis factor-alpha promoter increases the risk for severe sepsis after trauma. *J Trauma*. 2002;52(5):817–825.

94. Kim YH, Kim JS. The 2007 John Charnley Award: Factors leading to low prevalence of DVT and pulmonary embolism after THA. Analysis of genetic and prothrombotic factors. *Clin Orthop Relat Res*. 2007;465:33–39.

95. Elbuluk A, Deshmukh A, Inneh I, Iorio R. The present and future of genomics in adult reconstructive orthopaedic surgery. *JBJS Rev*. 2016;4(4):e61–e66.

2 Orthogenomics
Genome-Directed Therapies in Orthopedics

Joseph R. Veltmann, PhD, DCCN and
Roberta L. Kline, MD

From time to time, a research discovery or clinical project results in a paradigm shift in medicine. A recent example was the completion of the Human Genome Project in 2003 – it ushered in the era of personalized genomic medicine (1). In a very short period of time, the principles of genomic medicine have been applied across a wide range of medical specialties to personalize treatment strategies (2), individualize disease prevention programs (3), improve patient outcomes (4, 5), reduce health care costs (5, 6), and revolutionize medicine (7).

This chapter highlights recent advances in orthogenomics, the research and clinical science of applying genomics to care of patients with orthopedic conditions. Gene polymorphisms can impact a person's risk for two common orthopedic conditions: osteoarthritis and osteoporosis. Here we present the scientific research findings on the genomics of osteoarthritis and osteoporosis, followed by practice-ready, personalized prevention and treatment strategies using a patient's genomic map.

DIFFERENCE BETWEEN GENE MUTATIONS AND GENE POLYMORPHISMS IN A DISEASE PROCESS

While genomics is a branch of genetics, genetics operates in the realm of prediction, genomics in predisposition. It is important to understand the distinctions that exist between the two and how they impact health and disease. Genetic mutations typically follow well-established penetrance and inheritance patterns. Geneticists can use a person's genetic architecture or genotype to predict with considerable accuracy the impact and heredity risk of a rare, single gene mutation found in the germline. Inherited disorders such as Tay Sachs Syndrome, Hemophilia and Cystic Fibrosis fall into this category (8). Genetic testing enables identification of mutations that are linked to specific diseases, with the development of appropriate screening and treatment protocols. In most cases, however, there are no proactive steps available to mitigate or prevent the effects of the mutation.

In contrast, genomic polymorphisms do not follow specific and predictive patterns. Most chronic degenerative diseases are at the opposite end of the spectrum from inherited diseases (Figure 2.1). These chronic diseases are multi-factorial, polygenic disorders that result from interactions between gene polymorphisms and environmental factors (9, 10). Gene polymorphisms are changes in DNA nucleotide sequences that can lead to changes in gene function. Single nucleotide polymorphisms (SNPs) result from a change in one nucleotide sequence in a gene. This substitution of a single nucleotide in the DNA sequence of a gene can have varying effects, depending on the location. It may impact the functionality of the protein produced, alter protein synthesis on a quantitative level or have no impact at all (11). In contrast to genetic mutations, single gene polymorphisms typically have a small effect on phenotype, and multiple gene SNPs in a biochemical pathway or biological system can have an additive effect (12).

Adding to the complexity, environmental factors can interact with the effects of single or multiple gene polymorphism(s) in a biochemical or metabolic pathway. Therefore, a chronic disease process represents the unique interaction between a person's gene SNPs and environmental factors,

Effect Of DNA Sequence Change On Phenotype

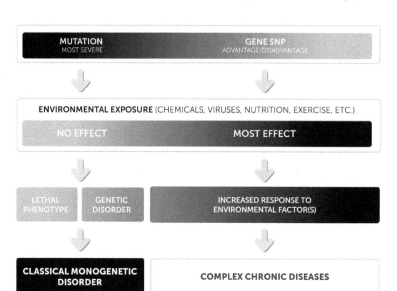

© GENOMA INTERNATIONAL—USED WITH PERMISSION

FIGURE 2.1   Spectrum of Impact from Genetic Mutations to Genomic SNPs.

which can vary from person to person, and by gender, ethnicity or even region of the world (13). The genomic diversity necessitates epidemiologic retooling to effectively address the current epidemic of polygenic, multi-factorial chronic diseases of the twenty-first century.

When genomic medicine and genomic testing are used in the early stages of osteoarthritis or osteopenia, orthogenomics provides a unique opportunity to uncover the molecular mechanism(s) associated with the disease process in each individual in order to stratify patients that need more aggressive therapies, and more effectively address a patient's co-morbidities. A clinician can then use evidenced-based, DNA-directed interventions to personalize prevention or treatment strategies to improve the phenotypic profile of each orthopedic patient.

IDENTIFYING GENE POLYMORPHISMS LINKED TO OSTEOARTHRITIS OR OSTEOPOROSIS

There are about 20,000 genes and more than 10 million gene polymorphisms in human DNA (14). Researchers currently use three main methods to find and identify the genes and gene SNPs linked to osteoarthritis and osteoporosis: candidate gene studies, genome-wide association studies (GWAS) and microarrays (15). A brief description, along with the advantages and disadvantages of each method, is provided to help clinicians know how best to interpret and translate genomic test results into action steps for a patient.

Candidate gene studies (CGS) use a case-control experimental design to determine whether one allele of a candidate gene is observed more frequently in a family member with a complex disease versus family members without the disease phenotype (16). An advantage to this approach is that researchers can focus on a single gene variant or multiple gene variants within a set of pre-selected genes associated with a disease phenotype, cutting down on costs and data analysis. However, the findings of CGS are often difficult to replicate in follow-up studies because chronic diseases are polygenic and multi-factorial, and prior knowledge about a gene's biological and functional impact on the disease phenotype is necessary.

In contrast, GWAS scans and compares the entire genome of individuals with and without the disease phenotype for differences among common gene variants (17). No prior knowledge about a gene's function is necessary, and GWAS is considered a non-candidate gene approach. However, in order to detect minor genotypic differences, many thousands of individuals need to be tested, driving up laboratory costs and requiring advanced bioinformatic systems to analyze and interpret the data. Some gene SNPs may also go undetected, depending on the frequency in the studied populations and the depth of the assay. The advantage is that meta-analysis of several GWAS studies can detect 10, 20 or even hundreds of loci associated with the identified disease phenotype and yield valuable information about the molecular mechanisms involved. For this reason, GWAS is often the first step in identifying genes that are candidates for further research by more detailed methods.

Microarray technology cuts costs, time and resources (18). Using a microchip-based testing platform enables many pieces of DNA to be analyzed at once using a high-volume, automated system. Nucleotide labels or probes on the microchip bind to specific chromosome regions, then analysis by a computer compares a patient's genes to a reference sample and gene polymorphisms are reported. Knowledge of specific genes and their functions is required. While the size of the microchip limits the number of nucleotide labels and the number of genes that can be evaluated, microarray technology is the method of choice by most clinical genomic testing laboratories due to its accuracy and high output with relatively low equipment and personnel costs.

ORTHOGENOMICS OF OSTEOARTHRITIS

Osteoarthritis (OA) is a multi-factorial, polygenic, chronic, degenerative joint disease that is a leading cause of disability in adult men and woman in populations around the world (19). The disease processes include degradation of articular cartilage and sclerosis, osteophyte formation, synovial membrane inflammation and involvement of tendon, ligaments and articular capsule (20). Currently there is no cure, nor are there effective treatments to arrest or slow the progression of the disease. Effective pain management with eventual joint replacement for advanced cases is the mainstay of treatment. Many options for pharmacological intervention can be used to alleviate pain, but these medications can result in severe adverse effects over time. Genomics may provide a more effective approach. Integrating a patient's pathophysiology with his or her orthogenomics for OA can lead to personalized prevention and treatment strategies, development of new and better biomarkers and therapeutic agents, risk stratification and construction of an OA genomic toolbox for clinicians.

OA is similar to other complex diseases, such as Alzheimer's disease, where early onset OA (EOOA) represents an inherited, monogenic Mendelian disease (21). EOOA is associated with rare mutations in SMAD3, TRPV4, ACAN, MATN3, COMP, GDF5, COL3A1 and MIR17HG and DIO2 (22). A hallmark of an EOOA mutation is its high penetrance in a small number of families. Thus, while the gene mutation is rare, it has a large physiological effect when it is present (23).

Late onset OA (LOOA) is the most common form of the disease, with a usual onset in individuals over 60 years of age. Interestingly, common polymorphisms for three of the genes involved in EOOA - GDF5, SMAD3 and DIO2, are associated with late onset OA in the joints of Caucasians and Asians (24). In contrast to EOOA, LOOA has low penetrance but its frequency in the population ranges between small to moderate. This is because polymorphisms are common variants with small effect (25). Candidate gene studies and genomic-wide-association studies are useful in identifying genes and gene variants that may be linked to the underlying molecular mechanisms of LOOA.

CANDIDATE GENE STUDIES AND MOLECULAR
MECHANISMS OF OA: MONOGENIC APPROACH

Candidate gene studies have uncovered different genes encoding for proteins that confer an increased susceptibility of hip or knee OA across a variety of molecular mechanisms. Examples are Wnt (wingless) cell signaling (FRZG) (26); extracellular proteins involved in cartilage anabolism (COL2A1, COL9A2, COL1A1, COL1A2 and COMP (27–31) and catabolism (MMP-3 and ADAMTS-5) (32, 33); programmed cell death (FAS and TNF) (34); as well as mitochondrial apoptosis (ANP32A) (35), alterations in estrogen receptor status (36) and vitamin D metabolism (GC, VDR) (37).

GENOME-WIDE ASSOCIATION STUDIES: POLYGENIC APPROACH

To overcome the inherent limitations in GWAS studies, meta-analysis of several osteoarthritis GWAS studies can improve statistical power to identify significant associations or develop odds ratios for a complex, polygenic disease like OA.

A recent meta-analysis of nine genome-wide association studies revealed more than 190 gene loci associated with OA across numerous biological pathways and molecular mechanisms that may contribute to the heterogeneity of the OA phenotype (38). Only two of the 190 gene OA loci showed a significant association, COL1A1 and VEGF. COL1A1 encodes for alpha chains of collagen 1A1, and a polymorphism associated with this gene is linked to lumbar disc herniation (39). VEGF encodes for vascular endothelial growth factor, a protein found in the synovial fluid. Carriers of a VEGF polymorphism produce a defective protein which is linked to increased severity in knee osteoarthritis (40).

Wang and his coworkers designed a meta-analysis of GWAS studies to pinpoint genes that confer an increased risk for OA for the hip, the knee or both (24). Tables 2.1 through 2.3 summarize the genes identified, as well as the metabolic system(s) associated with each gene, to illustrate the complex nature of OA. It is evident that there are multiple genotypes within the several subtypes of OA that play a prominent role in the pathogenesis of the disease across Asian and Caucasian populations.

MICROARRAY STUDIES

In orthopedic medicine, early screening for gene variants can alert a clinician to take proactive steps to mitigate their impact before the disease progresses to a more severe stage. Evidence-based nutrigenomic interventions have been shown to alter the disease process and improve patient outcomes across different medical specialties.

If GWAS evaluates the human genome at the 20,000-foot level, then microarray analysis evaluates genotypes at the 10-foot level to better understand molecular mechanisms for the many OA phenotypes. GWAS satisfies a researcher's curiosity globally about the etiology of OA, whereas microarray studies can help clinicians develop programs that can either prevent the disease or personalize treatment strategies. For example, a microarray analysis detected gene variants associated with cartilage metabolism (COL1A1, COL5A1, PLOD2 and LOX) that increase a person's risk for capsular fibrosis that can accompany OA – only one aspect of this disease (41). Other studies have identified more than a dozen additional gene SNPs as risk factors (42–44), but findings are inconsistent as impact varies among different ethnicities and gender, and with pathophysiology markers used. No clear interventions have been identified for many of these, making their clinical utility currently limited. However, SNPs in other genes, including IL-1B, IL-6, VDR and DIO2 have been identified as being relevant in OA (45), and have known nutritional genomic interventions.

CONSTRUCTION OF CLINICIAN'S GENOMIC TOOL
BOX: GENE-FUNCTION-ACTION STEP MATRIX

Given all the OA subtypes, their pathophysiology and their genomic diversity, constructing a clinically useful OA genomic tool box may appear to be a daunting task. For results to be most clinically useful, it is necessary to know not just what the potential impact of gene SNPs are, but also how to intervene and measure the effectiveness of the interventions.

TABLE 2.1

Genes Associated with Hip OA (GWAS)

Gene	Protein	Metabolic System(s)
ANP32A	Acidic Nuclear Phosphoprotein 32 Family Member A	Proliferation, differentiation, apoptosis
ASTN2	Astrotactin 2	Lipophilic membranes
CALM2	Calmodulin 2	Calcium, cell signaling, proliferation
CAMK2B	Calcium/Calmodulin Dependent Protein Kinase II Beta	Skeletal muscle
CHST11A1	Carbohydrate Sulfotransferase 11	Chondroitin sulfate
COL11A1	Collagen Type XI Alpha 1 Chain	Collagen fibrillogenesis
COL9A2	Collagen Type IX Alpha 2 Chain	Hyaline cartilage
DIO2	Iodothyronine Deiodinase 2	Thyroid hormone conversion (T3)
DNAH10	Dynein Axonemal Heavy Chain 10	Sperm motility
DOT1L	DOT1-Like Histone Lysine Methyltransferase	Histone methyltransferase
DYRK2	Dual Specificity Tyrosine Phosphorylation Regulated Kinase 2	Mitosis, proliferation, cytoskeleton, apoptosis
FILIP1	Filamin A Interacting Protein 1	Filamen A, cortical neuron, dendritic spine
HMGN3	High Mobility Group Nucleosomal Binding Domain 3	Thyroid hormone, transcription
IFRD1	Interferon-Related Developmental Regulator 1	Embryonic development and tissue regeneration
IGF1	Insulin-Like Growth Factor 1	Glucose transport in osteoblasts
IGFBP3	Insulin-Like Growth Factor Binding Protein 3	Insulin-like growth factor transport
KLHDC5	Kelch-Like Family Member 42	Mitosis
NACA2	Nascent Polypeptide Associated Complex Alpha Subunit 2	Endoplasmic reticulum
NCOA3	Nuclear Receptor Coactivator 3	Transcription, hormone receptors, histone acetyltransferase, NK-kappa-B activation
PHF2	PHD Finger Protein 2	Histone demethylation
SMAD3	SMAD Family Member 3	Wound healing, chondrogenesis, osteogenesis
VEGF	Vascular Endothelial Growth Factor A	Endothelial cell proliferation, cell migration, apoptosis

In our clinic, we have developed a Gene-Function-Action Step matrix when evaluating either single or multiple genes for chronic, degenerative diseases. Applying this process to OA, the Gene-Function-Action Step matrix helps sort gene SNPs based on their impact (low, moderate or high) on the disease process or pathophysiological trait, quantify and qualify how the gene variant(s) influences the molecular underpinnings of OA across various biological systems, and prioritize our nutritional genomic, lifestyle and pharmacological interventions.

CASE HISTORY 1: MONOGENIC EXAMPLE

For a monogenic example, let's consider a patient with OA who is in the early stages of the disease and is seeking therapies to mitigate its progress. She has a set of genomic test results from a commercial laboratory, revealing gene variants in the following single genes: COL1A1, IL-6 and DIO2. Interpretation of those results is crucial to not only identify genotypes but also to understand the potential qualitative and quantitative impact of the gene SNPs on one or more of the pathophysiological markers for OA. These include the severity of joint changes, capsular fibrosis, joint function, pain, cartilage loss, inflammation of synovial membrane, joint space narrowing, osteophyte formation and loss of bone contours based on single gene, evidenced-based studies in the literature.

TABLE 2.2

Genes Associated with Knee OA (GWAS)

Gene	Protein	Metabolic System(s)
ADAM12	ADAM Metallopeptidase Domain 12	Skeletal muscle regeneration, osteoclast formation
ADAMTS14	ADAM Metallopeptidase With Thrombospondin Type 1 Motif 14	Collagen formation
ASPN	Asporin	Chondrogenesis, cartilage homeostasis
COL9A3	Collagen Type IX Alpha 3 Chain	Hyaline cartilage
DUS4L	Dihydrouridine Synthase 4 Like	Transfer RNA
DVWA	Double von Willebrand factor A domains	Tubulin binding
ER-α	Estrogen Receptor 1	Estrogen receptor; sexual and reproductive; cell proliferation, bone homeostasis
ER-β	Estrogen Receptor 2	Estrogen receptor; cell growth, differentiation; skeletal, cardiovascular, nervous systems
GDF5	Growth Differentiation Factor 5	Growth factor, bone and cartilage formation
GPR22	G Protein-Coupled Receptor 22	Membrane protein
HIF1A	Hypoxia-Inducible Factor 1 Alpha Subunit	Transcription, cell metabolism, cell survival, angiogenesis
IL-1RN	Interleukin 1 Receptor Antagonist	Inflammatory response
IL-6	Interleukin 6	Inflammatory response, lipolysis, glucose homeostasis
IL-16	Interleukin 16	Chemoattractant, inflammatory response
IL-17A	Interleukin 17A	Inflammatory response, nitric oxide production
SMAD3	SMAD Family Member 3	Cell signaling, wound healing, chondrogenesis, osteogenesis
TP63	Tumor Protein P63	Transcription; ectoderm development; stem cell regulation; heart development

TABLE 2.3

Genes Associated with Both Hip and Knee OA (GWAS)

Gene	Protein	Metabolic System(s)
BAG6	BCL2 Associated Athanogene 6	Cytosolic protein formation and transport
C90RF3	Chromosome 9 Open Reading Frame 3	Protein formation
COX-2	Prostaglandin-Endoperoxide Synthase 2	Prostaglandin biosynthesis, apoptosis, tumor angiogenesis
GNL3	G Protein Nucleolar 3	Tumorigenesis, stem cell proliferation
IL-8	Interleukin 8	Chemotaxis, neutrophil activation
INSR	Insulin Receptor	Cell signaling, insulin and glucose homeostasis
LHCGR	Luteinizing Hormone/Choriogonadotropin Receptor	Receptor, luteinizing hormone and choriogonadotropin
LRCH1	Leucine Rich Repeats and Calponin Homology Domain Containing 1	Protein, function unclear
TGFβ1	Transforming Growth Factor Beta 1	Cell proliferation, differentiation; growth factor regulation; osteoblast
VDR Apal	Vitamin D Receptor	Receptor, vitamin D; transcription, mineral metabolism, inflammatory response

For this patient with early stage OA, the genomic testing laboratory identified that for the phenotypic trait – increased severity of OA over time – both IL-6 and DIO2 genotypes may have a high impact for her, while COL1A1 has a low or no impact. The report also identified how each SNP impacts the functionality of each gene, and provided evidenced-based nutrigenomic interventions and recommendations. A gene SNP on IL-6, for example, upregulates the synthesis of IL-6, a pro-inflammatory cytokine. Nutrigenomic interventions to downregulate IL-6 include supplementing the patient's diet with beta-sitosterol (46, 47) and having the patient be mindful of her stressors, since mental and emotional stress triggers IL-6 production (48).

A gene SNP on DIO2 decreases its enzyme activity (deiodinase 2), leading to reduced conversion of T4 to T3 in the peripheral tissues (49). Inadequate T3 levels can lead to poor cartilage metabolism in the joints. Pharmacological therapy (combination T4/T3) was added (50) and important dietary nutrient cofactors (iodine, zinc and selenium) were optimized in her diet to achieve thyroid hormone homeostasis (51).

CASE HISTORY 2: POLYGENIC EXAMPLE

For the polygenic example, let's consider a patient diagnosed with moderate to severe OA in his knees and hips. He is overweight, does not participate in outside activities, is sedentary, eats a Traditional American Diet (lots of carbohydrates, fat and sugar, little fiber and a moderate amount of deep fried chicken or fish) and takes no nutritional supplements. As you might expect, recent lab data showed a vitamin D deficiency (25 ng/mL).

In several microarray analyses, 25-hydroxy vitamin D status, along with several vitamin D receptors (ApaI and FokI), has demonstrated a significant role in the susceptibility to OA and progression of the disease (52). Low Vitamin D status has been linked with higher WOMAC pain scores, decreased joint function and poorer outcomes following total hip or knee replacement in patients with OA (52, 53).

Multiple genes encode for proteins that are essential for the synthesis of the active vitamin D molecule 1, alpha 25-dihydroxy vitamin D3. These proteins include enzymes, transport proteins and receptors. Polymorphisms associated with one of more of these genes in this metabolic pathway can alter vitamin D metabolism, leading to a vitamin D deficiency; the more gene SNPs in a single metabolic pathway, the greater the physiological impact (52). By evaluating a patient's gene SNPs associated with vitamin D metabolism, a clinician can uncover the underlying mechanism(s) for a vitamin D deficiency, provide effective and personalized strategies to improve vitamin D status, and potentially ameliorate OA pathophysiology now and in the future.

This patient's test results from a commercial genomic testing company showed gene variants for DHCR7, GC and VDR Fokl. The interpretative lab report informs us that he cannot effectively convert sunshine into vitamin D, transport of vitamin D and its metabolites is impaired, and binding of the active metabolite to the vitamin D receptor in the nucleus is also compromised. The latter is particularly important, since vitamin D acts through its vitamin D receptor to influence cell types and tissues important in OA – chondrocytes, osteoclasts and osteoblasts (54). The appropriate intervention for this OA patient is to encourage the consumption of vitamin D-rich foods and/or supplement with a vitamin D/K2 emulsion. His genomic test report also provides relevant biomarker testing recommendations. Monitoring his response to these interventions by testing both the 25-hydroxy and the 1,alpha 25-dihydroxy forms of vitamin D would be important for this patient.

CO-MORBIDITIES AND OA

Excess body weight, metabolic syndrome and prior injury are well-established risk factors for the development of OA (55). More effectively treating these existing conditions, or even preventing them in the first place, is another strategy in reducing the burden of OA. Comprehensive genomic testing can help identify people who are predisposed to obesity, metabolic syndrome or tendinopathies associated with physical activities. Genomic testing can also identify OA patients susceptible to an inherent excessive pro-inflammatory response and/or poor synthesis of endogenous antioxidants. With this information, personalized DNA-based strategies can be used to reduce the occurrence of these conditions or more effectively address existing comorbidities that can impact the OA disease process.

ORTHOGENOMICS OF OSTEOPOROSIS

Osteoporosis (OP) is a metabolic disease of the bone in which its micro architecture is disrupted, resulting in decreased bone mineral density and higher fracture risk (56). It is sometimes called the silent disease, because clinical manifestations of the disease are not apparent until fracture occurs, typically in the wrist, hip, humerus, tibia or vertebrae. Complications of these fractures can include intense pain, limited range of motion, deformity, loss of height and, in severe cases, death.

Bone is a metabolically dynamic tissue; it is being made and broken down at the same time. Osteoblasts and osteoclasts orchestrate this delicate balance with help of genes that encode for numerous hormones, micro environment factors, proinflammatory cytokines, cell signaling agents, along with the absorption, transport and utilization of dietary nutrients (57). As with OA, variations in a person's DNA can generate a wide range of phenotypes – from rare inherited mutations causing severe disease, to single or multiple SNPs in one or more biological systems predisposing an individual to OP over time depending on critical environmental factors.

CANDIDATE GENE STUDIES AND MOLECULAR MECHANISMS OF OP: MONOGENIC APPROACH

Candidate gene studies have discovered more than 38 inherited single gene mutations linked to osteoporosis (58). Some of the genes are related to collagen 1 biosynthesis (BMP2, COL1A1, COL1A2, CREB3L1, CRTAP, FDBP10, PLOD2, PPIB, SERPINH1), whereas others are related to osteoclast function (CA2, CCLNCN7, CTSK, OSTM1, PLEKHM1, SNX10, TC1RG1), osteoclast differentiation via NF-kB signaling (IKBKG, SQSTM1, TNFRSF 11A, TNFRSF11B, TNFSF11, VCP), and Wnt-regulated endochondral ossification (LRP4, LRP5, LRPS, SOST, WNT1, WTX). An inherited genetic mutation in one of these key genes can lead to severe bone diseases linked to either excessive bone formation or bone reabsorption such as osteogenesis imperfecta, osteopetrosis, sclerosis and autosomal recessive osteoporosis.

GENOME-WIDE ASSOCIATION STUDIES

Genome-wide association studies (GWAS) have successfully identified common gene variants linked with bone mineral density (BMD) and osteoporosis, with more than 100 loci reported using numerous meta-analyses (59). Thirty genes that are consistently reported in GWAS studies for osteoporosis are provided in Tables 2.4 through 2.6. As with OA, several genes appear both in the candidate gene studies and GWAS studies, reflecting how DNA changes in the same gene can impact an individual's phenotype differentially, with the magnitude depending on whether the change in person's DNA sequence is a mutation or a SNP.

TABLE 2.4

Gene SNPs (GWAS) Linked to Osteoclast Function and Osteoporosis Risk

Gene	Protein	Metabolic System
CLCN7	Chloride Voltage-Gated Channel 7	Osteoclast function, bone resorption

TABLE 2.5
Gene SNPs (GWAS) Linked to WNT Cell Signaling and Osteoporosis Risk

Gene	Protein	Metabolic System(s)
AXIN1	Axin 1	Wnt-signaling, phosphorylation and ubiquitination, cell growth, apoptosis
CTNNB1	Catenin Beta 1	Wnt-signaling, cell growth, actin cytoskeleton
DKK1	Dickkopf WNT Signaling Pathway Inhibitor 1	Wnt-signaling, embryonic development, bone formation
HOXC6	Homeobox C6	Wnt-signaling, anterior-posterior axis development
LRP4	LDL Receptor Related Protein 4	Wnt-signaling, bone formation, neuromuscular junction
LRP5	LDL Receptor Related Protein 5	Wnt-signaling, skeletal homeostasis
MEF2C	Myocyte Enhancer Factor 2C	Myogenesis, bone marrow B-lymphopoiesis
PIHLH	Parathyroid Hormone Like Hormone	Endochondral bone development
sFRP4	Secreted Frizzled Related Protein 4	Wnt-signaling, cell growth and differentiation, bone morphogenesis
SOST	Sclerostin	Wnt-signaling, bone formation
RPSO3	R-Spondin 3	Wnt-signaling, cell growth
WLS	Wntless Wnt Ligand Secretion Mediator	Wnt-signaling, anterior-posterior axis development
WNT3	Wnt Family Member 3	Wnt- signaling proteins, regulation of cell fate and patterning during embryogenesis
WNT4	Wnt Family Member 4	Wnt-signaling, tissue development.
WNT 16	Wnt Family Member 16	Wnt-signaling, regulation of cell fate and patterning during embryogenesis

TABLE 2.6
Gene SNPs (GWAS) Linked to Impaired Endochondral Ossification and Osteoporosis Risk

Gene	Protein	Metabolic System(s)
MEF2C	Myocyte Enhancer Factor 2C	Myogenesis, bone marrow B-lymphopoiesis
PIHLH	Parathyroid Hormone Like Hormone	This hormone, via its receptor, PTHR1, regulates endochondral bone development
RUNX2	Runt Related Transcription Factor 2	Osteoblastic differentiation, skeletal morphogenesis, skeletal gene expression
SOX4	SRY-Box 4	Apoptosis, bone development
SOX6	SRY-Box 6	Transcriptional activation, neurogenesis and skeleton formation
SOX9	SRY-Box 9	Skeletal development, chondrogenesis gene expression
SP7	Sp7 Transcription Factor	Transcriptional activation, osteoblast differentiation and bone formation
SPP1	Secreted Phosphoprotein 1	Attachment of osteoclasts to the mineralized bone matrix

MICROARRAY STUDIES

Microarray studies refine the broad scope of GWAS to identify clinically relevant gene SNPs that interact with environmental factors to impact the metabolic processes and specific pathophysiological endpoints of OP. This information can then be used by clinicians to develop prevention or treatment therapies, personalized to a person's unique genotype and phenotype. For example, it is well established that the lack of estrogen in menopausal women contributes to reduced BMD (60), but an individual's response is highly variable. Orthogenomics can provide information related to genotypes and molecular mechanisms that differentially affect this phenomenon. An estrogen deficiency promotes three gene-driven, metabolic processes related to increased activity of the RANKL (receptor activator of nuclear factor-kappa B ligand) gene, culminating in osteoclast generation and bone reabsorption (61). The first process is calcium metabolism, where higher renal excretion and reduced absorption of the mineral from the small intestine prompts a rise in parathyroid hormone (PTH). Increased PTH then upregulates the activity of the RANKL gene. T-cell activation is another consequence of an estrogen deficiency. Through various intermediates (IL-7, INF-gamma and MCH II), T-cell activation leads to increased RANKL activity. And, finally, estrogen deficiency promotes an increase in the expression of four pro-inflammatory genes (IL-1, IL-6, TNF-alpha and PGE2). Higher levels of these cytokines and prostaglandin E2 triggers an increase in the activity of the RANKL gene, leading to bone loss. A woman whose genotype consists of one or more polymorphisms in any one of these metabolic pathways can experience greater bone loss compared to someone without these DNA changes.

A proactive clinician can screen menopausal women for these gene SNPs and recommend evidenced-based, personalized interventions to improve calcium metabolism and mitigate the pro-inflammatory response, lessening the risk for osteopenia, osteoporosis and bone fractures induced by an estrogen deficiency.

CONSTRUCTION OF CLINICIAN'S GENOMIC TOOL BOX FOR OP: GENE-FUNCTION-ACTION STEP MATRIX

Orthogenomics helps to illuminate the interconnectedness between various seemingly unrelated biological systems that underlie the etiology and pathophysiology of OP. Genomic testing can unwrap these complicated and complex biological threads, as researchers continue to expand our knowledge with advances in genomics. Some of the more recent discoveries include gene SNPs linked to fat cell metabolism (PPAR-gamma) (62), growth factors (TGF Beta, VEGF) (63), cell signaling agents (NF-kappa B) (64), inflammation (IL-6) (65), nutrient utilization (DBP) (66), hormones (IGF) (67), hormonal receptors (ER-α, ER-ß) (68), stress response (COMT) (69), exercise regimen (ACTN) (70) and physical trauma (COL1A1) (71).

With this level of complexity, it is essential to use a comprehensive approach to genomic testing, with evaluation and interpretation of gene SNPs across these different biological systems grounded in clinical relevance. In addition, we use a Gene-Function-Action Step matrix in our clinic to map out the impact of a person's gene SNPs on osteoblast and osteoclast metabolism, micro architecture of bone and other metabolic aspects of OP. The matrix helps prioritize and personalize our evidenced-based and DNA-directed nutritional genomic, lifestyle and pharmacological interventions.

CASE HISTORY 3: MONOGENIC AND POLYGENIC EXAMPLE

Gina is a 39-year-old Caucasian woman who is concerned about her bone density. She had a hysterectomy with salpingo-oophorectomy at the age of 35 due to severe endometriosis, resulting in surgical menopause. She chose not to use hormone replacement therapy because of a strong family history of ER+ breast cancer.

She is mildly overweight, and her diet would be considered a traditional American diet: ample amounts of refined carbohydrates and animal protein, very few vegetables and fruits. She avoided dairy products due to lactose intolerance, and was not knowledgeable about other dietary sources of calcium. She did not take any nutritional supplements or prescribed medications. She played softball during the summer months, but the rest of the year she spent little time outdoors and led a sedentary lifestyle.

Initial lab results from a comprehensive metabolic panel, CBC and urinalysis were normal, but 25-OH vitamin D was low (30 ng/mL). Gina's DEXA scan showed osteopenia, with a T-score of −1.3 in the femoral neck and −1.1 in the lumbar spine. Genomic testing from a commercial lab evaluated genes related to bone mineral density and osteoporosis risk, including vitamin D metabolism.

The only gene SNP detected in her vitamin D metabolic pathway was VDR Bsml, which has been shown to alter receptor function for the active 1, alpha25-di-hydroxy vitamin D molecule (72). More recently, it has also been implicated in altered calcium absorption, independent of estrogen's effect (73). Gina was advised to increase her intake of vitamin D-rich foods and her sun exposure, since her genomic test results indicated she could readily convert the pre-vitamin D, 7-dehydrocholecalciferol, into the provitamin D molecule, cholecalciferol, a metabolic reaction facilitated by the sunlight. A vitamin D3/K2 emulsion was added to ensure adequate vitamin D intake during the winter months. Calcium intake was increased through the addition of a calcium/magnesium supplement.

While this example highlights the impact of one gene, VDR, on Gina's risk for osteoporosis, complex, chronic diseases are often the result of interactions between multiple genes in several biological systems and environmental factors. In our clinic, a polygenic model is used to explore these possibilities. Table 2.7 summarizes the different biological systems and multiple gene SNPs that may have also played a role in Gina's development of osteopenia. The Gene-Function-Action Step matrix helps prioritize the DNA-directed interventions associated with each biological system.

Inflammation is an independent risk factor for osteoporosis (74). Gina had SNPs in several of the pro-inflammatory genes evaluated (IL-1B, IL-6 and TNF-alpha) that increased the production of these cytokines, which over time could contribute to further bone loss. TNF-alpha has a potentially greater impact, as it triggers multiple proinflammatory pathways by activating intracellular nuclear factor NF-kappa B. Several plant-based compounds have been shown to suppress this TNF-alpha induced NF-kappa B activation, and were recommended to Gina to modulate her pro-inflammatory response. Biomarker testing for these pro-inflammatory cytokines is available through most commercial reference laboratories for assessment and monitoring the efficacy of the interventions.

The mechanical strain associated with physical activity benefits bone health and decreases the risk of osteoporosis (75). Gina's DNA-derived exercise recommendation was to combine endurance types of activities with weight training. Matching the type of exercise with her DNA ensures that she will sustain an effective exercise program throughout her life.

Gina was mildly overweight; her calculated BMI was 25. Adipose tissue can undergo lipid peroxidation, generating oxidative stress and activating the transcription factor, peroxisome proliferator-activated receptor-gamma or PPAR-gamma. Because PPAR-gamma has been shown to decrease osteoblast differentiation (62), a DNA-based, personalized weight reduction program was instituted to decrease her risk of further bone loss.

For a clinician, it is important to recognize that the same gene can impact two metabolic systems differently. This can be seen in Table 2.7 with IL-6 and VDR Bsml. A single intervention may have a desired biochemical or metabolic effect in multiple systems, or in just one biological system but not another. Understanding the underlying molecular mechanisms, biochemistry and physiology is crucial when interpreting genomic test results and applying interventions.

Gina instituted the DNA-directed changes and after 6 months her BMD was tested again on the same DEXA machine. Her T-score was −0.988, nearly a 25% increase in her BMD (76). Urinary markers confirmed the reversal of excessive bone turnover that had been noted at baseline. She was exercising regularly, had lost 15 pounds and overall had more energy.

PHARMACOGENOMICS

Drug metabolism is influenced by many factors, including genes, food and environmental factors in addition to other medications (77). Historically the focus has been on drug-drug interactions and the impact of substrates on cytochrome P450 enzymes (78). Today, advances in pharmacokinetics and pharmacogenomic testing help a clinician reduce the risk of drug-drug interactions and adverse effects, as well as maximize selection of effective medications (77).

To date, much of the research has focused on SNPs in single genes primarily involved in phase 1 metabolism by cytochrome P450 enzymes (CYP450). Six of these CYP450 enzymes are responsible for the metabolism of the majority of prescribed and over-the-counter medications (79). In fact,

TABLE 2.7
Summary of Gene SNPs and Interventions for Case History #3

Biological System	Gene	Intervention
Inflammation	IL-1B	EPA/DHA
	IL-6	Beta-sitosterol
	TNF-alpha	Curcumin, resveratrol
Exercise:	ACTN	⎫
Power versus	AGT	⎪
Endurance	ACE	⎪
Activity	eNOS3	Combination of endurance and power exercises
	COL5A1	⎪
	IL-6	⎪
	VDR	⎭
Fat Metabolism	PPAR-gamma	Weight reduction program
Vitamin D Metabolism	VDR Bsml	Vitamin K2/D3 emulsion
Calcium Absorption	VDR Bsml	Supplemental calcium and magnesium

two of these enzymes, CYP3A4 and CYP2D6, account for the metabolism of over 50% of pre-scribed drugs (70).

Until recently, pharmacogenomic research focused primarily on how a single drug is metabo-lized by a unique CYP450 enzyme. A more advanced polygenic approach is now being adopted to reflect more accurately what occurs for a patient on multiple drugs. In addition, pharmacogenomic research is evaluating how gene SNPs associated with drug absorption, transport, receptor function, utilization and excretion impact drug safety and efficacy. Understanding how a patient's genotype influences drug metabolism along with nutrient cofactors from the diet can go a long way in helping a clinician personalize drug use and improve predictability in clinical environment (77).

PHARMACOGENOMICS: OSTEOARTHRITIS

Many of the medications commonly used in osteoarthritis are related to pain control, primarily through the opioid or cyclooxygenase pathways. Knowledge of a patient's pharmacogenomic profile can assist in choosing the right medications.

Several commonly prescribed opioids exist as prodrugs and must be biotransformed to an active metabolite for maximal efficacy in treating pain. Codeine, oxycodone and hydrocodone all require metabolism by CYP2D6 into active morphine compounds (80). Poor metabolizer genotypes can result in decreased conversion to morphine, with insufficient pain relief at standard dosages. On the other hand, rapid metabolizer genotypes are at increased risk of toxicity due to increased conversion to morphine (77). For women who fall into this second category and are breastfeeding, there is an additional risk of neonatal respiratory depression (81).

Opioid receptors are another factor to consider, with OPRM1 being the most studied. OPRM1 is a *mu* opioid receptor that binds primarily morphine, fentanyl, methadone and oxyco-done (80). OPRM1 gene SNPs lead to decreased receptor function and can result in inadequate pain relief. Fentanyl also undergoes metabolism by CYP3A4 to inactive metabolites; a slow metabolizer genotype or concurrent use of drugs that inhibit this enzyme may increase the risk of toxicity (80).

COMT is involved in the dopaminergic pathway, and can influence the density of opioid recep-tors (82). Certain genotypes have been associated with the effectiveness of morphine for pain con-trol (83), and may have a synergistic effect with the OPRM1 genotype (82).

Many common nonsteroidal anti-inflammatory medications (NSAIDS) are metabolized by CYP2C9, including celecoxib, diclofenac and ibuprofen (84). A slow metabolizer genotype can result in a prolonged half-life with an increased risk of gastrointestinal bleeding (78). Celecoxib is metabolized mainly by CYP2C9 and, to a lesser extent, by CYP3A4. The therapeutic effect may depend on the ratio of metabolites produced between the two pathways; the rate may vary with the presence of other drugs or nutrients that interact with CYP2C9 or CYP3A4. It is important to note that celecoxib also inhibits the activity of CYP2D6 (85), and may impact metabolism of other drugs utilizing the CYP2D6 pathway.

Genes involving the cyclooxygenase pathway itself can also impact response to NSAIDs. The PTGS2 genotype, which encodes for the COX2 enzyme, has been associated with differential response to rofecoxib and ibuprofen (78).

PHARMACOGENOMICS: OSTEOPOROSIS

The pharmacogenomics of osteoporosis medications has been largely ignored, so there is very little data on which to base clinical recommendations (86). Bisphosphonates, the major class of medications used to treat osteoporosis, do not undergo appreciable metabolism, and are eliminated through the kidney. Preliminary research shows that transporter genes from the SLC22A, SLC17A and SLC13A families may be important in the distribution of bisphosphonates to certain tissues. Interestingly, two genes (COL1A1 and VDR) associated with bone metabolism may play a role in the efficacy of bisphosphonates in arresting osteopenia or osteoporosis (87).

The bone-forming hormone, calcitonin, undergoes renal excretion with no hepatic metabolism. Raloxifene is metabolized through phase 2 glucuronidation, and UGT1A1 polymorphisms have been shown to impact metabolism and response to treatment (88).

Hormone replacement therapy can be used as a secondary approach, but is often limited by the risk of breast cancer in women. Genomic testing can help identify those who may be at higher risk due to impaired phase 1 and/or phase 2 detoxification of estradiol. Nutrigenomic strategies can reduce the potential risks of estrogen or estrogen metabolite induced breast cancer (89).

Future pharmacogenomics research will continue to explore the polygenic drug model across more ethnically diverse populations as well as evaluate gene polymorphisms linked to drug-specific receptors, transporters, gastrointestinal absorption and even circadian rhythm (77, 90) to achieve personalized medicine in pharmacology.

SUMMARY

Genomic testing is a powerful tool to help clinicians personalize disease prevention and treatment programs. Orthogenomics is a new approach to orthopedic medicine that requires an understanding of the molecular mechanisms underlying a disease, how genes affect metabolic pathways, and how genes interact with environmental factors to contribute to a disease process. Pharmacogenomics impacts the efficacy and risk of adverse effects of medications commonly used in orthopedic medicine. With genomic testing and the deeper insight it provides, clinicians can now provide DNA-directed, individualized strategies to prevent or alter the course of disease and improve patient outcomes.

DISCLOSURE STATEMENT

Dr. Kline and Dr. Veltmann are cofounders of Genoma International, which provides genomic testing and education to clinicians. They are also cofounders of the GENESIS Center for Personalized Health, where they provide clinical genomic medicine services.

REFERENCES

1. Wilson, B. J. and Nicholls, S. G. 2015. The human genome project, and recent advances in personalized genomics. *Risk Manag. Healthc. Policy.* 8: 9–20.
2. Manolio, T. A., Chisholm RL, Ozenberger, B. et al. 2013. Implementing genomic medicine in the clinic: The future is here. *Genet. Med.* 15(4): 258–267.
3. McNally, E. M. 2017. Incorporating genetic testing into cardiovascular practice. *JAMA Cardiol.* Published online August 09. doi:10.1001/jamacardio.2017.2626.
4. Phillips, K. A., Deverka, P. A., Sox, H. C., et al. 2017. Making genomic medicine evidence-based and patient-centered: A structured review and landscape analysis of comparative effectiveness research. *Genet. Med.* Published online April 13. doi:10.1038/gim.2017.21.
5. Veltmann, J. R., 2009. Functional genomics 101: Its application to osteoporosis, hormone replacement, breast and prostate cancer. *Papers presented at Thinking Outside the Box: the Next Generation Conference.* October 3 and 4. Fort Lauderdale, FL.
6. Steinberg, G., Scott, A. Honcz, J., et al. 2015. Reducing metabolic syndrome risk using a personalized wellness program. *J. Occup. Env. Med.* 57 (12): 1269–1274.
7. Willard, H. F., Angrist, M., and Ginsburg, G. S. 2005. Genomic medicine: Genetic variation and its impact on the future of health care. *Philos. Trans. R. Soc. Lond. B: Biolo. Sci.* 360(1460): 1543–1550.
8. Chial, H. 2008. Rare genetic disorders: Learning about genetic disease through gene mapping, SNPs, and microarray data. *Nat. Ed.* 1(1): 192.
9. Lvovs, D., Favorova, O. O., and A. V. Favorov. 2012. A polygenic approach to the study of polygenic diseases. *Acta Naturae.* 4(3): 59–71.
10. Kincaid, E. 2016. Of mice and interaction: A new way to investigate complex genetic traits. *Nat. Med.* 22: 1065–1066.
11. Horner, S. M. and Gale M. Jr. 2013. Regulation of hepatic innate immunity by hepatitis C virus. *Nat. Med.* 19: 879–888.
12. Yang, J., Benyamin, B., McEvoy, B. P., et al. 2011. Common SNPs explain a large proportion of heritability for human height. *Nat. Genet.* 42(7): 565–569.
13. Mersha, T. B. and Abebe, T. 2015. Self-reporting race/ethnicity in the age of genomic research: Its potential impact on understanding of health disparities. *Hum. Genomics* 9(1): 1.
14. Venter, J. C., Adams, M. D., Myers, E. W., et al. 2001. The sequence of the human genome. *Science* 291(5507): 1304–1351.
15. Chang, C. Q., Yesupriya, A., Rowell, J. L., et al. 2014. A systematic review of cancer GWAS and candidate gene meta-analyses reveals limited overlap but similar effect sizes. *Eur. J. Hum. Genet.* 22: 402–408.
16. Tabor, H. K., Risch, N. J., and Myers, R. M. 2002. Candidate-gene approaches for studying complex genetic traits: Practical considerations. *Nature Rev. Genet.* 3: 391–397.
17. Riancho, J. A., 2012. Genome-wide association studies (GWAS) in complex diseases: Advantages and limitations. *Reumatol. Clin.* 8: 56–57.
18. Bumgarner, R., 2013. Overview of DNA microarrays: Types, applications and their future. *Curr. Protoc. Mol. Biol.* 101(1): 22.1.1–22.1.11.
19. Kraus, V. B., Blanco, F. J., Englund, M., et al. 2015. Call for standardized definitions of osteoarthritis and risk stratification for clinical trials and clinical use. *Osteoarthritis Cartilage* 23(8): 1233–1241.
20. Ashkavand, Z., Malekinejad, H., and Vishwanath, B. S. 2013. The pathophysiology of osteoarthritis. *J. Pharm. Res.* 7(1): 132–138.
21. Aury-Landas, J., Marcelli, C., Leclercq, S., et al. 2013. Genetic determinism of primary early-onset osteoarthritis. *Trends Mol. Med.* 22(1): 38–52.
22. Van Meurs, J. B. 2017. Osteoarthritis year in review 2016: genetics, genomics and epigenetics. *Osteoarthritis Cartilage* 25(2): 181–189.
23. Shawky, R., 2014. Reduced penetrance in human inherited disease. *Egypt. J. Med. Hum. Genet.* 15(2): 103–111.
24. Wang, T., Liang, Y., Li, H., et al. 2016. Single nucleotide polymorphisms and osteoarthritis. *Medicine* 95(7): e2811.
25. Bodmer, W. and Bonilla, C. 2008. Common and rare variants in multifactorial susceptibility to common diseases. *Nat. Genet.* 40(6): 695–701.
26. Kerkhof, J. M., Uitterlinden, A. G., Valdes, A. M., et al. 2008. Radiographic osteoarthritis at three joint sites and FRZB, LRB5 and LRP6 polymorphisms in two population-based cohorts. *Osteoarthritis Cartilage* 16: 1141–1149.

27. Mustafa, Z., Chapman, K., Irven, C., et al. 2000. Linkage analysis of candidate genes as susceptibility loci for osteoarthritis-suggestive linkage of COL9A1 to female hip osteoarthritis. *Rheumatology* 39(3): 299–306.

28. Zhai, G., Rivadeneira, F., Houwing-Duistermaat, J. J., et al. 2004. Insulin-like growth factor I gene promoter polymorphism, collagen type II alpha1 (COL2A1) gene, and the prevalence of radiographic osteoarthritis: The Rotterdam Study. *Ann. Rheum. Dis.* 63(5): 544–548.

29. Richards, A. J., Yates, J. R., Williams, R., et al. 1996. A family with Stickler syndrome type 2 has a mutation in the COL11A1 gene resulting in the substitution of glycine 97 by valine in alpha 1 (XI) collagen. *Hum. Mol. Genet.* 5(9): 1339–1343.

30. Loughlin, J., Irven, C., Mustafa, Z., et al. 1998. Identification of five novel mutations in cartilage oligomeric matrix protein gene in pseudoachondroplasia and multiple epiphyseal dysplasia. *Hum. Mutat.* 1(7): S10–S17.

31. Lian, K., Zmud, J. M., Nevitt, M. C., et al. 2005. Type I collagen alpha1 Sp1 transcription factor binding site polymorphism is associated with reduced risk of hip osteoarthritis defined by severe joint space narrowing in elderly women. *Arthritis Rheum.* 52(5): 1431–1436.

32. Nagase, H. and Kashiwagi, M. 2003. Aggrecanases and cartilage matrix degradation. *Arthritis Res. Ther.* 5: 94–103.

33. Rodriguez-Lopez, J., Mustafa, Z., Pombo-Suarez, M., et al. 2008. Genetic variation including nonsynonymous polymorphisms of a major aggrecanase, ADAMTS-5, in susceptibility to osteoarthritis. *Arthritis Rheum.* 58(2): 435–441.

34. Wei, L., Sun, X-J., Wang, Z., et al. 2006. CD95-induced osteoarthritic chondrocyte apoptosis and necrosis: Dependency on p38 mitogen-activated protein kinase. *Arthritis Res. Ther.* 8(2): R37.

35. Valdes, A. M., Lories, R. J., van Meurs, J. B., et al. (2009). Variation at the ANP32A gene is associated with risk of hip osteoarthritis in women. *Arthritis Rheum.* 60(7): 2046–2054.

36. Richette, P., Corvol, M., and Bardin, T. 2003. Estrogens, cartilage, and osteoarthritis. *Joint Bone Spine.* 70(4): 257–262.

37. Solovieva, S., Hirvonen, A., Siivola, P., et al. 2006. Vitamin D receptor gene polymorphisms and susceptibility of hand osteoarthritis in Finnish women. *Arthritis Res. Ther.* 8(1): R20.

38. Rodriguez-Fontenla, C., Calaza, M., Evangelou, E., et al. 2014. Assessment of osteoarthritis candidate genes in a meta-analysis of nine genome-wide association studies. *Arthritis Rheumatol.* 66(4): 940–949.

39. Mio, F., Chiba, K., Hirose, Y., et al. 2007. A functional polymorphism in COL11A1, which encodes the alpha 1 chain of type XI collagen, is associated with susceptibility to lumbar disc herniation. *Am. J. Hum. Genet.* 81(6): 1271–1277.

40. Sokolove, J. and Legus, C. M. 2013. The role of inflammation in the pathogenesis of osteoarthritis: Latest findings and interpretations. *Ther. Adv. Musculoskelet. Dis.* 5(2): 77–94.

41. Lambert, C., Dubuc, J. E., Montell, E., et al. 2014. Gene expression pattern of cells from inflamed and normal areas of osteoarthritis synovial membrane. *Arthritis Rheumatol.* 66(4): 960–968.

42. Chou, C. H., Wu, C. C., Song, I. W., et al. Genome-wide expression profiles of subchondral bone in osteoarthritis. *Arthritis Res. Ther.* 15(6): R190.

43. Schelbergen, R. F., de Munter, W. van den Bosch, M. H. et al. 2016. Alarmins S100A8/S100A9 aggravate osteophyte formation in experimental osteoarthritis and predict osteophyte progression in early human symptomatic osteoarthritis. *Ann. Rheum. Dis.* 75(1): 218–225.

44. Ramos, Y. F., Bos, S. D., Lakenberg, N., et al. 2014. Genes expressed in blood link osteoarthritis with apoptotic pathways. *Ann. Rheum. Dis.* 73(10): 1844–1853.

45. Tsezou, A. 2014. Osteoarthritis year in review 2014: Genetics and genomics. *Osteoarthritis Cartilage* 22: 2017e2024.

46. Hernandez-Valle, E. Herrera-Ruiz, M. Salgado, G. R., et al. 2014. Anti-inflammatory effect of 3-*O*-[(6'-*O*-palmitoyl)-β-glucopyranosyl sitosterol] from *Agave angustifolia* on ear edema in mice. *Molecules* 19: 15624–15637.

47. Lee, I-A., Kim, E-J, and Dim, D-H. 2012. Inhibitory effect of β-sitosterol on TNBS-induced colitis in mice. *Planta. Med.* 78 (08): 896–898.

48. Kiecolt-Glaser, J., Christian, L., Preston, H., et al. 2010. Stress, inflammation and yoga practice. *Psychosom. Med.* 72(2): 113.

49. McAninch, E. A., Jo, S., Preite, N. Z., et al., 2015. Prevalent polymorphism in thyroid hormone- activating enzyme leaves a genetic fingerprint that underlies associated clinical syndromes. *J Clin. Endocrinol. Metab.* 100: 920–933.

50. Panicker, V., Saravanan, P., Vaidya, B., et al. 2009. Common variation in the DIO2 gene predicts base-line psychological well-being and response to combination thyroxine plus triiodothyronine therapy in hypothyroid patients. *J. Clin. Endocrinol. Metab.* 94(5): 1623–1629.
51. Triggiani, V., Tafaro, E., Giagulli, V. A., et al. 2009. Role of iodine, selenium and micronutrients in thyroid function and disorders. *Endocr. Metab. Immune Disord. Drug Targets* 9(3): 277–294.
52. Mabey, T. and Honsawek, S. 2015. Role of vitamin D in osteoarthritis: Molecular, cellular and clinical perspectives. *Int. J. Endocrinol.* 2015: 383918.
53. Maniar, R. N., Patil, A. M., Maniar, A. R., et al. 2016. Effect of preoperative vitamin D levels on functional performance after total knee arthroplasty. *Clin. Orthop. Surg.* 8(2): 153–156.
54. Garfinkel, R. J., Dilisio, M. F., and Agrawal, D. K. 2017. Vitamin D and its effect on articular cartilage and osteoarthritis. *Orthop. J. Sports Med.* 5 (6): doi: 2325967117711376.
55. Malfait, A.-M., 2016. Osteoarthritis year in review 2015: Biology. *Osteoarthritis Cartilage* 24(1): 21–26.
56. Cosman, F., de Beur, S. J., Leboff, M. S., et al. 2014. The clinician's guide to prevention and treatment of osteoporosis. *Osteoporos. Int.* 25(10): 2359–2381.
57. Kruger, M. C. and Wolber, F. M. 2016. Osteoporosis: Modern paradigms for last century's bones. *Nutrients* 8(6): 376.
58. Rocha-Braz, M. G. and Ferraz-de-Souza, B. 2016. Genetics of osteoporosis: Searching for candidate genes for bone fragility. *Arch. Endocrinol. Metabol.* 60(4): 391–401.
59. Boudin, E., Fijalkowski, I., Hendrickx, G., et al. 2016. Genetic control of bone mass. *Mol. Cell. Endocrinol.* 432: 3–13.
60. Riggs, B. L., Khosla, S. and Melton L. J. 3rd. 1998. A unitary model for involutional osteoporosis: Estrogen deficiency causes both type I and type II osteoporosis in postmenopausal women and contributes to bone loss in aging men. *J. Bone Miner. Res.* 13(5): 763–773.
61. Patil, S. 2015. Denosumab-a new therapeutic option for osteoporosis. *World J Pharm Pharm Sci.* 4(12): 858–873.
62. Lecka-Czernik, B. 2010. PPARγ, an essential regulator of bone mass: Metabolic and molecular cues. *IBMS BoneKEy* 7: 171–181.
63. Fei, Y. and Hurley, M. M. 2012. Role of fibroblast growth factor 2 and Wnt signaling in anabolic effects of parathyroid hormone on bone formation. *J. Cell. Physiol.* 227(11): 3539–3545.
64. Abu-Amer, Y. 2013. NF-ƙB signaling and bone resorption. *Osteoporos. Int.* 24(9): 10.1007/s00198-013-2313-x.
65. Omoigui, S. 2007. The Interleukin-6 inflammation pathway from cholesterol to aging – role of statins, bisphosphonates and plant polyphenols in aging and age-related diseases. *Immun. Ageing* 4: 1.
66. Bhan, I. 2014. Vitamin D binding protein and bone health. *Int. J. Endocrinol.* Vol 2014, Article ID 561214, 5 pages.
67. Niu, T. and Rosen, C. J. 2005. The insulin-like growth factor-1 and osteoporosis. A critical appraisal. *Gene* 361: 38–56.
68. Gennari, L., Merlotti, D., De Paola, V., et al., 2005. Estrogen receptor gene polymorphisms and the genetics of osteoporosis: A HuGE review. *Am. J. Epidemiol.* 161(4): 307–320.
69. Lorentzon, M., Eriksson, A.-L., Mellstro, D., et al. 2004. The COMT val158met polymorphism is associated with peak BMD in men. *J. Bone Miner. Res.* 19(12): 2005–2011.
70. Min, S.-K., Lim, S.-T., and Kim, C.-S. 2016. Association of ACTN3 polymorphisms with BMD, and physical fitness of elderly women. *J. Phys. Ther. Sci.* 28(10): 2731–2736.
71. Goodlin, G. T., Roos, A. K., Roos, T. R., et al. 2015. Applying personal genetic data to injury risk assessment in athletes. *PLoS ONE* 10(4): e0122676.
72. Wu, J., Shang, D-P., Yang, S., et al. 2016. Association between the vitamin D receptor gene polymorphism and osteoporosis. *Biomed. Rep.* 5(2): 233–236.
73. Laaksonen, M., Karkkainen, M. and Outila, T. 2002. Vitamin D receptor gene *Bsm*I-polymorphism in Finnish premenopausal and postmenopausal women: Its association with bone mineral density, markers of bone turnover, and intestinal calcium absorption, with adjustment for lifestyle factors. *J. Bone Miner. Met.* 20(6): 383–390.
74. Mundy, G. R. 2007. Osteoporosis and inflammation. *Nutr. Rev.* 65(12 Pt 2): S147–S151.
75. Kelley, G. A., Kelley, K. S., and Kohrt, W. M. 2013. Exercise and bone mineral density in premenopausal women: A meta-analysis of randomized controlled trials. *Int. J. Endocrinol.* 2013: 741639.
76. Veltmann, J. R. and Kline, R. L. 2015. Functional genomics beyond MTHFR: Nutrigenomics in a clinical practice in the prevention and/or treatment of chronic diseases and cancer. *Keynote Presentation 10th Annual National Association of Nutrition Professionals Conference.* May 1. St. Paul, MN.

77. Tannenbaum, C. and Sheehan, N. 2014. Understanding drug-drug and drug-gene interactions. *Expert Rev. Clin. Pharmacol.* 7(4): 533–544.

78. Kapur, B. M., Lala, P. K., and Shaw, J. L. 2014. Pharmacogenetics of chronic pain management. *Clin. Biochem.* 47: 1169–1187.

79. English, B. A., Dortch, M., Ereshefsky, L., et al. 2012. Clinically significant psychotropic drug-drug interactions in the primary care setting. *Curr. Psychiatry Rep.* 14(4): 376–390.

80. Trescot, A. M. 2016. Opioid pharmacology and pharmacogenetics. In *Controlled Substance Management in Chronic Pain*, ed. P. S. Staats and S. S. Silverman, 45–62. Switzerland: Springer International Publishing.

81. FDA Health Advisory: Food and Drug Administration. 2007. Public Health Advisory: Use of codeine by some breastfeeding mothers may lead to life-threatening side effects in nursing babies. Available online www.fda.gov/drugs/drugsafety/postmarketdrugsafetyinformationforpatientsandproviders.

82. Reyes-Gibby, C. C., Shete, S., Rakvag, T., et al. 2007. Exploring joint effects of genes and the clinical efficacy of morphine for cancer pain: OPRM1 and COMT gene. *Pain* 130: 25–30.

83. Rakvag, T. T., Klepstad, P., Baar, C., et al. 2005. The val158met polymorphism of the human catechol-O-methyltransferase (COMT) gene may influence morphine requirements in cancer pain patients. *Pain* 116: 73–78.

84. Stamer, U. M and Stuber, F. 2007. The pharmacogenetics of analgesia. *Expert Opin. Pharmac.* 8: 2235–2245.

85. Wyatt, J. E., Pettit, W. L., and Harirforoosh, S. 2012. Pharmacogenetics of nonsteroidal anti-inflammatory drugs. *Pharmacogenomics J.* 12: 462–467.

86. Marini, F. and Brandi, M. L. 2010. Pharmacogenetics of osteoporosis. *F1000 Biol. Rep.* 2: 63.

87. Gonga, L., Altmana, R. B., and Klein, T. E. 2011. Bisphosphonates pathway. *Pharmacogenet. Genomics* 21(1): 50–53.

88. Trontelz, J., Marc, J., Zavrtnik, A., et al. 2009. Effects of UGT1A1*28 polymorphism on raloxifene pharmacokinetics and pharmacodynamics. *Br. J. Clin. Pharmacol.* 67(4): 437–444.

89. Cerne, J. Z., Novakovic, S., Frkovic-Grazio, S., et al. 2011. Estrogen metabolism genotypes, use of long-term hormone replacement therapy and risk of postmenopausal breast cancer. *Onco. Rep.* 26: 479–485.

90. Ferrell, J. M. and Chiang, J. Y. L. 2015. Circadian rhythms in liver metabolism and disease. *Acta Pharm. Sin. B.* 5(2): 113–122.

3 Predictive Biomarkers in Personalized Laboratory Diagnoses and Best Practices Outcome Monitoring for Musculoskeletal Health

Russell Jaffe MD, PhD, CCN and Jayashree Mani, MS, CCN

INTRODUCTION

Musculoskeletal disorders are not just conditions affecting bones and joints, but have a systemic impact on muscles, nerves, adjoining ligaments, tendons, and blood vessels. Pain and inflammation due to repair deficits are strong co-factors in these conditions. In fact in 2012, according to CDC statistics, more than 50% of American adults had musculoskeletal pain disorders [1].

DEFINING THE TERM "BIOMARKER"

National Institutes of Health: "A characteristic that is objectively measured and evaluated as an indicator of normal biological processes, pathogenic processes, or pharmacologic responses to therapeutic intervention." [2]

U.S. Food and Drug Administration: "Any measurable diagnostic indicator that is used to assess the risk or presence of disease." [3]

Health Studies Collegium Working Group: "A measurable functional indicator that accesses individual validated risk or change in risk over time."

Chronic health issues, including those pertaining to the musculoskeletal system, precipitate from a myriad of origins. They share three common underlying causes:

- Cumulative repair deficits in essential nutrients and neurohormonal distress
- Oxidative damage due to antioxidant and buffering mineral unmet needs
- Metabolic acidosis due to cell mineral deficits that reduce cell energetics

This chapter presents eight biomarkers for these three causes of musculoskeletal dysfunction.

BACKGROUND ON PREDICTIVE BIOMARKERS

The chapter's predictive biomarkers (PBs) were developed on the premise that epigenetics influence 92% and genetics influence the remaining 8% of health [4,5]. Each PB covers an aspect of epigenetics and is an all-cause mortality predictor adding ten or more years of survival regardless of geographic, ethnic, and socioeconomic factors. Collectively the assays cover the 92% of conditions and diseases that are due to a lifetime of habits and lifestyle choices.

These PBs are different from most laboratory tests physicians would generally order. They are an interdependent suite of tests referenced to best outcome goal values rather than usual or normal statistical ranges. "Least risk, most gain" goal values for each test can be directly translated into quality years of life conserved. The chapter's selected predictive biomarkers add 10 or more years of quality life to best outcome goal values or ranges.

The technologic advance for the treatment of musculoskeletal conditions is the interrelation of the assays. They are the first synergistic combination of tests that can result in a comprehensive, personalized lifestyle action plan based on quantitative risk reduction. This proactive approach is evidence-based and has been shown to lower costs while enhancing individual outcomes when compared to current best standards of care, reducing risks, and adding "years to life and life to years."

These predictive biomarkers intended to better health and better care have also been demonstrated to lower projected medical costs through prevention and early treatment. Musculoskeletal diseases cost $796.3 billion dollars in 2011, 5.7% of the annual U.S. gross domestic product (GDP) [6]. Table 3.1 illustrates mortality measured both by final diagnosis and by underlying fundamental cause [7].

SELECTION CRITERIA FOR PREDICTIVE BIOMARKERS

Standards are rigorous for inclusion as a PB. Each PB is an all-cause morbidity and mortality indicator. Each is interdependent with the other predictive biomarkers in assessing or measuring aspects of epigenetics. All PBs are applicable to improving outcomes at lower costs based on a robust published literature of molecular and clinical outcome studies. This is a shift from comparing values

TABLE 3.1

Mortality Measured both by Final Diagnosis and Underlying Fundamental Cause

Cause of Death (Final Diagnosis)	Annual Deaths	Underlying Fundamental Causes			
		Diabetes	Mood Disorder	Malnutrition	Environment or Other
Heart Disease	620,000	320,000	60,000	80,000	160,000
Cancer	600,000	15,000	150,000	100,000	435,000
Respiratory	150,000	10,000	30,000	20,000	90,000
Stroke	140,000	75,000		10,000	55,000
Accidents[a]	120,000	10,000	40,000	10,000	60,000
Alzheimer's	85,000	10,000	30,000	5,000	25,000
Diabetes	70,000	70,000			
Kidney	50,000	10,000	20,000	5,000	15,000
Pneumonia	50,000	10,000	20,000	5,000	15,000
Suicide	40,000			15,000	25,000
Top 10 Causes	1,925,000	500,000	250,000	250,000	865,000
Other	675,000	Lives savable	Lives savable	Lives savable	unknown
Total Deaths	2,600,000				

Source: CDC Centers for Disease Control and Prevention, *National Center for Health Statistics*, "Table 18: Years of potential life lost before age 75 for selected causes of death, by sex, race, and Hispanic origin: United States selected years 1980–2014," https://www.cdc.gov/nchs/hus/contents2015.htm#018. [adapted] [7].

Notes: *National Center for Health Statistics data re-examined by fundamental cause by Health Studies Collegium Task Force on Sustainable Health.*; Legend: Predictive, proactive, personalized primary prevention saves lives at low cost compared to current best standards of disease care.

[a] Accidents (includes homicide)

to a statistical range to using best outcome values to assess individual risk. This shift turns concern into clinical opportunity to reduce risks and improve outcomes by meeting metabolic needs and enhancing restorative habits.

Every test has a standard deviation or range within which the value exists. Typical variance for most classic ELISA-based tests is 20% or more. This means that a value of 6 from a given specimen will cluster values around 6, with a large range of values from 4.8 to 7.2.

For predictive biomarker tests, a variance of 5% or less is desirable. The less the variance, the more predictive is the observed value. By example, if the "true" value is 6, and the test technology allows for better precision with a resulting 3% variance, a single test value *actually* exists between a narrow range of 5.92 and 6.18. In contrast, a 15+% variance offers limited individual applicability of results.

Usual (Statistical, "Normal") Test Results vs. Predictive (Best Outcome, Anticipatory) Goal Value Results

Conventional clinical lab tests provide information about "usual" or "normal" statistical ranges of a particular item analyzed. They are useful for population studies, yet are not individually predictive [8]. By contrast, specific PB tests provide information that allows the patient to implement individual habit changes based on the PB tests results that can bring about health improvements and changes in lab tests within just a few months. This approach builds upon the concept of "optimum" or "high-level health" reference ranges and the biochemical individuality concept pioneered by Roger Williams, Emanuel Cheraskin and colleagues [9], in which therapy, practice, and health standards must be tailored to individual's metabolic requirements [10].

The goal values recommended here for each predictive biomarker are designed to improve precision in practice and are defined as the least risk or highest gain value or range for each PB. When predictive biomarker tests are at their goal value, all-cause morbidity and mortality are at their best outcome value; quality of life and lifespan are optimized; and net costs of care are reduced. Table 3.2 gives an overview of the selected predictive biomarkers with their clinical significance.

These biomarkers do not depend on age providing an advantage. *Usual*, or statistically *normal* ranges, for biomarkers are based on age and gender-calculated statistical ranges where higher proportions of unwell people are represented. This means that because there are more deficient and distressed people, and thus more unhealthy people in the population as it ages, statistical ranges are unhelpful in individual cases.

Age-conditional *usual* lab ranges drift toward the less well with advancing longevity. Age, however, is a contingent variable. The significant variable is how many unhealthy people are present at each age. Chronology is fixed, yet most of function is choice, based on habits of daily living that can be relearned particularly when appropriate incentives are applied.

PREDICTIVE BIOMARKER 1:
GLYCOSYLATED HEMOGLOBIN (HEMOGLOBIN A1C)

There is a known direct relationship with increased glycemia and increased musculoskeletal issues complicating metabolic syndrome and diabetes [12]. Similarly, high blood sugar levels are associated with increased pain [13]. Elevated blood glucose levels mean progressively increasing levels of advanced glycation end products (AGEs). AGEs result from an antioxidant deficit in granulocytes and oxidative free radical damage that harms the delicate endothelial lining of blood vessels. AGEs indicate cumulative repair deficits in turn due to immune defense and repair overload. The most common sources of increased immune defense work are digestive remnants, aero-allergens, and environmental chemicals [14].

Fasting and two-hour post-prandial glucose levels have long been measured to get information about levels at specific times of the day. Insulin and glucose/insulin ratios were developed more recently (HOMA, glycemic index).

TABLE 3.2

Predictive Biomarkers and Significance for Musculoskeletal Dysfunction

Predictive Biomarker Test (PB)	Best Outcome Goal Value	Measures	Significance
Hgb A1c, HbA1c (Hemoglobin A1c)	< 5%	Blood sugar, diabetic risk, and insulin resistance	Highly predictive of certain aspects of physiology having to do with sugar metabolism and insulin functions, which in turn are linked to cell energy status, metabolism, weight and related chronic health conditions such as metabolic syndrome, diabetes, cardiovascular disease, and bone- and collagen-related conditions
hsCRP (high sensitivity C-reactive protein)	< 0.5 mg/L	Repair and inflammation status	Highly predictive of repair deficits, connected with pain in several musculoskeletal conditions
Homocysteine (high sensitivity homocysteine)	< 6 μmol/L	Methylation, detoxification, cardiovascular risk	Helps to measure adequate methylation, sulfur metabolism, detoxification, and epigenetic modulation
hs LRA by ELISA/ACT	No delayed allergies	Immune tolerance to foods and chemicals	*LRA* measures immune defense and repair tolerance and intolerance across all delayed allergy pathways.
First AM Urine pH	6.5–7.5	Mineral need assessment and cellular acid/alkaline balance	Measurement after six hours rest reflects net acid excess and metabolic acidosis. Consequences of metabolic acidosis include hormonal changes, insulin resistance, loss of bone and muscle protein degradation
Vitamin D (25-OH cholecalciferol)	50–80 ng/mL	Cellular equilibrium and communication	Vitamin D pleiotropic functions dictate cellular function, physiology and proliferation—crucial for immune health, bone metabolism, neurological and cognitive function
Omega-3 Index	> 8%	Omega-3 level of oxidative stress	Reflects the relative amount of omega -3 fatty acids within red blood cell membranes and expressed as percentage of total fatty acids—useful in predicting oxidative stress
DNA Oxidative Stress (8-OHdG)	<5 ng/mg creatinine	Oxidative stress and nuclear antioxidant status	DNA oxidative stress marker that can be a predictor of repair deficit and risk of conditions like diabetes and atherosclerosis

Source: R Jaffe and J Mani, *Polyphenols in Human Health and Disease*, Academic Press, 2014 [11].

Hgb A1c is the current reference standard analyte to determine average "sugar" related risks. Of all measures of excess average sugar in the body, hemoglobin A1c is the best studied and the most validated and widely available.

Day-to-day blood sugar levels are influenced by exercise, meal timings, mood, and/or medications. In contrast, Hgb A1c provides the average blood sugar over the last three months and prevails over these variables, uncovering pre-diabetic states accurately and giving a more reliable indication of current and future sugar related risk [15, 16]. Hgb A1c/PB1 measures are also strongly linked to inflammation (hsCRP/PB2), immune tolerance (LRA/PB4), and oxidative stress (8-OHdG/PB8). Hgb A1C is a PB that anticipates chronic, degenerative, inflammatory, and autoimmune disease risks.

Insulin has been known to contribute to the bone remodeling process for a number of years [17]. But when insulin is present in excessive amounts (as in insulin resistance and type 2 diabetes), bone resorption and circulating levels of osteocalcin both decrease within hours of an insulin surge, according to a recent study [18]. Collagen renewal is reduced when average blood sugar is increased, resulting in weaker bones and higher fracture incidences.

The following graphs (Figures 3.1 and 3.2) represent the correlation between Hgb A1c levels, blood glucose levels, and 10+ year survival probability.

When Hgb A1c levels and blood glucose levels are above goal value, an immunotolerant diet of whole foods enriched with nutrient-dense super foods is appropriate. In addition, advanced supplements with enhanced uptake and chaperoned delivery of essential nutrients are shown to improve stability of energy, reduce average blood glucose, and improve insulin sensitivity. Being active physically and mentally is an integral part of this approach to evoke healing responses.

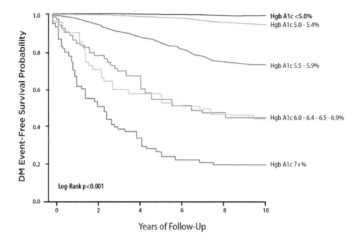

FIGURE 3.1 Hgb A1c levels and extent of 10-year survival probability. (From Peiyao Cheng, et al., *Diabetes Care*, 34, 610–15, 2011 [19].) Source: *DM – Diabetes Mellitus. Diabetes is linked to accelerated loss of bone, joint, and lean muscle. This graph highlights the link between the HgbA1c level and 10+ year all cause morbidity and mortality risk.

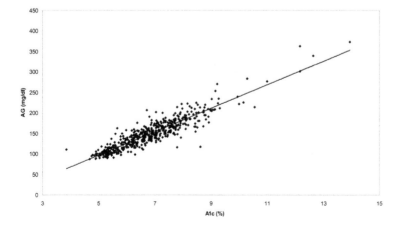

FIGURE 3.2 Correlation of Hgb A1c levels with average blood glucose. (From David M. Nathan, et al., *Diabetes Care*, 31, 1473–8, 2008 [15].) Source: Each dot represents one individual. The linear regression analysis represented in this graph confirms that HgbA1c correlates tightly with average glucose (AG).

For example, since researchers have found that constant sitting has as much disease risk as smoking, an exercise routine is critical. Walking for an aggregate of 45+ minutes per day or being physically active for five minutes for each hour at a desk can dramatically reduce risk as documented by improved Hgb A1c. Practicing abdominal breathing and relaxation response mindfulness practice also favorably affects this and other PB measures.

A *Hgb A1c of <5% is the desired or goal value* and reflects a 99% probability of living ten+ years and also reflects efficient use of sugar to regulate cell growth and energy.

PREDICTIVE BIOMARKER 2:
HIGH SENSITIVITY C-REACTIVE PROTEIN (hsCRP)

A healthy body repairs itself from injury or from wear and tear promptly, efficiently, and effectively. When health is compromised, the body's attempt to heal or repair itself falls short, resulting in a repair deficit, otherwise known as inflammation. The process of defense and repair is a complex one involving many cells and enzymes. Inducible proteins for example, are a family of mostly liver-derived glycoproteins that, in aggregate, are the body's cry for help to induce cells and systems to effect repair and heal.

When repair deficits persist, inflammation puts a metabolic burden on the body's organ systems, especially the immune system. Unmet repair needs and too much defense work slowly wear down immune functions, taking a toll on daily quality of life, increasing risk for disease, and reducing survival [20].

The musculoskeletal system is especially vulnerable to inflammation. Inflammation is connected to increased oxidative stress, which produces Reactive Oxygen Species (ROS). ROS plays a crucial role in cartilage homeostasis [21] and has been implicated in bone loss even while having a role in bone remodeling [22].

C-reactive protein (CRP) is a measure of inflammation—the liver produces more CRP when inflamed. High sensitivity C-reactive protein (hsCRP), however, is more precise and predictive than regular CRP [23] and is known as a predictive marker of inflammation systemically, particularly in connection with the cardiovascular risks.

Figures 3.3 and 3.4 illustrate the correlation between hsCRP, Framingham 10-year CVD risk scores, and 10-year survival probability.

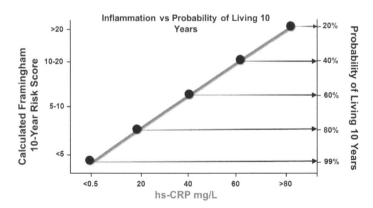

FIGURE 3.3 High sensitivity C-reactive protein (hsCRP) measurements and Framingham risk score. (From Paul Ridker, et al., *Arch Intern Med*, 166, 1327–8 [24].) Source: Inflammation is repair deficit. The hsCRP test correlates best with degree of repair deficit/inflammation and has been validated as an all cause morbidity/mortality parameter. Repair of the musculoskeletal system depends upon essential nutrients to prevent hsCRP from being induced by repair deficit. In this linear regression analysis, it is evident that the probability of living longer is indirectly proportional to the calculated cardiovascular Framingham risk score and increased hsCRP levels.

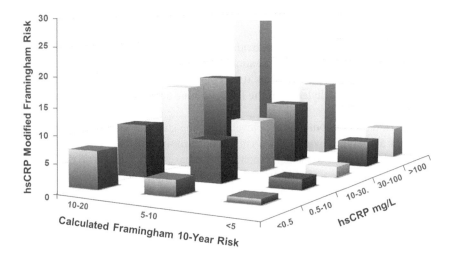

FIGURE 3.4 3-D presentation of Framingham data demonstrates the combined effect of high sensitivity C-reactive protein (hsCRP) measurements and 10-year survival. (From PM Ridker, PWF Wilson, and SM Grundy, *Circulation*, 109, 2818–925, 2004 [25].)

HsCRP correlates with clinical activity of other inflammatory, autoimmune diseases, from rheumatoid to juvenile arthritis, lupus (SLE), diabetes, vasculitis, psoriasis, eczema, asthma, and multiple sclerosis. Levels of hsCRP rise in proportion to the need for repair. Persisting elevations of hsCRP indicate overload in the innate immune system, fatigue in phagocytic functions, and increased host hospitality to chronic infection or autoimmune self-attack.

Higher levels of hsCRP are associated with increased fracture risk. The SWAN (Study of Women's Health Across the Nation) study [26] showed that bone strength significantly declines with increased inflammation. Higher hsCRP measurements also indicate disease progression in osteoarthritis, reflecting synovial inflammation in such patients, perhaps by means of increased synovial IL-6 production [27].

GOAL VALUE FOR HSCRP OF <0.5 MG/L

An hsCRP of less than 0.5 mg/L indicates the individual has tamed inflammation risk. Recommended nutrients to accomplish this goal include antioxidants like fully buffered l-ascorbate, polyphenolics (particularly quercetin dehydrate and soluble OPC), magnesium and choline citrate and ubiquinone (CoEnzyme Q10) that can dramatically alter the state of inflammation and improve hsCRP levels by potentiating much-needed cellular repair.

PREDICTIVE BIOMARKER 3: HOMOCYSTEINE (HCY)

A healthy body requires the correct ratio of methionine to homocysteine since HCY is an important predictor of long-term survival for all-cause morbidity and mortality. The usual lab values for HCY range from 5–15 µmol/L, and most practitioners take action when values are above 15 µmol/L. To predict better lifetime health, the goal value for HCY is to be less than 6 µmol/L. At this homocysteine level, the methionine to homocysteine ratio favors healthy methylation, robust, self-renewing vascular and tissue infrastructure, and sulfur-based detoxification.

Methylation controls many aspects of cell function, including DNA and RNA expression of genes and helps to transport or deposit proteins as needed. When methylation is impaired, e.g., when methylation regulators like C complex, magnesium, and trimethylglycine (TMG) are deficient, homocysteine levels increase, and methionine decreases, reflecting defects in sulfur metabolism, detoxification, and methyl group transfer.

Elevated homocysteine levels result in oxidative stress that is linked to increased risk of heart attacks, strokes, senility, systemic inflammation, osteoporosis, and autoimmune diseases [28]. For example, in osteoporosis and osteoarthritis (two epigenetically modulated conditions) it is important to note how impaired methylation of the DNA of bone cells and cartilage is part of the disease process [29].

In osteoporosis, elevated homocysteine levels alter the structure of collagen cross-linking, thus affecting stability and mineralization occurring in bone tissue [30]. Similarly, elevated homocysteine levels have been shown to cause corresponding decreases in bone mineral density [31].

As a measure of all-cause morbidity and mortality, homocysteine is definitely an important predictor of long-term survival. Healthier people have adequate dietary sulfur sources to produce higher MET and lower HCY as indicated in Figures 3.5 and 3.6.

If homocysteine levels are above the goal value, our recommendation includes an immunotolerant whole foods diet, with an emphasis on sulfur rich super foods such as ginger, garlic, onions, brassica sprouts, and eggs. It is important to include sufficient intake of buffered ascorbate, vitamin B12 (hydroxocobalamin) natural folate, vitamin B6 (natural forms preferred), magnesium, and trimethylglycine (TMG; betaine HCl) [34].

In addition, any system that brings together movement and conscious breathing is recommended to evoke healing responses, including meditation, Hatha Yoga, Qigong, or even walking. Alternating practices that involve gentle stretching exercises and cardio or weight-bearing activities are also highly beneficial, since muscles and bones equally benefit from exercise to evoke healing responses.

The good news is that as homocysteine levels come back into a more normal range and methylation functions normally, risk for serious health conditions can be reduced in a few short months.

GOAL VALUES FOR HCY

The goal value of less than 6 µmol/L for HCY predicts better lifetime health. While the usual lab values range for HCY is 5–15 µmol/L, most practitioners take action when values are above 15 µmol/L. When the patient achieves an HCY under 6 µmol/L, the methionine to homocysteine

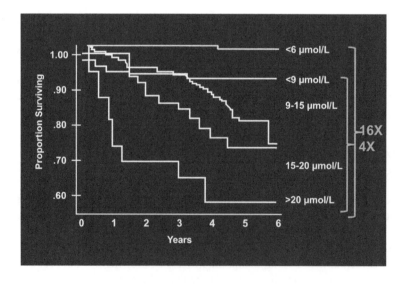

FIGURE 3.5   Homocysteine <6 µmol/L is Predictive Biomarker. (From O Nygård, et al., *NEJM*, 337, 230–6, 1997 [32].) Source: This is a survival plot and shows the percentage of survival (proportion surviving) starting from 100 and declining as homocysteine levels rise.

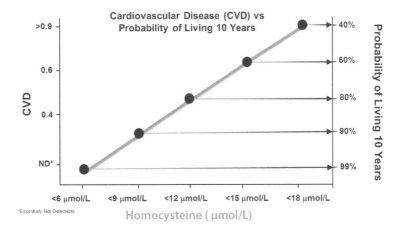

FIGURE 3.6 Homocysteine level, cardiovascular disease, and 10-year survival probability. (From AG Bostom, et al., *Arch Intern Med*, 159, 1077–80, 1999 [33].) Source: This regression analysis illustrates the probability of living 10+ years, increasing with decreasing homocysteine levels and lower incidence of cardiovascular disease, confirming the value of homocysteine as an important all cause morbidity/mortality parameter.

ratio favors methionine to support healthy methylation, robust, self-renewing vascular and tissue infrastructure, and sulfur-based detoxification.

PREDICTIVE BIOMARKER 4: IMMUNE TOLERANCE CELL CULTURES LYMPHOCYTE RESPONSE ASSAY (LRA)

The lymphocyte response assay (LRA) determines individual reactive foods and/or chemicals that can impair immune system functions. A healthy immune system is tolerant. This means that the innate immune first-line cells are able to handle defense, repair, and deletion of abnormal cells. When the immune system attacks rather than defends *and* repairs, a condition called inflammation and/or autoimmunity (AI) is present.

AI conditions are widely prevalent. Autoimmunity means loss of immune tolerance and self-restoring homeostasis. Examples range from diabetes to thyroiditis and arthritis, to migraine headaches, eczema, and psoriasis. Concurrent presence of multiple AI syndromes is common [35], and while it may not seem immediately apparent, the immune system is closely involved in so many conditions associated with the musculoskeletal system, especially rheumatic conditions such as rheumatoid arthritis, multiple sclerosis, polymyalgia rheumatica, temporal arteritis, and systemic lupus [36].

Highlighting the importance of the immune system is a recent study by stem cell scientists from Harvard University who have shown that regulatory T cells (Tregs) that temper immune responses increase in muscular dystrophy cases and actually could be utilized to heal wounds and improve disease outcome [37].

When routine wear-and-tear is *not* repaired, the integrity of the extracellular connective tissue scaffolding is impaired [38]. Increase in tissue permeability ensues, setting the stage for AI. This can be provoked by a variety of external or internal antigens perceived as foreign that preoccupy the immune system with excess defense burden [39]. Initially, this increase in tissue permeability results in the entry of larger plasma proteins and platelets, dendritic cells, and lymphocytes all seeking to induce repair, i.e., to "put things right" [40]. Fibromyalgia is a classic example. Leaky gut syndrome is another common clinical term for incomplete repair. Too often, the lack of essential nutrients and/or excess defense burdens on the immune system prevent repair of cells from being completed [41].

Causes of repair deficit, also known as inflammation, can be summarized as:

1. Chronic deferral of necessary routine repair due to distress (neurohormone imbalance) [42–44], toxin excess (impaired detoxification), or lack of essential nutrients needed for the immune defense and repair systems to function;
2. Depletion of buffering reserve (particularly magnesium) resulting in intracellular acidosis, loss of the proton gradient, and mitochondrial shutdown [45];
3. Immunologic overload from repeated digestive, respiratory, and/or auto-antigen exposure resulting in loss of tolerance and development of B and T cell delayed allergy responses;
4. Adequate activity patterns to move fluids and help maintain a healthy digestive transit time (since long-term sitting can lead to as much disease as smoking); and
5. Lack of learned stress resilience based on relaxation response practices.

The LRA measures all three delayed allergy pathways *ex vivo* while avoiding false positives that are common in other types of delayed allergy tests according to the Gel and Coombs organization of immune responses:

- Type II: Reactive antibody (IgA, IgM, and IgG) meaning the distinction between protective, neutralizing, and harmful symptom-provoking antibodies
- Type III: Immune complexes: IgM anti-IgG-antigen complex
- Type IV: Direct T-cell activation: no antibodies, yet direct activation

Figure 3.7 illustrates the immune response mechanism.

Identifying the patient's specific sensitivities and delayed allergies that burden the immune system can result in a clinical breakthrough. Patients often experience sustained remission when using an alkalinizing, immune tolerant diet and targeted supplementation, as well as changes in lifestyle habits and attitude.

Tolerance can be restored as part of a proactive prevention lifestyle. If reactions are found by LRA tests, substitution of reactive foods can be initiated. Eating whole foods that can be digested,

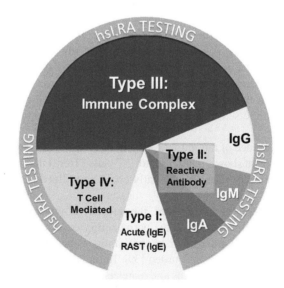

FIGURE 3.7 Wheel of immune response mechanism. (From PG Gel, et al., *Clinical Aspects of Immunology*, Hoboken, NJ: Wiley-Blackwell, 1975 [46].) Source: hsLRA- high sensitivity Lympocyte Response Assay; Ig-Immunoglobulin of E, G, A and M types.

assimilated, and eliminated without immune burden is recommended. The plan includes high-nutrient-dense, easily digested super foods and targeted supplementation to promote repair and rebalance mental as well as physical reserves, while evoking healing responses.

LRA by ELISA/ACT cell cultures are reproducible [47] with a variance of less than 3% for over 30 years on consecutive blind split samples such as the consecutive data presented at the American Society for Investigative Pathology (ASIP) conference in 2016 (Table 3.3).

Common conventional practice today includes therapies assessing immune intolerance based only on antibodies. The assumption is that *any* antibody is harmful, and some combination of immune suppressive therapies results. This approach lacks solid research support and clinical evidence.

LRA GOAL VALUE

The *healthy goal value is immune tolerance, with no LRA reactions*, which confirms innate and adaptive immune tolerance and functional resilience in the immune defense and repair system. Using LRA tests and developing an associated immune enhancement program can help restore immune competence, tolerance, and resilience.

TABLE 3.3
Consecutive Blind Split LRA Samples Showing High Reproducibility

# Items Tested	# Items Matched	# Items Unmatched	% Items Matched	% Items Unmatched	Time (Years)
4138	4050	88	97.60 ± 3.00	2.25 ± 2.75 Split variance	2011–14

Source: AE Lynch and R Jaffe, Lymphocyte response assay: Report on precision of novel cell culture test, experimental biology, *Poster presented at the American Society for Investigative Pathology Conference*, San Diego, CA, 2016 [47].

Legend: Test precision is measured best by consecutive blind split samples analyzed over at least two years as shown in this table. By contrast other cell culture methods that assess lymphocytic white blood cell function report 15%–30% variance. LRA by this method is a documented advance in precision, sensitivity, specificity and predictive significance.

PREDICTIVE BIOMARKER 5: URINE PH AFTER 6+ HOURS REST

Diet-induced cell acidosis has been shown to create changes in the body that have fundamental effects on the degree of oxidative stress, free radical activity, cell energetics (ATP/ADP ratio), and osteoclastic activity in bone, and on possible tumor progression [48].

The pH of urine after six hours of rest reflects equilibration with kidney and bladder cells. Levels below 6.5 indicate metabolic acidosis inside cells, as is indicated in Figure 3.8. Low pH suggests mineral deficits. Minerals tend to get pulled from bone and body fluids to neutralize metabolic acids that can form faster than the intake of buffering minerals and alkalinizing nutrients. [49]

Tiny changes in cell pH have deep implications for metabolism. Life exists poised exquisitely just above the pH neutral point of 7.0. Levels of urine pH above 7.5 can indicate presence of catabolic illness in which amino acids are used as energy sources. When net acid excess is expressed in urine, changes in diet, supplements, activity, attitude (mental and emotional health) are needed to restore acid-alkaline balance.

Figure 3.9 outlines foods based on their acidifying and alkalinizing capabilities.

Checking the pH level each day provides ongoing monitoring to see whether acid-alkaline balance is present.

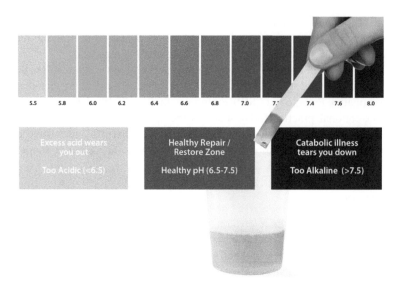

FIGURE 3.8 First morning urine pH levels and health status. (From R Jaffe and S Brown, *Intl J Integrative Med*, 2, 7–18, 2000 [49].)

Goal Value for Urine pH

The pH value in urine is more accurate when the urine is fresh. Cells and bacteria in urine shift pH over time due to their metabolic products.

The predictive *goal value range for urine pH is 6.5–7.5* after six or more hours of rest, typically checked first thing in the morning.

PREDICTIVE BIOMARKER 6: VITAMIN D

It is estimated that anywhere from 30% to 50% of Americans, depending upon their age and community living environments, are deficient in Vitamin D. Vitamin D is a neurohormone. Functionally, this nutrient is important in regulating mineral uptake and regulating cell proliferation.

Vitamin D levels play a significant role in numerous systems in the body, including immune and neurological regulation and bone health. Less than healthy levels increase risks of obesity, cancer, heart disease, inflammatory, autoimmune disorders, and psychiatric and mood disorders [50].

Healthy vitamin D levels:

- Are protective against musculoskeletal disorders (muscle weakness, falls, fractures), multiple sclerosis, rheumatoid arthritis, type 1 and type 2 diabetes, cardiovascular diseases, neurocognitive dysfunction, and others;
- Allow vitamin D to function successfully as a hormone, moderating cell division, providing vital communication links between cells, normalizing cell growth, and avoiding aggressive cell production;
- Improve immune status and protect against autoimmune disorders; and
- Reduce inflammation in the brain and nervous system—this is particularly important since brain repair depends on an energetic, tolerant immune system.

Vitamin D deficiency/insufficiency is associated with all-cause mortality [51].

GOAL VALUE RANGE FOR VITAMIN D

Knowing the status of vitamin D levels in the body is helpful to determine if supplementation is required. Less than 5% of Americans have adequate vitamin D levels. The preferred test to assess vitamin D levels involves the measurement of 25 hydroxycholecalciferol (25 OH-D). The best outcome *goal value range for 25-OH D is 50–80 ng/ml.*

PREDICTIVE BIOMARKER 7: OMEGA 3 TEST

Most Americans have low omega-3 levels and excess omega-6 fat intake. People pay a substantial metabolic price for this imbalance in essential oils. Omega-3 fats are an integral part of cell membranes throughout the body and affect the function of the cell receptors in these membranes. They provide the starting point for making hormones that regulate blood clotting, contraction and relaxation of artery walls, and inflammation. By greatly tuning down inflammatory signaling, omega 3 fats send osteoclasts home, preventing excessive bone loss. They also increase the action of osteoblasts and give them enough time to lay down new bone. The attainment of peak bone mass in adolescence, increased bone mineral density and the prevention of age-related osteoporosis are positive effects of omega 3 fatty acids [52].

The omega-3 test is a measure of the active omega-3 fatty acids, eicosapentanaeoic acid (EPA) + docosahexaenoic acid (DHA), in red blood cells. Levels of omega-3 are predictive of coronary heart disease (CHD) risk and are important for brain and joint health [53]. Low levels of omega-3s are also related to increased risk for fatal heart attack, depression, and possibly dementia [54, 55].

While deficiency in omega-3 fats is too common, excess of omega-6 fats is equally prevalent. In essence, omega-3 fats enhance, repair, and soothe the body, while omega-6 fats stimulate and activate the body. We need both in balance. Recent studies, such as NHANES IV [56] suggest typical Americans take in 20 to 100 times more omega-6 than omega-3, mostly due to the high consumption of vegetable oils and practices like frying and high-heat cooking. Cooking with broth and wine and minimizes the use of edible oils. Salads can be enjoyed with a drizzle of vinegar, fresh ground pepper, and sea salt rather than with added oils.

Whole foods like deep sea, cold water fish, nuts and seeds, and greens have balanced omega-3 to omega-6 fats. Whole foods also contain protective antioxidants so that easily damaged fats do not become rancid, a common problem when oils are isolated and separated from their source.

An omega-3 index of <8% indicates an increase in the intake of EPA and DHA through food and supplements is needed. The amount of EPA/DHA needed to raise the omega-3 index to the target range is individual and is based on current levels of active omega-3 fatty acids, EPA + DHA, and how much the individual takes in through their diet.

An index of 4% or less (common in the US) indicates the highest risk [57]. *The goal value for the omega-3 test is 8% and above,* a level associated with the lowest risk of death from coronary heart disease.

PREDICTIVE BIOMARKER 8: 8-OXOGUANINE OR 8-OHDG (8-HYDROXYGUANINE, 8-OXO-GUA, OR OH⁸GUA)

Oxidative stress describes the injury caused to cells resulting from increased formation of free radicals and/or decreased antioxidant reserve. Oxidative stress can define bone cell behavior [58] and is seen to play a crucial role in the development of conditions like osteopenia [59], diabetes, and cardiovascular disease. Testing for 8-oxoguanine provides important information about oxidative

MORE ACID
(Consume Less)

Food Category				
Citrus Fruit Fruit		Cranberry Pomegranate	Plum Prune Tomato	Coconut Fig Guava Persimmon Juice Cherimoya Date Dry Fruit
Bean Vegetable Legume Pulse Root	Soybean Carob	Pea Green/Snow Peanut Legumes (other) Carrot Chick Pea/Garbanzo	Bean Pinto/White/Navy/Red/Aduki/Lima or Mung Chard Split Pea	Bean Fava/Kidney/Black-eyed/String/Wax Spinach Zucchini Chutney Rhubarb
Grain Cereal Grass	Barley *Processed Flour*	Corn Rye Oat Bran	Wheat Semolina/Spelt, teff/Kamut White Rice Buckwheat	Triticale Brown Rice Millet Kasha
Fowl	Pheasant	Chicken	Goose/Turkey	Wild Duck
Meat Game Fish/Shell Fish	Beef Shell Fish (Processed) Lobster	Pork/Veal Mussel/Squid	Lamb/Mutton Game Meat Shell Fish (Whole)	Gelatin/Organs Venison Fish
Egg				Egg, Chicken
Processed Dairy Cow/Human Soy Goat/Sheep	*Processed Cheese* Ice Cream	Casein Cottage Cheese Milk, Soy	Milk; Goat, Cow, Sheep	Cream/Butter Yogurt Cheese; Goat, Sheep
Oil Seed/Sprout Nut	*Cottonseed Oil/Meal* *Fried Food* Hazelnut Walnut Brazil Nut	Oil Chestnut/Palm Kernel Lard Pistachio Seed Pecan	Oil Almond/Sesame/Safflower Tapioca Seitan or Tofu	Oil Canola/Pumpkin Seed/Grape Seed/Sunflower Pine Nut
Beverage Preservative Sweetner Vinegar	*Beer* *"Soda"* *Table Salt* *Yeast/Hops/Malt* *Sugar/Cocoa* *White/Acetic Vinegar*	Coffee Aspartame Saccharin Red Wine Vinegar	*Alcohol* *Black Tea* *Benzoate* *Balsamic Vinegar*	*Kona Coffee* *MSG* *Honey/Maple Syrup* *Rice Vinegar*
Spice/Herb	Pudding/Jam/Jelly	Nutmeg	Vanilla Stevia	Curry
Therapeutic	*Antibiotics*	*Psychotropics*	*Antihistamines*	

FIGURE 3.9 Food and chemical effects on acid/alkaline body chemical balance.

>>>>> MORE ALKALINE
(Consume More)

✚	✚✚	✚✚✚	✚✚✚✚	Food Category
Orange Banana Blueberry Raisin, Grapes Currant Strawberry	Lemon Pear Avocado Apple Blackberry Cherry Peach	Grapefruit Canteloupe Honeydew Olive Mango Citrus Loganberry	Lime Nectarine Raspberry Watermelon Tangerine Pineapple	Citrus Fruit Fruit
Brussel Sprout Beet Chive/Scallion Celery/Cilantro Squash Artichoke Lettuce Jicama Turnip Greens	Potato/Bell Pepper Mushroom/Fungi Cauliflower Cabbage Eggplant Pumpkin Collard Greens	Kohlrabi Parsnip/Taro Garlic Asparagus Kale/Parsley Endive/Arugula Jerusalem Artichoke Ginger Root Broccoli	Lentil Brocoflower Seaweed Noril|Kombu| Wakame|Hijiki Onion/Miso Daikon/Taro Root Sea Vegetables Burdock/Lotus Root Sweet Potato/Yam	Bean Vegetable Legume Pulse Root
Quinoa Wild Rice Oat				Grain Cereal Grass
				Fowl
				Meat Game Fish/Shell Fish
Egg, Duck	Egg, Quail			Egg
Ghee Human Breast Milk				Processed Dairy Cow/Human Soy Goat/Sheep
Oil Avocado Coconut Olive/Macadamia Linseed/Flax Seeds (most)	Oil Cod Liver Primrose Sesame Seed Almond Sprout	Poppy Seed Pepper Chestnut Cashew	Pumpkin Seed	Oil Seed/Sprout Nut
Ginger Tea *Sulfite* Sucanat Umeboshi vinegar	Green or Mu Tea Rice syrup Apple Cider Vinegar	Kambucha Molasses Soy Sauce	Mineral Water Sea Salt	Beverage Preservative Sweetner Vinegar
White Willow Bark Slippery Elm Artemesia Annua	Herbs Aloe Vera Nettle	Spices/Cinnamon Valerian Licorice Agave	Baking Soda	Spice/Herb
Algae, Blue Green	Sake		Umeboshi Plum	Therapeutic

Italicised items are NOT recommended

stress and its effects on DNA and the genetic sequence. The test is well validated as a measure of nuclear and mitochondrial DNA oxidative stress and is well supported in the research literature [60].

This predictive biomarker focuses on the acceleration of age-related decline due to DNA status, particularly telomere length, and is an effective way to evaluate the success of an intervention, whether it involves dietary change or essential nutrients. When antioxidant levels are sufficient, oxidative damage from free radicals does not occur.

Tracking the results of this test provides an indication of:

1. Risks due to oxidative stress in the DNA of both mitochondria and cell nuclei that particularly increase cardiovascular disease; and
2. Benefit or lack of benefit from therapies designed to reduce DNA oxidative distress to reduce future disease risks.

GOAL VALUE FOR 8-OXOGUANINE

The *goal for 8-oxoguanine we suggest is a value of <5 ng/mg of creatinine*, indicating adequate DNA antioxidant protection and efficient DNA repair from oxidative stresses. To achieve goal values, we recommend antioxidants such as ascorbate, polyphenolics, micellized ubiquinone, mixed natural carotenoids and tocopherols, which stimulate efficient energy production.

DISCUSSION AND CONCLUSION

When one biomarker is no longer at best outcome goal value, the entire organism is distressed, less resilient, and more at risk. Homeostasis is reduced; impaired functions are likely. This loss of homeostasis is captured by the biomarkers because they are *interdependent*. When all eight are interpreted together, their predictive power increases, together covering the 92% of lifetime health conditions and diseases determined by choice and habit. And though each biomarker is a separate marker of specific aspects of physiology, human systems are interdependent.

The biomarkers are *responsive*. Changes in daily lifestyle habits, diet, and stress levels return markers back to or toward the goal or best outcome value. The biomarkers are *not age dependent*. Healthy people at any age have best outcome values for these predictive biomarker tests; outcome goal values for PB are *not* dependent on age or gender. What is known as aging is more accurately understood as having more unwell people as age advances.

Each biomarker has biologic plausibility and elucidated metabolic pathways. At times for clinical efficiency physicians may wish to select biomarkers to evaluate a suspected disturbance in one particular pathway. Four essential predictive biomarkers that should make the list are HgbA1c, homocysteine, hsCRP and Lymphocyte Response Assay (Table 3.2). These biomarkers provide the practitioner with a window into glucose, inflammation, methylation, and immune status of an individual.

The PBs are most meaningful when pre-analytic variables can be improved. A superior assay is one that provides accurate measurement. For that, it is important to reduce any interfering substances used in the assay, e.g., glass versus plastic. The conditions involved in the analysis are equally crucial and any compromise there can skew the assay accuracy. Last of all, the curve of the assay is critical in making sure that the assay conveys an accurate measurement.

As a result, the predictive significance of any specific value becomes much greater if the analysis is scientifically sound Predictive biomarkers are timely. An increasing number of healthcare consumers are interested in predictive, proactive, personalized primary prevention. They are careful of information found on health websites and books (and even from their healthcare providers) and are more inclined to verify that tests and procedures are effective and applicable to themselves. Those of us who are evidence-based clinicians have an obligation to integrate advances in informatics, human behavior, technology, and mind and body techniques into our practices, with a focus on predictive biomarkers.

Lastly, predictive biomarkers can help healthcare practitioners fulfill an inner calling. We can help our patients avert the tragic cycle explained by the 14th Dalai Lama [61].

Sometimes people sacrifice their health to gain wealth only to later sacrifice their wealth to regain their health. You can help those whose health forces them to live in the past or in the future. As health care practitioners, we are uniquely placed to help return individuals to vibrant living in the present moment.

ACKNOWLEDGMENTS AND DISCLOSURES

The authors wish to acknowledge their affiliation with ELISA/ACT Biotechnologies, LLC and PERQUE Integrative Health.

REFERENCES

1. Tainya C. Clarke, et al., Use of complementary health approaches for musculoskeletal pain disorders among adults, *National Health Statistics Reports*, *National Institutes of Health*, United States Number 98 (October 12, 2016), https://www.cdc.gov/nchs/data/nhsr/nhsr098.pdf.
2. NIH Biomarker Working Group, *Clin Pharmacol Ther* 69 (2001): 89–95.
3. S Gutman and LG Kessler, The US Food and Drug Administration perspective on cancer biomarker development, *Nat Rev Cancer* 6 (2006): 565–71.
4. Donald Fredrickson, Task force on genetic factors in atherosclerotic disease, National Heart and Lung Institute, 1974–1975 [subseries], *Report from the National Heart and Lung Institute*, 1974–1975.
5. JB Stanbury, JB Wyngaarden, DS Fredrickson, eds., *The Metabolic Basis of Inherited Disease* (New York, Toronto, and London: McGraw-Hill, 1960).
6. Edward H. Yelin, Miriam Cisternas, Sylvia I. Watkins-Castillo, Musculoskeletal Disease Burden, *The Burden of Musculoskeletal Disease Prevalence, Bone and Joint Initiative* (2013 to 2017), http://www.boneandjointburden.org/2014-report/xb0/musculoskeletal-disease-prevalence.
7. CDC Centers for Disease Control and Prevention, *National Center for Health Statistics*, Table 18: Years of potential life lost before age 75 for selected causes of death, by sex, race, and Hispanic origin: United States selected years 1980–2014, https://www.cdc.gov/nchs/hus/contents2015.htm#018. [adapted].
8. RS Galen and SR Gambino, *Beyond Normality: The Predictive Value and Efficiency of Medical Diagnosis* (New York, NY: Wiley, 1975), 10–40.
9. E Cheraskin, WM Ringsdorf, Jr., and JW Clark, *Diet and Disease* (Emmaus, PA: Rodale Books, 1968).
10. Roger J. Williams, et al., *The Wonderful World Within You*, 3rd Edition (Biocommunications, 1998).
11. R Jaffe and J Mani, Polyphenolics evoke healing responses: Clinical evidence and role of predictive biomarkers, in *Polyphenols in Human Health and Disease*, eds. RR Watson, et al. (Academic Press, 2014), Oxford, UK, 695–705.
12. ME Larkin, et al., Musculoskeletal complications in type 1 diabetes, *Diabetes Care*, 37 (July 2014): 1863–69, http://dx.doi.org/10.2337/dc13-2361.
13. MS Herbert, et al., Association of pain with HbA1c in a predominantly black population of community-dwelling adults with diabetes: A cross-sectional analysis, *Diabet Med* 12 (December 2013): 1466–71, doi:10.1111/dme.12264.
14. R. Jaffe, *The Alkaline Way in Digestive Health in Bioactive Food as Dietary Interventions in Liver and Gastrointestinal Disease*, eds. Ronald Ross Watson and Victor Preedy (Academic Press, 2013), 1–21.
15. David M. Nathan, et al., Translating the A1C assay into estimated average glucose values, *Diabetes Care* 31 no. 8 (August 2008): 1473–8.
16. W Zhao, et al., HbA$_{1c}$ and coronary heart disease risk among diabetic patients, *Diabetes Care* 37 no. 2 (February 2014): 428–35.
17. CJ Rosen and KJ Motyl, No bones about it: Insulin modulates skeletal remodeling, *Cell* 142 no. 2 (July 23, 2010): 198–200, doi:10.1016/j.cell.2010.07.001.
18. K Ivaska, et al., The effects of acute hyperinsulinemia on bone metabolism, *Endocr Connect* 4 no. 3 (September 1, 2015): 155–62.
19. Peiyao Cheng, et al., Hemoglobin A$_{1c}$ as a predictor of incident diabetes, *Diabetes Care* 34 no. 3 (March 2011): 610–15.

20. R Jaffe and J Mani, Rethink health: Inflammation is actually repair deficit: Using physiology first to achieve better outcomes, part 1: Value and importance of understanding inflammation as repair deficit, *Townsend Letter for Doctors and Patients* 359 (2013): 68–74.

21. Y Henrotin, B Kurz, and T Aigner, Oxygen and reactive oxygen species in cartilage degradation: Friends or foes? *OsteoArthritis Cartilage* 13 no. 8 (August 2005): 643–54, http://www.oarsijournal.com/article/S1063-4584(05)00098-1/pdf.

22. G Banfi, EL Iorio, and MM Corsi, Oxidative stress, free radicals, and bone remodeling, *Clin Chem Lab Med.* 46 no. 11 (2008): 1550–5, doi:10.1515/CCLM.2008.302.

23. D Silva and A Pais de Lacerda, high-sensitivity C-reactive protein as a biomarker of risk in coronary artery disease, *Rev Port Cardiol* 31 (2012): 733–45.

24. Paul Ridker, et al., C-reactive protein and cardiovascular risk in the Framingham study, *Arch Intern Med* 166 no. 12: 1327–8.

25. PM Ridker, PWF Wilson, and SM Grundy, Should C-reactive protein be added to metabolic syndrome and to assessment of global cardiovascular risk? *Circulation* 109 (2004): 2818–925.

26. Ishii Shinya, C-reactive protein, bone strength, and nine-year fracture risk: Data from the Study of Women's Health Across the Nation (SWAN), *J Bone Miner Res* 28 no. 7 (July 2013): 10.1002, doi: 10.1002/jbmr.1915.

27. AD Pearle, et al., Elevated high-sensitivity C-reactive protein levels are associated with local inflammatory findings in patients with osteoarthritis, *Osteoarthritis Cartilage*, Open Archive, 15 no. 5 (May 2007): 516–23. doi:http://dx.doi.org/10.1016/j.joca.2006.10.010.

28. RJ Schulz, Homocysteine as a biomarker for cognitive dysfunction in the elderly, *Curr Opin Clin Nutr Metab Care* 10 no. 6 (2007): 718–23.

29. Sjur Reppe, Harish Datta, and Kaare M. Gautvik, The influence of DNA methylation on bone cells, *Curr Genomics* 16 no. 6 (December 2015): 384–92. doi:10.2174/1389202916666150817202913

30. M Fayman, The relation of plasma homocysteine to radiographic knee osteoarthritis, *Osteoarthritis Cartilage* 17 no. 6 (June 2009): 766–71. Published online 2008 Nov 30, doi:10.1016/j.joca.2008.11.015.

31. MO Ebesunun, et al., Plasma homocysteine, B vitamins and bone mineral density in osteoporosis: A possible risk for bone fracture, *Afr J Med Med Sci* 43 no. 1 (March 2014): 41–7. https://www.ncbi.nlm.nih.gov/pubmed/25335377.

32. O Nygård, et al., Plasma homocysteine levels and mortality in patients with coronary artery disease, *NEJM* 337 no. 4 (1997): 230–6.

33. AG Bostom, et al., Nonfasting plasma total homocysteine levels in all-cause and cardiovascular disease mortality in elderly Framingham men and women, *Arch Intern Med* 159 no. 10 (1999): 1077–80.

34. R Jaffe, Bioactive food as dietary interventions in cardioprotective nutrients, in *Bioactive Food as Dietary Interventions*, eds. RR Watson and VR Preedy (San Diego, CA: Academic Press, 2013), 103–19.

35. PA Deuster and RA Jaffe, A novel treatment for fibromyalgia improves clinical outcomes in a community based study, *J Musculo Pain* 6 (1998): 133–49.

36. Rula A. Hajj-ali, Introduction to autoimmune rheumatic disorders, in *Merck Manual Professional Version* (June 2013).

37. New research implicates immune system cells in muscle healing, *The President and Fellows of Harvard College Accessibility Report*, (December 20, 2013), Harvard Stem Cell Institute, https://hsci.harvard.edu/news/new-research-implicates-immune-system-cells-muscle-healing.

38. CF Franzblau, et al., Chemistry and biosynthesis of cross-links in elastin, in *Chemistry and Molecular Biology of the Extracellular Matrix*, ed. Ed Balazs (Academic Press, 1970): 617–41.

39. R Jaffe and D Deykin, Evidence for the structural requirement for the aggregation of platelets by collagen, *J Clin Invest* 53 (1974): 875–83.

40. SS Pullamsetti, et al., Inflammation, immunological reaction and role of infection in pulmonary hypertension, *Clin Microbial Infect* 17 no.1 (January 2011): 7–14.

41. JM Wan, MP Haw, and GL Blackburn, Nutrition, immune function, and inflammation: An overview, *Proc Nutr Soc* 48 no. 3 (September 1989): 315–35.

42. J Gill, M Vythilingam, and GG Page, Low cortisol, high DHEA, and high levels of stimulated TNFα, and IL-6 in women with PTSD, *J Trauma Stress* 21 no. 6 (2008): 530–9.

43. IJ Elenkov and GP Chrousos, Stress system – organization, physiology and immunoregulation, *Neuroimmunomodulation* 13 Nos. 5–6 (2006): 257–67.

44. C Franceschi, et al., Genes involved in immune response/inflammation, IGF1/insulin pathway and response to oxidative stress play a major role in the genetics of human longevity: The lesson of centenarians, *Mech Ageing Dev* 126 no. 2 (2005): 351–61.

45. LA Frassetto and A Sebastian, How metabolic acidosis and oxidative stress alone and interacting may increase the risk of fracture in diabetic subjects, *Med Hypotheses* 79 no. 2 (2012): 189–92.

46. PG Gel, RR Coombs, and PJ Lachman, *Clinical Aspects of Immunology*, (Hoboken, NJ: Wiley-Blackwell, 1975), 1399–404.

47. AE Lynch and R Jaffe, Lymphocyte response assay: Report on precision of novel cell culture test, experimental biology, *Poster presented at the American Society for Investigative Pathology Conference*, San Diego, CA, 2016.

48. IF Robey, Examining the relationship between diet induced acidosis and cancer, *Nutrition & Metabolism* 9 (2012): 72.

49. R Jaffe and S Brown, Acid-alkaline balance and its effect on bone health, *Intl J Integrative Med* 2 no. 6 (2000): 7–18.

50. M Pereira-Santos, et al., Obesity and vitamin D deficiency: A systematic review and meta-analysis, *Obes Rev* 16 no. 4 (2015): 341–9.

51. Pawel Pludowski, et al., Vitamin D effects on musculoskeletal health, immunity, autoimmunity, cardiovascular disease, cancer, fertility, pregnancy, dementia and mortality—A review of recent evidence, *Autoimmunity Reviews* 12 no. 6 (August 2013): https://doi.org/10.1016/j.autrev.2013.02.004.

52. M Hogstrom, P Nordstrum and A Nordstrom, n-3 Fatty acids are positively associated with peak bone mineral density and bone accrual in healthy men: The NO_2 Study, *Am J Clin Nutr* 85 no.3 (2007): 803–7.

53. BN Justin, Michele Turek, and Antoine M. Hakim, Heart disease as a risk factor for dementia, *Clin Epidemiol* 5 (2013): 135–45.

54. Liana C. Del Gobbo, et al., ω-3 polyunsaturated fatty acid biomarkers and coronary heart disease pooling project of 19 cohort studies, *JAMA Intern Med* 176 (2016): 1155–66.

55. B Hallahan, Efficacy of omega-3 highly unsaturated fatty acids in the treatment of depression, *Br J Psychiatry* 209 (2016): 192–201.

56. Yanni Papanikolaou, et al., U.S. adults are not meeting recommended levels for fish and omega-3 fatty acid intake: Results of an analysis using observational data from NHANES 2003–2008, *Nutr J* 13 (2014): 31.

57. Clemens von Schacky, Omega-3 index and cardiovascular health, *Nutrients* 6 no. 2 (Feb 2014): 799–814.

58. Claire Philippe and Yohann Wittrant, Oxidative stress in musculoskeletal disorders – bone disease, in *Systems Biology of Free Radicals and Antioxidants*, ed. I Laher (Berlin: Springer-Verlag, 2014), 1–2. https://link.springer.com/referenceworkentry/10.1007%2F978-3-642-30018-9_125.

59. Carlo Cervellati, et al., Higher urinary levels of 8-Hydroxy-2′-deoxyguanosine are associated with a worse RANKL/OPG ratio in postmenopausal women with osteopenia, *Oxidative Medicine and Cellular Longevity* 2016 (2016): open access, 8 pages, http://dx.doi.org/10.1155/2016/6038798.

60. V Humphreys, et al., Age-related increases in DNA repair and antioxidant protection: A comparison of the Boyd Orr Cohort of elderly subjects with a younger population sample, *Age Ageing* 36 no. 5 (2007): 521–52.

61. Jaffe A S, personal communication from HH the 14th Dalai Lama.

4 Veterinary Medicine's Advances in Regenerative Orthopedics

Sophie H. Bogers, BVSc, MVSc, PhD and
Jennifer G. Barrett, DVM, PhD

OVERVIEW

The link between human and animal disease, together with the widespread use of regenerative therapies in veterinary medicine has created an invaluable repository of data and biological understanding that can be used for the development of human orthopedic therapies. In this chapter, we focus on the current use of regenerative therapies in horses and dogs, which are the species with diseases, lifestyles and access to advanced orthopedic healthcare most similar to us. Similar to in human medicine, osteoarthritis and tendinopathy are the two orthopedic diseases most commonly treated with regenerative therapies in our veterinary patients. The chapter synthesizes the experimental and clinical research findings, and how these advances can be applied to human pathophysiology.

INTRODUCTION

The synthesis of human medicine with veterinary medicine, and its corresponding benefit to all species, is a hallmark of the "One Health" concept. This concept is not new; in the 19th century, Dr. Rudolf Virchow recognized that although human and veterinary doctors work on different species, there exists a single "basis of all medicine" (Schultz, 2008). The concept of having "no dividing lines" between animal and human medicine developed into One Medicine in the 20th century, and One Health in the 21st century. In less than a decade, the US Centers for Disease Control has moved One Health from a concept into a multi-national effort that saves both human and animal lives through collaborative centers and integrative research (CDC, 2016). Within the framework of One Health, comparative medicine and translational medicine have been identified as crucial partners in furthering our ability to treat orthopedic diseases and injuries in man and animal (Lerner and Berg, 2015).

Dogs and horses are the most commonly treated veterinary species for orthopedic disease and injury. Canine and equine athletes suffer from similar sports injuries as humans, including chronic conditions such as desmopathy and tendinopathy, as well as acute traumatic injuries such as ruptured tendons and ligaments. Additionally, companion and working animals' increased lifespan and lifestyle-related health conditions have increased the incidence of osteoarthritis in dogs and horses, comparable to their human counterparts. Animal owners' high expectations, increasing incomes and desire for the latest innovations in orthopedics means that equine and canine patients have access to advanced diagnostics similar to human patients, such as CT-guided fracture repair in horses (Perrin et al., 2011; Gasiorowski and Richardson, 2015). Figure 4.1 demonstrates relevant similarities between humans, horses and dogs. These factors, together with the high monetary and/or sentimental value of veterinary patients, have pushed orthopedic therapeutics beyond what is typically performed in human medicine, specifically in the field of veterinary regenerative medicine.

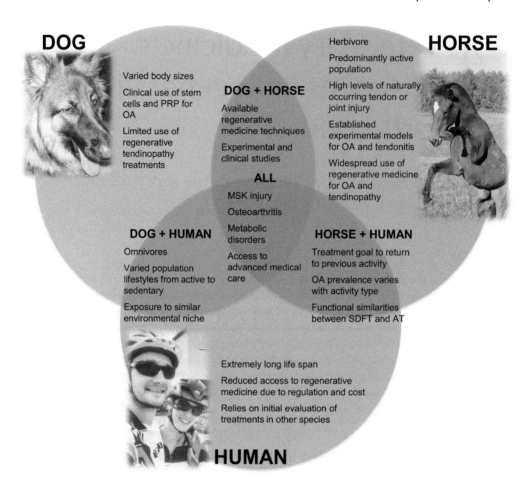

FIGURE 4.1 Venn diagram showing common and unique elements of orthopedic disease and regenerative therapies in humans and companion animals.

Regenerative medicine aims to harness the body's own anti-inflammatory and regenerative machinery to (1) reduce inflammation and scarring to treat conditions due to chronic inflammation and (2) promote healing in sites that have poor regenerative capacity. As such, the main strategy in regenerative medicine is to isolate a biologic, such as blood, cells, tissue, proteins or extracellular matrix, and either use that substance in an area where it is usually absent, use it at a higher dose than is normally present, or treat the biologic substance to enhance its natural regenerative properties. Therapies include platelet-rich plasma (PRP), autologous conditioned serum (ACS) and mesenchymal stem cells (MSCs), all of which are in wide clinical use for canine and equine orthopedic disease. Table 4.1 summarizes regenerative products currently available for clinical use in veterinary species.

The therapies mentioned above are similar to those used in human medicine, but the economic and regulatory landscapes differ and influence clinical use. Many major medical veterinary insurance plans cover the use of PRP and ACS (i.e. IRAP I™, IRAP II™), especially in the equine market where there are specific insurance plans for lameness related to orthopedic disease and injury. From the regulatory perspective, the FDA requires that veterinary biologic therapies undergo a thorough pre-market review of experimental data to ensure that the product is safe, effective and high quality (FDA, 2017). Where regulations differ from human use is that using devices to make the biologic therapies for PRP and ACS does not require pre-market approval (FDA, 2016). The nuanced difference in current regulations and the affordability and availability together have allowed PRP and ACS to quickly become ubiquitous for treatment of equine and canine orthopedic disease. Regardless of how clinically effective the different therapies are, the broad veterinary use can be analyzed to inform future human applications.

COMPARATIVE ORTHOPEDICS

OSTEOARTHRITIS

Osteoarthritis (OA) is a progressive disease of diarthrodial joints that represents the failed repair of joint damage resulting from stresses in any of the synovial joint tissues. It ultimately results in the breakdown of cartilage and bone leading to pain, stiffness and functional disability (Lane et al., 2011). The disease process is a whole organ disease, involving all tissues of the joint: articular cartilage, subchondral bone, synovium, joint capsule and ligaments (Dequeker and Luyten, 2008). Osteoarthritis affects all species and is a key disease where regenerative therapies have been used for horses and dogs.

OA incurs a significant economic cost to both human health and the equine industry. The collective economic burden to human patients with osteoarthritis is $36.1 billion in out-of-pocket treatment costs and $10.3 billion in lost earnings and due to absenteeism (Kotlarz et al., 2010; Kotlarz et al., 2009). OA is also the leading cause of financial loss and loss of use in Thoroughbred racehorses (Bailey et al., 1998).

Beyond financial implications, there are many parallels in the epidemiology and pathophysiology of osteoarthritis in humans and companion animals. Epidemiology in both populations depends on specific joints under investigation and characteristics of the population in question. Prevalence for knee OA in humans depends upon population demographics such as whether the population is predominantly suburban (Felson et al., 1995) or rural (Jordan et al., 1997) since this affects types of physical activities, and therefore types of joint injuries that occur. Likewise for horses, the prevalence of OA varies with horse use, for example, 54% of Thoroughbred racehorses admitted to a university hospital in the United Kingdom had evidence of OA (Todhunter and Lust, 1992) but 10%–19% of Quarter Horses used for Western Sports that were also admitted for lameness examination had OA (Dabareiner et al., 2005a,b). Post-traumatic osteoarthritis (PT-OA) is a sub-group of OA that develops as a result of trauma to any of the joint tissues. Human PT-OA patients are 10–15 years younger than primary OA patients, but incur an equally debilitating disease (Brown et al., 2006). Up to a third of Thoroughbred racehorses are affected by osteoarthritis by the time they are 2–3 years old (Neundorf et al., 2010), largely due to a high incidence of intra-articular injuries (Reed et al., 2012).

Meta-analysis of case-control or cohort studies have found that the main risk factors for the development of knee OA in humans are age, previous joint injury (pooled OR 3.86, 95% CI 2.61–5.70) and obesity (pooled OR 2.63, 95% CI 2.28–3.05) (Blagojevic et al., 2010). There are no similar case-control or cohort studies for horses; however, joint injury, age, overuse, conformational defects and developmental orthopedic disease have all been implicated as risk factors (McIlwraith, 1996). Like humans, OA in horses has increased prevalence with age, affecting 83.5% ≥15-year-olds (Ireland et al., 2012). Obesity is of increasing concern for modern society, and the likelihood of acquiring OA increases with increasing BMI in a dose-response manner (Grotle et al., 2008). The effect of obesity on equine OA has not been investigated; however, the prevalence of equine obesity (BCS ≥ 7–8/9) is 18.7%–35% depending on study location (Giles et al., 2014; Thatcher et al., 2012), and it is likely that this will be an area of future research due to increasing awareness of equine metabolic disease. The effect of obesity is twofold; (1) increased biomechanical stressors on the articular cartilage (Guilak and Hung, 2005; Arokoski et al., 2000) and (2) the production of pro-inflammatory cytokines by adipose tissue and adipocytes in such as IL-1β, TNFα (Hotamisligil et al., 1995;

TABLE 4.1

Regenerative Medicine Products used in Dog and Horse for Osteoarthritis and Tendinopathy

Category	Description	U.S. Veterinary Suppliers/Product	Effects in Osteoarthritis	Effects in Tendinopathy
Autologous conditioned serum	Autologous blood product that increases anti-inflammatory cytokines including IL-1Ra	IRAP (Dechra/Orthokine); IRAP II (Arthrex); MediVet; Biologics; EC-ACS (Vetlinebio)	Improved lameness, synovial thickness and cartilage fibrillation[1,2]	Reduction in lameness and improved ultrasound appearance when administered early after injury[3]
Platelet-rich plasma	Autologous blood product that contains growth factors including IGF-1 and PDGF	MediVet; VetStem; Osteokine (Dechra); Arthrex ACP; V-Pet (Pall Life Sciences); PRPKits. com; DrPRP USA; RegenKit-BCT (RegenLab); E-Pet (V-Care); V-PET (Nupsala)	Variable response to intra-articular injection in horses, some show reduction in lameness and joint effusion[4-6]. In dogs has a pain- relieving effect that is slower onset but similar effect compared to corticosteroid injection[7,8]	Experimental studies in horses show improved angiogenesis and histologic organization, but in naturally occurring disease treated and control horses had similar rates of return to work as each other[9]
Autologous protein solution	Autologous blood product that contains both growth factors and ant-inflammatory cytokines via a two-step process	Pro-Stride; N-Stride	Reduced clinical signs of pain and lameness in dogs at 12 weeks[10] and horses at 14 days and 12 weeks via client assessment[11]	N/A
Adipose-derived stromal vascular fraction	Digest of autologous adipose tissue that contains ~1%–2% of CFU-fibroblasts	VetStem (Biopharma)	Subjectively less effective than cultured bone marrow–derived stem cells when compared to placebo for experimental OA in horses[12]. Functional improvements in naturally occurring and induced canine OA, with some evidence of improvement when paired with PRP[13,14]	Improved histologic appearance in experimentally induced equine tendinopathy[15]
Mesenchymal stem cells	Autologous or allogeneic plastic adherent cells that are commonly isolated from bone marrow or fat. Capable of differentiating into osteogenic, chondrogenic or adipogenic cell lines	Variable - stem cell therapy may be offered by comparative orthopedic research laboratories	Bone marrow–derived mesenchymal stem cells showed no significant effects for naturally occurring OA; however, can improve return to work of horses with intra-articular soft tissue injury[16]. Canine studies using adipose- derived mesenchymal stem cells show improved functional outcomes, their effect may be complemented when PRP is used as a vehicle[17]	Improved histologic outcome with no change in ultrasonographic appearance[18-20]. Does not decrease the time of healing, but reduces re-injury rate by approximately half compared to conservative management[21]

IL-1Ra, interleukin-1 antagonist protein; IGF-1, insulin-like growth factor-1; PDGF, platelet-derived growth factor; CFU-fibroblasts, colony-forming unit fibroblasts.

References:

1 Frisbie DD, Kawcak CE, Werpy NM, Park RD, McIlwraith CW. Clinical, biochemical, and histologic effects of intra-articular administration of autologous conditioned serum in horses with experimentally induced osteoarthritis. Am J Vet Res 2007;68(3):290–296.

2 Lasarzik J, Bondzio A, Rettig M, Estrada R, Klaus C, Ehrle A, Einspanier R, Lischer C. Evaluation of two protocols using autologous conditioned serum for intra-articular therapy of equine osteoarthritis–A pilot study monitoring cytokines and cartilage-specific biomarkers. J Equine Vet Sci 2016;In Press.

3 Geburek F, Lietzau M, Beineke A, Rohn K, Stadler PM. Effect of a single injection of autologous conditioned serum (ACS) on tendon healing in equine naturally occurring tendinopathies. Stem Cell Res Ther 2015;6:126.

4 Mirza MH, Bommala P, Richbourg HA, Rademacher N, Kearney MT, Lopez MJ. Gait changes vary among horses with naturally occurring osteoarthritis following intra-articular administration of autologous platelet-rich plasma. Front Vet Sci 2016;3:29.

5 Tyrnenopoulou P, Diakakis N, Karayannopoulou M, Savvas I, Koliakos G. Evaluation of intra-articular injection of autologous platelet lysate (PL) in horses with osteoarthritis of the distal interphalangeal joint. Vet Q 2016;36(2):56–62.

6 Carmona JU, Argüelles D, Climent F, Prades M. Autologous platelet concentrates as a treatment of horses with osteoarthritis: A preliminary pilot clinical study. J Equine Vet Sci 2007;27(4):167–170.

7 Fahie MA, Ortolano GA, Guercio V, Schaffer IA, Johnston G, Au J, Hettlich BA, Phillips T, Allen MJ, Bertone AL. A randomized controlled trial of the efficacy of autologous platelet therapy for the treatment of osteoarthritis in dogs. J Am Vet Med Assoc 2013;243(9):1291–1297.

8 Franklin SP, Cook JL. Prospective trial of autologous conditioned plasma versus hyaluronan plus corticosteroid for elbow osteoarthritis in dogs. Can Vet J 2013;54(9):881–884.

9 Geburek F, Gaus M, van Schie HT, Rohn K, Stadler PM. Effect of intralesional platelet-rich plasma (PRP) treatment on clinical and ultrasonographic parameters in equine naturally occurring superficial digital flexor tendinopathies - a randomized prospective controlled clinical trial. BMC Vet Res 2016;12(1):191.

10 Wanstrath AW, Hettich BF, Su L, Smith A, Zekas LJ, Allen MJ, Bertone AL. Evaluation of a single intra-articular injection of autologous protein solution for treatment of osteoarthritis in a canine population. Vet Surg 2016;45(6):764–774.

11 Bertone AL, Ishihara A, Zekas LJ, Wellman ML, Lewis KB, Schwarze RA, Barnaba AR, Schmall ML, Kanter PM, Genovese RL. Evaluation of a single intra-articular injection of autologous protein solution for treatment of osteoarthritis in horses. Am J Vet Res 2014;75(2):141–151.

12 Frisbie DD, Kisiday JD, Kawcak CE, Werpy NM, McIlwraith CW. Evaluation of adipose-derived stromal vascular fraction or bone marrow-derived mesenchymal stem cells for treatment of osteoarthritis. J Orthop Res 2009;27(12):1675–1680.

13 Upchurch DA, Renberg WC, Roush JK, Milliken GA, Weiss ML. Effects of administration of adipose-derived stromal vascular fraction and platelet-rich plasma to dogs with osteoarthritis of the hip joints. Am J Vet Res 2016;77(9):940–951.

14 Yun S, Ku SK, Kwon YS. Adipose-derived mesenchymal stem cells and platelet-rich plasma synergistically ameliorate the surgical-induced osteoarthritis in Beagle dogs. J Orthop Surg Res 2016;11:9.

15 Nixon AJ, Dahlgren LA, Haupt JL, Yeager AE, Ward DL. Effect of adipose-derived nucleated cell fractions on tendon repair in horses with collagenase-induced tendinitis. Am J Vet Res 2008;69(7):928–937.

16 Ferris DJ, Frisbie DD, Kisiday JD, McIlwraith CW, Hague BA, Major MD, Schneider RK, Zubrod CJ, Kawcak CE, Goodrich LR. Clinical outcome after intra-articular administration of bone marrow-derived mesenchymal stem cells in 33 horses with stifle injury. Vet Surg 2014;43(3):255–265.

17 Vilar JM, Morales M, Santana A, Spinella G, Rubio M, Cuervo B, Cugat R, Carrillo JM. Controlled, blinded force platform analysis of the effect of intraarticular injection of autologous adipose-derived mesenchymal stem cells associated to PRGF-Endoret in osteoarthritic dogs. BMC Vet Res 2013;9:131.

18 Schnabel LV, Lynch ME, van der Meulen MC, Yeager AE, Kornatowski MA, Nixon AJ. Mesenchymal stem cells and insulin-like growth factor-I gene-enhanced mesenchymal stem cells improve structural aspects of healing in equine flexor digitorum superficialis tendons. J Orthop Res 2009;27(10):1392–1398.

19 Crovace A, Lacitignola L, Rossi G, Francioso E. Histological and immunohistochemical evaluation of autologous cultured bone marrow mesenchymal stem cells and bone marrow mononucleated cells in collagenase-induced tendinitis of equine superficial digital flexor tendon. Vet Med Int 2010;2010:250978.

20 Carvalho A, Alves A, de Oliveira P, Alvarez L, Amorim R, Hussni C, Deffune E. Use of adipose tissue-derived mesenchymal stem cells for experimental tendinitis therapy in equines. J Equine Vet Sci 2011;31.

21 Godwin E, Young N, Dudhia J, Beamish I, Smith R. Implantation of bone marrow-derived mesenchymal stem cells demonstrates improved outcome in horses with overstrain injury of the superficial digital flexor tendon. Equine Vet J 2012;44(1):25–32.

Kern et al., 1995; Montague et al., 1998) and IL-6 (Purohit et al., 1995; Fried et al., 1998). In rabbits, high-fat diets cause decreased glycosaminoglycan content and aggrecan expression regardless of body weight (Brunner et al., 2012). The parallels between human and companion animal lifestyles will continue to shed light on the pathophysiology of shared orthopedic disease and allow cross-species approaches to treatment.

TENDINOPATHY

The superficial digital flexor tendon (SDFT) in the horse is functionally analogous to the Achilles tendon (AT) in man and both structures store high amounts of energy during locomotion. The SDFT traverses the posterior (caudal) aspect of the equine limb, and reaches a strain of 11%–16%, which is close to its functional limit of 12%–21% when the limb is in weight-bearing position during gallop (Crevier et al., 1996; Dowling et al., 2002; Wilson and Goodship, 1991; Stephens et al., 1989; Riemersma and Schamhardt, 1985). Functionally, the SDFT stores around 40% of energy at gallop (Biewener, 1998), which is similar to that in the AT of a human running (Alexander and Bennet-Clark, 1977). In both humans and horses, the location and extent of the injury is dependent on the activity type (Chesen et al., 2009; Tipton et al., 2013; Ristolainen et al., 2010).

The pathophysiology of SDFT injury has elements that are reflected in both traumatic AT rupture as well as Achilles tendinopathy. While SDFT injuries appear to be as a result of overstrain during strenuous activity, age and cumulative load-associated degradation predispose the SDFT to injury. Most SDFT injuries are found in horses over 3 years of age and this is significantly increased after 5 years of age (Pool, 1996; Perkins et al., 2005). Cumulative load is also an important factor for AT injury, which is prone to core lesions with overstrain, and most commonly in males >45 years old (Kujala et al., 2005; Longo et al., 2009). Additionally, core hyperthermia has been implicated as a potential risk factor for injury in both humans and horses (Farris et al., 2011; Wilson and Goodship, 1994). SDFT re-injury rates in Thoroughbred racehorses are as high as 44% (Dyson, 2004), and are up to 31% for AT injury in humans (Lopes et al., 2012; van der Eng et al. 2013; Raikin et al., 2013). The horse poses an excellent model of tendon injury because of the similarities in SDFT and AT tendon structure, function and pathophysiology. Due to the high re-injury rates, economic impact and loss of use of athletic horses, SDFT injury has been the focus of intense research for regenerative therapies. Figure 4.2 shows a core lesion in an equine SDFT.

In canine patients, supraspinatus tendinopathy, akin to human rotator cuff injuries, occurs in the shoulder region of young to middle-aged large-breed dogs. Sporting dogs make up the majority of patients with this problem (Canapp et al., 2016b), especially those that jump, including agility and flygility (a combination of fly ball and agility) dogs, likely due to increased shoulder muscle activation and landing loads at jump (Cullen et al., 2017). The injury is less common in non-jumping sporting dogs, such as Iditarod sledding dogs; however, shoulder injury still accounts for approximately 30% of dogs that drop out of racing (von Pfeil et al., 2015). Although the pathophysiology and etiology are less defined than that of equine SDF tendinopathy, it is likely due to a similar cycle of repetitive strain injury and microdamage. Supraspinatus tendinopathy is induced experimentally in small lab animals, including rats and rabbits, using a treadmill overuse model to mimic human tendinopathy (Lui et al., 2011).

Achilles tendon injuries in humans are sustained from trauma and can be precipitated by aging (Fahlström et al., 2003; Holmes and Lin, 2006; Frey and Zamora, 2007). Similarly, dogs who are aging or obese can also experience tendinopathy. In this way, dogs demonstrate the link between metabolic state, diet and orthopedic disease. Experimental canine models are currently used to investigate effects of weight-loss surgery, obesity-related insulin resistance, heart disease and aging (Head, Cabrol et al., 1998; Vegesna et al., 2009; Broussard et al., 2016). The rate of canine obesity in the US in 2006 was 34% (Lund et al., 2006) and is a problem internationally (Mao et al., 2013; McGreevy et al., 2005). Obese canines obesity may be predisposed to orthopedic diseases such as anterior (cranial) cruciate ligament rupture (Lampman et al., 2003; Duval et al., 1999).

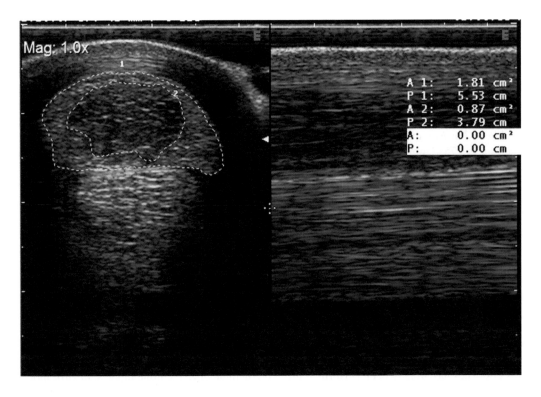

FIGURE 4.2 Core lesion of the superficial digital flexor tendon (SDFT) in a horse, 14 cm distal to the accessory carpal bone. Note that the outer-margin of the SDFT (1) is enlarged and the core lesion (2) is greater than 50% of the total tendon cross-sectional area.

VETERINARY SPECIES AS MODELS FOR HUMAN ORTHOPEDIC DISEASE

MODELS FOR OSTEOARTHRITIS

While *in vitro* models are valuable for investigating specific pathways altered by a therapeutic intervention, they are limiting when understanding systemic influences on therapeutic efficacy. OA initiation and progression is multifactorial and involves all of the joint tissues with complex cytokine-cell, cell-extracellular matrix and cell-cell interactions. Therefore, *in vivo* models give a more accurate understanding of how a therapy interacts under complex disease conditions. OA can be induced *in vivo* by creating joint instability (Hayami et al., 2006; Brandt et al., 1991; Little et al., 1997), intra-articular trauma to the subchondral bone (Mrosek et al., 2006) and/or cartilage (Bolam et al., 2006; Mastbergen et al., 2006b; Furman et al., 2007), animals that naturally develop OA (Jimenez et al., 1997), transgenic models (Helminen et al., 2002) or through intra-articular injection of cytokines or other inflammatory stimulant (Ross et al., 2012; Palmer and Bertone, 1994; Todhunter et al., 1996). It is important for the researcher to choose the model that best represents the aspects of the disease that are being altered with therapy, particularly with biologic therapies that are multimodal and are affected by the disease environment. For example, the anterior cruciate ligament transection/medial meniscectomy model was used to test the effects of bone marrow-derived stem cells (BMSCs) in goats and concluded that the amelioration of OA was due to reduced articular cartilage degeneration, subchondral bone sclerosis and osteophytes (Murphy et al., 2003). However, it is now known that a key effect of BMSCs in this model is to regenerate intra-articular tissues; therefore, the improved hallmarks of OA were likely due to increased stabilization compared to the control. Similarly, intra-articular injection of a cytokine or inflammatory stimulant such as LPS causes intense synovial and chondrocyte inflammation that is supra-physiologic compared to OA (de Grauw et al., 2009b; Ross et al., 2012; Palmer et al., 1996).

Horses represent a relevant model species for human OA due to their size, lifestyle and the abundance of OA drugs that have already been tested under different *in vivo* conditions (McIlwraith et al., 2012b). Compared to other model species commonly used to test OA therapies, such as rodents and rabbits, equine joint anatomy is more similar to humans in terms of size and articular cartilage thickness. For example, human articular cartilage thickness is approximately 2.2–2.5 mm, and in horses it is 1.75–2 mm thick (Grässel and Lorenz, 2014). Additionally, ample synovial fluid can be collected via arthrocentesis enabling a wide range of cellular, molecular and biochemical assays from each sample. Like humans, horses suffer from OA and their use as athletes requires OA treatment and the return of joint function, which is a treatment goal for human OA (Dabareiner et al., 2005a,b, Neundorf et al., 2010). Objective and subjective return of joint function can be determined through lameness examination with semi-quantitative grading, kinematic analysis, inertial sensors, force plate meters, joint flexion tests or goniometry (Keegan, 2007; Bell et al., 2016; Keegan et al., 2012; Fuller et al., 2006). The horse also provides an animal model with similar degrees of lifestyle variation to people, so that long-term efficacy of treatments of OA can be performed in a "real-world" setting prior to investigation of a treatment for use in people. Their ability to perform high-intensity exercise also makes them a sensitive model for the effects of symptom-modifying treatments on cartilage health; for example, the negative effects of corticosteroids on cartilage metabolism were highlighted in a treadmill-exercised equine model (Knych et al., 2017; Murray et al., 1998). Furthermore, due to the value of horses as competition athletes, testing of various OA drugs has already been performed using predictable *in vivo* equine models. *In vitro* models have also been established for investigating underlying mechanisms of action (Johnson et al., 2016; McIlwraith et al., 2012b).

Experimental *in vivo* models of equine OA have been developed with predictable levels of inflammation, cartilage matrix degradation and orthopedic pain or "lameness" (McIlwraith et al., 2012b). The most widely used models are the carpal osteochondral fragment (COF) model and the LPS-induced synovitis model. The COF model mimics post-traumatic OA and involves the arthroscopic creation of an 8 mm osteochondral fragment on the distal dorsal aspect of the radial carpal bone with consistent treadmill exercise and treatment initiated 2 weeks after surgery (Frisbie et al., 2008). This model has been used to investigate the effects of intra-articular or systemic pharmaceuticals (Frisbie, et al., 2009a,c; Frisbie et al., 2016; McIlwraith et al, 2012a; Kawcak et al., 1997) as well as biologic therapies including stem cells (Frisbie et al., 2009b), autologous conditioned serum (Frisbie et al., 2007) and gene therapy (Frisbie et al., 2002). Additionally, the pathological response over time has been analyzed and inflammation levels are as low as to be expected with OA (Frisbie et al., 2008). The LPS-induced synovitis model involves the intra-articular injection of 0.5 ng LPS per joint, which is the level determined not to cause systemic endotoxemia (Palmer and Bertone, 1994). Like the COF model, it has been used to test the anti-inflammatory effects of intra-articular and systemic pharmaceuticals (van de Water et al., 2016; de Grauw et al., 2009a; Lindegaard et al., 2010; Morton et al., 2005; Owens et al., 1996; White et al., 1994) as well as biologics (Williams et al., 2016); and the pathologic events over time have been characterized (de Grauw et al., 2009b; Palmer et al., 1996). The synovitis lasts for up to 72 hours and horses recover without lasting deleterious effects (de Grauw et al., 2009b; Palmer and Bertone, 1994).

Most *in vivo* canine models of OA are induced by creating joint instability, such as cranial cruciate transection and/or meniscectomy (Lindhorst et al., 2000). Interpretation of the efficacy of regenerative therapeutics is complicated in models that rely on instability to induce OA due to the potential regeneration of these soft tissue structures. The canine "groove" model was developed to overcome these concerns (Marijnissen et al., 2002a; Marijnissen et al., 2002b, Mastbergen et al. 2006a). Longitudinal cartilage defects are created in the medial femoral condyle followed by progressive loading of the joint. This model results in similar radiographic, biochemical and histological changes as seen in the cruciate ligament transection models without inducing joint instability (Marijnissen et al., 2002a). For veterinary medicine, once pre-clinical *in vivo* models suggest safety and efficacy, treatment of spontaneously occurring OA in our companion animal population becomes an ethical source of treatment-response information and long-term efficacy for regenerative therapies, albeit in a less controlled manner.

MODELS FOR TENDINOPATHY

The pathophysiology of equine SDFT injury has been widely studied and the drive to improve healing in equine athletes has driven the development of established models to test regenerative therapies. Models using the equine SDFT have been developed to monitor the pathophysiology of tendon healing, as well as investigate new therapies. Due to practical and economic considerations, exercise-induced models of tendinopathy have not been developed in the horse. Instead, enzymatic and surgical models have been developed. The enzymatic model was first developed in 1983, by injecting the SDFT with collagenase (Silver et al., 1983). This method is limited because the enzymatic damage can vary between individuals, it does not mimic the slow degradation that precedes equine tendinopathy, and can cause widespread tendon damage (Williams et al., 1984; Birch et al., 1998). Recently, consistency of the collagenase model has been improved with the creation of a needle tract and use of collagenase gel, thus creating a more focal lesion with no disruption to the epitenon (Watts et al., 2012).

The earliest surgical model of creating tendinopathy involved removal of a small square of paratendon and tendon (Watkins et al., 1985; Watkins et al., 1985). The limitation is that this disrupted the paratendon, which does not occur in naturally occurring disease. Since then, a surgical method of localizing the lesion to the tendon core has been developed using a motorized synovial resector (Schramme et al., 2010). The high degree of inflammation induced in most collagenase models and the acute nature of surgically induced models do not mimic the preceding slow degradation in the tendon. Therefore, more research needs to be performed on the temporal patterns of SDF tendinopathy so that realistic models can be produced. Although the collagenase gel model causes upregulation of genes associated with tendon matrix breakdown while preserving the epitenon and paratendon (Watts et al., 2012), the most realistic method for assessing intralesional tendon therapies is to assess equine patients with naturally occurring tendinopathy in a prospective, controlled, blinded manner.

Despite natural tendinopathy occurring in dogs, there are currently no well-established models of tendinopathy used experimentally. So far, research into regenerative treatments for canine tendinopathy is limited. Given that dogs share many lifestyle factors with humans and the similarities of supraspinatus tendinopathy with tendinopathy in sedentary individuals, this is an area that is open for regenerative medicine innovation.

REGENERATIVE THERAPIES USED CLINICALLY IN DOGS AND HORSES FOR OSTEOARTHRITIS

INTRODUCTION TO AUTOLOGOUS BLOOD-DERIVED PRODUCTS FOR VETERINARY PATIENTS

Autologous blood-derived products include autologous conditioned serum (ACS), platelet-rich plasma (PRP) and platelet and leukocyte-rich plasma (L-PRP). These products are all commonly produced using a kit sold as a veterinary "device", thus avoiding the need for pre-market approval as described previously (FDA, 2016). However, the final product varies in cytokine and anabolic factor levels between and within preparation types because they are influenced by patient factors and preparation method. ACS, such as IRAP I™ (Dechra/ Orthokine) and IRAP II™ (Arthrex), use whole blood that is incubated with chromium sulfate-treated glass beads to increase the production of anti-inflammatory cytokines, such as interleukin-1 receptor antagonist (IL-1Ra), by direct physico-chemical induction (Meijer et al., 2003). In comparison, an L-PRP preparation such as Pro-Stride™ (Biomet Biologics), firstly isolates white blood cells, platelets and plasma, then in a second step desiccates the product (Bertone et al., 2014). This results in both platelet- and plasma-derived growth factors as well as cytokines such as IL-1Ra and IL-10 and does not need an incubation period (Bertone et al., 2014). However, the concomitant concentrating of pro-inflammatory cytokines and white blood cells has unknown effects. PRP is made by concentrating platelets in plasma obtained from whole blood. Growth factors are released upon activation of the platelets, either endogenously when administered into the disease environment (collagen induces this process), or exogenously by the addition of thrombin or $CaCl_2$. When platelets are concentrated other blood cells, such as leukocytes and erythrocytes, are also concentrated. Therefore, PRP can further be defined as "pure" PRP, which is defined as leukocyte-reduced over whole blood, or leukocyte- and platelet-rich plasma (L-PRP). PRP can also be referred to as autologous platelet concentrate in the literature; however, usually, the term platelet concentrate is reserved for platelets that are maximally concentrated, unlike PRP.

AUTOLOGOUS CONDITIONED SERUM FOR OSTEOARTHRITIS IN VETERINARY PATIENTS

The initial description of human ACS production measured a 140-fold increase in IL-1Ra, which is a protein that competes with IL-1 for binding to the IL-1 receptor thus antagonizing the inflammatory effects of IL-1 (Meijer et al., 2003). Additionally, the anti-inflammatory cytokines IL-10 and IL-4 were increased approximately 2-fold with no increase in the inflammatory cytokines IL-1β and TNFα (Meijer et al., 2003). The preparation technique (Hraha et al., 2011; Rutgers et al., 2010; Carlson et al., 2013; Sawyere et al., 2016) and individual variations (Fjordbakk et al., 2015; Huggins et al., 2015) alter the bioactive composition of equine and canine ACS. The two main systems of ACS production for horses are IRAP I™ (Dechra Veterinary Products, previously Orthokine) and IRAP II™ (Arthrex). IRAP II™ achieves a higher IL-1Ra:IL-1 ratio than IRAP I™ (Hraha et al., 2011). Pro-inflammatory cytokines IL-1β and TNFα are also increased with ACS preparation (Hraha et al., 2011; Rutgers et al., 2010); therefore, the ratio of anti-inflammatory to pro-inflammatory cytokines may be important for a therapeutic effect (Hraha et al., 2011). Horses that have undergone surgical stress produce ACS with reduced IL-1Ra and TGF-β levels that are lower with higher levels of post-operative systemic inflammation (Fjordbakk et al., 2015); therefore, the timing of ACS collection may be important in horses undergoing surgical treatment.

Clinical results for the treatment of equine OA with ACS have been promising; however, it is a combinatorial substance, and the precise mechanisms of action remain incompletely understood. Treatment of a carpal osteochondral fragment model of equine OA with IRAP I™ injected four times at weekly intervals, found improved lameness, synovial thickness and cartilage fibrillation compared to saline-treated controls (Frisbie et al., 2007). The injection frequency of ACS is likely important. Horses with arthroscopically defined OA treated with three injections of IRAP II™ at 2-day intervals had significantly lower levels of IL-1β, biomarkers of cartilage degradation and IL-1Ra 42 days after treatment initiation compared to horses injected at 7 -day intervals (Lasarzik et al., 2016). Despite clinical improvements, *in vitro* studies have not shown chondroprotective effects. Although ACS (IRAP II™) increased IL-1Ra and IGF-1 in equine cartilage explants treated with IL-1β, there was no significant difference in MMP-3 production and proteoglycan loss or synthesis between ACS and serum-treated samples (Carlson et al., 2013). The ability of ACS to provide chondroprotection and mechanisms of action remain incompletely understood, so its efficacy is currently based on improvements in clinical signs and symptoms. Autologous blood products that concentrate platelets, such as PRP and L-PRP, are mostly used in canine OA; however, it has been established that canine ACS has increased IL-1Ra:IL-1β ratios compared to plasma, and the IL-1Ra levels are comparable to equine and human products (Sawyere et al., 2016; Huggins et al., 2015).

Platelet-Rich Plasma for Osteoarthritis in Veterinary Patients

The minimum platelet concentration that defines human PRP is >1 million platelets per µL (Filardo et al., 2010); however, there are no minimum platelet concentrations or fold increases over the systemic platelet count defined for equine or canine PRP. When platelets in PRP are activated by the disease environment or prior to injection through the use of $CaCl_2$, thrombin or a combination, the alpha granules release growth factors and cytokines. The two main growth factors in PRP are PDGF and TGF-β1; however, there are also VEGF and IGF-1 (Textor, 2011). Human studies have shown that TGF-β1 and IGF-1 stimulate extracellular matrix synthesis from chondrocytes (Sun et al., 2010; Fan et al., 2010) and IGF-1 decreases synovial inflammation (Rogachefsky et al., 1993); however, TGF-β1 has undesirable effects on the synovium including increased leukocyte infiltration, synovial fibrosis and osteophyte formation (Bakker et al., 2001). Another mechanism of action is PRP stimulation of synoviocytes to produce hyaluronic acid (Anitua et al., 2007), which may be more important in early OA as no differences were found between people treated with PRP or hyaluronic acid (Filardo et al., 2012), except if cartilage degeneration was present (Raeissadat et al., 2015; Filardo et al., 2012). A potential limitation of PRP is that inflammatory cytokines including IL-1β, IL-6 and IL-8 have been found using different preparation techniques with human blood (Sundman et al., 2011; Wadhwa et al., 1996). However, inflammatory cytokines are related to leukocyte content and can be reduced by leukocyte depletion (Sundman et al., 2011).

PRP use for equine OA has shown some success in clinical studies; however, production and activation techniques differ. PRP improved lameness and effusion scores in a pilot study of four horses (Carmona et al., 2007), PRP with pre-activation of platelets via freeze-thaw improved lameness associated with distal interphalangeal joint OA compared to a saline control (Tyrnenopoulou et al., 2016), while a larger study for equine OA using a derivative of PRP, APS, that undergoes a two-step process to increase platelet concentration and cytokines also found improved lameness scores (Bertone et al., 2014). The main limitation is that there was either little or incomplete analysis of the growth factor and cytokine profiles of the products tested. This is an issue because of high variability associated with preparation systems (Rios et al., 2015), platelet activation (Textor et al., 2013) and individual horse factors (Textor, 2011) that could affect the clinical response to PRP treatment. Leukocytes are also concentrated during equine PRP processing, and the quantity of leukocytes affects the ability of PRP to ameliorate inflammation from equine synoviocytes (Rios et al., 2015). Additionally, there is variation in the ability to concentrate platelets of available systems currently used for horses, which influences growth factor levels (Hessel et al., 2015). The largest source of variation lies in the activation method; although thrombin-activated PRP has higher levels of growth factors, when injected into healthy metacarpo-/metatarsophalangeal joints it caused joint effusion (Textor and Tablin, 2013) with increased synovial fluid TNFα and IL-6 (Textor et al., 2013). No controlled clinical investigation of PRP for OA treatment in horses has been performed, and so far clinical improvement after injection is variable (Mirza et al., 2016; Tyrnenopoulou et al., 2016). Further research to ascertain the efficacy of PRP products derived from various systems needs to be performed prior to widespread use for OA, and the use of bovine thrombin for intra-articular use should be avoided.

In contrast to horses, more research has been performed for the intra-articular use of PRP in dogs. In patients with OA, a single intra-articular PRP treatment decreases objective and subjective lameness and comfort scores compared to baseline or placebo controls (Fahie et al., 2013) and the pain-relieving effects were not significantly different from the traditional intra-articular therapy of corticosteroid and hyaluronic acid (Franklin and Cook, 2013). The difference between PRP and traditional therapy is that maximum pain-relieving response is seen at approximately 1 week with traditional therapy, but is most prominent after 6 weeks with PRP therapy (Franklin and Cook, 2013). A slow onset of maximum therapeutic response was also seen when PRP was combined with AdMSCs (Vilar et al., 2013). Experimental canine models using PRP suggest that a reduction in synovitis, as well as, reduced collagen breakdown and matrix metalloproteinase activity could be responsible for positive therapeutic responses (Xie et al., 2013; Cook et al., 2016).

MESENCHYMAL STEM CELLS

Stem cells are adult or embryonic in origin. Adult stem cells do not have telomerase so they undergo senescence in 30–40 population doublings; however, this gives them clinical advantages such as reduced tumorogenicity when used *in vivo* (Zimmermann et al., 2003; Bernardo et al., 2007). MSCs have regenerative, anti-inflammatory, immunomodulatory and trophic functions (Shi et al., 2010). As a result of the multifaceted nature of stem cell function, they are being investigated in the treatment of a wide range of diseases. Bone marrow-derived MSCs (BMSCs) and adipose-derived MSCs (AdMSCs) are the most common sources for clinical use, with BMSCs dominating equine veterinary medicine and AdMSCs dominating canine veterinary medicine. In horses, BMSCs are harvested from the sternum or ileum (Kasashima et al., 2011; Lombana et al., 2015; Arnhold et al., 2007) and AdMSCs from adjacent to the tail head (de Mattos Carvalho et al. 2009). Mesenchymal stem cells have been used successfully for the treatment of various equine musculoskeletal diseases including tendinopathy (Godwin et al., 2012; Pacini et al., 2007; Smith, 2008), intra-articular soft tissue injury (Barker et al., 2013) and cartilage regeneration (Wilke et al, 2007; McIlwraith et al., 2011).

The use of BMSCs for equine cartilage resurfacing of osteochondral defects has been investigated; however, the results vary because some studies fail to use an adequate control, or the treatment effect occurs over a defined time period. For example, positive results that included reduced initial PGE_2, total nucleated cell count (TNCC) and improved histological and functional quality of repair tissue were reported using AdMSCs in fibrin glue, but these were compared to no treatment controls (Yamada et al., 2013). In contrast, when compared to autologous platelet-enriched fibrin alone, the addition of BMSCs did not alter the biomechanical properties of cartilage at 1 year. In fact, grafts with BMSCs had increased bone edema and some horses had ectopic bone formation (Goodrich et al., 2016). This example highlights the need for controlling for scaffold when performing cartilage-resurfacing studies. Resurfacing studies have also found that treatment effects either occur early or are delayed. For example, BMSC implantation in a fibrin gel glue improved cartilage defect healing 30 days after surgery; however, there was no prolonged benefit at 8 months (Wilke et al., 2007). In comparison, scaffold-free BMSCs injected intra-articular 30 days after creating an osteochondral defect and treating with microfracture improved tissue repair, quality and firmness at 6–12 months (McIlwraith et al., 2011). The success of the second approach may be due to the trophic effects of MSCs on already forming fibrocartilage.

Scaffold-free intra-articular injection of MSCs has been investigated in both naturally occurring and experimental equine OA. A summary of clinical trials using MSCs for equine OA and tendinopathy is found in Table 4.2. Results have been variable; which may be an indicator that the degree of inflammatory environment varies significantly between models, follow-up time, MSC dose and source, as well as inter-observer differences in subjective outcome parameters. MSCs respond to inflammatory milieu by becoming "cytokine licensed", which enables them to have an anti-inflammatory and immunomodulatory effect. The equine studies demonstrate that MSCs exposed to non-inflamed, healthy joints cause significant inflammation, evident as synovitis and increased total protein (TP), TNCC and inflammatory cytokines (Carrade et al., 2011; Pigott et al., 2013; Ardanaz et al., 2016; Williams et al., 2016). In contrast, the most severe model for intra-articular inflammation, LPS-induced synovitis, showed reduced TNCC compared to LPS used alone, demonstrating modulation of the inflammatory response to LPS (Williams et al., 2016). Studies with variable or low intra-articular inflammation show a variable response to MSC treatment. For example, BMSC treatment 14 days after surgery in the COF model did not result in appreciable levels of reduced inflammation aside from reduction in PGE_2 (Frisbie et al., 2009b); and out of 165 horses with OA, synovitis occurred in 1.8% and there was high variability in response to treatment

TABLE 4.2

Clinical Trials using Mesenchymal Stem Cells for Osteoarthritis (OA) and Tendinopathy in Horses

Disease	Stem Cell Type	Dose	Vehicle	Control	Results	References
OA – Tarsometatarsal joint	Auto-AdMSC	5×10^6	Saline	Betamethasone No treatment	No change in lameness at 30 days but reduced at 60 days. 180 days improvement remained in MSC group but not betamethasone group. Decreased neutrophil count at 90 days in MSC and betamethasone compared to pre-injection	Nicpon et al. (2013)
OA – Stifle, fetlock, pastern, coffin joints	Allo- peripheral blood MSCs Native or chondrogenic induction	Not stated	PRP	None	1.8% (of 165 horses) synovitis in the first week, improved return to work at 18 weeks compared to 6 weeks, chondrogenic MSCs resulted in a higher return to work in distal limb joints but not stifle joints	Broeckx et al. (2014)
OA – due to Meniscal, ligament, cartilage injury	Auto-BMSC + arthroscopy	$15–20 \times 10^6$	Autologous serum/5% DMSO+HA	Results compared to previous literature	Unilateral affected horses 45% return to previous work, 23% return to work, 32% failure to return to work. In comparison to previous studies without MSCs, more meniscal injuries returned to work/ previous level of work. 3/33 horses had acute joint inflammation after MSC injection	Ferris et al., (2014)
SDF tendinopathy	Auto-BMSCs	9.5×10^6	1.5 mL autologous serum	No treatment	9/11 horses returned to previous use no injury 9–12 months after injection All control horses re-injured 4–12 months. Treatment failure horse received $<1 \times 10^6$ BMSCs	Pacini et al., (2007)
SDF tendinopathy	Auto-BMSCs	$2–10 \times 10^6$	Bone marrow supernatant 5×10^6cells/mL	Results compared to previous literature	27.4% of horses re-injured the treated tendon, re-injury rate significantly lower than for conservative management (~50% re-injury rate)	Godwin et al., (2012)

(Continued)

TABLE 4.2 (CONTINUED)

Clinical Trials using Mesenchymal Stem Cells for Osteoarthritis (OA) and Tendinopathy in Horses

Disease	Stem Cell Type	Dose	Vehicle	Control	Results	References
SDF tendinopathy	Auto-BMSCs Allogeneic amniotic derived MSCs	5×10^6	1 mL autologous plasma	BMSCs compared to amniotic derived MSCs	Amniotic derived MSCs had 4% re-injury rate, significantly lower than BMSCs 23%. Recovery time in both groups ~4 months	Lange-Consiglio et al. (2013a)
SDF tendinopathy	Allogeneic AdMSCs	2×10^6 cells/mL	2–6mL PRP 1×10^9 platelets/ mL	Results compared to previous literature	No adverse reactions, 89% resumed previous activity, 11% re-injury rate. Re-injury rates not significantly different to studies using BMSCs ± PRP but was different compared to conservative management	Ricco et al., (2013)
SDF tendinopathy	Auto-BMSCs	10×10^6	2 mL citrated BM supernatant	Saline	Significantly decreased stiffness in treated tendon vs. control, trend for higher elastic modulus. Improved histologic organization in treated tendon. Reduced sGAG levels in treated group, more similar to uninjured tendon. Reduced MMP-13 activity in treated tendon	Smith et al., (2013)

OA, osteoarthritis; SDF, superficial digital flexor; AdMSC, adipose-derived mesenchymal stem cells; Allo-, allogeneic; Auto-, autologous; BMSC, bone marrow-derived mesenchymal stem cell; MSC, mesenchymal stem cell; PRP, platelet-rich plasma; DMSO, dimethyl sulfoxide; HA, hyaluronic acid; BM, bone marrow; sGAG, sulfated glycosaminoglycans; MMP-13, matrix metalloproteinase-13.

(Broeckx et al., 2014). Two equine studies report improved lameness results; however, this was either a delayed response with no degree of improvement reported (Nicpon et al., 2013), or did not have a control for comparison with high variability between joints treated (Broeckx et al., 2014). Given that the other studies report no improvement in lameness, further controlled studies are needed with subjective and objective lameness assessment to prove efficacy. Overall, the functional outcomes for horses (lameness) seem to be less consistent than those observed in the human clinical trials, which may be due to increased pain and OA progression in human compared to equine patients and the high standard of pain relief needed for horses to return to the previous level of use. It is clear that MSC treatment for horses could be optimized to improve functional and pathobiologic outcomes in horses with joint disease.

In contrast to horses, the majority of research for canine OA has investigated the use of AdMSCs and shown improved functional outcomes. Improved functional outcome has been reported using adipose-derived stromal vascular fraction (AdSVF) and cultured AdMSCs for the treatment of elbow and coxofemoral OA (Black et al., 2007a,b; Guercio et al., 2012; Vilar et al., 2013; Cuervo et al., 2014; Upchurch et al., 2016). These therapies have had a considerable effect on the subjective measurement of lameness, pain in manipulation and range of motion (Black et al., 2007a), improved objective lameness measurements (Vilar et al., 2013; Upchurch et al., 2016) and overall client satisfaction with treatment (Black et al., 2007a; Vilar et al., 2013; Cuervo et al., 2014). The results of one study comparing AdMSCs to PRP suggest that, although both treatments improved functional outcomes compared to the baseline, the AdMSC group had improved outcomes compared to PRP (Cuervo et al., 2014). Canine OA MSC studies vary significantly in their preparation of MSCs and the vehicle for injection ranges from hyaluronic acid to PRP to saline (Black et al., 2007a; Guercio et al., 2012; Vilar et al., 2013; Cuervo et al., 2014). Experimental studies suggest that both these factors can influence clinical outcomes (Yun et al., 2016). Canine preparations of AdSVF are reported to contain 1.72% of CFU-fibroblasts, which are the MSC-like fraction proposed to be active in the product (Black et al., 2007a); however, the differences between the therapeutic activity of CFU-fibroblasts and MSCs as well as effective cellular doses are unknown. Although there are a limited number of studies comparing vehicles for AdMSC injection, there is some evidence that PRP has complimentary activity. In clinical canine patients with hip OA, a single intra-articular injection of cultured AdMSCs in PRP (Vilar et al., 2013) or AdSVF in PRP (Upchurch et al., 2016) improves objective lameness data compared to baseline and placebo. This clinical data is partially supported by experimental evidence of improved lameness, cartilage compressive strength and cartilage histology in patients treated with AdMSCs in PRP compared to AdMSCs alone, PRP alone or saline control in a canine cranial cruciate transection model of OA (Yun et al., 2016). This comparison needs to be performed in patients with OA due to confounding factors associated with models using injury of intra-articular soft tissue structures for MSC studies.

REGENERATIVE THERAPIES USED CLINICALLY IN DOGS AND HORSES FOR TENDINOPATHY

Horses dominate as the species for clinical and research applications of veterinary regenerative therapies for tendinopathy. In contrast, little controlled clinical research has been performed for canine tendinopathy. This section will largely focus on horses, with canine applications discussed at the end.

STEM CELLS FOR TREATMENT OF EQUINE TENDINOPATHY

The regenerative capacity of MSCs was the first to be investigated, and has been applied extensively to SDFT healing in both naturally occurring and experimentally induced disease. There are two approaches to MSC-derived tissue regeneration: (1) the application of cells that will remain and differentiate to form part of the recipient tissue, (2) the application of cells that will have trophic effects on endogenous stem and immune cells to speed endogenous tissue repair. Autologous and allogeneic equine BMSCs mainly stay at the site of injection and can integrate into the healing tendon tissue (Guest et al., 2008). However, the survival rate of MSCs in SDFT lesions is less than 10% by day 10 (Guest et al., 2010) and initial persistence after intralesional injection is around 25% after 24 hours (Sole et al., 2013). Therefore, trophic effects on tendon healing may be the key mechanism in MSC therapy for equine tendinopathy. This was demonstrated by decreased tendon re-injury rate and a similar clinical and ultrasonographic course of healing injection in patients with tendinopathy injected with culture media conditioned by MSCs compared to whole cells (Lange-Consiglio et al., 2013a,b). Despite these findings, the persistence and regenerative effects at a delivery site can be dependent on specific stem cell factors and the injury environment encountered. In contrast to MSCs, more than about 60% of embryonic stem cells survived intralesional injection after 10 days (Guest et al., 2010). The stem cell niche is the microenvironment that interacts with the stem cell. Key niche factors at SDFT injury sites include immune/inflammatory cells, soluble factors, signaling receptors, biomechanical forces and extracellular matrix interactions (Moore and Lemischka, 2006; Shi and Gronthos, 2003; Méndez-Ferrer et al., 2010). The biomechanical niche is particularly important for equine and human MSCs to differentiate into tenocytes (Kuo and Tuan, 2008; Subramony et al., 2013; Youngstrom et al., 2015). Within this niche, equine stem cells isolated from bone marrow had an improved ability to form a tenocyte-like phenotype *in vitro* compared with AdMSCs (Youngstrom et al., 2016).

Clinically, horses with tendon injury are most commonly treated with BMSCs administered via intralesional injection at multiple sites to gain even distribution along the tendon lesion. Intralesional injection of BMSCs results in the highest number of cells in experimentally induced SDFT lesions compared with intravenous or intra-arterial regional limb perfusion after 24 hours (Sole et al., 2013). Although there is an initial reduction of injected stem cells by 75%–95% (Becerra et al., 2013; Guest et al., 2010), the remaining intralesional stem cells persist up to 8 weeks for allogeneic umbilical cord-derived MSCs in naturally occurring lesions (Berner et al., 2016), up to 24 weeks for autologous AdMSCs in collagenase gel-induced lesions (Burk et al., 2016) and up to 9 weeks for AdMSCs in surgically induced lesions (Geburek et al., 2016b). BMSCs stay at the intralesional injection site, rather than migrate to other injured parts of the tendon (Guest et al., 2008 and 2010). The reduction of BMSCs at the lesion site after 10 days may be attributed to cell death or migration into the peripheral vasculature (Guest et al., 2010; Carvalho et al., 2014). However, despite evidence of BMSCs entering the peripheral blood from an injected injury site within the first 24 hours (Carvalho et al., 2014; Burk et al., 2016), it is unclear if they are able to home to other sites of injury. One study found no evidence of migration to contralateral limb injuries treated with DMEM media (Carvalho et al., 2014), while another found evidence of AdMSCs into lesions injected with serum (Burk et al., 2016). In this case, trophic factors in the serum or differences in sensitivity of labeling techniques could be responsible for the discrepancy. Intralesional injection of tendon lesions is performed under ultrasound guidance with a 19–22 gauge needle; needle diameters equal to or less than 25 g are not recommended due to decreased BMSC viability (Lang et al., 2017).

In vivo studies using either experimentally induced or naturally occurring tendon injury have shown that stem cell treatment improves the histologic appearance of the healed tissue by increasing promotion of linear fiber pattern, promoting increased collagen type 1 and alignment of fibroblasts compared with placebo control (Crovace et al., 2007; Schnabel et al., 2009; Crovace et al., 2010; Carvalho et al., 2011; Carvalho et al., 2013; Smith et al., 2013). Clinically, there is no difference in the ultrasonographic appearance of lesions and stem cell treated tendons take the same time course to heal (Schnabel et al., 2009; Crovace et al., 2010; Carvalho et al., 2011; Carvalho et al., 2013). However, one study showed that early injection of stem cells prevented an enlargement of lesion size 2–6 weeks after collagenase-induced tendinopathy (Carvalho et al., 2013). Although most studies have waited at least 2–4 weeks prior to stem cell treatment, and a delay is common in clinical cases, there are no controlled studies of the effect of treatment timing, or stem cell dose. One study that compared allogeneic amnion-derived stem cells to autologous fresh BMSCs showed improved results in the amnion-derived group (Lange-Consiglio et al., 2013b). This could be as a result of a shorter time to treatment in the "off-the-shelf" allogeneic cells. So far, differences in outcome have not been found between stem cells derived from bone marrow, or bone marrow-derived mononuclear cells (Crovace et al., 2007; Crovace et al., 2010), or with the addition of growth factors or PRP (Schnabel et al., 2009; Ricco et al., 2013); however, direct comparison has not been performed. Additionally, the optimum injection volume, dose concentration or total dose have not been determined. Thus, clinical practices vary, with the authors' preference to use 10×10^6 BMSCs in PRP at a concentration of $2.5–5 \times 10^6$ cells/mL depending on lesion size. Figure 4.3 shows how ultrasound guidance using orthogonal images is used to place the injection into the core lesion.

Aside from improved histologic appearance, a key advantage of stem cell therapy over conventional rest and rehabilitation protocols is that stem cell treated tendons have a reduced risk of re-injury. A study that compared BMSC treatment to conservative management found that re-injury rates dropped to 27.4% from around 50% in racehorses (Godwin et al., 2012), and studies in sport horses have found re-injury rates that range from 4% to 23% depending on the treatment type and horse use (Lange-Consiglio et al., 2013b; Ricco et al., 2013). Despite this clinical data, few studies have investigated if a true biomechanical improvement in healed tissue results from stem cell treatment. One study found a decreased stiffness and improved elastic modulus with stem cell therapy (Smith et al., 2013), which is in line with improved crimp pattern seen histologically in other studies (Schnabel et al., 2009; Crovace et al., 2010; Carvalho et al., 2011). However, other results are conflicting, finding either an increased stiffness in treated tendons (Schnabel et al., 2009), or no difference in collagen fiber size (Caniglia et al., 2012), which has been linked to biomechanical properties.

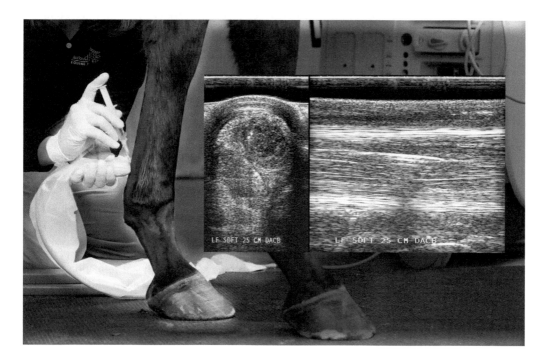

FIGURE 4.3 Injection of lesions of the superficial digital flexor tendon is performed with ultrasound guidance for accurate placement of the biological therapy. Orthogonal views (inserts) taken in cross (left insert) and transverse (right insert) sections allow accurate placement.

PLATELET-RICH PLASMA

Platelet-rich plasma increases growth factors, such as TGFβ and PDGF by triggering their release from concentrated platelets. TGFβ-1 increases extracellular matrix deposition in healing tendons; however over-expression can lead to scar tissue formation, while PDGF is released early during tendon injury and enhances the expression of other growth factors necessary in the repair phase of tendon healing (Klein et al., 2002; Tsubone et al., 2006; Hou et al., 2009). Equine PRP has the highest levels of TGFβ-1 and PDGF compared to whole blood, plasma, platelet-poor plasma or bone marrow aspirate and enhances the gene expression of SDFT matrix molecules *in vitro* (Schnabel et al., 2007). However, the concentration of platelets and leukocytes likely affects the ability for PRP to positively influence tendon healing. Leukocyte reduction of PRP reduces the amount of pro-inflammatory cytokines in tendon explants (McCarrel et al., 2012) and could decrease a prolonged inflammatory phase and subsequent scar tissue during the repair phase. Increasing the platelet concentration, and subsequently the amount of growth factors, may in fact reduce the ability of tendon to heal by decreasing the synthesis of type I and II collagen (Boswell et al., 2014).

In vivo PRP may promote equine SDFT healing through multimodal effects including promotion of angiogenesis (Bosch et al., 2011), histologic organization (Maia et al., 2009; Bosch et al., 2010) and biomechanical properties (Bosch et al., 2010). The limitation to equine studies investigating PRP is that there are a small amount of studies and each uses different experimental models of injury induction and PRP preparation. Additionally, due to the expense of live horse studies, there is a lack of complete control groups to completely assess the benefits of PRP on tendon healing in *in vivo* studies (Maia et al., 2009; Bosch et al. 2010). There are not enough studies currently to give definitive evidence that the beneficial effects of PRP seen in experimental studies transfer somewhat into the naturally occurring disease. Recently, Geburek et al. (2016a) demonstrated that PRP injected into patients with tendinopathy allowed 80% of the horses to return to previous levels at work after 12 months, compared with 50% of horses treated with saline placebo. However, the benefits may be short-lived or not as important as prolonged rest and controlled exercise because by 24 months horses at previous levels of activity had reduced to 60% in the PRP-treated group and remained at 50% in the placebo group.

REGENERATIVE MEDICINE APPROACHES TO CANINE TENDINOPATHY

Regenerative medicine approaches to canine tendon degeneration and injury have only been published in the last 2 years (Canapp et al., 2016a; Ho et al., 2015). The first study in 2015 treated ten dogs for supraspinatus tendinopathy with ultrasonographic changes including core lesions as well as disrupted fiber pattern and altered echogenicity. In the study, 3 mL of PRP was injected into each lesion with subjectively improved ultrasound appearance in six dogs and improved comfort assessment by the owners in four dogs (Ho et al., 2015). Canapp et al. (2016a) recently reviewed 55 patients with canine supraspinatus tendinopathy treated with 5×10^6 autologous AdMSCs in 1mL of PRP via intralesional injection (Canapp et al., 2016a). Figure 4.4 shows the performance of a supraspinatus injection with a dog under sedation. The study showed a significant reduction in tendon cross-sectional area, with 82% of cases reaching the size of their contralateral uninjured tendon, as well as significant improvements in objective lameness evaluation, with 88% of dogs reaching relative soundness. These findings are in contrast with an earlier study on the surgical management of the same condition, in which 50% of dogs with non-mineralized tendinopathy had improved outcome following surgery (Lafuente et al., 2009). Such findings, as well as evidence that mineralization and lameness can recur with surgery (Laitinen and Flo, 2000), warrant continued investigation using placebo-controlled, blinded studies of the beneficial effects of regenerative therapies for canine tendinopathies.

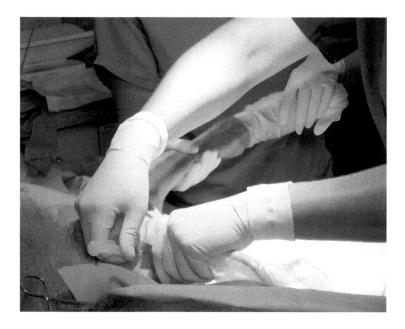

FIGURE 4.4 Ultrasound guidance of stem cells into the supraspinatus tendon of a dog is performed under heavy sedation with manual restraint. Note that the dog is in a lateral recumbent position compared to the horse in Figure 4.3, in which injection is performed under standing sedation.

OTHER CONSIDERATIONS IN THE USE OF REGENERATIVE THERAPIES IN VETERINARY ORTHOPEDICS

STEM CELL TISSUE SOURCE

Bone marrow-derived MSCs (BMSCs) and adipose-derived MSCs (AdMSCs) are the most common sources for clinical use in dogs and horses. In horses, BMSCs are harvested from the sternum or ileum (Kasashima et al., 2011; Lombana et al., 2015; Arnhold et al., 2007) and AdMSCs from adjacent to the tail head (de Mattos Carvalho et al. 2009). BMSCs derived from the sternum and ileum have no difference in differentiation ability, markers of stemness (Lombana et al., 2015), cell counts and growth rates (Adams et al., 2013), number of BMSCs or ability to form colony-forming units (Kisiday et al., 2013). However, a study using horses ≤5 years old found that ileal BMSCs had slightly more population doublings per 24 hours than sternal BMSCs (Kisiday et al., 2013), but sternal aspirates had a higher yield of total BMSCs than ileal aspirates in 13-year-old geldings (Delling et al., 2012).

Equine BMSCs and AdMSCs show inherent differences in differentiation potential, senescence and immunophenotype/stem cell markers. Equine BMSCs (eBMSCs) have increased expression of osteogenic markers compared to AdMSCs when stimulated to undergo osteogenic differentiation, but there is no difference in calcium deposition and ALP activity (Toupadakis et al., 2010). Chondrogenesis was found to be more efficient in BMSCs compared with AdMSCs (Vidal et al., 2008). BMSCs senesce after fewer population doublings, with senescence at 30 population doublings (~10th passage), whereas AdMSCs senesced at around 70 population doublings (Vidal et al., 2011). Osteonectin, a genetic marker for osteogenic differentiation, was expressed in both AdMSCs and BMSCs as they underwent senescence and was increased at passages 3–4 in BMSCs (Vidal et al., 2011). Therefore, use of low passage BMSCs may reduce the chance of osteogenic differentiation: however, there are no reports of heterotopic calcification in horses attributed to BMSCs treatment in studies using serial ultrasonography (Pacini et al., 2007; Smith et al., 2013; Smith, 2008).

BMSCs remain the MSC source with the widest use and most research for equine orthopedic disease, while AdMSCs are predominant in canine, with no direct comparisons to AdMSCs for efficacy in specific disease conditions or species.

There are inter-donor differences in MSC ability to differentiate, proliferate and in stem cell markers (Phinney, 2012). Inter-donor variation was a higher source of variation than the difference between stem cell sources in one study of equine stem cells (Barberini et al., 2014). These differences have also been shown in human (Phinney et al., 1999b) and murine (Phinney et al., 1999a) BMSCs. Donors can also have significant therapeutic implications during allogeneic MSC treatment. Variation between healthy human BMSC donors (18–45 years old) in a rodent model of spinal cord transection was responsible for variation in axon growth and the degree of recovery in behavioral tests (Neuhuber et al., 2005). However, specific age-matched studies have not been performed so the scope of phenotypic or therapeutic inter-donor variation of BMSCs is not fully understood.

Autologous versus Allogeneic Use

MSCs can be used therapeutically in an autologous or allogeneic manner. Autologous therapy uses MSCs derived from the tissue of the recipient or patient, in contrast to allogeneic treatment that uses a different donor tissue than that of the recipient, but is the same species. Currently, autologous use is most common in equine medicine as the perceived risk of immune rejection is lower, although this remains unconfirmed in the current literature. Allogeneic MSCs can decrease proliferation of T cells, alter the phenotype of macrophages and cause a reduction in inflammatory cytokines in humans and horses in a similar manner to autologous MSCs (Colbath et al., 2017; Ardanaz et al., 2016; Kol et al. 2015; Griffin et al., 2010). In a study that used allogeneic hematopoietic MSCs in humans, no antibodies to the MSCs were found, but there were antibodies to the fetal bovine serum that the cells were cultured in (Sundin et al., 2007). In contrast, use of allogeneic BMSCs and AdMSCs in horses caused the detection of alloantibodies (Owens et al., 2016). MSC's are classified as lacking MHC II; however, some conditions can cause MHC II expression (Schnabel et al., 2014), if this occurs and donor and recipient MHC II and MHC I are mismatched, there is a higher chance of immune reaction in horses (Schnabel et al., 2014). Despite these findings, allogeneic MSCs have been successfully used *in vivo* without immune rejection in equine tendinopathy (Guest et al., 2008) and synovitis (Williams et al., 2016). Allogeneic MSCs provides off-the-shelf treatment, as currently the propagation of autologous MSCs is prolonged (3–4 weeks), and does not allow clinicians to take advantage of the inflammatory niche in the acute to subacute period after injury. Additionally, allogeneic use allows harvest from a younger or non-diseased donor and may increase therapeutic efficacy. Understanding the biological and therapeutic differences between autologous and allogeneic therapies is important for future optimization of MSC-based therapies.

SUMMARY OF THE IMPORTANCE OF REGENERATIVE THERAPIES IN VETERINARY MEDICINE

One Medicine and One Health are examples of existing infrastructure to foster collaborative learning across human and veterinary medicine. Within the specialty of orthopedics, horses and dogs are clinical models for orthopedic injuries. These animals acquire osteoarthritis and tendonopathies both as athletes with overuse injuries and with aging or obesity. OA and tendon research in animals have specifically assisted in understanding the pathophysiology of the disease. Now economic and regulatory parameters have hastened the clinical uptake of regenerative orthopedic therapies among horses and dogs. Human orthopedics is gaining from clinical trial outcomes in veterinary medicine, especially in regards to emerging metabolic therapies such as regenerative orthopedics.

REFERENCES

Adams, M. K., L. R. Goodrich, S. Rao, F. Olea-Popelka, N. Phillips, J. D. Kisiday, and C. W. McIlwraith. 2013. Equine bone marrow-derived mesenchymal stromal cells (BMDMSCs) from the ilium and sternum: Are there differences? *Equine Veterinary Journal* 45 (3):372–375. doi:10.1111/j.2042-3306.2012.00646.x.

Alexander, R. McN. and HC Bennet-Clark. 1977. Storage of elastic strain energy in muscle and other tissues. *Nature* 265 (5590):114–117.

Anitua, E., M Sánchez, A. T. Nurden, M. M. Zalduendo, M. De La Fuente, J. Azofra, and I. Andía. 2007. Platelet-released growth factors enhance the secretion of hyaluronic acid and induce hepatocyte growth factor production by synovial fibroblasts from arthritic patients. *Rheumatology* 46 (12):1769–1772.

Ardanaz, N., F. J. Vazquez, A. Romero, A. R. Remacha, L. Barrachina, A. Sanz, B. Ranera, A. Vitoria, J. Albareda, M. Prades, P. Zaragoza, I. Martin-Burriel, and C. Rodellar. 2016. Inflammatory response to the administration of mesenchymal stem cells in an equine experimental model: Effect of autologous, and single and repeat doses of pooled allogeneic cells in healthy joints. *BMC Veterinary Research* 12:65. doi:10.1186/s12917-016-0692-x.

Arnhold, S. J., I. Goletz, H. Klein, G. Stumpf, L. A. Beluche, C. Rohde, K. Addicks, and L. F. Litzke. 2007. Isolation and characterization of bone marrow-derived equine mesenchymal stem cells. *American Journal of Veterinary Research* 68 (10):1095–1105. doi:10.2460/ajvr.68.10.1095.

Arokoski, J. P. A., J. S. Jurvelin, U. Väätäinen, and H. J. Helminen. 2000. Normal and pathological adaptations of articular cartilage to joint loading. *Scandinavian Journal of Medicine and Science in Sports* 10 (4):186–198.

Bailey, C. J., W. J. Reid, D. R. Hodgson, J. M. Bourke, and R. J. Rose. 1998. Flat, hurdle and steeple racing: Risk factors for musculoskeletal injury. *Equine Veterinary Journal* 30 (6):498–503. doi:10.1111/j.2042-3306.1998.tb04525.x.

Bakker, A. C., F. A. J. van de Loo, H. M. Van Beuningen, P. Sime, P. L. E. M. van Lent, P. M. Van der Kraan, C. D. Richards, and W. B. Van Den Berg. 2001. Overexpression of active TGF-beta-1 in the murine knee joint: Evidence for synovial-layer-dependent chondro-osteophyte formation. *Osteoarthritis and Cartilage* 9 (2):128–136.

Barberini, D. J., N. P. P. Freitas, M. S. Magnoni, L. Maia, A. J. Listoni, M. C. Heckler, M. J. Sudano, et al., 2014. Equine mesenchymal stem cells from bone marrow, adipose tissue and umbilical cord: Immunophenotypic characterization and differentiation potential. *Stem Cell Research and Therapy* 5 (1):1–11.

Barker, W. H., M. R. Smith, G. J. Minshall, and I. M. Wright. 2013. Soft tissue injuries of the tarsocrural joint: A retrospective analysis of 30 cases evaluated arthroscopically. *Equine Veterinary Journal* 45 (4):435–441. doi:10.1111/j.2042-3306.2012.00685.x.

Becerra, P., M. A. Valdes Vazquez, J. Dudhia, A. R. Fiske-Jackson, F. Neves, N. G. Hartman, and R. K. Smith. 2013. Distribution of injected technetium(99m)-labeled mesenchymal stem cells in horses with naturally occurring tendinopathy. *Journal of Orthopaedic Research* 31 (7):1096–1102. doi:10.1002/jor.22338.

Bell, R. P., S. K. Reed, M. J. Schoonover, C. T. Whitfield, Y. Yonezawa, H. Maki, P. F. Pai, and K. G. Keegan. 2016. Associations of force plate and body-mounted inertial sensor measurements for identification of hind limb lameness in horses. *American Journal of Veterinary Research* 77 (4):337–345. doi:10.2460/ajvr.77.4.337.

Bernardo, M. E., N. Zaffaroni, F. Novara, A. M. Cometa, M. A. Avanzini, A. Moretta, D. Montagna, R. Maccario, R. Villa, and M. G. Daidone. 2007. Human bone marrow-derived mesenchymal stem cells do not undergo transformation after long-term in vitro culture and do not exhibit telomere maintenance mechanisms. *Cancer Research* 67 (19):9142–9149.

Berner, D., W. Brehm, K. Gerlach, C. Gittel, J. Offhaus, F. Paebst, D. Scharner, and J. Burk. 2016. Longitudinal cell tracking and simultaneous monitoring of tissue regeneration after cell treatment of natural tendon disease by low-field magnetic resonance imaging. *Stem Cells International* 2016:1207190. doi:10.1155/2016/1207190.

Bertone, A. L., A. Ishihara, L. J. Zekas, M. L. Wellman, K. B. Lewis, R. A. Schwarze, A. R. Barnaba, M. L. Schmall, P. M. Kanter, and R. L. Genovese. 2014. Evaluation of a single intra-articular injection of autologous protein solution for treatment of osteoarthritis in horses. *American Journal of Veterinary Research* 75 (2):141–151. doi:10.2460/ajvr.75.2.141.

Biewener, A. A. 1998. Muscle-tendon stresses and elastic energy storage during locomotion in the horse. *Comparative Biochemistry and Physiology B* 120 (1):73–87. doi:10.1016/S0305-0491(98)00024-8.

Birch, H. L., A. J. Bailey, and A. E. Goodship. 1998. Macroscopic 'degeneration' of equine superficial digital flexor tendon is accompanied by a change in extracellular matrix composition. *Equine Veterinary Journal* 30 (6):534–539.

Black, L. L., J. Gaynor, D. Gahring, C. Adams, D. Aron, S. Harman, D. A. Gingerich, and R. Harman. 2007a. Effect of adipose-derived mesenchymal stem and regenerative cells on lameness in dogs with chronic osteoarthritis of the coxofemoral joints: A randomized, double-blinded, multicenter, controlled trial. *Veterinary Therapeutics* 8 (4):272–284.

Black, L. L., J. Gaynor, C. Adams, S. Dhupa, A. E Sams, R. Taylor, S. Harman, D. A Gingerich, and R. Harman. 2007b. Effect of intraarticular injection of autologous adipose-derived mesenchymal stem and regenerative cells on clinical signs of chronic osteoarthritis of the elbow joint in dogs. *Veterinary Therapeutics: Research in Applied Veterinary Medicine* 9 (3):192–200.

Blagojevic, M., C. Jinks, A. Jeffery, K. P. Jordan. 2010. Risk factors for onset of osteoarthritis of the knee in older adults: A systematic review and meta-analysis. *Osteoarthritis and Cartilage* 18 (1):24–33. doi:http://dx.doi.org/10.1016/j.joca.2009.08.010.

Bolam, C. J., M. B. Hurtig, A. Cruz, and B. J. McEwen. 2006. Characterization of experimentally induced post-traumatic osteoarthritis in the medial femorotibial joint of horses. *American Journal of Veterinary Research* 67(3):433–447.

Bosch, G., H. T. van Schie, M. W. de Groot, J. A. Cadby, C. H. van de Lest, A. Barneveld, and P. R. van Weeren. 2010. Effects of platelet-rich plasma on the quality of repair of mechanically induced core lesions in equine superficial digital flexor tendons: A placebo-controlled experimental study. *Journal of Orthopaedic Research* 28 (2):211–217. doi:10.1002/jor.20980.

Bosch, G., M. Moleman, A. Barneveld, P. R. van Weeren, and H. T. van Schie. 2011. The effect of platelet-rich plasma on the neovascularization of surgically created equine superficial digital flexor tendon lesions. *Scandinavian Journal of Medicine and Science in Sports* 21 (4):554–561. doi:10.1111/j.1600-0838.2009.01070.x.

Boswell, S. G., L. V. Schnabel, H. O. Mohammed, E. A. Sundman, T. Minas, and L. A. Fortier. 2014. Increasing platelet concentrations in leukocyte-reduced platelet-rich plasma decrease collagen gene synthesis in tendons. *American Journal of Sports Medicine* 42 (1):42–49. doi:10.1177/0363546513507566.

Brandt, K. D., E. M. Braunstein, D. M. Visco, B. O'Connor D. Heck, and M. Albrecht. 1991. Anterior (cranial) cruciate ligament transection in the dog: A bona fide model of osteoarthritis, not merely of cartilage injury and repair. *The Journal of Rheumatology* 18 (3):436–446.

Broeckx, S., M. Suls, C. Beerts, A. Vandenberghe, B. Seys, K. Wuertz-Kozak, L. Duchateau, and J. H. Spaas. 2014. Allogenic mesenchymal stem cells as a treatment for equine degenerative joint disease: A pilot study. *Current Stem Cell Research and Therapy* 9 (6):497–503.

Broussard, J. L., M. D. Nelson, C. M. Kolka, I. A. Bediako, R. L. Paszkiewicz, L. Smith, E. W. Szczepaniak, D. Stefanovski, L. S. Szczepaniak, and R. N. Bergman. 2016. Rapid development of cardiac dysfunction in a canine model of insulin resistance and moderate obesity. *Diabetologia* 59 (1):197–207. doi:10.1007/s00125-015-3767-5.

Brown, T. D., R. C. Johnston, C. L. Saltzman, J. L. Marsh, and J. A. Buckwalter. 2006. Posttraumatic osteoarthritis: A first estimate of incidence, prevalence, and burden of disease. *Journal of Orthopaedic Trauma* 20 (10):739–744. doi:10.1097/01.bot.0000246468.80635.ef.

Brunner, A. M., C. M. Henn, E. I. Drewniak, A. Lesieur-Brooks, J. Machan, J. J. Crisco, and M. G. Ehrlich. 2012. High dietary fat and the development of osteoarthritis in a rabbit model. *Osteoarthritis and Cartilage* 20 (6):584–592.

Burk, J., D. Berner, W. Brehm, A. Hillmann, C. Horstmeier, C. Josten, F. Paebst, G. Rossi, S. Schubert, and A. B. Ahrberg. 2016. Long-term cell tracking following local injection of mesenchymal stromal cells in the equine model of induced tendon disease. *Cell Transplantation* 25 (12):2199–2211.

Cabrol, P., M. Gallnier, J. Fourcade, P. Léger, J. L. Montastruc, J. P. Bounhoure, J. M. Fauvel, and J. M. Sénard. 1998. Failing of left ventricular β adrenergic affinity in a canine model of obesity-hypertension. *Journal of the American College of Cardiology* 31:444. doi:http://dx.doi.org/10.1016/S0735-1097(98)80277-5.

Canapp, S. O., Jr., D. A. Canapp, V. Ibrahim, B. J. Carr, C. Cox, and J. G. Barrett. 2016a. The use of adipose-derived progenitor cells and platelet-rich plasma combination for the treatment of supraspinatus tendinopathy in 55 dogs: A retrospective study. *Frontiers in Veterinary Science* 3:61. doi:10.3389/fvets.2016.00061.

Canapp, S. O., D. A. Canapp, B. J. Carr, C. Cox, and J. G. Barrett. 2016b. Supraspinatus tendinopathy in 327 dogs: A retrospective study. *Veterinary Evidence* 1 (3). doi:10.18849/ve.v1i3.32.

Caniglia, C. J., M. C. Schramme, and R. K. Smith. 2012. The effect of intralesional injection of bone marrow derived mesenchymal stem cells and bone marrow supernatant on collagen fibril size in a surgical model of equine superficial digital flexor tendonitis. *Equine Veterinary Journal* 44 (5):587–593. doi:10.1111/j.2042-3306.2011.00514.x.

Carlson, E. R., A. A. Stewart, K. L. Carlson, S. S. Durgam, and H. C. Pondenis. 2013. Effects of serum and autologous conditioned serum on equine articular chondrocytes treated with interleukin-1beta. *American Journal of Veterinary Research* 74 (5):700–705. doi:10.2460/ajvr.74.5.700.

Carmona, J. U., D. Argüelles, F. Climent, and M. Prades. 2007. Autologous platelet concentrates as a treatment of horses with osteoarthritis: A preliminary pilot clinical study. *Journal of Equine Veterinary Science* 27 (4):167–170. doi:10.1016/j.jevs.2007.02.007.

Carrade, D. D., S. D. Owens, L. D. Galuppo, M. A. Vidal, G. L. Ferraro, F. Librach, S. Buerchler, M. S. Friedman, N. J. Walker, and D. L. Borjesson. 2011. Clinicopathologic findings following intra-articular injection of autologous and allogeneic placentally derived equine mesenchymal stem cells in horses. *Cytotherapy* 13 (4):419–430. doi:10.3109/14653249.2010.536213.

Carvalho, A., A. Alves, P. de Oliveira, L. Alvarez, R. Amorim, C. Hussni, and E. Deffune. 2011. Use of adipose tissue-derived mesenchymal stem cells for experimental tendinitis therapy in equines. *Journal of Equine Veterinary Science* 31 (1):26–34. doi:10.1016/j.jevs.2010.11.014.

Carvalho, A. M., P. R. Badial, L. E. C. Álvarez, A. L. M. Yamada, A. S. Borges, E. Deffune, C. A. Hussni, and A. L. G. Alves. 2013. Equine tendonitis therapy using mesenchymal stem cells and platelet concentrates: A randomized controlled trial. *Stem Cell Research and Therapy* 4 (4):85. doi:10.1186/scrt236.

Carvalho, A. M., A. L. Yamada, M. A. Golim, L. E. Alvarez, C. A. Hussni, and A. L. Alves. 2014. Evaluation of mesenchymal stem cell migration after equine tendonitis therapy. *Equine Veterinary Journal* 46 (5):635–638. doi:10.1111/evj.12173.

CDC. 2016. Timeline: People and Events in One Health. Centers for Disease Control and Prevention, Last Modified 10.25.16 Accessed June 1, 2017. https://www.cdc.gov/onehealth/basics/history/index.html.

Chesen, A. B., R. M. Dabareiner, M. K. Chaffin, and G. K. Carter. 2009. Tendinitis of the proximal aspect of the superficial digital flexor tendon in horses: 12 cases (2000–2006). *Journal of the American Veterinary Medical Association* 234 (11):1432–1436.

Colbath, A. C., S. W. Dow, J. N. Phillips, C. W. McIlwraith, and L. R. Goodrich. 2017. Autologous and allogeneic equine mesenchymal stem cells exhibit equivalent immunomodulatory properties in vitro. *Stem Cells and Development* 26 (7):503–511. doi:10.1089/scd.2016.0266.

Cook, J. L., P. A. Smith, C. C. Bozynski, K. Kuroki, C. R. Cook, A. M. Stoker, and F. M. Pfeiffer. 2016. Multiple injections of leukoreduced platelet rich plasma reduce pain and functional impairment in a canine model of ACL and meniscal deficiency. *Journal of Orthopaedic Research* 34 (4):607–615. doi:10.1002/jor.23054.

Crevier, N., P. Pourcelot, J. M. Denoix, D. Geiger, C. Bortolussi, X. Ribot, and M. Sanaa. 1996. Segmental variations of in vitro mechanical properties in equine superficial digital flexor tendons. *American Journal of Veterinary Research* 57 (8):1111–1117.

Crovace, A., L. Lacitignola, R. De Siena, G. Rossi, and E. Francioso. 2007. Cell therapy for tendon repair in horses: An experimental study. *Veterinary Research Communications* 31 (Suppl 1):281–283. doi:10.1007/s11259-007-0047-y.

Crovace, A., L. Lacitignola, G. Rossi, and E. Francioso. 2010. Histological and immunohistochemical evaluation of autologous cultured bone marrow mesenchymal stem cells and bone marrow mononucleated cells in collagenase-induced tendinitis of equine superficial digital flexor tendon. *Veterinary Medicine International* 2010:250978. doi:10.4061/2010/250978.

Cuervo, B., M. Rubio, J. Sopena, J. M. Dominguez, J. Vilar, M. Morales, R. Cugat, and J. M. Carrillo. 2014. Hip osteoarthritis in dogs: A randomized study using mesenchymal stem cells from adipose tissue and plasma rich in growth factors. *International Journal of Molecular Sciences* 15 (8):13437–13460. doi:10.1016/j.joca.2011.12.003.

Cullen, K. L., J. P. Dickey, S. H. Brown, S. G. Nykamp, L. R. Bent, J. J. Thomason, and N. M. Moens. 2017. The magnitude of muscular activation of four canine forelimb muscles in dogs performing two agility-specific tasks. *BMC Veterinary Research* 13 (1):68. doi:10.1186/s12917-017-0985-8.

Dabareiner, R. M, D. M. Cohen, G. K. Carter, S. Nunn, and W. Moyer. 2005a. Lameness and poor performance in horses used for team roping: 118 cases (2000–2003). *Journal of the American Veterinary Medical Association* 226 (10):1694–1699. doi:10.2460/javma.2005.226.1694.

Dabareiner, R. M., D. M. Cohen, G. K. Carter, S. Nunn, and W. Moyer. 2005b. Musculoskeletal problems associated with lameness and poor performance among horses used for barrel racing: 118 cases (2000–2003). *Journal of the American Veterinary Medical Association* 227 (10):1646–1650. doi:10.2460/javma.2005.227.1646.

de Grauw, J. C., C. H. van de Lest, P. A. J. Brama, B. P. B. Rambags, and P. R. van Weeren. 2009a. In vivo effects of meloxicam on inflammatory mediators, MMP activity and cartilage biomarkers in equine joints with acute synovitis. *Equine Veterinary Journal* 41 (7):693–699. doi:10.2746/042516409x436286.

de Grauw, J. C., C. H. van de Lest, and P. R. van Weeren. 2009b. Inflammatory mediators and cartilage bio-markers in synovial fluid after a single inflammatory insult: A longitudinal experimental study. *Arthritis Research and Therapy* 11 (2):R35. doi:10.1186/ar2640.

de Mattos Carvalho, A., A. L. Alves, M. A. Golim, A. Moroz, C. A. Hussni, P. G. de Oliveira, and E. Deffune. 2009. Isolation and immunophenotypic characterization of mesenchymal stem cells derived from equine species adipose tissue. *Veterinary Immunology and Immunopathology* 132 (2–4):303–6.

Delling, U., K. Lindner, I. Ribitsch, H. Jülke, and W. Brehm. 2012. Comparison of bone marrow aspiration at the sternum and the tuber coxae in middle-aged horses. *Canadian Journal of Veterinary Research* 76 (1):52–6.

Dequeker, J. and F. P. Luyten. 2008. The history of osteoarthritis-osteoarthrosis. *Annals of the Rheumatic Diseases* (67):5–10.

Dowling, B. A., A. J. Dart, D. R Hodgson, R. J. Rose, and W. R. Walsh. 2002. Recombinant equine growth hormone does not affect the in vitro biomechanical properties of equine superficial digital flexor tendon. *Veterinary Surgery* 31 (4):325–330.

Duval, J. M., S. C. Budsberg, G. L. Flo, and J. L. Sammarco. 1999. Breed, sex, and body weight as risk factors for rupture of the cranial cruciate ligament in young dogs. *Journal of the American Veterinary Medical Association* 215 (6):811–814.

Dyson, S. J. 2004. Medical management of superficial digital flexor tendonitis: A comparative study in 219 horses (1992–2000). *Equine Veterinary Journal* 36 (5):415–419.

Fahie, M. A., G. A Ortolano, V. Guercio, J. A. Schaffer, G. Johnston, J. Au, B. A. Hettlich, T. Phillips, M. J. Allen, and A. L. Bertone. 2013. A randomized controlled trial of the efficacy of autologous platelet therapy for the treatment of osteoarthritis in dogs. *Journal of the American Veterinary Medical Association* 243 (9):1291–1297.

Fahlström, M., P. Jonsson, R. Lorentzon, and H. Alfredson. 2003. Chronic achilles tendon pain treated with eccentric calf-muscle training. *Knee Surgery, Sports Traumatology, Arthroscopy* 11 (5):327–333.

Fan, H., H. Tao, Y. Wu, Y. Hu, Y. Yan, and Z. Luo. 2010. TGF-β3 immobilized PLGA-gelatin/chondroitin sulfate/hyaluronic acid hybrid scaffold for cartilage regeneration. *Journal of Biomedical Materials Research Part A* 95 (4):982–992.

Farris, D. J., G. Trewartha, and M. P. McGuigan. 2011. Could intra-tendinous hyperthermia during running explain chronic injury of the human Achilles tendon? *Journal of Biomechanics* 44 (5):822–826.

Ferris, D. J., D. D. Frisbie, J. D. Kisiday, C. W. McIlwraith, B. A. Hague, M. D. Major, R. K. Schneider, C. J. Zubrod, C. E. Kawcak, and L. R. Goodrich. 2014. Clinical outcome after intra-articular administration of bone marrow derived mesenchymal stem cells in 33 horses with stifle injury. *Veterinary Surgery* 43 (3):255–265. doi: 10.1111/j.1532-950X.2014.12100.x.

FDA. 2016. How FDA regulates veterinary devices. U.S. Food & Drug Administration, Last Modified 7.14.16 Accessed February 21, 2017. https://www.fda.gov/AnimalVeterinary/ResourcesforYou/ucm047117.htm.

FDA. 2017. What are veterinary biologics (including vaccines) and is FDA responsible for these products?. U.S. Food & Drug Administration, Last Modified 1.24.17 Accessed February 21, 2017. https://www.fda.gov/AboutFDA/Transparency/Basics/ucm193868.htm.

Felson, D. T., Y. Zhang, M. T Hannan, A. Naimark, B. N. Weissman, P. Aliabadi, and D. Levy. 1995. The incidence and natural history of knee osteoarthritis in the elderly, the framingham osteoarthritis study. *Arthritis and Rheumatology* 38 (10):1500–1505.

Filardo, G., E. Kon, A. Di Martino, B. Di Matteo, M. L. Merli, A. Cenacchi, P. M. Fornasari, and M. Marcacci. 2012. Platelet-rich plasma vs hyaluronic acid to treat knee degenerative pathology: Study design and preliminary results of a randomized controlled trial. *BMC Musculoskeletal Disorders* 13:229. doi:10.1186/1471-2474-13-229.

Filardo, G., E. Kon, R. Buda, A. Timoncini, A. Di Martino, A. Cenacchi, P. M. Fornasari, S. Giannini, and M. Marcacci. 2010. Platelet-rich plasma intra-articular knee injections for the treatment of degenerative cartilage lesions and osteoarthritis. *Knee Surgery, Sports Traumatology, Arthroscopy* 19 (4):528–35.

Fjordbakk, C. T., G. M. Johansen, A. C. Lovas, K. L. Oppegard, and A. K. Storset. 2015. Surgical stress influences cytokine content in autologous conditioned serum. *Equine Veterinary Journal* 47 (2):212–217. doi:10.1111/evj.12277.

Franklin, S. P. and J. L. Cook. 2013. Prospective trial of autologous conditioned plasma versus hyaluronan plus corticosteroid for elbow osteoarthritis in dogs. *Canadian Veterinary Journal* 54 (9):881–884.

Frey, C. and J. Zamora. 2007. The effects of obesity on orthopaedic foot and ankle pathology. *Foot and Ankle International* 28 (9):996–999.

Fried, S. K., D. A. Bunkin, and A. S. Greenberg. 1998. Omental and subcutaneous adipose tissues of obese subjects release interleukin-6: Depot difference and regulation by glucocorticoid 1. *The Journal of Clinical Endocrinology and Metabolism* 83 (3):847–850.

Frisbie, D. D., S. C. Ghivizzani, P. D. Robbins, C. H. Evans, and C. W. McIlwraith. 2002. Treatment of experimental equine osteoarthritis by in vivo delivery of the equine interleukin-1 receptor antagonist gene. *Gene Therapy* 9 (1):12–20. doi:10.1038/sj.gt.3301608.

Frisbie, D. D., F. Al-Sobayil, R. C. Billinghurst, C. E. Kawcak, and C. W. McIlwraith. 2008. Changes in synovial fluid and serum biomarkers with exercise and early osteoarthritis in horses. *Osteoarthritis Cartilage* 16 (10):1196–1204. doi:10.1016/j.joca.2008.03.008.

Frisbie, D. D., C. E. Kawcak, N. M. Werpy, R. D. Park, and C. W. McIlwraith. 2007. Clinical, biochemical, and histologic effects of intra-articular administration of autologous conditioned serum in horses with experimentally induced osteoarthritis. *American Journal of Veterinary Research* 68 (3):290–296. doi:10.2460/ajvr.68.3.290.

Frisbie, D. D., C. E. Kawcak, C. W. McIlwraith, and N. M. Werpy. 2009a. Evaluation of polysulfated glycosaminoglycan or sodium hyaluronan administered intra-articularly for treatment of horses with experimentally induced osteoarthritis. *American Journal of Veterinary Research* 70 (2):203–209. doi:10.2460/ajvr.70.2.203.

Frisbie, D. D., J. D. Kisiday, C. E. Kawcak, N. M. Werpy, and C. W. McIlwraith. 2009b. Evaluation of adipose-derived stromal vascular fraction or bone marrow-derived mesenchymal stem cells for treatment of osteoarthritis. *Journal of Orthopaedic Research* 27 (12):1675–1680. doi:10.1002/jor.20933.

Frisbie, D. D., C. W. McIlwraith, C. E. Kawcak, N. M. Werpy, and G. L. Pearce. 2009c. Evaluation of topically administered diclofenac liposomal cream for treatment of horses with experimentally induced osteoarthritis. *American Journal of Veterinary Research* 70 (2):210–215. doi:10.2460/ajvr.70.2.210.

Frisbie, D. D., C. W. McIlwraith, C. E. Kawcak, and N. M. Werpy. 2016. Efficacy of intravenous administration of hyaluronan, sodium chondroitin sulfate, and N-acetyl-d-glucosamine for prevention or treatment of osteoarthritis in horses. *American Journal of Veterinary Research* 77 (10):1064–1070. doi:10.2460/ajvr.77.10.1064.

Fuller, C. J., B. M. Bladon, A. J. Driver, and A. R. Barr. 2006. The intra- and inter-assessor reliability of measurement of functional outcome by lameness scoring in horses. *Veterinary Journal* 171 (2):281–286. doi:10.1016/j.tvjl.2004.10.012.

Furman, B. D., J. Strand, W. C. Hembree, B. D. Ward, F. Guilak, and S. A. Olson. 2007. Joint degeneration following closed intraarticular fracture in the mouse knee: A model of posttraumatic arthritis. *Journal of Orthopaedic Research* 25 (5):578–592. doi:10.1002/jor.20331.

Gasiorowski, J. C. and D. W. Richardson. 2015. Clinical use of computed tomography and surface markers to assist internal fixation within the equine hoof. *Veterinary Surgery* 44 (2):214–222. doi:10.1111/j.1532-950X.2014.12253.x.

Geburek, F., M. Gaus, H. T. van Schie, K. Rohn, and P. M. Stadler. 2016a. Effect of intralesional platelet-rich plasma (PRP) treatment on clinical and ultrasonographic parameters in equine naturally occurring superficial digital flexor tendinopathies - a randomized prospective controlled clinical trial. *BMC Veterinary Research* 12 (1):191. doi:10.1186/s12917-016-0826-1.

Geburek, F., K. Mundle, S. Conrad, M. Hellige, U. Walliser, H. T. M. van Schie, R. van Weeren, T. Skutella, and P. M. Stadler. 2016b. Tracking of autologous adipose tissue-derived mesenchymal stromal cells with in vivo magnetic resonance imaging and histology after intralesional treatment of artificial equine tendon lesions-a pilot study. *Stem Cell Research and Therapy* 7 (1):21.

Giles, S. L., S. A. Rands, C. J. Nicol, and P. A. Harris. 2014. Obesity prevalence and associated risk factors in outdoor living domestic horses and ponies. *Peer-Reviewed Journal* 2:e299. doi:10.7717/peerj.299.

Godwin, E. E., N. J. Young, J. Dudhia, I. C. Beamish, and R. K. W. Smith. 2012. Implantation of bone marrow-derived mesenchymal stem cells demonstrates improved outcome in horses with overstrain injury of the superficial digital flexor tendon. *Equine Veterinary Journal* 44 (1):25–32.

Goodrich, L. R., A. C. Chen, N. M. Werpy, A. A. Williams, J. D. Kisiday, A. W. Su, E. Cory, P. S. Morley, C. W. McIlwraith, R. L. Sah, and C. R. Chu. 2016. Addition of mesenchymal stem cells to autologous platelet-enhanced fibrin scaffolds in chondral defects: Does it enhance repair? *Journal of Bone and Joint Surgery* 98 (1):23–34. doi:10.2106/JBJS.O.00407.

Grässel, S. and J. Lorenz. 2014. Tissue-engineering strategies to repair chondral and osteochondral tissue in osteoarthritis: Use of mesenchymal stem cells. *Current Rheumatology Reports* 16 (10):1–16.

Griffin, M. D., T. Ritter, and B. P. Mahon. 2010. Immunological aspects of allogeneic mesenchymal stem cell therapies. *Human Gene Therapy* 21 (12):1641–1655. doi:10.1089/hum.2010.156.

Grotle, M., K. B. Hagen, B. Natvig, F. A. Dahl, and T. K. Kvien. 2008. Obesity and osteoarthritis in knee, hip and/or hand: An epidemiological study in the general population with 10 years follow-up. *BMC Musculoskeletal Disorders* 9 (1):132.

Guercio, A., P. Marco, S. Casella, V. Cannella, L. Russotto, G. Purpari, S. Bella, and G. Piccione. 2012. Production of canine mesenchymal stem cells from adipose tissue and their application in dogs with chronic osteoarthritis of the humeroradial joints. *Cell Biology International* 36 (2):189–194.

Guest, D. J., M. R. Smith, and W. R. Allen. 2008. Monitoring the fate of autologous and allogeneic mesen-chymal progenitor cells injected into the superficial digital flexor tendon of horses: Preliminary study. *Equine Veterinary Journal* 40 (2):178–181. doi:10.2746/042516408X276942.

Guest, D. J., M. R. W. Smith, and W. R. Allen. 2010. Equine embryonic stem-like cells and mesenchymal stromal cells have different survival rates and migration patterns following their injection into damaged superficial digital flexor tendon. *Equine Veterinary Journal* 42 (7):636–642.

Guilak, F. and C. T. Hung. 2005. Physical regulation of cartilage metabolism. In *Basic Orthopaedic Biomechanics and Mechanobiology 3*, edited by V. C. Mow and R. Huiskes, 179–207. Philadelphia, PA: Lipincott Williams & Wilkins.

Hayami, T., M. Pickarski, Y. Zhuo, G. A. Wesolowski, G. A. Rodan, and L. T. Duong. 2006. Characterization of articular cartilage and subchondral bone changes in the rat anterior cruciate ligament transection and meniscectomized models of osteoarthritis. *Bone* 38 (2):234–243.

Head, E. 1998. A canine model of human aging and Alzheimer's disease. *Biochimica et Biophysica Acta. Molecular Basis of Disease* 1832 (9):1384–1389. doi:10.1016/j.bbadis.2013.03.016.

Helminen, H. J., A. M. Säämänen, H. Salminen, and M. M. Hyttinen. 2002. Transgenic mouse models for studying the role of cartilage macromolecules in osteoarthritis. *Rheumatology* 41 (8):848–856.

Hessel, L. N., G. Bosch, P. R. van Weeren, and J. C. Ionita. 2015. Equine autologous platelet concentrates: A comparative study between different available systems. *Equine Veterinary Journal* 47 (3):319–325. doi:10.1111/evj.12288.

Ho, L. K., W. I. Baltzer, S. Nemanic, and S. M. Stieger-Vanegas. 2015. Single ultrasound-guided platelet-rich plasma injection for treatment of supraspinatus tendinopathy in dogs. *Canadian Veterinary Journal* 56 (8):845–849.

Holmes, G. B. and J. Lin. 2006. Etiologic factors associated with symptomatic achilles tendinopathy. *Foot and Ankle International* 27 (11):952–959.

Hotamisligil, G. S, P. Arner, J. F. Caro, R. L. Atkinson, and B. M. Spiegelman. 1995. Increased adipose tissue expression of tumor necrosis factor-alpha in human obesity and insulin resistance. *Journal of Clinical Investigation* 95 (5):2409.

Hou, Y., Z. Mao, X. L. Wei, L. Lin, L. Chen, H. Wang, X. Fu, J. Zhang, and C. Yu. 2009. The roles of TGF-β1 gene transfer on collagen formation during Achilles tendon healing. *Biochemical and Biophysical Research Communications* 383 (2):235–239.

Hraha, T. H., K. M. Doremus, C. W. McIlwraith, and D. D. Frisbie. 2011. Autologous conditioned serum: The comparative cytokine profiles of two commercial methods (IRAP and IRAP II) using equine blood. *Equine Veterinary Journal* 43 (5):516–521. doi:10.1111/j.2042-3306.2010.00321.x.

Huggins, S. S., J. S. Suchodolski, R. N. Bearden, J. M. Steiner, and W. B. Saunders. 2015. Serum concentrations of canine interleukin-1 receptor antagonist protein in healthy dogs after incubation using an autologous serum processing system. *Research in Veterinary Science* 101:28–33. doi:10.1016/j.rvsc.2015.05.012.

Ireland, J. L., P. D. Clegg, C. M. McGowan, S. A. McKane, K. J. Chandler, and G. L. Pinchbeck. 2012. Disease prevalence in geriatric horses in the United Kingdom: Veterinary clinical assessment of 200 cases. *Equine Veterinary Journal* 44 (1):101–106. doi:10.1111/j.2042-3306.2010.00361.x.

Jimenez, P. A., S. S Glasson, O. V. Trubetskoy, and H. B. Haimes. 1997. Spontaneous osteoarthritis in Dunkin Hartley guinea pigs: Histologic, radiologic, and biochemical changes. *Comparative Medicine* 47 (6):598–601.

Johnson, C. I., D. J. Argyle, and D. N. Clements. 2016. In vitro models for the study of osteoarthritis. *Veterinary Journal* 209:40–9. doi:10.1016/j.tvjl.2015.07.011.

Jordan, J. M., G. Luta, J. Renner, A. Dragomir, M. C. Hochberg, and J. Fryer. 1997. Knee pain and knee osteo-arthritis severity in self-reported task specific disability: The Johnston County Osteoarthritis Project. *The Journal of Rheumatology* 24 (7):1344–1349.

Kasashima, Y., T. Ueno, A. Tomita, A. E. Goodship, and R. K. Smith. 2011. Optimisation of bone marrow aspiration from the equine sternum for the safe recovery of mesenchymal stem cells. *Equine Veterinary Journal* 43 (3):288–294. doi:10.1111/j.2042-3306.2010.00215.x.

Kawcak, C. E, D. D Frisbie, G. W. Trotter, C. W. McIlwraith, S. M. Gillette, B. E. Powers, and R. M. Walton. 1997. Effects of intravenous administration of sodium hyaluronate on carpal joints in exercising horses after arthroscopic surgery and osteochondral fragmentation. *American Journal of Veterinary Research* 58 (10):1132–1140.

Keegan, K. G. 2007. Evidence-based lameness detection and quantification. *Veterinary Clinics of North America: Equine Practice* 23 (2):403–423. doi:10.1016/j.cveq.2007.04.008.

Keegan, K. G., C. G. MacAllister, D. A. Wilson, C. A. Gedon, J. Kramer, Y. Yonezawa, H. Maki, and P. F. Pai. 2012. Comparison of an inertial sensor system with a stationary force plate for evaluation of horses with bilateral forelimb lameness. *American Journal of Veterinary Research* 73 (3):368–374. doi:10.2460/ajvr.73.3.368.

Kern, P. A., M. Saghizadeh, J. M. Ong, R. J. Bosch, R. Deem, and R. B. Simsolo. 1995. The expression of tumor necrosis factor in human adipose tissue. Regulation by obesity, weight loss, and relationship to lipoprotein lipase. *Journal of Clinical Investigation* 95 (5):2111.

Kisiday, J. D., L. R. Goodrich, C. W. McIlwraith, and D. D. Frisbie. 2013. Effects of equine bone marrow aspirate volume on isolation, proliferation, and differentiation potential of mesenchymal stem cells. *American Journal of Veterinary Research* 74 (5):801–807. doi:10.2460/ajvr.74.5.801.

Klein, M. B., N. Yalamanchi, H. Pham, M. T. Longaker, and J. Chan. 2002. Flexor tendon healing in vitro: Effects of TGF-β on tendon cell collagen production. *The Journal of Hand Surgery* 27 (4):615–620.

Knych, H. K., M. A. Vidal, N. Chouicha, M. Mitchell, and P. H. Kass. 2017. Cytokine, catabolic enzyme and structural matrix gene expression in synovial fluid following intra-articular administration of triamcinolone acetonide in exercised horses. *Equine Veterinary Journal* 49 (1):107–115. doi:10.1111/evj.12531.

Kol, A., J. A. Wood, D. D. Carrade Holt, J. A. Gillette, L. K. Bohannon-Worsley, S. M. Puchalski, N. J. Walker, K. C. Clark, J. L. Watson, and D. L. Borjesson. 2015. Multiple intravenous injections of allogeneic equine mesenchymal stem cells do not induce a systemic inflammatory response but do alter lymphocyte subsets in healthy horses. *Stem Cell Research and Therapy* 6:73. doi:10.1186/s13287-015-0050-0.

Kotlarz, H., C. L. Gunnarsson, H. Fang, and J. A. Rizzo. 2009. Insurer and out-of-pocket costs of osteoarthritis in the US: Eevidence from national survey data. *Arthritis and Rheumatism* 60 (12):3546–3553. doi:10.1002/art.24984.

Kotlarz, H., C. L Gunnarsson, H. Fang, and J. A. Rizzo. 2010. Osteoarthritis and absenteeism costs: Evidence from US National Survey Data. *Journal of Occupational and Environmental Medicine* 52 (3):263–268.

Kujala, U. M., S. Sarna, and J. Kaprio. 2005. Cumulative incidence of achilles tendon rupture and tendinopathy in male former elite athletes. *Clinical Journal of Sport Medicine* 15 (3):133–135.

Kuo, C. K. and R. S. Tuan. 2008. Mechanoactive tenogenic differentiation of human mesenchymal stem cells. *Tissue Engineering Part A* 14 (10):1615–1627.

Lafuente, M. P., B. A. Fransson, J. D. Lincoln, S. A. Martinez, P. R. Gavin, K. K. Lahmers, and J. M. Gay. 2009. Surgical treatment of mineralized and nonmineralized supraspinatus tendinopathy in twenty-four dogs. *Veterinary Surgery* 38 (3):380–387. doi:10.1111/j.1532-950X.2009.00512.x.

Laitinen, O. M. and G. L. Flo. 2000. Mineralization of the supraspinatus tendon in dogs: A long-term follow-up. *Journal of the American Animal Hospital Association* 36 (3):262–267.

Lampman, T. J., E. M. Lund, and A. J. Lipowitz. 2003. Cranial cruciate disease: Current status of diagnosis, surgery, and risk for disease. *VCOT Archive* 16 (3):122.

Lane, N. E., K. Brandt, G. Hawker, E. Peeva, E. Schreyer, W. Tsuji, and M. C. Hochberg. 2011. OARSI-FDA initiative: Defining the disease state of osteoarthritis. *Osteoarthritis Cartilage* 19 (5):478–482. doi:10.1016/j.joca.2010.09.013.

Lang, H. M., L. V. Schnabel, J. M. Cassano, and L. A. Fortier. 2017. Effect of needle diameter on the viability of equine bone marrow derived mesenchymal stem cells. *Veterinary Surgery* 46 (5):731–737. doi:10.1111/vsu.12639.

Lange-Consiglio, A., D. Rossi, S. Tassan, R. Perego, F. Cremonesi, and O. Parolini. 2013a. Conditioned medium from horse amniotic membrane-derived multipotent progenitor cells: Immunomodulatory activity in vitro and first clinical application in tendon and ligament injuries in vivo. *Stem Cells and Development* 22 (22):3015–3024. doi:10.1089/scd.2013.0214.

Lange-Consiglio, A., S. Tassan, B. Corradetti, A. Meucci, R. Perego, D. Bizzaro, and F. Cremonesi. 2013b. Investigating the efficacy of amnion-derived compared with bone marrow-derived mesenchymal stromal cells in equine tendon and ligament injuries. *Cytotherapy* 15 (8):1011–1020. doi:10.1016/j.jcyt.2013.03.002.

Lasarzik, J., A. Bondzio, M. Rettig, R. Estrada, C. Klaus, A. Ehrle, R. Einspanier, and C. J. Lischer. 2016. Evaluation of two protocols using autologous conditioned serum for intra-articular therapy of equine osteoarthritis-a pilot study monitoring Cytokines and Cartilage-specific biomarkers. *Journal of Equine Veterinary Science* 60:34–42. doi:10.1016/j.jevs.2016.09.014.

Lerner, H. and C. Berg. 2015. The concept of health in One Health and some practical implications for research and education: What is One Health? *Infection Ecology and Epidemiology* 5 (1):25300.

Lindegaard, C., K. B. Gleerup, M. H. Thomsen, T. Martinussen, S. Jacobsen, and P. H. Andersen. 2010. Anti-inflammatory effects of intra-articular administration of morphine in horses with experimentally induced synovitis. *American Journal of Veterinary Research* 71 (1):69–75. doi:10.2460/ajvr.71.1.69.

Lindhorst, E., T. P. Vail, F. Guilak, H. Wang, L. A. Setton, V. Vilim, and V. B. Kraus. 2000. Longitudinal characterization of synovial fluid biomarkers in the canine meniscectomy model of osteoarthritis. *Journal of Orthopaedic Research* 18 (2):269–280. doi:10.1002/jor.1100180216.

Little, C., S. Smith, P. Ghosh, and C. Bellenger. 1997. Histomorphological and immunohistochemical evaluation of joint changes in a model of osteoarthritis induced by lateral meniscectomy in sheep. *The Journal of Rheumatology* 24 (11):2199–2209.

Lombana, K. G., L. R. Goodrich, J. N. Phillips, J. D. Kisiday, A. Ruple-Czerniak, and C. W. McIlwraith. 2015. An investigation of equine mesenchymal stem cell characteristics from different harvest sites: More similar than not. *Frontiers in Veterinary Science* 2:67. doi:10.3389/fvets.2015.00067.

Longo, U. G., J. Rittweger, G. Garau, B. Radonic, C. Gutwasser, S. F. Gilliver, K. Kusy, et al., 2009. No influence of age, gender, weight, height, and impact profile in achilles tendinopathy in masters track and field athletes. *The American Journal of Sports Medicine* 37 (7):1400–1405.

Lopes, A. D., L. C. Hespanhol, S. S. Yeung, and L. O. P. Costa. 2012. What are the main running-related musculoskeletal injuries? *Sports Medicine* 42 (10):891–905.

Lui, P. P., N. Maffulli, C. Rolf, and R. K. Smith. 2011. What are the validated animal models for tendinopathy? *Scandinavian Journal of Medicine and Science in Sports* 21 (1):3–17. doi:10.1111/j.1600-0838.2010.01164.x.

Lund, E. M, P. J. Armstrong, C. A. Kirk, and J. S. Klausner. 2006. Prevalence and risk factors for obesity in adult dogs from private US veterinary practices. *International Journal of Applied Research in Veterinary Medicine* 4 (2):177.

Maia, L., M. V. de Souza, J. I. R. Júnior, A. C. de Oliveira, G. E. S. Alves, L. dos Anjos Benjamin, Y. F. R. S. Silva, Bruna Mota Zandim, and José do Carmo Lopes Moreira. 2009. Platelet-rich plasma in the treatment of induced tendinopathy in horses: Histologic evaluation. *Journal of Equine Veterinary Science* 29 (8):618–626. doi:10.1016/j.jevs.2009.07.001.

Mao, J., Z. Xia, J. Chen, and J. Yu. 2013. Prevalence and risk factors for canine obesity surveyed in veterinary practices in Beijing, China. *Preventive Veterinary Medicine* 112 (3):438–442.

Marijnissen, A. C., P. M. van Roermund, N. Verzijl, J. M. Tekoppele, J. W. J. Bijlsma, and F. P. J. G. Lafeber. 2002a. Steady progression of osteoarthritic features in the canine groove model. *Osteoarthritis and Cartilage* 10 (4):282–289. doi:http://dx.doi.org/10.1053/joca.2001.0507.

Marijnissen, A. C., P. M. van Roermund, J. M. TeKoppele, J. W. Bijlsma, and F. P. Lafeber. 2002b. The canine 'groove' model, compared with the ACLT model of osteoarthritis. *Osteoarthritis Cartilage* 10 (2):145–155. doi:10.1053/joca.2001.0491.

Mastbergen, S. C., A. C. Marijnissen, M. E. Vianen, P. M. van Roermund, J. W. Bijlsma, and F. P. Lafeber. 2006a. The canine 'groove' model of osteoarthritis is more than simply the expression of surgically applied damage. *Osteoarthritis Cartilage* 14 (1):39–46. doi:10.1016/j.joca.2004.07.009.

Mastbergen, S. C., A. C. Marijnissen, M. E. Vianen, P. M. van Roermund, J. W. Bijlsma, and F. P. Lafeber. 2006b. The canine 'groove'model of osteoarthritis is more than simply the expression of surgically applied damage. *Osteoarthritis and Cartilage* 14 (1):39–46.

McCarrel, T. M., T. Minas, and L. A. Fortier. 2012. Optimization of leukocyte concentration in platelet-rich plasma for the treatment of tendinopathy. *Journal of Bone and Joint Surgery* 94 (19):e143(1–8). doi:10.2106/JBJS.L.00019.

McGreevy, P. D., P. C. Thomson, C. Pride, A. Fawcett, T. Grassi, and B. Jones. 2005. Prevalence of obesity in dogs examined by Australian veterinary practices and the risk factors involved. *Veterinary Record-English Edition* 156 (22):695–701.

McIlwraith, C. W. 1996. General pathobiology of the joint and response to injury. *Joint Disease in the Horse*, Oct 30, 40.

McIlwraith, C. W., D. D. Frisbie, and C. E. Kawcak. 2012a. Evaluation of intramuscularly administered sodium pentosan polysulfate for treatment of experimentally induced osteoarthritis in horses. *American Journal of Veterinary Research* 73 (5):628–633. doi:10.2460/ajvr.73.5.628.

McIlwraith, C. W., D. D. Frisbie, and C. E. Kawcak. 2012b. The horse as a model of naturally occurring osteoarthritis. *Bone and Joint Research* 1 (11):297–309. doi:10.1302/2046-3758.111.2000132.

McIlwraith, C. W., D. D. Frisbie, W. G. Rodkey, J. D. Kisiday, N. M. Werpy, C. E. Kawcak, and J. R. Steadman. 2011. Evaluation of intra-articular mesenchymal stem cells to augment healing of microfractured chondral defects. *Arthroscopy* 27 (11):1552–1561. doi:10.1016/j.arthro.2011.06.002.

Meijer, H., J. Reinecke, C. Becker, G. Tholen, and P. Wehling. 2003. The production of anti-inflammatory cytokines in whole blood by physico-chemical induction. *Inflammation Research* 52 (10):404–407. doi:10.1007/s00011-003-1197-1.

Méndez-Ferrer, S., T. V. Michurina, F. Ferraro, A. R. Mazloom, B. D. MacArthur, S. A. Lira, D. T. Scadden, A. Ma'ayan, G. N. Enikolopov, and P. S. Frenette. 2010. Mesenchymal and haematopoietic stem cells form a unique bone marrow niche. *Nature* 466 (7308):829–834.

Mirza, M. H., P. Bommala, H. A. Richbourg, N. Rademacher, M. T. Kearney, and M. J. Lopez. 2016. Gait changes vary among horses with naturally occurring osteoarthritis following intra-articular administration of autologous platelet-rich plasma. *Frontiers in Veterinary Science* 3:29. doi:10.3389/fvets.2016.00029.

Montague, C. T., J. B. Prins, L. Sanders, J. Zhang, C. P. Sewter, J. Digby, C. D. Byrne, and S. O'Rahilly. 1998. Depot-related gene expression in human subcutaneous and omental adipocytes. *Diabetes* 47 (9):1384–1391.

Moore, K. A. and I. R. Lemischka. 2006. Stem cells and their niches. *Science* 311 (5769):1880–1885. doi:10.1126/science.1110542.

Morton, A. J., N. B. Campbell, J. M. Gayle, W. R. Redding, and A. T. Blikslager. 2005. Preferential and non-selective cyclooxygenase inhibitors reduce inflammation during lipopolysaccharide-induced synovitis. *Research in Veterinary Science* 78 (2):189–192. doi:10.1016/j.rvsc.2004.07.006.

Mrosek, E. H., A. Lahm, C. Erggelet, M. Uhl, H. Kurz, B. Eissner, and J. C. Schagemann. 2006. Subchondral bone trauma causes cartilage matrix degeneration: An immunohistochemical analysis in a canine model. *Osteoarthritis Cartilage* 14 (2):171–178. doi:10.1016/j.joca.2005.08.004.

Murphy, J. M., D. J. Fink, E. B. Hunziker, and F. P. Barry. 2003. Stem cell therapy in a caprine model of osteo-arthritis. *Arthritis and Rheumatism* 48 (12):3464–3474. doi:10.1002/art.11365.

Murray, R. C., R. M. DeBowes, E. M. Gaughan, C. F. Zhu, and K. A. Athanasiou. 1998. The effects of intra-articular methylprednisolone and exercise on the mechanical properties of articular cartilage in the horse. *Osteoarthritis Cartilage* 6 (2):106–114. doi:10.1053/joca.1997.0100.

Neuhuber, B., B. T. Himes, J. S. Shumsky, G. Gallo, and I. Fischer. 2005. Axon growth and recovery of function supported by human bone marrow stromal cells in the injured spinal cord exhibit donor variations. *Brain Research* 1035 (1):73–85. doi:10.1016/j.brainres.2004.11.055.

Neundorf, R. H., M. B. Lowerison, A. M. Cruz, J. J. Thomason, B. J. McEwen, and M. B. Hurtig. 2010. Determination of the prevalence and severity of metacarpophalangeal joint osteoarthritis in Thoroughbred racehorses via quantitative macroscopic evaluation. *American Journal of Veterinary Research* 71 (11):1284–1293. doi:10.2460/ajvr.71.11.1284.

Nicpon, J., K. Marycz, and J. Grzesiak. 2013. Therapeutic effect of adipose-derived mesenchymal stem cell injection in horses suffering from bone spavin. *Polish Journal of Veterinary Sciences* 16 (4):753–754. doi:10.2478/pjvs-2013-0107.

Owens, J. G., Kammerling, S. G., Stanton S. R., Keowen M. L., Prescott-Mathews J. S. 1996. Effects of pre-treatment with ketoprofen and phenylbutazone on experimentally induced synovitis in horses. *American Journal of Veterinary Research* (57):866–874.

Owens, S. D., A. Kol, N. J. Walker, and D. L. Borjesson. 2016. Allogeneic mesenchymal stem cell treatment induces specific alloantibodies in horses. *Stem Cells International* 2016:5830103. doi:10.1155/2016/5830103.

Pacini, S., S. Spinabella, L. Trombi, R. Fazzi, S. Galimberti, F. Dini, F. Carlucci, and M. Petrini. 2007. Suspension of bone marrow-derived undifferentiated mesenchymal stromal cells for repair of superficial digital flexor tendon in race horses. *Tissue Engineering* 13 (12):2949–2955. doi:10.1089/ten.2007.0108.

Palmer, J. L. and A. L. Bertone. 1994. Experimentally-induced synovitis as a model for acute synovitis in the horse. *Equine Veterinary Journal* 26 (6):492–495. doi:10.1111/j.2042-3306.1994.tb04056.x.

Palmer, J. L., A. L. Bertone, C. J. Malemud, and J. Mansour. 1996. Biochemical and biomechanical altera-tions in equine articular cartilage following an experimentally-induced synovitis. *Osteoarthritis and Cartilage* 4 (2):127–137. doi:10.1016/s1063-4584(05)80321-8.

Perkins, N. R., S. W. J. Reid, and R. S. Morris. 2005. Risk factors for injury to the superficial digital flexor ten-don and suspensory apparatus in Thoroughbred racehorses in New Zealand. *New Zealand Veterinary Journal* 53 (3):184–192.

Perrin, R. A. R., M. T. Launois, L. Brogniez, P. D. Clegg, R. P. C. Coomer, F. G. Desbrosse, and J. M. E. F. Vandeweerd. 2011. The use of computed tomography to assist orthopaedic surgery in 86 horses (2002–2010). *Equine Veterinary Education* 23 (6):306–313.

Phinney, D. G. 2012. Functional heterogeneity of mesenchymal stem cells: Implications for cell therapy. *Journal of Cellular Biochemistry* 113 (9):2806–2812. doi:10.1002/jcb.24166.

Phinney, D. G., G. Kopen, R. L. Isaacson, and D. J. Prockop. 1999a. Plastic adherent stromal cells from the bone marrow of commonly used strains of inbred mice: Variations in yield, growth, and differentiation. *Journal of Cellular Biochemistry* 72 (4):570–585.

Phinney, D. G., G. Kopen, W. Righter, S. Webster, N. Tremain, and D. J. Prockop. 1999b. Donor variation in the growth properties and osteogenic potential of human marrow stromal cells. *Journal of Cellular Biochemistry* 75 (3):424–436.

Pigott, J. H., A. Ishihara, M. L. Wellman, D. S. Russell, and A. L. Bertone. 2013. Inflammatory effects of autologous, genetically modified autologous, allogeneic, and xenogeneic mesenchymal stem cells after intra-articular injection in horses. *Veterinary and Comparative Orthopaedics and Traumatology* 26 (6):453–460. doi:10.3415/VCOT-13-01-0008.

Pool, R. R. 1996. Pathologic changes in tendonitis of athletic horses. Dubai Equine International Symposium Proceedings.

Purohit, A., M. W. Ghilchik, L. Duncan, D. Y. Wang, A. Singh, M. M. Walker, and M. J. Reed. 1995. Aromatase activity and interleukin-6 production by normal and malignant breast tissues. *The Journal of Clinical Endocrinology and Metabolism* 80 (10):3052–3058.

Raeissadat, S. A., S. M. Rayegani, H. Hassanabadi, M. Fathi, E. Ghorbani, M. Babaee, and K. Azma. 2015. Knee osteoarthritis injection choices: Platelet- Rich Plasma (PRP) Versus Hyaluronic Acid (A one-year randomized clinical trial). *Clinical Medicine Insights: Arthritis and Musculoskeletal Disorders* 8:1–8. doi:10.4137/CMAMD.S17894.

Raikin, S. M., D. N. Garras, and P. V. Krapchev. 2013. Achilles tendon injuries in a United States population. *Foot and Ankle International* 34 (4):475–480.

Reed, S. R., B. F. Jackson, C. W. Mc Ilwraith, I. M. Wright, R. Pilsworth, S. Knapp, J. L. Wood, J. S. Price, and K. L. Verheyen. 2012. Descriptive epidemiology of joint injuries in Thoroughbred racehorses in training. *Equine Veterinary Journal* 44 (1):13–19. doi:10.1111/j.2042-3306.2010.00352.x.

Ricco, S., S. Renzi, M. Del Bue, V. Conti, E. Merli, R. Ramoni, E. Lucarelli, G. Gnudi, M. Ferrari, and S. Grolli. 2013. Allogeneic adipose tissue-derived mesenchymal stem cells in combination with platelet rich plasma are safe and effective in the therapy of superficial digital flexor tendonitis in the horse. *International Journal of Immunopathology and Pharmacology* 26 (1 Suppl):61–68.

Riemersma, D. J. and H. C. Schamhardt. 1985. In vitro mechanical properties of equine tendons in relation to cross-sectional area and collagen content. *Research in Veterinary Science* 39 (3):263–270.

Rios, D. L., C. Lopez, and J. U. Carmona. 2015. Platelet-rich gel supernatants stimulate the release of anti-inflammatory proteins on culture media of normal equine synovial membrane explants. *Veterinary Medicine International* 2015:547052. doi:10.1155/2015/547052.

Ristolainen, L., A. Heinonen, H. Turunen, H. Mannström, B. Waller, J. A. Kettunen, and U. M. Kujala. 2010. Type of sport is related to injury profile: A study on cross country skiers, swimmers, long-distance runners and soccer players. A retrospective 12-month study. *Scandinavian Journal of Medicine and Science in Sports* 20 (3):384–393.

Rogachefsky, R. A., D. D. Dean, D. S. Howell, and R. D. Altman. 1993. Treatment of canine osteoarthritis with insulin-like growth factor-1 (IGF-1) and sodium pentosan polysulfate. *Osteoarthritis and Cartilage* 1 (2):105–114.

Rolf, C. and T. Movin. 1997. Etiology, histopathology, and outcome of surgery in achillodynia. *Foot and Ankle International* 18 (9):565–569.

Ross, T. N., J. D. Kisiday, T. Hess, and C. W. McIlwraith. 2012. Evaluation of the inflammatory response in experimentally induced synovitis in the horse: A comparison of recombinant equine interleukin 1 beta and lipopolysaccharide. *Osteoarthritis Cartilage* 20 (12):1583–1590. doi:10.1016/j.joca.2012.08.008.

Rutgers, M., D. B. F. Saris, W. J. A. Dhert, and L. B. Creemers. 2010. Cytokine profile of autologous conditioned serum for treatment of osteoarthritis, *in vitro* effects on cartilage metabolism and intra-articular levels after injection. *Arthritis Research and Therapy* 12 (3):R114.

Sawyere, D. M., O. I. Lanz, L. A. Dahlgren, S. L. Barry, A. C. Nichols, and S. R. Werre. 2016. Cytokine and growth factor concentrations in Canine Autologous Conditioned Serum. *Veterinary Surgery* 45 (5):582–586. doi:10.1111/vsu.12506.

Schnabel, L. V., H. O. Mohammed, B. J. Miller, W. G. McDermott, M. S. Jacobson, K. S. Santangelo, and L. A. Fortier. 2007. Platelet rich plasma (PRP) enhances anabolic gene expression patterns in flexor digitorum superficialis tendons. *Journal of Orthopaedic Research* 25 (2):230–240. doi:10.1002/jor.20278.

Schnabel, L. V., M. E. Lynch, M. C. van der Meulen, A. E. Yeager, M. A. Kornatowski, and A. J. Nixon. 2009. Mesenchymal stem cells and insulin-like growth factor-I gene-enhanced mesenchymal stem cells improve structural aspects of healing in equine flexor digitorum superficialis tendons. *Journal of Orthopaedic Research* 27 (10):1392–1398. doi:10.1002/jor.20887.

Schnabel, L. V., L. M. Pezzanite, D. F. Antczak, M. J. Felippe, and L. A. Fortier. 2014. Equine bone marrow-derived mesenchymal stromal cells are heterogeneous in MHC class II expression and capable of inciting an immune response in vitro. *Stem Cell Research and Therapy* 5 (1):13.

Schramme, M., S. Hunter, N. Campbell, A. Blikslager, and R. Smith. 2010. A surgical tendonitis model in horses: Technique, clinical, ultrasonographic and histological characterisation. *Veterinary and Comparative Orthopaedics and Traumatology* 23 (4):231–239. doi:10.3415/VCOT-09-10-0106.

Schultz, M. 2008. Rudolf virchow. *Emerging Infectious Diseases* 14 (9):1480.

Shi, S. and S. Gronthos. 2003. Perivascular niche of postnatal mesenchymal stem cells in human bone marrow and dental pulp. *Journal of Bone and Mineral Research* 18 (4):696–704.

Shi, Y., G. Hu, J. Su, W. Li, Q. Chen, P. Shou, C. Xu et al., 2010. Mesenchymal stem cells: A new strategy for immunosuppression and tissue repair. *Cell Research* 20 (5):510–518.

Silver, I. A., P. N. Brown, A. E. Goodship, L. E. Lanyon, K. G. McCullagh, G. C. Perry, and I. F. Williams. 1983. A clinical and experimental study of tendon injury, healing and treatment in the horse. *Equine Veterinary Journal. Supplement* (1):1–43.

Smith, R. K. 2008. Mesenchymal stem cell therapy for equine tendinopathy. *Disability and Rehabilitation* 30 (20–22):1752–1758. doi:10.1080/09638280701788241.

Smith, R. K., N. J. Werling, S. G. Dakin, R. Alam, A. E. Goodship, and J. Dudhia. 2013. Beneficial effects of autologous bone marrow-derived mesenchymal stem cells in naturally occurring tendinopathy. *PloS one* 8 (9):e75697.

Sole, A., M. Spriet, K. A. Padgett, B. Vaughan, L. D. Galuppo, D. L. Borjesson, E. R. Wisner, and M. A. Vidal. 2013. Distribution and persistence of technetium-99 hexamethyl propylene amine oxime-labelled bone marrow-derived mesenchymal stem cells in experimentally induced tendon lesions after intratendinous injection and regional perfusion of the equine distal limb. *Equine Veterinary Journal* 45 (6):726–731.

Stephens, P. R., D. M. Nunamaker, and D. M. Butterweck. 1989. Application of a Hall-effect transducer for measurement of tendon strains in horses. *American Journal of Veterinary Research* 50 (7):1089–1095.

Subramony, S. D., B. R. Dargis, M. Castillo, E. U. Azeloglu, M. S. Tracey, A. Su, and H. H. Lu. 2013. The guidance of stem cell differentiation by substrate alignment and mechanical stimulation. *Biomaterials* 34 (8):1942–1953.

Sun, Y., Y. Feng, C. Q. Zhang, S. B. Chen, and X. G. Cheng. 2010. The regenerative effect of platelet-rich plasma on healing in large osteochondral defects. *International Orthopaedics* 34 (4):589–597.

Sundin, M., O. Ringden, B. Sundberg, S. Nava, C. Gotherstrom, and K. Le Blanc. 2007. No alloantibodies against mesenchymal stromal cells, but presence of anti-fetal calf serum antibodies, after transplantation in allogeneic hematopoietic stem cell recipients. *Haematologica* 92 (9):1208–1215. doi:10.3324/haematol.11446.

Sundman, E. A., B. J. Cole, and L. A. Fortier. 2011. Growth factor and catabolic cytokine concentrations are influenced by the cellular composition of platelet-rich plasma. *American Journal of Sports Medicine* 39 (10):2135–2140. doi:10.1177/0363546511417792.

Textor, J. 2011. Autologous biologic treatment for equine musculoskeletal injuries: Platelet-rich plasma and IL-1 receptor antagonist protein. *Veterinary Clinics of North America: Equine Practice* 27 (2):275–298. doi:10.1016/j.cveq.2011.05.001.

Textor, J. A., N. H. Willits, and F. Tablin. 2013. Synovial fluid growth factor and cytokine concentrations after intra-articular injection of a platelet-rich product in horses. *Journal of Veterinary* 198 (1):217–223. doi:10.1016/j.tvjl.2013.07.020.

Textor, J. and F. Tablin. 2013. Intra-articular use of a platelet-rich product in normal horses: Clinical signs and cytologic responses. *Veterinary Surgery* 42 (5):499–510.

Thatcher, C. D., R. S. Pleasant, R. J. Geor, and F. Elvinger. 2012. Prevalence of overconditioning in mature horses in southwest Virginia during the summer. *Journal of Veterinary Internal Medicine* 26 (6):1413–1418. doi:10.1111/j.1939-1676.2012.00995.x.

Tipton, T. E., C. S. Ray, and D. R. Hand. 2013. Superficial digital flexor tendonitis in cutting horses: 19 cases (2007–2011). *Journal of the American Veterinary Medical Association* 243 (8):1162–1165.

Todhunter, R. J. and G. Lust. 1992. Synovial joint anatomy, biology and pathobiology. In *Equine Surgery*, edited by J. A. Auer, 844–866. Philadelphia, PA: W.B. Saunders Co.

Todhunter, P. G., S. A. Kincaid, R. J. Todhunter, J. R. Kammermann, B. Johnstone, A. N. Baird, R. R. Hanson, J. M. Wright, H. C. Lin, and R. C. Purohit. 1996. Immunohistochemical analysis of an equine model of synovitis-induced arthritis. *American Journal of Veterinary Research* 57 (7):1080–1093.

Toupadakis, C. A., A. Wong, D. C. Genetos, W. K. Cheung, D. L. Borjesson, G. L. Ferraro, L. D. Galuppo, J. K. Leach, S. D. Owens, and C. E. Yellowley. 2010. Comparison of the osteogenic potential of equine mesenchymal stem cells from bone marrow, adipose tissue, umbilical cord blood, and umbilical cord tissue. *American Journal of Veterinary Research* 71 (10):1237–1245. doi:10.2460/ajvr.71.10.1237.

Tsubone, T., S. L. Moran, M. Subramaniam, P. C. Amadio, T. C. Spelsberg, and K. N. An. 2006. Effect of TGF-β inducible early gene deficiency on flexor tendon healing. *Journal of Orthopaedic Research* 24 (3):569–575.

Tyrnenopoulou, P., N. Diakakis, M. Karayannopoulou, I. Savvas, and G. Koliakos. 2016. Evaluation of intra-articular injection of autologous platelet lysate (PL) in horses with osteoarthritis of the distal interphalangeal joint. *Vet Q* 36 (2):56–62. doi:10.1080/01652176.2016.1141257.

Upchurch, D. A., W. C. Renberg, J. K. Roush, G. A. Milliken, and M. L. Weiss. 2016. Effects of administration of adipose-derived stromal vascular fraction and platelet-rich plasma to dogs with osteoarthritis of the hip joints. *American Journal of Veterinary Research* 77 (9):940–951. doi:10.2460/ajvr.77.9.940.

van der Eng, D. M., T. Schepers, J. C. Goslings, and N. W. L. Schep. 2013. Rerupture rate after early weight-bearing in operative versus conservative treatment of Achilles tendon ruptures: A meta-analysis. *The Journal of Foot and Ankle Surgery* 52 (5):622–628.

van de Water, E., M. Oosterlinck, M. Dumoulin, N. M. Korthagen, P. R. van Weeren, J. van den Broek, H. Everts, F. Pille, and D. A. van Doorn. 2016. The preventive effects of two nutraceuticals on experimentally induced acute synovitis. *Equine Veterinary Journal* Accessed Aug 24. doi:10.1111/evj.12629.

Vegesna, A. K., M. I. Ramashesai Besetty, L. T. Tiwana A. K. Bright, M. April, A. Agelan, and L. S. Miller. 2009. Pyloric suture narrowing trial to treat obesity (a canine model). *Gastrointestinal Endoscopy* 69 (5):AB259. doi:http://dx.doi.org/10.1016/j.gie.2009.03.674.

Vidal, M. A., S. O. Robinson, M. J. Lopez, D. B. Paulsen, O. Borkhsenious, J. R. Johnson, R. M. Moore, and J. M. Gimble. 2008. Comparison of chondrogenic potential in equine mesenchymal stromal cells derived from adipose tissue and bone marrow. *Veterinary Surgery* 37 (8):713–724. doi:10.1111/j.1532-950X.2008.00462.x.

Vidal, M. A., N. J. Walker, E. Napoli, and D. L. Borjesson. 2011. Evaluation of senescence in mesenchymal stem cells isolated from equine bone marrow, adipose tissue, and umbilical cord tissue. *Stem Cells and Development* 21 (2):273–283. doi:10.1089/scd.2010.0589.

Vilar, J. M., M. Morales, A. Santana, G. Spinella, M. Rubio, B. Cuervo, R. Cugat, and J. M. Carrillo. 2013. Controlled, blinded force platform analysis of the effect of intraarticular injection of autologous adipose-derived mesenchymal stem cells associated to PRGF-Endoret in osteoarthritic dogs. *BMC Veterinary Research* 9:131. doi:10.1186/1746-6148-9-131.

von Pfeil, D. J. F., W. D. Liska, S. Nelson, S. Mann, and J. J. Wakshlag. 2015. A survey on orthopedic injuries during a marathon sled dog race. *Veterinary Medicine: Research and Reports*:329. doi:10.2147/vmrr.s88276.

Wadhwa, M., M. J. Seghatchian, A. Lubenko, M. Contreras, P. Dilger, C. Bird, and R. Thorpe. 1996. Cytokine levels in platelet concentrates: Quantitation by bioassays and immunoassays. *British Journal of Haematology* 93 (1):225–234.

Watkins, J. P., J. A. Auer, S. Gay, and S. J. Morgan. 1985. Healing of surgically created defects in the equine superficial digital flexor tendon: Collagen-type transformation and tissue morphologic reorganization. *American Journal of Veterinary Research* 46 (10):2091–2096.

Watkins, J. P., J. A. Auer, S. J. Morgan, and S. Gay. 1985. Healing of surgically created defects in the equine superficial digital flexor tendon: Effects of pulsing electromagnetic field therapy on collagen-type transformation and tissue morphologic reorganization. *American Journal of Veterinary Research* 46 (10):2097–2103.

Watts, A. E., A. J. Nixon, A. E. Yeager, and H. O. Mohammed. 2012. A collagenase gel/physical defect model for controlled induction of superficial digital flexor tendonitis. *Equine Veterinary Journal* 44 (5):576–586. doi:10.1111/j.2042-3306.2011.00471.x.

White, G. W., E. W. Jones, J. Hamm, and T. Sanders. 1994. The efficacy of orally administered sulfated glycosaminoglycan in chemically induced equine synovitis and degenerative joint disease. *Journal of Equine Veterinary Science* 14 (7):350–353. doi:10.1016/s0737-0806(06)81744-2.

Wilke, M. M., D. V. Nydam, and A. J. Nixon. 2007. Enhanced early chondrogenesis in articular defects following arthroscopic mesenchymal stem cell implantation in an equine model. *Journal of Orthopaedic Research* 25 (7):913–925. doi:10.1002/jor.20382.

Williams, I. F., K. G. McCullagh, A. E. Goodship, and I. A. Silver. 1984. Studies on the pathogenesis of equine tendonitis following collagenase injury. *Research in Veterinary Science* 36 (3):326–338.

Williams, L. B., J. B. Koenig, B. Black, T. W. Gibson, S. Sharif, and T. G. Koch. 2016. Equine allogeneic umbilical cord blood derived mesenchymal stromal cells reduce synovial fluid nucleated cell count and induce mild self-limiting inflammation when evaluated in an lipopolysaccharide induced synovitis model. *Equine Veterinary Journal* 48 (5):619–625. doi:10.1111/evj.12477.

Wilson, A. M. and A. E. Goodship. 1991. Mechanical properties of the equine superficial digital flexor tendon (SDFT). *Journal of Biomechanics* 24 (6):474.

Wilson, A. M. and A. E. Goodship. 1994. Exercise-induced hyperthermia as a possible mechanism for tendon degeneration. *Journal of Biomechanics* 27 (7):899903–901905.

Xie, X., H. Wu, S. Zhao, G. Xie, X. Huangfu, and J. Zhao. 2013. The effect of platelet-rich plasma on patterns of gene expression in a dog model of anterior cruciate ligament reconstruction. *Journal of Surgical Research* 180 (1):80–88. doi:10.1016/j.jss.2012.10.036.

Yamada, A. L. M., A. M. Carvalho, A. Moroz, E. Deffune, M. J. Watanabe, C. A. Hussni, C. A. Rodrigues, and A. L. G. Alves. 2013. Mesenchymal stem cell enhances chondral defects healing in horses. *Stem Cell Discovery* 03 (04):218–225. doi:10.4236/scd.2013.34027.

Youngstrom, D. W., I. Rajpar, D. L. Kaplan, and J. G. Barrett. 2015. A bioreactor system for in vitro tendon differentiation and tendon tissue engineering. *Journal of Orthopaedic Research* 33 (6):911–918.

Youngstrom, D. W., J. E. LaDow, and J. G. Barrett. 2016. Tenogenesis of bone marrow-, adipose-, and tendon-derived stem cells in a dynamic bioreactor. *Connective Tissue Research* 57 (6):454–465. doi:10.3109/03008207.2015.1117458.

Yun, S., S. K. Ku, and Y. S. Kwon. 2016. Adipose-derived mesenchymal stem cells and platelet-rich plasma synergistically ameliorate the surgical-induced osteoarthritis in Beagle dogs. *Journal of Orthopaedic Surgery and Research* 11:9. doi:10.1186/s13018-016-0342-9.

Zimmermann, S., M. Voss, S. Kaiser, U. Kapp, C. F. Waller, and U. M. Martens. 2003. Lack of telomerase activity in human mesenchymal stem cells. *Leukemia* 17 (6):1146–1149.

5 Biotensegrity
How Ultrasound Diagnostics Guide Regenerative Orthopedic Therapies to Restore Biomechanical Function

Bradley D. Fullerton, MD

INTRODUCTION

A convergence of knowledge, both old and new, holds great promise in reducing the burden of musculoskeletal pain and dysfunction. This potential has been demonstrated through centuries of manual therapies and 80 years of clinical experience in prolotherapy (i.e. injection to stimulate repair at ligament and tendon entheses), yet it has been limited by a mechanistic understanding of orthopedic pathology. Biotensegrity, a new form of functional anatomic modeling, and ultrasonography, high-resolution dynamic imaging of living tissue, now provide us with the vision of a path forward in nonsurgical, interventional orthopedics. Two case studies will illustrate this shift.

CASE #1 A MIDDLE-AGED ATHLETE WITH A WEAK PAINFUL KNEE AFTER TRAUMA

A 40-year-old male presents with a 14-month history of anterior knee pain and weakness that began after a skateboarding accident. He initially fell with impact at the anterior patella resulting in a nondisplaced patellar fracture, which was treated conservatively with resolution of the fracture. Despite his excellent overall fitness, extensive physical therapy has not improved his quadriceps strength. An MRI shows a region of cartilage loss at the trochlear groove and patellar tendinopathy with partial tear. Treatment with an injection of dextrose and platelet-rich plasma (PRP) resolved the tendon tear (Figure 5.1) and improved overall strength and stability, yet he continues to have anterior knee pain and describes his knee as having a "lack of structural strength and integrity." Though a surgeon has not recommended it, he states "I may just have to resort to surgery. There's something wrong with the knee; maybe a piece of cartilage is floating around."

- Does he need exploratory surgery?
- Can we understand the cause of his knee pain through a better anatomic understanding of his injury?

CASE #2 A TEENAGER WITH A DISEASE OF MIDDLE AGE

A 15-year-old competitive swimmer presents with a 2-year history of progressive shoulder pain and "popping" that she relates to a mild injury incurred while playing badminton prior to the onset of symptoms. Despite various anti-inflammatory treatments, extensive physical therapy and rest, she is not able to swim due to pain and lack of range of motion. She has seen two orthopedic surgery consultants and received sub-acromial corticosteroid injections which provided temporary relief of symptoms. Clinically, she continues to decline in function. Magnetic resonance imaging (MRI) reveals infraspinatus and supraspinatus tendinopathy with moderate subacromial, subdeltoid

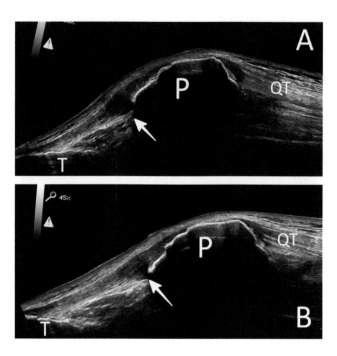

FIGURE 5.1 Ultrasound images of patellar tendinopathy with tear (arrows) – before (A) and 3 months after (B) injection with dextrose and low WBC/low RBC PRP. (T) – tibial tuberosity. (P) – patella. (QT) – quadriceps tendon.

bursitis. Ultrasonography shows the dynamic bony impingement of the bursa and supraspinatus tendon (Figure 5.2, Video 5.1).

- Why is an adolescent athlete developing metabolic tissue changes that are commonly associated with middle age?
- Do corticosteroid injections address the primary pathology?

PERSPECTIVE

> *What he saw as One was*
> *One, and what he saw*
> *as not One was also One.*
> *In that he saw the unity,*
> *he was of God; in that*
> *he saw the distinctions,*
> *he was of man.*

– Laotse [1]

The fruits of scientific knowledge are proliferating at such a rate that there is no way for any physician to keep up. As the details multiply, physicians necessarily become more and more specialized. As we become more specialized, patient care becomes more disconnected from the patient. Patients and physicians alike become more disenchanted. We know, somehow, that the solution involves not losing sight of the forest for the trees. We know that we must oscillate from seeing the details of patient pathology (i.e. Laotse's "distinctions") to seeing the patient as a whole, integrated human being (i.e. Laotse's "One"). In this era of information overload, we long for a simplicity that

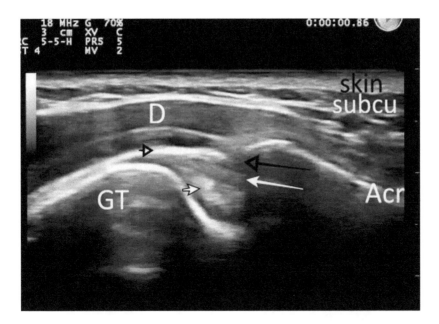

FIGURE 5.2 Ultrasonography showing dynamic impingement of the rotator cuff in a 15-year-old female swimmer. The short, white arrow is located at the tendon insertion and points to a region of normal tendon. The long, white arrow deep to the acromion points to a region of hypoechoic tendinopathy due to impingement. The black arrow points to the thickened, impinged region of bursitis, while the open black arrowhead points to the bright white layer of normal bursa. (D) – deltoid muscle. (GT) – greater tuberosity of the humerus. (Acr) – acromion.

can keep us centered on the patient in front of us, while not oversimplifying the amazing details of knowledge available to us. Biotensegrity is such a concept.

THE MISFRAMING OF ANATOMY

Our understanding of the body begins before we enter medical training. As preschoolers, we see skeletons at Halloween or Dia de los Muertos celebrations. As young students, we often learn of ancient civilizations through the bones they left behind. As young people, we see our most common and earliest imaging modality, X-rays, with the bones clear to even the untrained. These events prepare us all to see the skeleton as the frame of our body, the reference point for all of the other tissues in our "musculoskeletal system." Whether medically educated or not, this frame is so ingrained in our unconscious that we resist any other way of seeing our body structure, even when the known frame leads us astray. So, the tissue that resists compression becomes the focal point of our understanding, and the specialty that focuses on bones naturally sits at the center of musculoskeletal medicine.

Anatomy and biomechanics, then, are based on this frame. In fact, muscles are defined by what they do to bones. To understand muscle function, we learn origins and insertions on bones. As the muscle contracts and shortens, one bone moves in relation to another at a joint space. To control joint movement, we need rapid feedback from receptors in the tissue with rapid signaling back to the muscles to control how the bones move. This framing of the bones as the primary reference point persists even though it is demonstrably false. For example, the vastus lateralis muscle of the quadriceps is described as originating from the femur and inserting at the patella via the quadriceps tendon. Therefore, vastus lateralis is a knee extensor. Yet, a muscle twitch observed on dynamic ultrasonography (Figure 5.3 and Video 5.2) shows that part of the muscle "originates" at the lateral intermuscular septum. This part of the muscle is not pulling on a bone; it is pulling on connective tissue that also distorts other muscles. So, how do we understand movement now? To complicate

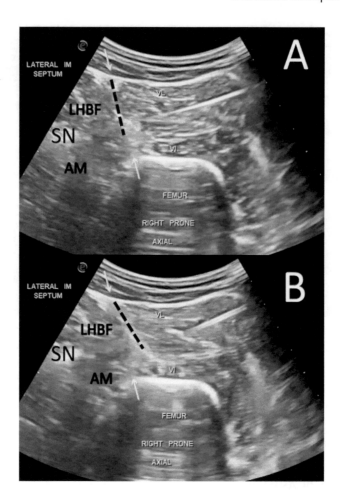

FIGURE 5.3 Ultrasonography of twitch response in the vastus lateralis (VL) muscle with line of force pulling on the lateral intermuscular septum of the thigh (dashed line). Parts A and B are still images from Video 5.2. A is just before the muscle twitch; B is during the twitch. The green arrows point at the septum dividing quadriceps on the right with long head biceps femoris (LHBF) and adductor magnus (AM) on the left. SN is sciatic nerve.

matters further, the inferior gluteus maximus also tensions the lateral intermuscular septum [2]; so, two muscles shown as separate in standard anatomy texts are actually part of the same myofascial continuity (Figure 5.4).

The framing of anatomy by the bones is also shown to be false when we consider embryology. In utero, we all start as soft bodied organisms, stable and dynamic, even without calcification. We are actually taught (and often quickly forget) a more accurate frame in embryology and histology courses, where we learn that bone is actually a specialized connective tissue. The connective tissue is the frame that exists before specialization into bone. Yet, we forget this as we try to understand biomechanics. Biomechanics is all about forces that can be diagramed and measured, via lever mechanics, ground reaction forces, force transmission. For most physicians and researchers, this reinforces the unconscious notion that movement is all about where the bones are moved by forces that are external to the bones. Without the bones as the frame, it is difficult to visualize what is happening as we move. We need to be able to visualize the body in a way that honors our embryologic origin and the actual complexity of muscles, which often transmit forces via fascial sheets, rather than bone [3].

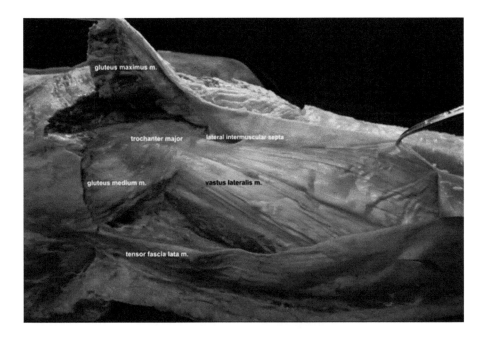

FIGURE 5.4 Fresh cadaver dissection showing myofascial continuity of the inferior gluteus maximus to vastus lateralis of the quadriceps via the lateral intermuscular septum.

TENSEGRITY: THE TENSION IS THE FRAME

The term *tensegrity*, a combination of tension and integrity, was introduced by Buckminster Fuller when he observed the early sculptures of Kenneth Snelson. Snelson's sculptures exhibit what he calls "floating compression" [4]; the solid elements, which resist compression, float in a continuous network of tension (Figure 5.5). Fuller's term emphasizes that the integrity of the structure depends upon the continuity of the tension. The tension is stored energy in the form of pre-stress applied to the network of cables. Snelson vividly describes this storing of energy during the installation of *New Dimension*, a tensegrity sculpture in Berlin. "As many as six men fought with the forces in *New Dimension* while it was going up. It is like taking on a colossal, dead weight wrestler....Until the piece is put together the forces are not there. The forces are introduced as things are added piece-by-piece. Finally, when the last cable is attached, the closed system of forces is complete" [4] (Figure 5.6).

Appropriately, Snelson also described his work as "forces made visible" [5]. If the continuity of tension (i.e. pre-stress) is compromised, the structure changes shape and loses stability [6].

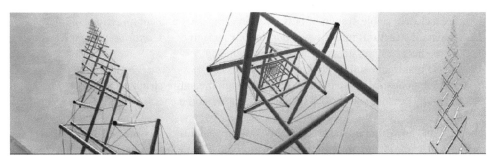

FIGURE 5.5 Tensegrity sculpture: *Needle Tower* (1968) by Kenneth Snelson. Photographs by the author at the Hirshhorn Museum and Sculpture Garden in Washington D.C., United States.

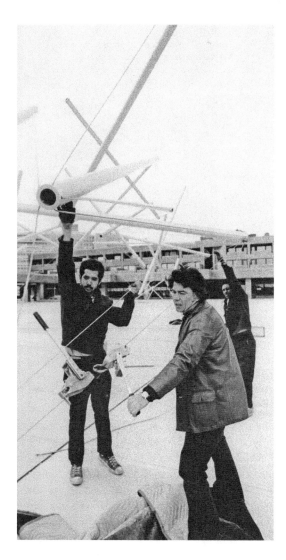

FIGURE 5.6 "Assembling *Free Ride Home* at Waterside Plaza, 1974, New York, NY." In this picture from *Art and Ideas*, Kenneth Snelson is using muscle energy to install tension (and store energy) in the form of pre-stress to cables. Snelson described his tensegrity sculptures as "organizations of forces in space."

Tensegrity Structures…

1. …are a closed, stable system of only two forces: tension and compression.
2. …maintain structural integrity via *continuous* tension & *discontinuous* compression.
3. …store energy as pre-stress in the tension elements.
4. …create maximum stability with minimal mass.
5. …instantaneously diffuse outside forces through the entire structure.
6. …naturally produce oscillations without dissipating stored energy (Figure 5.7 and Video 5.3).

Stephen Levin, an orthopedic surgeon and systems scientist, has argued that only tensegrity modeling can explain dynamic stability in biology [7]. Levin coined the term *biotensegrity* to emphasize differences with engineering-based (i.e. human-made) tensegrity models, which inevitably compromise the unique qualities of biologic structures. He states that in biology, "there are no shears, bending moments or levers, just simple tension and compression, in a

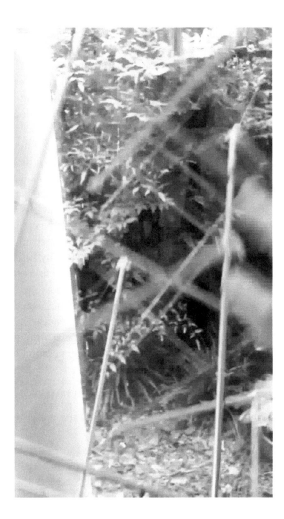

FIGURE 5.7 Tensegrity oscillations introduced with the flick of finger. The energy stored in the tension fibers sustains the oscillation, yet it does not dissipate with the motion. A model of biologic movement with minimal energy input (See Video 5.3).

self-organizing, hierarchical, load distributing, low energy consuming structure [8]." In fact, to more closely imitate the adaptive, stable movement of nature, the National Aeronautics Space Administration (NASA) [9] now incorporates tensegrity modeling into robot development. Ingber was inspired by tensegrity to advance the field of mechanobiology and, more specifically, *mechanotransduction*: "how physical forces regulate cellular biochemical responses" [10]. Biotensegrity then becomes the *structure* of homeostasis in biology. Physical trauma that damages structure clearly alters metabolic processes, as in the normal inflammatory response at a site of injury. Could the altered dynamics of past injury lead to altered metabolics remote from the site of injury?

BIOTENSEGRITY-BASED ANATOMY AND BIOMECHANICS: BONES FLOAT AND FASCIA COMMUNICATES

Scarr has described the concepts of biotensegrity from geometric first principles as learned from Levin [11] and has used biotensegrity modeling to reexamine the elbow [12]. If the human body is a tensegrity structure, the continuous fascial system is the tensional network, and the bones float in that network. In this construct, all bones are sesamoid bones, fully suspended and discontinuous; they float even at joint spaces, where we are accustomed to imagining cartilage surfaces touching.

Tensegrity structures are fully structurally integrated, so that an external force will instantaneously change the shape of the entire structure. This allows for instantaneous body-wide communication via the tensional continuity. This insight has been eloquently communicated in terms of *haptic perception* [13] – our ability to perceive objects and our environment through touch. It seems obvious that this ability would be determined by our sensory nervous system. However, if your eyes are closed and a tennis racquet is placed in your hand, you will quickly surmise that it is a tennis racquet. Without opening your eyes, you would likely be able to use your other hand to touch near the sweet spot on the face of the racquet. There is an instantaneous perception of the shape of the object by holding it. Turvey and Fonseca have hypothesized that this ability is a function of the body-wide tensegrity system composed of "connective tissue and the conjunction of muscular, connective tissue net, and skeletal (MCS) as the body's proper characterization [14]."

These tissues, which develop from the mesoderm, are structurally linked as a tensegrity system; thus, Levin and Scarr have proposed the term "mesokinetic system as the 'organ of movement'" [10]. The muscle cells within this fascial continuity then are seen as the fine-tuning mechanism of movement rather than the prime movers. The energy stored in the fascial system provides the primary oscillating mechanism of movement, without dissipating energy as occurs with muscle contraction. The energy contained in the pre-stressed fascia dissipates only via aging or trauma (acute or repetitive); the energy may only be restored via repair or regeneration of collagen.

BIOTENSEGRITY-BASED ANATOMY AND BIOMECHANICS: A SUMMARY

1. The most rapid communication in the body occurs via the pre-stressed collagen fibers of the myofascial system.
2. Muscles are *not* structures that "pull" on bones to cause movement.
3. Bones float in a *variable tension network* consisting of muscle and fascial elements.
4. Fascial continuity provides *passive* tension and stored energy in the form of pre-stress.
5. Muscle fibers within the fascial continuity provide *dynamic* tension.
6. Thus, bones move (or, in the setting of outside forces, remain stable) when the tension around them changes.

CLINICAL APPLICATION OF BIOTENSEGRITY PRINCIPLES IN REGENERATIVE ORTHOPEDICS: A SUMMARY

1. Construct: Focus on tensional continuity, which provides instantaneous, body-wide communication.
2. History: Past trauma (acute or repetitive) is a loss of pre-stress in the tensegrity system.
3. Signs/Symptoms: A loss of pre-stress results in muscle dysfunction (e.g. spasm, poor control, inability to strengthen, development of trigger point) as the body attempts to compensate.
4. Diagnosis: Use dynamics (in physical exam and ultrasonography) to find a loss of tensional continuity in the myofascia.

BIOTENSEGRITY-BASED DIAGNOSTICS: "FORCES MADE VISIBLE"

Over the past 100+ years, osteopathic and chiropractic physicians have practiced a holistic art requiring advanced palpatory diagnostics and treatment developed over years of practice and mentorship. These professions have developed through the use of the examiner's own haptic perception, i.e. through the practitioner's own tensegrity system. This appears wholly subjective to basic science; however, the osteopathic manual method actually integrates the scientific process into each encounter, repetitively hypothesizing a structural dysfunction then testing the diagnosis with a manual intervention such as muscle energy techniques or manipulation.

Allopathic physicians, on the other hand, have focused on scientific reductionism to produce clear evidence of tissue pathology, imaging diagnostics and predictable pharmaceutical and surgical interventions. Allopathic medicine tends to restrict the scientific *process* only to the research setting, forbidding it from the exam room. In orthopedics, MRIs can easily become the diagnosis in our mind before we've examined the patient, even though MRIs are static imaging while most pain occurs with motion. Clinical research is now showing that static, structural imaging can lead to misuse of surgery in conditions such as degenerative meniscus [15]. Likewise, a focus only on biochemistry and objective lab testing can lead to overuse of corticosteroids in degenerative joint disease [16] and tendinopathy [17], where inflammation does not explain the full clinical picture.

These fields of medicine have historically been in conflict [18] and remain remarkably suspicious of each other at times. A focus on touch for diagnosis risks subjectivity, while a focus on objective testing risks objectifying the patient in the exam room.

Biotensegrity can serve as model that pushes us to integrate all of these disparate viewpoints, reminding us to use palpation/touch in every appointment as a connection to the whole patient and as a quick assessment of connective tissue integrity via haptic perception. Often a visual overview of posture will reveal a distortion of the myofascial system, such as prominent paraspinal muscles unilaterally. Then, upon palpation in the area, the patient recalls a forgotten injury (e.g. "oh, that's right where I hit that tree in my mountain bike wreck a few years back"). In short order, a presenting complaint of hip pain with a normal X-ray and MRI could be a soft-tissue injury in the low back with trigger-point referral from a muscle such as quadratus lumborum [19].

Biotensegrity also emphasizes dynamics, as in the term *mesokinetic* system described above. Ultrasonography provides excellent visualization of dynamics in soft tissue, as in echocardiography. While echocardiography has extensive research and clinical experience, the dynamic utilization of ultrasound in the musculoskeletal system is still lacking in both research and clinical experience. That is changing quickly as multiple specialties have adopted this modality [20]. Naturally, each sees the use of ultrasonography from its own vantage point and with its own diagnostic considerations. Rheumatologists will evaluate more consistently for the acute inflammatory changes of autoimmune disease, while sports medicine specialists will more consistently evaluate for acute muscle strains. If biotensegrity is a familiar model, ultrasonography will be used dynamically to evaluate for a loss of pre-stress in the myofascial system, which includes muscles, tendons, ligaments, aponeuroses, raphes and previously unrecognized fascial insertions of muscles.

CLINICAL APPLICATION OF BIOTENSEGRITY: BROADENING OUR DIFFERENTIAL DIAGNOSIS

Case #1 A Middle-Aged Athlete with a Weak Painful Knee after Trauma; What Are We Missing?

Clearly, the energy transferred to his patella at impact damaged the bone, which healed through a normal inflammatory, healing cascade of cytokine and cellular responses. The patellar and quadriceps tendons, however, did not fully heal and remained a source of chronic pain. They were tender to palpation prior to treatment with dextrose/PRP injection; the nociceptive signals were theoretically limiting the patient's ability to strengthen the quadriceps. After injection, the tissue structure improved and the tendons were no longer tender to palpation, yet he still could not strengthen the quadriceps. With trauma localized to the knee, sensation of instability localized to the knee and MRI findings of cartilage damage localized to the knee, it is logical that he is still looking toward exploratory arthroscopy of the knee as the solution.

We know that tensegrity structures diffuse forces broadly; perhaps the force of impact at the patella actually injured myofascial structures at a distance from the joint. If biotensegrity modeling is accurate, the femur and patella float in a continuity of tension, and the force of impact could have caused a loss of pre-stress anywhere in that continuity, with the extensor mechanism the most likely candidate. A single-leg squat provides a quick assessment of the mechanism (Figure 5.8 and Video 5.4) and reveals dynamic patella baja (i.e. the patella floats low/too far distal as compared to the uninjured side). Why?

In supine, knee extension produces a synchronized contraction of the four quadriceps muscle on the normal right side. On the injured left side, the four quadriceps contract asynchronously (Video 5.5). In the biotensegrity model, this asynchronous contraction would be related to the past trauma, which has caused a loss of pre-stress in the fascial network of the quadriceps muscle. This loss of stored tension is reflected by laxity in the *relaxed* muscle, similar to a loose rigging on a sail without wind. When the wind blows, the lax sail will not move the boat as well as the taut sail. Muscle laxity at baseline would alter the length–tension ratio, which is crucial in the function of mechanoreceptors and muscle recruitment.

Sonographic palpation then becomes a crucial tool to identify the part of the muscle that has been injured. It is important to understand that I am not necessarily looking for a clear tear in the muscle that could be identified in an MRI. I am looking for a loss of tension that may be subtler than a clear visual tear. This is where the dynamics of ultrasound become irreplaceable. Muscle, like any tensegral structure, should become stiffer and more stable as force is applied through the ultrasonography probe. At the anterolateral thigh, the deepest layer of the quadriceps, the vastus intermedius, collapses under the probe and translates medially, while the overlying vastus lateralis resists the compression and becomes more well defined (Figure 5.9 and Video 5.6).

Now we have a plausible explanation for his loss of control and sense of instability at the knee. Later, we will test the hypothesis with a treatment.

Case #2 A Teenager with a Disease of Middle Age

Rotator cuff tendinopathy and associated subacromial bursitis are recognized clinical diagnoses, attributed to impingement of these structures between the greater tuberosity of the humerus and the overlying acromion. This diagnosis has been confirmed by MRI and ultrasonography in this 15-year-old patient; however, many questions remain. Why is a 15-year-old developing a degenerative process usually found in an aging population? Why is the contralateral shoulder unaffected in

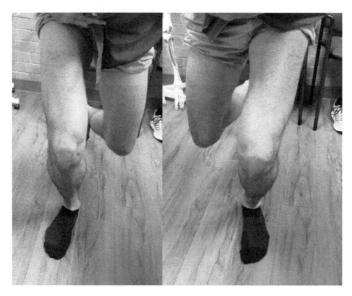

FIGURE 5.8   Still images of single-leg squat on normal right and abnormal left. Note the low-riding patella baja on the left. After this dynamic physical exam (see Video 5.4), loss of tensional integrity at the vastus intermedius in the thigh was found via dynamic ultrasonography.

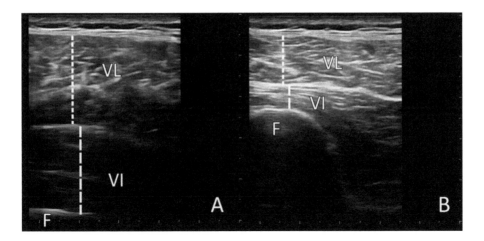

FIGURE 5.9   Still images from Video 5.6: Dynamic compression (i.e. sonographic palpation) to identify a muscle with a loss of pre-stress. A is uncompressed; B is compressed. The vastus intermedius (VI) is hypoechoic and thickened. With compression, the muscle collapses easily, losing about ¾ of its thickness (long dash line). The deep layer of the overlying vastus lateralis (VL) is hypoechoic as well, yet the muscle is more resistant to compression, losing less than ½ of its thickness with compression (short dash line).

this athlete, who is involved in swimming, a sport of symmetric movement? Does "overuse" and microtrauma in a young athlete actually explain this unilateral disease? On physical examination, her left scapula is more protracted with glenoid depressed, and the inferior angle more lateral as compared to the right. Speed's, Neer Impingement, O'Brien's and Empty-can tests were all positive. With active range of motion, there is mild scapular dyskinesis (i.e. altered scapular motion and position) on the left with limited active abduction to 145° and limited flexion to 160°.

Levin has argued that the scapula is a sesamoid bone, floating in a continuous tensional system of soft tissue [21]. As described above, biotensegrity leads to the conclusion that all bones float, including the adjacent humerus. As you lift your hand to reach for an object, your body dynamically maintains the subacromial space within millimeters to avoid impingement of the rotator cuff tendons and overlying bursa. This remarkably complex coordination occurs without conscious effort. When this coordination fails, physical therapy (PT) uses conscious and specific strengthening exercises to address abnormal scapular muscle control. Unfortunately, this approach has not improved our patient's symptoms. While PT has become a primary form of treatment in rotator cuff impingement syndromes, the cause of the scapular dyskinesis has been elusive [22]. A syndrome of scapular muscle detachment (involving the rhomboids and lower trapezius) from high-force trauma has been described, and a surgical treatment has been developed. Yet, even these "detached" muscles appear normal on MRI [23]. These injuries can be visualized by dynamic ultrasonography; myofascial continuity likely explains the lack of retraction in these significant tears [24].

If high-force trauma can functionally detach rhomboid and lower trapezius muscles, perhaps lower-force trauma could cause a smaller injury to these same muscles. Our 15-year-old patient identifies the start of her shoulder issues as the minor injury she suffered while playing badminton at the age of 13. She describes rapidly throwing her arm to the left in effort to strike the shuttlecock. She felt a "pop" at the medial scapular border. From that time forward, swimming became gradually more difficult and painful until she could only swim 10 minutes at a time. Careful palpation along the medial scapular border revealed subtle crepitus and tenderness. Tenderness was also found at the left side of the thoracic posterior spinous processes, yet not the right. Prone strength testing of middle and lower trapezius was 2+/5, less than antigravity. Ultrasound examination of the scapular muscles revealed a small tear at the junction of left rhomboid major/minor (Figure 5.10/Video 5.7) at the medial scapular border and stretch injury to the lower trapezius/latissimus dorsi (Figure 5.11).

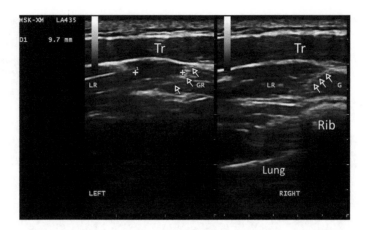

FIGURE 5.10   Sagittal images just medial to the scapula showing the fascial junction between rhomboid major (also known as greater rhomboid – GR) and rhomboid minor (also known as lesser rhomboid – LR). Hypoechoic region (compressible as seen in Video 5.7) at left LR is the region of tear. Tr – trapezius.

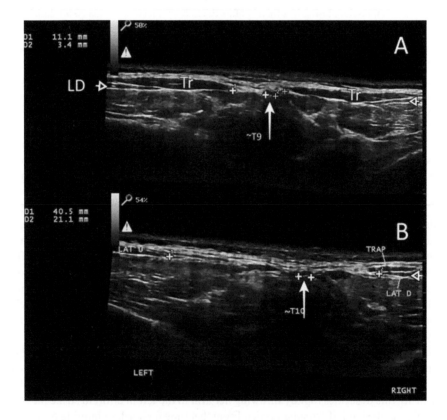

FIGURE 5.11   Stretch injury to left upper extremity muscles of the trunk (see embryology discussion in the text). Extended field of view (EFOV) ultrasound images in the axial plane at T9 (A) and T10 (B). Solid arrows indicate midline location of posterior spinous process. Note lower trapezius (TR) is partially pulled away from the spinous process at T9. TR muscle fibers are absent at T10 on the left; they are visible on the uninjured right side. TR and latissimus dorsi (LD) insert into the posterior layer of the thoracolumbar fascia (PLF), which extends between the calipers indicated by D1 on left and D2 on right.

The embryology of these muscles is interesting to consider in light of her mechanism of injury. Each of the myofascial structures that appear abnormal on ultrasound (rhomboids, lower trapezius and latissimus dorsi) emerged as part of the limb bud lateral to the midline [25]. During development, each of these migrated to the midline (anterior muscles such as pectoralis major also migrate to the midline) and attached to the posterior spinous processes. This helps us visualize how the upper extremity is a continuity that embraces our trunk during development. The acting of "throwing" the upper extremity away from body could have resulted in a stretch injury to this continuity.

BIOTENSEGRITY-BASED INTERVENTIONS: RESTORE MOTION OR RESTORE PRE-STRESS?

Biotensegrity-based interventions focus on restoring balanced and continuous tension throughout the body. When viewed through the lens of basic science, this appears to be a vague and unattainable goal. Yet, for millennia, manual therapists (i.e. "body workers") have provided relief of musculoskeletal symptoms without clear diagnosis as required in the medical model. Manual therapies seek to restore function by addressing restrictions in movement that distort the continuity of connective tissue. These restrictions are colloquially referred to as "scar" or "adhesions," and, in some cases, these are likely accurate terms. Yet, the science of these felt restrictions is far more complex than a simple scar. Structural integration (founded by Ida Rolf and often referred to as "Rolfing") is a whole-body, manual therapy that seeks to balance forces in the body to restore freedom of movement. The Ida P. Rolf Research Foundation has been instrumental in advancing the science of all manual therapies via the Fascia Research Society and the Fascia Research Congress [26]. Since 2007, these meetings have brought together manual practitioners of all disciplines with basic science researchers. Much of this science is discussed in Chapter 21, by David Lesondak, which also includes a case study illustrating the clinical efficacy of manual treatment informed by biotensegrity. Manual techniques clearly improve mobility and can be near curative of chronic pain, as illustrated by the case study.

Similarly, manipulation and joint mobilization also seek to restore lost motion through physical forces. Yet, a need for chronic treatment with manual therapies or manipulation likely indicates a loss of tensional continuity, as described in the cases described in this chapter. Rather than a restriction that requires loosening, these cases display a laxity that requires tightening, specifically, a tightening that "re-stores" energy in the form of collagen.

WHAT IS PROLOTHERAPY?

In 1937, Gedney [27] and Schultz [28] began experimenting with sclerosing agents to treat unstable joints diagnosed by physical exam. In the late 1950s, Schultz [29] reported on 20 years of successful treatment of loose temperomandicular joints (TMJ) using sclerosant injections of the joint capsule. In 1955, Hackett [30], a general surgeon in Ohio, published histological studies of tissue response to sclerosant injection of tendons; this included a discussion of clinical applications in ligament laxity related to chronic pain. He felt that the evidence showed proliferation of normal tissue rather than scar; thus, he introduced the term *prolotherapy*. Hackett defined prolotherapy as an injection technique for strengthening "the weld of disabled ligaments and tendons to bone by stimulating the production of new bone and fibrous tissue cells" (Hackett 1958 [31]). He was inspired by Kellgren's report [32] of sciatic-like pain referral patterns from interspinous ligaments to document similar patterns from iliolumbar, sacroiliac and hip ligaments.

Hackett began injecting bony insertions (i.e. entheses) of ligaments and tendons in 1939 and quickly became convinced that the majority of chronic low back pain was due to weakening of these structures. Hackett reported that 82% of his patients with chronic musculoskeletal pain considered themselves cured after treatment with prolotherapy (Hackett 1958 [30]. This led to a tradition of extensive needling and injection at entheses of the spine and peripheral joints to treat chronic pain and instability. Treatment location was most often guided by anatomic knowledge of ligament structure, pain referral patterns, pain to palpation at enthesis and subtle crepitus found on detailed palpation reminiscent of osteopathic examination methods. Yet the extensive injection patterns appeared too invasive for holistic practitioners, while appearing too imprecise for the serious science of allopathic medicine. Without established scientific evidence of a regenerative response to these injections or even the pathology being treated at these locations, prolotherapy existed on the periphery of medicine for decades. The most common injectant used in prolotherapy during this time was hypertonic dextrose (usually 15%–25%); the basic science and research-supported, clinical applications of dextrose prolotherapy were recently reviewed [33].

THE LATE DAWNING OF REGENERATIVE ORTHOPEDICS

The burgeoning science of platelet-rich plasma, stem cell manipulation and the overall field of "bio-orthopedics" have now brought regenerative orthopedics to the forefront [34]. The fundamental importance of integrated structure and function demonstrated in the clinical practice of prolotherapy, however, has, thus far, been lost on many in the field of regenerative orthopedics. Use of biotensegrity modeling can be essential for the clinical effectiveness of regenerative injection, as demonstrated in our case examples.

CLINICAL APPLICATION OF BIOTENSEGRITY: REGENERATIVE INJECTION TO RESTORE TENSIONAL CONTINUITY

Case #1 A Middle-Aged Athlete with a Weak Painful Knee after Trauma

Based on our patient's history, physical exam and dynamic ultrasound findings, prolotherapy was applied at a distance from the perceived pain and dysfunction. Ultrasound guidance facilitates treatment at entheses, as has been the tradition in prolotherapy training; it also expands our ability to locations other than the bony insertion, such as muscle and fascial planes. In this case, injection of 10–15 ml solution (0.3% lidocaine/15% dextrose) was performed at the origin and substance of the vastus intermedius from the anterolateral femur (Figure 5.12 and Video 5.8) and the fascial plane adjoining rectus femoris and vastus lateralis. Quadriceps contraction and single-leg squat were repeated and the patient reported "it's stronger; feels solid." The same locations were then injected with 6 ml of the patient's low WBC-low RBC PRP made from 60 ml whole blood.

At 2-month phone follow-up, the patient reported "The treatment to the thigh really, really helped. It gave it a lot more ability for the quad to activate." At 3-month follow-up, quadriceps bulk and activation had improved, single-leg squat was normal (Figure 5.13 and Video 5.9) and ultrasound examination showed improved VI definition and resistance to compression (Video 5.10). The patient was no longer considering surgery. At 22-month phone follow-up, he reported that he had no difficulty with deep squats and the left quads were now larger than the right, as they had been prior to the accident. He cycles regularly to maintain fitness.

Case #2 A Teenager with a Disease of Middle Age

In this 15-year-old swimmer, abnormal metabolic processes are reflected in the tendon degeneration and bursitis seen on MRI and ultrasound. Yet, this "disease" is caused by altered dynamics; treating the metabolic changes with corticosteroid only provides temporary relief and may worsen the tendinopathy in the long run [17]. Treating the altered scapular dynamics with PT has not improved symptoms. Based on the diagnosis of a loss of pre-stress due to injury of rhomboids at the scapula and the PLF insertions of the lower trapezius and latissimus dorsi, dextrose prolotherapy is applied to these structures using palpation guidance (i.e. traditional prolotherapy technique/injection only at enthesis). A total of 12–18 ml solution (0.3% lidocaine and 15% dextrose) was injected via a

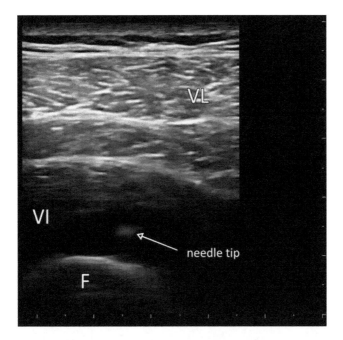

FIGURE 5.12 Ultrasound guided injection at the femoral origin of vastus intermedius (VI). VL – vastus lateralis. F – femur.

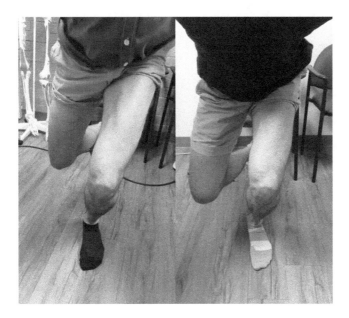

FIGURE 5.13 Single-leg squat test before (left) and 3 months after (right) dextrose/PRP prolotherapy to the quadriceps. Note the return of quadriceps muscle bulk, improved femoral–tibial alignment and resolution of patella baja on the right image (see Video 5.9).

27-gauge, 1.25 inch needle at scapular spine, medial scapular border and left side of thoracic spinous processes, the dose being 0.5–1 ml per injection site. Treatment was repeated at 3 and 6 weeks after initial session.

At follow-up 2 months after the third treatment, the patient reported 70%–75% improvement in pain and 100% improvement in active range of motion (confirmed on exam). Speed's and Empty-can tests were normal; O'Brien's test was still positive. Prone middle trapezius strength improved to 4/5 and lower trapezius to 3+/5. Fascial definition of lower trapezius and latissimus dorsi is markedly improved (Figure 5.14). Dynamic impingement shown on ultrasound was also clearly improved (Figure 5.15 and Video 5.11).

The patient received two more dextrose prolotherapy treatments, one month apart, and her pain resolved. Phone follow-up 4 years, 9 months after the last treatment confirmed that she had returned to full function and required no other form of treatment after her prolotherapy.

CONCLUSION

The biotensegrity model inspires us to examine anatomy and biomechanics with new eyes and to consider the source of biomechanical dysfunction in tissues we have traditionally ignored; this expands our differential diagnosis in interesting directions. Dynamic ultrasonography now provides

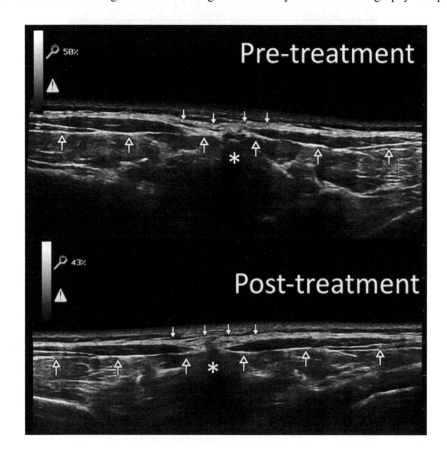

FIGURE 5.14 EFOV ultrasound images in the axial plane at T9 pre and post-dextrose prolotherapy. Note the improved tension (pre-stress) in the fascial layer indicated by the large, open arrows. The untreated right side also shows improvement, possibly related to midline injections performed in traditional prolotherapy. The small, closed arrows point to bridging fascia across the midline, which also markedly improved after treatment.

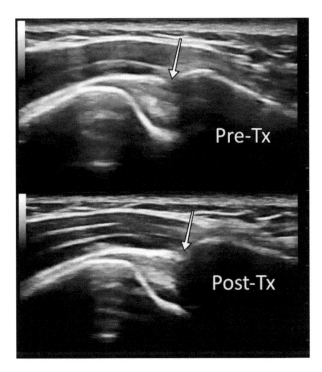

FIGURE 5.15   Still images from dynamic impingement test before and after dextrose prolotherapy to scapular and thoracic entheses only. Arrows indicate location of impingement by the acromion. Note the indention of bursa and supraspinatus tendon before treatment and lack of impingement after (see Video 5.11).

diagnostic confirmation of pathology that had been intuited by the clinical experience of prolotherapists, and it provides a method of guiding injections to the damaged tissue. Combined with the dawning science of cellular medicine, these developments will inevitably provide improved diagnosis and treatment of chronic musculoskeletal pain.

LIST OF VIDEOS

Full videos can be found at www.BetterOrthopedics.com.

VIDEO 5.1   Dynamic subacromial impingement of the supraspinatus tendon in a 15-year-old swimmer. See Figure 5.2 in the text to identify structures in the video. Notice the deformation of the bursa and superficial tendon during scapular plane abduction of the shoulder.

VIDEO 5.2   Twitch response in the vastus lateralis during needling. See Figure 5.3 in the text to identify structures. The muscle contraction pulls on the lateral intermuscular septum of the thigh, confirming that muscles do not insert only at bone.

VIDEO 5.3   The natural oscillation of tensegrities demonstrated in a sculpture built by Bruce Hamilton of Tension Designs. A small outside force produces an oscillation of movement and eventual return to a steady state without a loss of pre-stress in the tension elements.

VIDEO 5.4   Video of single-leg squat on normal right and abnormal left. Note the low-riding patella baja on the left. After this dynamic physical exam, loss of tensional integrity at the vastus intermedius in the thigh was found via dynamic ultrasonography.

VIDEO 5.5   In supine, knee extension produces a synchronized contraction of the four quadriceps muscles on the normal right side. On the injured left side, the four quadriceps contract asynchronously.

VIDEO 5.6   Dynamic compression (i.e. sonographic palpation) to identify a muscle with a loss of pre-stress. In this case, the vastus intermedius overlying the surface of the femur collapses easily with compression, while the overlying vastus lateralis becomes more resistant as force is applied (see Figure 5.9).

VIDEO 5.7 Dynamic compression showing collapsing tear in the lesser rhomboid (LR).

VIDEO 5.8 Ultrasound guided injection at the femoral origin of vastus intermedius. Note the easy flow of fluid at the myo-osseous origin of this muscle.

VIDEO 5.9 Single-leg squat test before (left) and 3 months after (right) dextrose/PRP prolotherapy to the quadriceps (see Figure 5.13).

VIDEO 5.10 Dynamic compression of the quadriceps after treatment. Compare to Video 5.6 and note the improved resistance to compression and lack of muscle translation in the VI.

VIDEO 5.11 Dynamic supraspinatus impingement test 2 months after third dextrose prolotherapy. Compare to Video 5.1 and note resolution of impingement (see Figure 5.15).

REFERENCES

1. Laotse. (1948) *The Wisdom of Laotse*. New York, NY: Random House.
2. Stecco, A., Gilliar, W., Hill, R., Fullerton, B., and Stecco, C. (2013) The anatomical and functional relation between gluteus maximus and fascia lata. *Journal of Bodywork and Movement Therapies*, 17 (4): 512–517. doi:10.1016/j.jbmt.2013.04.004.
3. Stecco, C. (2015) *Functional Atlas of the Human Fascial System*. London: Churchill Livingstone.
4. Snelson, K. *Art and Ideas*. Kenneth Snelson in association with Marlborough Gallery, New York, NY.
5. Heartney, E. (2009) *Kenneth Snelson: Forces Made Visible*. Burlington, VT: Hudson Hills Publishers.
6. Snelson, K. Frequently asked questions: What happens if a wire is cut? www.kennethsnelson.net/faqs/faq.htm (accessed July 25, 2017).
7. Levin, S. M. (2016) Tensegrity: The new biomechanics. In: Hutson, M. and Ellis, R. eds, *Textbook of Musculoskeletal Medicine*, New York, NY: Oxford University Press, 150–162.
8. Levin, S. M., Biotensegrity: A new way of modeling biologic forms. http://www.biotensegrity.com (accessed July 12, 2017).
9. Sunspiral, V. SUPERball: A Biologically Inspired Robot for Planetary Exploration. https://www.nasa.gov/ames/ocs/2016-summer-series/vytas-sunspiral (accessed July 10, 2018).
10. Ingber, D. E., Wang, N., and Stamenovic, D. (2014). Tensegrity, cellular biophysics, and the mechanics of living systems. *Reports on Progress in Physics Physical Society (Great Britain)*, 77 (4): 46603. doi:10.1088/0034-4885/77/4/046603.
11. Scarr, G. (2014) *Biotensegrity: The Structural Basis of Life*. Pencaitland, Scotland: Handspring Publishing.
12. Scarr, G. (2012) A consideration of the elbow as a tensegrity structure. *International Journal of Osteopathic Medicine*, 15 (2): 53–65. doi:10.1016/j.ijosm.2011.11.003.
13. Perceivingacting. Michael Turvey – Haptic perception and tensegrity. https://www.youtube.com/watch?v=BLR7ZTSel9M (accessed August 5, 2017).
14. Turvey, M. T. and Fonseca, S. T. (2014) The medium of haptic perception: A tensegrity hypothesis. *Journal of Motor Behavior*, 46 (3): 143–187. doi:10.1080/00222895.2013.798252.
15. Sihvonen, R., Paavola, M., Malmivaara, A., Itälä, A., Joukainen, A., Nurmi, H., Kalske J., and Järvinen, T. L. N. (2013) Arthroscopic partial meniscectomy versus sham surgery for a degenerative meniscal tear. *New England Journal of Medicine* 369 (26): 2515–2524. doi:10.1056/NEJMoa1305189.
16. McAlindon, T. E., LaValley, M. P., Harvey, W. F., Price, L. L., Driban, J. B., Zhang, M., and Ward, R. J. (2017) Effect of intra-articular triamcinolone vs saline on knee cartilage volume and pain in patients with knee osteoarthritis: A randomized clinical trial. *JAMA* 317 (19): 1967–1975. doi:10.1001/jama.2017.5283.
17. Abate, M., Salini, V., Schiavone, C., and Andia, I. (2017) Clinical benefits and drawbacks of local corticosteroids injections in tendinopathies. *Expert Opinion on Drug Safety*, 16 (3): 341–349. doi:10.1080/14740338.2017.1276561.
18. Gevitz, N. (1989) The chiropractors and the AMA: Reflections on the history of the consultation clause. *Perspectives in Biology and Medicine*, 32 (2): 281–299.
19. Travell, J. G. and Simons, D. G. (1999) *Myofascial Pain and Dysfunction: The Trigger Point Manual. Vol. 2, The Lower Extremities*. Baltimore, MA: Williams & Wilkins, pp. 28–30.
20. Berko, N. S., Goldberg-Stein, S., Thornhill, B. A., and Koenigsberg, M. (2016) Survey of current trends in postgraduate musculoskeletal ultrasound education in the United States. *Skeletal Radiology*, 45 (4): 475–482. doi:10.1007/s00256-015-2324-0.
21. Levin, S. M. (2005) The scapula is a sesamoid bone. *Journal of Biomechanics* 38 (8): 1733.

22. Kibler, W. B., Ludewig, P. M., McClure, P. W. et al., (2013) Clinical implications of scapular dyskinesis in shoulder injury: The 2013 consensus statement from the 'scapular summit'. *Br J Sports Med*, 47: 877–885.

23. Kibler, W. B. and Sciascia, A. D. (2009) Scapular muscle detachment: Clinical presentation and results of treatment. *Journal of Orthopaedic and Sports Physical*, 39 (11): A13.

24. Fullerton, B. (2016). Embryology, anatomy and ultrasonography of scapular dyskinesis. *Platform Presentation at Annual Meeting of the American Academy of Physical Medicine and Rehabilitation*, New Orleans, LA.

25. Willard, F. H. (2012) Somatic fascia. In: Schleip, R., Findley, T.W., Chaitow, L., and Huijing, P. A. (eds) *Fascia: Tensional Network of the Human Body*, 11–17. New York: Elsevier.

26. Findley, T and Schleip, R. (2007) *"Fascia research." Basic Science and Implication for Conventional and Complementary Health Care*. Munich, Germany: Elsevier Health Sciences.

27. Gedney, E. H. (1937) Hypermobile joint. *Osteopathic Profession*, 4 (9): 30–31.

28. Schultz, L. W. (1937) A treatment for subluxation of the temporomandibular joint. *Journal of the American Medical Association*, 109 (13): 1032–1035.

29. Schultz, L. W. (1956) Twenty years' experience in treating hypermobility of the temporomandibular joints. *The American Journal of Surgery* 92 (6): 925–928.

30. Hackett, G. S. and Henderson, D. G. (1955) Joint stabilization: An experimental, histologic study with comments on the clinical application in ligament proliferation. *The American Journal of Surgery*, 89 (5): 968–973.

31. Hackett, G. S. (1958) *Ligament and Tendon Relaxation Treated by Prolotherapy*, 3rd edn. (eds) Springfield, I. L. and Thomas, C. C, p. 51.

32. Kellgren, J. H. (1939) On the distribution of pain arising from deep somatic structures with charts of segmental pain areas. *Clinical Science*, 4: 35.

33. Reeves, K. D., Sit, R. W. S., and Rabago, D. P. (2016) Dextrose prolotherapy: A narrative review of basic science, clinical research, and best treatment recommendations. *Physical Medicine and Rehabilitation Clinics of North America*, Regenerative Medicine, 27 (4) 783–823. doi:10.1016/j.pmr.2016.06.001.

34. ISAKOS. (2017) *Bio-Orthopaedics – A New Approach*. Berlin, Heidelberg: Springer-Verlag.

6 Photobiomodulation Therapy in Orthopedics
Metabolic Effects

Michael R. Hamblin, PhD

INTRODUCTION TO PHOTOBIOMODULATION

Photobiomodulation (PBM) also known as low-level laser (light) therapy (LLLT) is approaching its 50th anniversary [1]. LLLT was originally discovered by Endre Mester working in Hungary, who was trying to repeat an experiment described by Paul McGuff in Boston. McGuff had used the newly discovered ruby laser to cure experimental tumors implanted in Syrian hamsters [2, 3]. However, Mester's laser only had a small fraction of the power possessed by McGuff's laser and was insufficient to cure any tumors. Nevertheless Mester observed that the skin wounds that had been made during implantation of the tumors healed better in laser treated animals [4, 5]. Since those early days, LLLT has become gradually more accepted in scientific, medical and popular circles, especially as the number of peer-reviewed papers has grown.

For much of this time, lasers were thought to have special biological properties due to their coherence and monochromaticity [6], and the field was sometimes called "laser biostimulation" [7]. However in recent years it has become clear that non-coherent light-emitting diodes (LEDs) perform equally to medical lasers, with the added advantage of being much less expensive and having fewer safety concerns [8]. The first lasers to be used generally emitted red light. The ruby (694 nm) and HeNe (633 nm) lasers were popular, but after the introduction of diode lasers, many more wavelengths became available including several in the near-infrared region (780–940 nm).

In 2016 there was an international consensus to change the terminology away from LLLT and the old term "low-level", and instead use the new term "photobiomodulation" [9]. The reasons for this decision were several-fold: (1) nobody had any idea exactly what "low-level" actually meant; (2) the term laser was inappropriate as LEDs are rapidly taking over; (3) due to the biphasic dose response, PBM can have inhibitory or stimulatory effects even at the same wavelength with just the use of a much higher energy density.

One feature of PBM that is becoming appreciated is the biphasic dose response [10, 11] (also known as the Arndt-Schulz law) [12]. This states that a very low dose of light often has no effect, a somewhat bigger dose has a positive effect, until eventually a plateau is reached. If the light dose is increased beyond that point the benefit progressively decreases, until the baseline (no effect) is reached, and further increases will actually start to have damaging effects on the tissue. This curve is well known in the field of toxicology, where the phenomenon is called "hormesis" [13]. Part of the explanation of this "U" or "J" shaped curve is that small doses of a potentially toxic drug or harmful intervention, can induce expression inside the cells of a range of protective factors such as antioxidant enzymes and anti-apoptotic proteins that will enhance normal function and protect against subsequent lethal challenges [14].

BACKGROUND ON CHROMOPHORES

The first law of photobiology states that photons of light must be absorbed by some molecule (called a chromophore) located within the tissue to have any biological effect.

MITOCHONDRIAL CHROMOPHORES

Tiina Karu working in Russia and Salvatore Passarella in Italy were the first to suggest that one of the principal chromophores responsible for the beneficial effects of LLLT was located inside mitochondria [15]. Previously Britton Chance had observed that the mitochondrial fraction accounted for 50 % of the optical absorption of blood-free rat liver [16] at 780 nm. Although hemoglobin and myoglobin have high absorption coefficients in the visible spectral regions (blue, green and red), their absorption in the NIR region, (where PBM is highly effective) is not very high. The purified enzyme, cytochrome c oxidase (CCO) was shown to be activated in vitro by red laser (633 nm) [17]. CCO is unit IV of the mitochondrial respiratory chain and is a complex molecule with 13 separate protein subunits. CCO contains two different copper centers Cu_A and Cu_B and two heme centers, heme-a and heme-$a3$. All these centers can be in a reduced or an oxidized state giving a total of 16 possibilities. CCO transfers four protons to molecular oxygen to form two water molecules using the electrons from reduced cytochrome c. The proton gradient so formed drives the activity of ATP synthase. Several investigators have reported that the action spectra (relative efficiency of different wavelengths for mediating aspects of the PBM process) correspond to the absorption spectrum of CCO [18, 19]. The leading hypothesis to explain how exactly light increases CCO enzyme activity is that nitric oxide (a molecule that is known to inhibit CCO by non-covalently binding between heme-$a3$ and Cu_B [20], can be photodissociated by absorption of a photon of red or NIR light [21]. One theory to explain why PBM appears to have greater effects in diseased or damaged cells and tissues, and to not dramatically affect healthy cells, is that unhealthy or hypoxic cells are more likely to have inhibitory concentrations of NO. This proposed mechanism is illustrated in Figure 6.1.

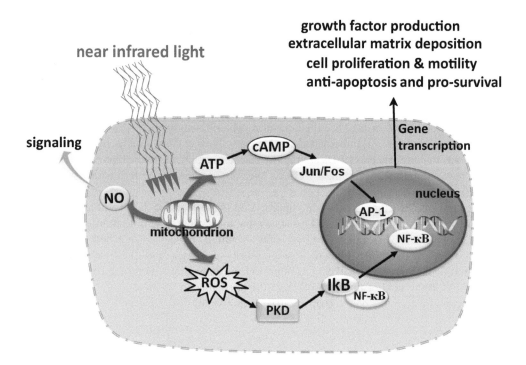

FIGURE 6.1 Mitochondrial mechanisms of PBM. Red and NIR light (up to 940 nm) is primarily absorbed by cytochrome c oxidase (CCO) in the mitochondrial respiratory chain of all mammalian cells. Nitric oxide is dissociated and respiration increases leading to more adenosine triphosphate (ATP) being produced. Released NO, a brief burst of reactive oxygen species (ROS), and ATP leading to cAMP, can all lead to activation of transcription factors.

LIGHT/HEAT GATED ION CHANNELS

An important discovery was made by Hardie and Minke working with the fruit fly *Drusophila melanogaster* in 1992 [22]. A spontaneous mutation (later found to be in the *trp* gene) led to a blind mutant, even though the flies were exposed to intense light. A combination of electrophysiological, biochemical, calcium measurements, combined with genetic studies in these flies, and eventually in other invertebrates finally showed that TRP was a novel phosphoinositide-regulated calcium permeable ion channel [23]. The underlying mechanism of vision is quite different in insects (relying on TRP channels) and mammalian organisms (relying on rhodopsin photoreceptors) [24].

Transient receptor potential (TRP) channels are now known to be pleiotropic cellular sensors mediating the response to a wide range of external stimuli (heat, cold, pressure, taste, smell) and involved in many different cellular processes [25]. Activation of TRP causes non-selective permeabilization (mainly of the plasma membrane) to calcium, sodium and magnesium [26]. Interestingly, it was recently reported that TRP channels were involved in sensing the "redox status" [27].

It is now known that TRP channel proteins are conserved throughout evolution and are found in most organisms, tissues and cell types. The TRP channel superfamily is now classified into seven related subfamilies: TRPC, TRPM, TRPV, TRPA, TRPP, TRPML and TRPN [28]. Light-sensitive ion channels are based on an opsin chromophore (isomerization of a cis-retinal molecule to the trans configuration) as illustrated in *Drusophila* photorecelptors [29].

GREEN AND BLUE-LIGHT CHROMOPHORES

It is possible that blue light interacts with mitochondrial chromophores in the same way as red/NIR light since heme centers that are widespread in cytochromes have a significant absorption peak that coincides with the Soret band of porphyrins. However, there are several other plausible chromophores for blue light (and to a lesser extent green light). It should be noted that the term "blue light" can refer to a relatively wide range of wavelengths such as violet (390–425 nm), indigo (425–450 nm), royal blue (450–475 nm), blue green (475–500 nm). Because of the width of a typical absorption band (30 nm full width half maximum), it is theoretically possible that blue light could be absorbed by several distinct chromophores. For blue light these potential chromophores are in order of increasing wavelength: (A) tryptophan that can be photo-oxidized to form 6-formylindolo[3,2-b] carbazole (FICZ) that acts as an endogenous ligand of the aryl-hydrocarbon receptor (AhR) [30, 31]. The shortest wavelength blue light (380–400 nm) would be optimal here, as in general UV wavelengths are thought to be responsible for trytptophan photodegradation. (B) Next is the Soret band of heme groups (400 nm) where presumably similar processes are initiated as have been proposed for red/NIR light. Cytochromes b and a/a(3) were found to be responsible for the inhibitory effects of blue light on yeast [32]. (C) Wavelengths in the 440 nm range have been found to be optimal for activation of cryptochromes [33]. Cryptochromes are blue-light sensitive flavoproteins that have wide applications in plants and lower life-forms, mediating such functions as photomorphogenesis [34]. Cryptochromes are thought to play a role in entraining circadian rhythms [35] and may even be involved in sensing of magnetic fields in fruit flies [36]. Cryptochromes have recently been found to be expressed in some mammalian cells and tissues [37] and also to have activity in regulating circadian rhythms [38]. (D) The family of opsins are light-sensitive G-protein coupled receptors that rely on isomerization of cis-retinal. The wavelength maximum can range from UVA all the way to the green and red, but melanopsin (OPN4) has a λ_{max} of 479 nm [39]. The signaling pathways differ between different opsins. Opsins signal via two main pathways depending on the type of G-protein they are coupled with [40, 41]. Those opsins (OPN1, OPN2, OPN3, OPN5) that are coupled with G_o, G_i, G_t, G_s proteins, signal via a pathway involving cyclic nucleotides (cAMP and cGMP). On the other hand, OPN4 (melanopsin) is coupled to Gq and signals via the phospholipase C pathway leading to production of inositol triphosphate and di-acylglycerol. These signaling pathways are shown in Figure 6.2. It is known that activation of retinal opsins by blue light can generate ROS, which is partly responsible for ocular phototoxicity caused by violet and blue light [42].

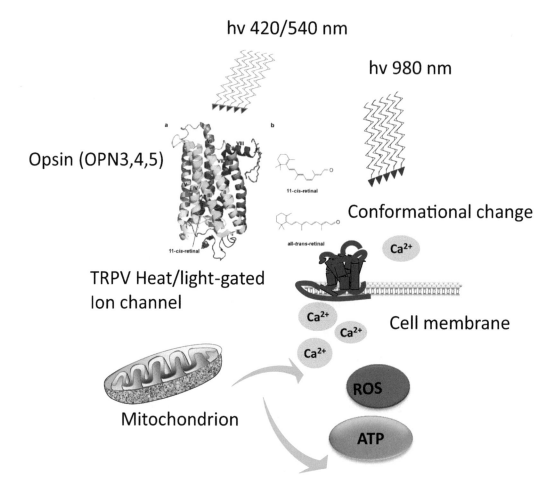

FIGURE 6.2   Opsins and ion channels as chromophores for PBM. Blue and green light are primarily absorbed by opsins (cis-retinal-containing) signaling proteins. Longer wavelength NIR light (980 nm, 1064 nm) is primarily absorbed by water and protein conformation can be altered. The chief target of both these pathways is transient receptor potential ion channels, that chiefly affect calcium signaling, but produce comparable effects to the CCO mechanisms.

METABOLIC EFFECTS OF PHOTOBIOMODULATION

The wide range of downstream effects that PBM can exert on all the different cells and tissues that make up the body is summarized in Figure 6.3.

OXIDATIVE STRESS

One of the most frequently observed changes when PBM experiments are conducted in vitro has been modulation of levels of reactive oxygen species (ROS) [43]. ROS have particularly been reported to be produced by large doses of light, and even more particularly by blue light. The production of modest amounts of ROS by red/NIR light being absorbed in the mitochondria is reasonably well established [44]. It is known that mitochondria are one of the most important sources of ROS in mammalian cells [45]. Leakage of electrons leads to production of superoxide anion that is then removed by manganese-dependent superoxide dismutase (MnSOD) [46].

The mitochondrial membrane potential (MMP) is increased by PBM, leading to increased electron transport. Classically it is believed that increased MMP will produce increased ROS [47].

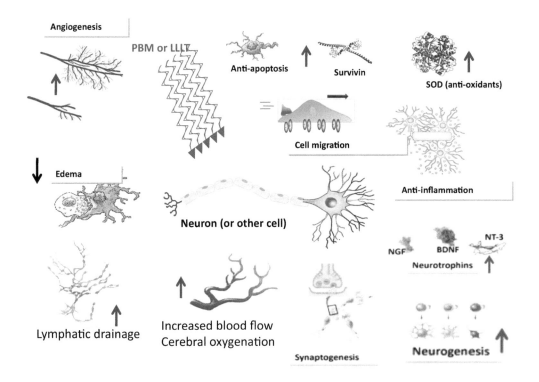

FIGURE 6.3 Downstream mechanisms of PBM. The gene transcription process described in Figures 6.1 and 6.2 can lead to decreases in apoptosis and excitotoxicity, and lessening of inflammation and reduction of edema due to increased lymphatic flow, which together with protective factors such as antioxidants, will all help to reduce progressive damage to the brain and other tissues. Increases in angiogenesis, expression of neurotrophins leading to activation of neural progenitor cells and more cell migration, and increased synaptogenesis may all contribute to the brain repairing itself from damage sustained in the trauma.

However, it is also well known that dysfunctional mitochondria also produce ROS. This process is characterized by a self-amplifying feedback loop called "ROS-induced ROS release" (RIRR) [48]. Under conditions such as exposure to excessive or prolonged oxidative stress, the increase in ROS may reach a threshold level that triggers the opening of a mitochondrial channel such as the mitochondrial permeability transition (MPT) pore, or the mitochondrial inner membrane anion channel (IMAC). Activation of these channels in turn leads to the simultaneous collapse of MMP and increased ROS generation by the electron transport chain [49]. Production of a large enough burst of ROS to flood the cytosol could potentially function as a "second messenger" to activate RIRR in neighboring mitochondria, which could then act as another damaging feedback loop to increase cellular damage [50].

We first showed that PBM with 810 nm laser (3 J/cm^2) could activate NF-kB in embryonic fibroblasts isolated from NF-kB luciferase reporter mice [43]. We showed that ROS were generated inside the cells, and ATP production was increased. Interestingly, addition of the anti-oxidant N-acetylcysteine abrogated the activation of NF-kB by quenching the ROS, but had no effect on the increase in ATP (Figure 6.4). The explanation for these observations is that PBM raised MMP leading to more ATP production, and at the same time produced a burst of ROS that activated NF-kB, probably by activation of protein kinase D [51].

We next went on to show that PBM (810 nm laser) had biphasic dose-response effects in primary cultured cortical neurons from embryonic mouse brains [52]. Using a wide range of energy densities (0.03–30 J/cm^2) we found a maximum effect at 3 J/cm^2 on MMP and intracellular calcium. Higher doses of light (10 or 30 J/cm^2) had lower effects and 30 J/cm^2 actually lowered the MMP below

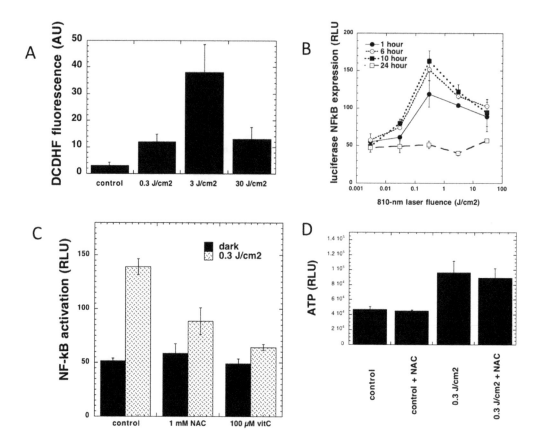

FIGURE 6.4 NFkB is activated by PBM induced ROS in embryonic fibroblasts. (A) Intracellular ROS measured by DCDHF fluorescence; (B) NF-kB activation measured by a luciferase assay; (C) NF-kB activation is inhibited by antioxidants; (D) ATP increase is not affected by antioxidants. (Adapted from data in Chen, A.C., et al., *PLoS ONE*, 6(7), e22453, 2011.)

baseline. When we looked at intracellular ROS production we found a double peak. The first peak was at $3\,J/cm^2$ while there was a second peak at $30\,J/cm^2$ (Figure 6.5). We interpret these data to mean that ROS were produced from mitochondria by raising MMP above baseline at $3\,J/cm^2$, and also by lowering the MMP below baseline at $30\,J/cm^2$.

Next we asked what would happen when PBM was delivered to cells that had already been subjected to oxidative stress [53]. Using the same cultured cortical neurons, we applied three different chemical treatments that were all designed to cause oxidative stress as shown by increases in

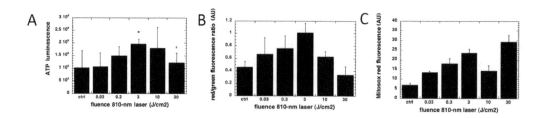

FIGURE 6.5 Dose response of 810 nm laser in cortical neurons. (A) ATP production as a function of fluence; (B) mitochondrial membrane potential (JC1 red/green ratio); (C) mitochondrial ROS. (Adapted from data in Sharma, S.K., et al., *Lasers Surg Med*, 43(8), 851–859, 2011.)

intracellular ROS. These were cobalt chloride (activation of hypoxia-inducible factor 1), rotenone (complex 1 inhibitor), or hydrogen peroxide. All these chemicals led to reductions in MMP and ATP production, as well as increased intracellular ROS. PBM (810 nm laser, 3 J/cm²) led to increased MMP and ATP and reduced ROS, while by contrast control cells (no oxidative stress) had a small increase in ROS accompanied by increases in MMP and ATP above baseline levels (Figure 6.6). We interpret these results to mean that PBM tends to increase MMP back towards baseline thereby reducing ROS production.

In contrast to NIR light, the mechanisms for production of ROS by blue light are less well established. Using adipose-derived stem cells, we showed that blue light (415 nm) produced a linear dose-dependent increase in ROS accompanied by reductions in ATP and MMP and inhibition of proliferation (submitted for publication). However, 810 nm (and 660 nm) gave a biphasic dose-dependent increase in proliferation and ATP accompanied by a rise in MMP and a rise in ROS that was less than that found with blue light. Interesting many of the effects of blue light (including ROS generation) could be at least partly blocked by the TRPV ion channel inhibitor capsazepine (Figure 6.6).

One intriguing question is how PBM generated ROS can apparently be both beneficial and detrimental. If superoxide is produced inside mitochondria and is then dismutated to hydrogen peroxide by MnSOD then the uncharged H_2O_2 is free to diffuse outside the mitochondria where it can take part in many signaling pathways [54]. This manageable level of H_2O_2 has recently been termed "oxidative eustress" [55]. However, if the levels of superoxide within the mitochondria exceed the capacity of MnSOD to detoxify it then the charged $O_2^{-\bullet}$ may accumulate within the mitochondrial matrix and cause damage [56]. The ability of MnSOD to detoxify superoxide may depend on the rate at which $O_2^{-\bullet}$ is produced, which in turn may depend on the rate at which light is delivered, i.e. the power density. This consideration may explain some observations that have been made where the biological effects of PBM depended on the power density of the light (mW/cm²), and not on the total dose (J/cm²) [57–59].

SYNERGY WITH EXERCISE

There are several similarities between the systemic effects of PBM and those of physical exercise. Both appear to cause a brief increase in ROS, but in the long term can increase anti-oxidant

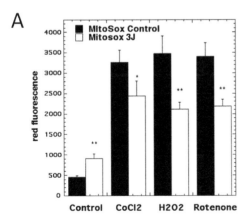
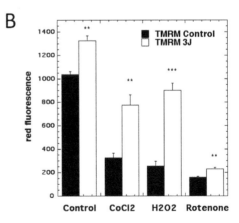

FIGURE 6.6 PBM reduces oxidative stress in cortical neurons. Oxidative stress was induced by three different treatments (cobalt chloride, hydrogen peroxide, rotenone) and cells were treated with 3 J/cm² 810 nm. (A) Mitochondrial ROS, (B) mitochondrial membrane potential (tetramethylrhodamine methyl ester). (Adapted from data in Huang, Y.Y., et al., Low-level laser therapy (LLLT) reduces oxidative stress in primary cortical neurons in vitro. *J Biophotonics*, 2012.)

defenses. A highly cited paper [60] reported that administration of vitamins C and E abrogated the health-promoting effects of exercise training in healthy young men, as measured by insulin sensitivity and anti-oxidant defenses. On the other hand, PBM appears to combine well with exercise. One report showed that TBARS were reduced, while glutathione (GSH), superoxide dismutase (SOD) and catalase (CAT) were increased in muscle tissue from rats that underwent daily swimming training for 6 weeks combined with PBM, compared to either exercise or PBM alone [61].

Mitochondria are generated by the expression of genes on both nuclear and mitochondrial genomes. Mitochondrial biogenesis is highly responsive to cellular demands for energy and environmental stimuli [62]. The mechanistic target of rapamycin (mTOR) pathway regulates mitochondrial biogenesis to co-ordinate energy homeostasis with cell growth [63]. It is well known that exercise induces the proliferation of mitochondria within the cells, particularly mitochondrial biogenesis within muscle cells [64]. A recent paper [65] reviewed the new subject of "exercise mimetics" in other words, pharmacological substances (aminoimidazole carboxamide ribonucleotide (AICAR), endurobol, irisin, resveratrol, (–)epicatechin) that can duplicate many of the physiological effects of exercise without actually doing any. PGC-1α (peroxisome proliferator-activated receptor γ coactivator 1α) is a master transcriptional coactivator regulating oxidative metabolism in skeletal muscle [66, 67]. Many of these 'exercise mimetics" can activate PGC-1α. Moreover, research is progressing into dietary modifications that can stimulate PGC-1α [68]. One paper showed that PGC-1α mRNA was increased in rat gastrocnemius muscle using PBM ($3.75 J/cm^2$ of 810 nm). It is highly likely that in some circumstances PBM can be considered to act like an "exercise mimetic", but further work is needed to fully corroborate this hypothesis.

AICAR can activate adenosine monophosphate (AMP)-activated kinase (AMPK) and was shown to improve exercise performance (running endurance of untrained mice) by 45 % [69]. AMPK acts as an "energy sensor" and constitutes an important regulator of cellular metabolism. It is activated in states of ATP depletion such as excessive training, hypoxia/ischemia, heat stress and starvation [70]. Activation of AMPK leads to processes that inhibit ATP consumption, such as gluconeogenesis in the liver and fatty acid release in liver and adipose cells. A recent study [71] found that AMPK activation can promote mitochondrial biogenesis by phosphorylating the epigenetic factors DNMT1, RBBP7 and HAT1, leading to increased expression of PGC-1α, transcription factor A (Tfam) and uncoupling proteins 2 and 3 (UCP2 and UCP3). Zhang et al. showed that PBM (810 nm, $3 J/cm^2$) could promote mitochondrial biogenesis in megakayrocytes (MKs) [72]. Four hours after PBM there was upregulation of PGC-1α followed by increases in Tfam, dynamin-related protein (Drp1), mitochondrial fission 1 protein (Fis1) and mitochondrial fission factor (Mff). The role of PGC-1α was confirmed by the finding that PBM on MKs sorted from PGC-1α +/– heterozygous transgenic mice produced only a 10 % rise in mitochondrial mass, while wild-type MKs showed an 87 % increase in mitochondrial mass.

Interestingly, another compound that has been shown to act (at least partly) by activation of AMPK and PGC-1α is the TRPV1 ion channel agonist capsaicin (CAP) [73]. CAP has been shown to increase mitochondrial biogenesis [74], and in addition dietary supplementation reduces physical fatigue and improves exercise performance in mice [75]. We have previously shown that PBM can activate TRPV1 channels in a similar manner to capsaicin [76, 77].

Animal experiments have shown that exercise and PBM combine very well together. Aquino and colleagues reported that PBM combined with swimming exercise improved the lipid profiles in rats fed a high-fat high-cholesterol diet better than either PBM or exercise alone [78].

PBM can clearly function as a performance-enhancing intervention in athletic activity, and to enhance response to sports training regimens [79, 80]. This has been shown in individual athletes (for instance an elite runner [81]) and in sports teams such as a volleyball team in a National Championship in Brazil [82]. However, since at present there is no conceivable biochemical assay for having exposed oneself to light, it cannot be outlawed by the World Anti-Doping Agency (WADA).

SYSTEMIC EFFECTS OF PHOTOBIOMODULATION

Another important question that remains to be settled is the degree to which PBMT is a localized therapy, and to what extent it has systemic effects. In other words, does the principal therapeutic response happen in the tissue that receives the light? However, multiple publications report substantial systemic effects of PBMT, both in experimental animals and in humans. One example is from the Mitrofanis laboratory where they studied transcranial PBM for Parkinson's disease in mouse models [83]. Having established the effectiveness of shining light on the head, they proceeded to cover up the head with aluminum foil and shine light on the rest of the mouse body [84]. There was still a significant benefit on the brain (although not as pronounced as transcranial light delivery). They called this phenomenon an "abscopal neuroprotective effect". Another example is from a human clinical trial of wound healing [85]. These workers carried out a randomized, triple-blind, placebo-controlled trial with 22 healthy subjects who received a partial thickness abrasion on each forearm. They received either real or sham PBM to one of the two wounds. At days 6, 8 and 10 the real PBM group had smaller wounds than the sham group for both the treated and the untreated wounds ($P < .05$). A third example is the growing popularity of intravenous laser therapy [67, 86, 87]. Conditions treated include type 2 diabetes, fibromyalgia/chronic pain and shoulder pain. It has emerged that many of the mechanistic pathways for mediating the biological effects of PBM do in fact involve ROS. This came as somewhat of a surprise originally, as many people believed that ROS and oxidative stress were entirely harmful. However, the prevailing view on the merits of limited levels of ROS and brief bouts of oxidative stress has changed away from a black and white dogma [88, 89]. Now it is accepted that ROS can have both good and bad sides depending on the magnitude and duration [55].

EFFECTS OF PHOTOBIOMODULATION ON STEM CELLS

PBM has been widely studied in connection with stem cells [90]. It has been shown that shining light on the legs (for instance) in order to irradiate the bone marrow can have remarkable effects. Damage sustained after a heart attack [91] or ischemic kidney injury [92], and defects in memory and spatial learning in Alzheimer's disease [93], all in experimental animal models, can be ameliorated by PBM delivered to the bone marrow. PBM delivered to the bone marrow can improve thrombocytopenia caused by gamma-irradiation [72] or by immune-mediated platelet destruction [94] in mouse models.

EFFECTS OF PHOTOBIOMODULATION ON INFLAMMATION

Although it is widely known that PBM has a pronounced anti-inflammatory effect, the situation is not exactly as simple as that. As we see below, in normal cells that have not been activated by any inflammatory stimulus, PBM can have what appears to be a brief pro-inflammatory effect. In fact, this observation also appears to apply to clinical PBM treatments, where practitioners have observed that sometimes the inflammation seems to get worse in the short-term before it gets better.

PBM ACTIVATES NF-κB IN NORMAL CELLS

As mentioned above we found [44] that PBM ($3 J/cm^2$ of 810 nm laser) activated NF-kB in embryonic fibroblasts isolated from mice that had been genetically engineered to express firefly luciferase under control of an NF-kB promoter. Although it is well-known that NF-kB functions as a pro-inflammatory transcription factor, it is also well known that in clinical practice or in laboratory animal studies PBM has a profound anti-inflammatory effect in vivo. This gives rise to another apparent contradiction that must be satisfactorily resolved.

PBM Reduces Levels of Pro-inflammatory Cytokines in Activated Inflammatory Cells

Part of the answer to the apparent contradiction highlighted above was addressed in a subsequent paper [95]. We isolated primary bone marrow-derived dendritic cells (DCs) from the mouse femur and cultured them with GM-CSF. When these cells were activated with the classical toll-like receptor (TLR) agonists, LPS (TLR4) and CpG oligodeoxynucleotide (TLR9), they showed upregulation of cell-surface markers of activation and maturation such as MHC class II, CD86 and CD11c as measured by flow cytometry. Moreover, IL12 was secreted by CpG-stimulated DCs. PBM (0.3 or 3 J/cm² of 810 nm laser) reduced all the markers of activation and also the IL12 secretion (Figure 6.7).

Yamaura et al. [96] tested PBM (810 nm, 5 or 25 J/cm²) on synoviocytes isolated from rheumatoid arthritis patients. They applied PBM before or after addition of tumor necrosis factor-α (TNF-α). mRNA and protein levels of TNF-α and interleukins (IL)-1beta and IL-8 were reduced (especially by 25 J/cm²).

Hwang et al. [97] incubated human annulus fibrosus cells with conditioned medium obtained from macrophages (THP-1 cells) containing proinflammatory cytokines IL1β, IL6, IL8 and TNF-α. They compared 405, 532 and 650 nm at doses up to 1.6 J/cm². They found that all wavelengths reduced IL8 expression and 405 nm also reduced IL6.

The "Super-Lizer" is a Japanese device that emits linear polarized infrared light. Imaoka et al. [98] tested it against a rat model of rheumatoid arthritis involving immunizing the rats with bovine type II collagen, after which they develop autoimmune inflammation in multiple joints. The found reductions in IL20 expression in histological sections taken from the PBM-treated joints and also in human rheumatoid fibroblast-like synoviocyte (MH7A) stimulated with IL1β.

Lim et al. [99] studied HGF treated with lipopolysaccharides (LPS) isolated from *Porphyromonas gingivalis*. They used PBM mediated by a 635 nm LED and irradiated the cells + LPS directly or indirectly (transferring medium from PBM treated cells to other cells with LPS). Both direct and indirect protocols showed reductions in inflammatory markers (cyclooxygenase-2 (COX2), prostaglandin E2 (PGE2), granulocyte colony-stimulating factor (G-CSF), regulated on activated normal T-cell expressed and secreted (RANTES), and CXCL11). In the indirect irradiation group, phosphorylation of C-Raf and Erk1/2 increased. In another study [100] the same group used a similar system (direct PBM on HGF + LPS) and showed that 635 nm PBM reduced IL6, IL8, p38 phosphorylation and increased JNK phosphorylation. They explained the activation of JNK by the growth promoting effects of PBM. Sakurai et al. reported [101] similar findings using HGF treated with *Campylobacter rectus* LPS and PBM (830 nm up to 6.3 J/cm²) to reduce levels of COX2 and PGE2. In another study [102] the same group showed a reduction in IL1β in the same system.

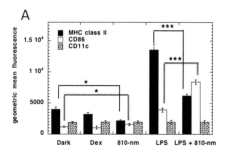
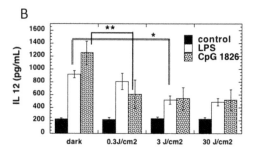

FIGURE 6.7 PBM reduces inflammatory markers in activated murine DCs in vitro. (A) Flow cytometry was used to measure MHC class II, CD86, CD11c (dexamethasone was used as positive control); (B) secreted IL12 measured by ELISA. (Adapted from data in Chen, A.C., et al., *Photomed Laser Surg*, 29(6), 383–389, 2011.)

EFFECTS OF PBM ON MACROPHAGE PHENOTYPE

Another very interesting property of PBM is its ability to change the phenotype of activated cells of the monocyte or macrophage lineage. These cells can display two very different phenotypes depending on which pathological situation the cells are faced with. The M1 phenotype (classically activated) applies to macrophages that are faced with a situation in which bacteria or other pathogens need to be killed, or alternatively tumor cells need to be destroyed. Inducible nitric oxide synthase is a hallmark of the M1 phenotype and nitric oxide secretion is often measured. On the other hand, the M2 phenotype (alternatively activated) applies to macrophages that are involved in disposal of cellular or protein debris and stimulation of healing by angiogenesis. The M2 phenotype produces arginase, an enzyme that inhibits NO production and allows them to produce ornithine, a precursor of hydroxyproline and polyamines [103]. The markers of these two phenotypes of activated macrophage have some aspects in common, but also show many aspects that are very different [104]. It should be noted that this concept of M1 and M2 activation states, applies to other specialized macrophage type cells that are resident in different tissues, such as microglia in brain [105], alveolar macrophages in lung [106], Kuppfer cells in liver [107] etc.

Fernandes et al. used J774 macrophage-like cells activated with interferon-γ and LPS to produce a MI phenotype and compared 660 and 780 nm laser. They found that both wavelengths reduced TNF-α, COX-2 and iNOS expression, with the 780 nm being somewhat better [108]. Silva et al. used RAW264.7 macrophages to test two wavelengths (660 and 808 nm) at a range of fluences (11–214 J/cm^2) [109]. They found increases in NO release with 660 nm at the higher fluences. von Leden et al. carried out an interesting study looking at the effects of PBM on microglia and their interaction with cortical neurons [110]. They used both primary microglia isolated from mouse brains and the BV2 mouse microglial cell line and compared four fluences (0.2, 4, 10, and 30 J/cm^2, at 808 nm). Fluences between 4 and 30 J/cm^2 induced expression of M1 markers in microglia. Markers of the M2 phenotype, including CD206 and TIMP1, were observed at lower energy densities of 0.2–10 J/cm^2. In addition, co-culture of PBM or control-treated microglia with primary neuronal cultures demonstrated a dose-dependent effect of PBM on microglial-induced neuronal growth and neurite extension. This suggests that the benefits of PBM on neuroinflammation may be more pronounced at lower overall doses.

EFFECT OF PBM ON AUTOIMMUNE DISEASES AND T-CELLS

PBM has been extensively used to treat autoimmune diseases, both in experimental animals and in humans. Lyons and her team have published several papers looking at the effects of PBM a mouse model of multiple sclerosis called experimental autoimmune encephalomyelitis (EAE). EAE is the most commonly studied animal model of multiple sclerosis (MS), a chronic autoimmune demyelinating disorder of the central nervous system. Immunomodulatory and immunosuppressive therapies currently approved for the treatment of MS slow disease progression, but do not prevent it. Lyons et al. [111] studied a mouse model of EAE involving immunization with myelin oligodendrocyte glycoprotein (MOG35-55). They treated the female C57BL/6 mice with PBM (670 nm) for several days in different regimens. In addition to improved muscular function, they found downregulation of inducible nitric oxide synthase (iNOS) gene expression in the spinal cords of mice as well as an upregulation of the Bcl-2 anti-apoptosis gene, an increased Bcl-2: Bax ratio and reduced apoptosis within the spinal cord of animals over the course of disease. 670 nm light therapy failed to ameliorate MOG-induced EAE in mice deficient in iNOS, confirming a role for remediation of nitrosative stress in the amelioration of MOG-induced EAE by 670 nm mediated photobiomodulation.

The most studied human application of PBM for autoimmune disease was by Chavantes and Chammas in Brazil who studied PBM for chronic autoimmune thyroiditis. An initial pilot trial [112] used 10 applications of PBM (830 nm, 50 mW, 38–108 J/cm^2) twice a week, using either the punctual technique (8 patients) or the sweep technique (7 patients). Patients required a lower dosage of levothyroxine and showed an increased echogenicity by ultrasound. The next study [113] was a randomized, placebo-controlled trial of 43 patients with a 9-month follow-up. In addition to improved thyroid function they found reduced autoimmunity evidenced by lower thyroid peroxidase antibodies (TPOAb) and thyroglobulin antibodies (TgAb). A third study [114] used color Doppler ultrasound to show improved normal vascualrization in the thyroid parenchyma. Finally, [115] they showed a statistically significant increase in serum TGF-β1 levels 30 days post-intervention in the PBM group, thus confirming the anti-inflammatory effect.

PBM AND TRAUMATIC BRAIN INJURY

Perhaps one of the most exciting applications of PBM is its effects on the brain. The first applications were for acute stroke, but then its use spread to acute and chronic TBI, neurodegenerative diseases (dementia, Alzheimer's and Parkinson's) and to a range of psychiatric disorders. Given the clinical frequency with which traumatic brain injury (TBI) accompanies orthopedic conditions, photobiomodulation's effects on the brain are presented here.

There have been a number of studies looking at the effects of PBM in animal models of TBI. Oron's group was the first [116] to demonstrate that a single exposure of the mouse head to a NIR laser (808 nm) a few hours after creation of a TBI lesion could improve neurological performance and reduce the size of the brain lesion. A weight-drop device was used to induce a closed-head injury in the mice. An 808 nm diode laser with two energy densities (1.2–2.4 J/cm^2 over 2 minutes of irradiation with 10 and 20 mW/cm^2) was delivered to the head 4 hours after TBI was induced. Neurobehavioral function was assessed by the neurological severity score (NSS). There were no significant difference in NSS between the power densities (10 vs 20 mW/cm^2) or significant differentiation between the control and laser treated group at early time points (24 and 48 hours) post TBI. However, there was a significant improvement (27 % lower NSS score) in the PBM group at times of 5 days to 4 weeks. The laser treated group also showed a smaller loss of cortical tissue than the sham group [116].

Hamblin's laboratory then went on (in a series of papers [116]) to show that 810 nm laser (and 660 nm laser) could benefit experimental TBI both in a closed head weight drop model [117], and also in controlled cortical impact model in mice [118]. Wu et al. [117] explored the effect that varying the laser wavelengths of LLLT had on closed-head TBI in mice. Mice were randomly assigned to LLLT treated group or to sham group as a control. Closed-head injury (CHI) was induced via a weight drop apparatus. To analyze the severity of the TBI, the neurological severity score (NSS) was measured and recorded. The injured mice were then treated with varying wavelengths of laser (665, 730, 810 or 980 nm) at an energy level of 36 J/cm^2 at 4 hours directed onto the scalp. The 665 and 810 nm groups showed significant improvement in NSS when compared to the control group at day 5–28. Results are shown in Figure 6.8. Conversely, the 730 and 980 nm groups did not show a significant improvement in NSS and these wavelengths did not produce similar beneficial effects as in the 665 and 810 nm LLLT groups [117]. The tissue chromophore cytochrome c oxidase (CCO) is proposed to be responsible for the underlying mechanism that produces the many PBM effects that are the byproduct of LLLT. COO has absorption bands around 665 and 810 nm while it has low absorption bands at the wavelength of 730 nm [119]. It should be noted that this particular study found that the 980 nm did not produce the same positive effects as the 665 and 810 nm wavelengths did; nevertheless, previous studies did find that the 980 nm wavelength was an active one for LLLT. Wu et al. proposed these dissimilar results may be due to the variance in the energy level, irradiance etc. between the other studies and this particular study [117].

Ando et al. [118] used the 810 nm wavelength laser parameters from the previous study and varied the pulse modes of the laser in a mouse model of TBI. These modes consisted of either pulsed wave at 10 Hz or at 100 Hz (50 % duty cycle) or continuous wave laser. For the mice, TBI was induced with a controlled cortical impact device via open craniotomy. A single treatment with an 810 nm Ga-Al-As diode laser with a power density of 50 mW/m^2 and an energy density of 36 J/cm^2

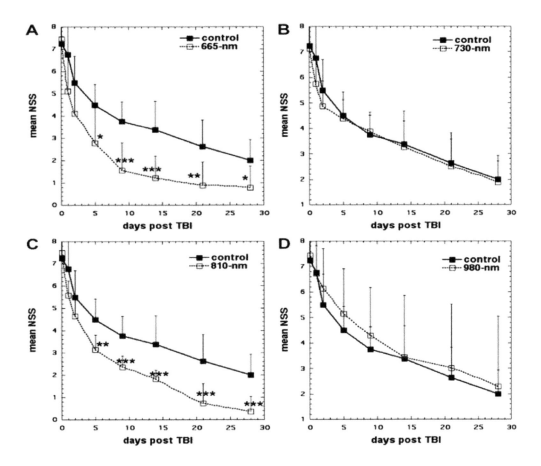

FIGURE 6.8 Effect of different laser wavelengths of tPBM in closed-head TBI in mice. (A) Sham-treated control versus 665 nm laser. (B) Sham-treated control versus 730 nm laser. (C) Sham-treated control versus 810 nm laser. (D) Sham-treated control versus 980 nm laser. Points are means of 8 to 12 mice and bars are SD. *$P < 0.05$; **$P < 0.01$; ***$P < 0.001$ (one-way ANOVA). (Reprinted with permission from Wu, Q., et al., *Lasers Surg Med*, 44, 218–226, 2012 [170].)

was given via tPBM to the closed head in mice for a duration of 12 minutes at 4 hours post CCI. At forty-8 hours to 28 days post TBI, all laser treated groups had significant decreases in the measured neurological severity score (NSS) when compared to the control (Figure 6.9A). Although all laser treated groups had similar NSS improvement rates up to day 7, the PW 10 Hz group began to show greater improvement beyond this point as seen in Figure 6.4. At day 28, the forced swim test for depression and anxiety was used and showed a significant decrease in the immobility time for the PW 10 Hz group. In the tail suspension test which measures depression and anxiety, there was also a significant decrease in the immobility time at day 28, and this time also at day 1, in the PW 10 Hz group.

Studies using immunofluorescence of mouse brains showed that tPBM increased neuroprogenitor cells in the dentate gyrus (DG) and subventricular zone at 7 days after the treatment [120]. The neurotrophin called brain derived neurotrophic factor (BDNF) was also increased in the DG and SVZ at 7 days, while the marker (synapsin-1) for synaptogenesis and neuroplasticity was increased in the cortex at 28 days but not in the DG, SVZ or at 7 days [121] (Figure 6.9B). Learning and memory as measured by the Morris water maze was also improved by tPBM [122]. Whalen's laboratory [123] and Whelan's laboratory [124] also successfully demonstrated therapeutic benefits of tPBM for TBI in mice and rats respectively.

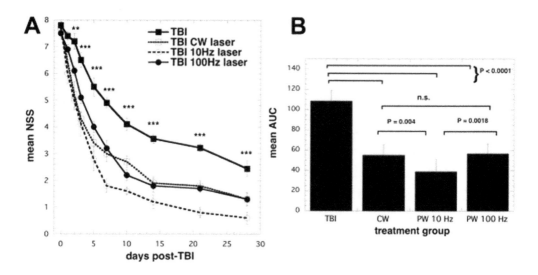

FIGURE 6.9 Effects of pulsing in tPBM for CCI-TBI in mice. (A) Time course of neurological severity score (NSS) of mice with TBI receiving either control (no laser-treatment), or 810 nm laser (36 J/cm² delivered at 50 mW/cm² with a spot size of 0.78 cm² in either CW, PW 10 Hz or PW 100 Hz modes. Results are expressed as mean +/– S.E.M ***$P < 0.001$ vs. the other conditions. (B) Mean areas under the NSS-time curves in the two-dimensional coordinate system over the 28–day study for the four groups of mice. Results are means +/– SD ($n = 10$). (Reprinted from Ando, T., et al., *PLoS ONE*, 6(10), e26212–e26220, 2011. [171] (open access).)

Zhang et al. [125] showed that secondary brain injury occurred to a worse degree in mice that had been genetically engineered to lack "Immediate Early Response" gene X-1 (IEX-1) when exposed to a gentle head impact (this injury is thought to closely resemble mild TBI in humans). Exposing IEX-1 knockout mice to PBM 4 hours post injury, suppressed proinflammatory cytokine expression of interleukin (IL)-Iβ and IL-6, but upregulated TNF-α. The lack of IEX-1 decreased ATP production, but exposing the injured brain to PBM elevated ATP production back to near normal levels.

Dong et al. [126] even further improved the beneficial effects of PBM on TBI in mice, by combining the treatment with metabolic substrates such as pyruvate and/or lactate. The goal was to even further improve mitochondrial function. This combinatorial treatment was able to reverse memory and learning deficits in TBI mice back to normal levels, as well as leaving the hippocampal region completely protected from tissue loss; a stark contrast to that found in control TBI mice that exhibited severe tissue loss from secondary brain injury.

Margaret Naeser and collaborators have tested PBM in human subjects who had suffered TBI in the past [127]. Many sufferers from severe or even moderate TBI have very long-lasting and even life-changing sequelae (headaches, cognitive impairment and difficulty sleeping) that prevent them working or living any kind or normal life. These individuals may have been high achievers before the accident that caused damage to their brain [128]. Initially, Naeser published a report [129] describing two cases she treated with PBM applied to the forehead twice a week. A 500 mW continuous wave LED source (mixture of 660 nm red and 830 nm NIR LEDs) with a power density of 22.2 mW/cm² (area of 22.48 cm²) was applied to the forehead for a typical duration of 10 minutes (13.3 J/cm²). In the first case study the patient reported that she could concentrate on tasks for a longer period of time (the time able to work at a computer increased from 30 minutes to 3 hours). She had a better ability to remember what she read, decreased sensitivity when receiving haircuts in the spots where PBM was applied and improved mathematical skills after undergoing PBM. The second patient had statistically significant improvements compared to prior neuropsychological tests after 9 months of treatment. The patient had a two standard deviation (SD) increase on tests of inhibition and inhibition accuracy (9th percentile to 63rd percentile on the Stroop test for executive function and a one SD increase on the Wechsler Memory scale test for the logical memory test (83rd percentile to 99th percentile) [130].

Naeser et al. then went on to report a case series of a further 11 patients [131]. This was an open protocol study that examined whether scalp application of red and near infrared (NIR) light could improve cognition in patients with chronic, mild traumatic brain injury (mTBI). This study had 11 participants ranging in age from 26 to 62 (6 males, 5 females) who suffered from persistent cognitive dysfunction after mTBI. The participants' injuries were caused by motor vehicle accidents, sports-related events and, for 1 participant, an improvised explosive device (IED) blast. tPBM consisted of 18 sessions (Monday, Wednesday and Friday for 6 weeks) and commenced anywhere from 10 months to 8 years post-TBI. A total of 11 LED clusters (5.25 cm in diameter, 500 mW, 22.2 mW/cm^2, 13 J/cm^2) were applied for about 10 minutes per session (five or six LED placements per set, Set A and then Set B, in each session). Neuropsychological testing was performed pre-LED application and 1 week, 1 month and 2 months after the final treatment. Naeser and colleagues found that there was a significant positive linear trend observed for the Stroop Test for executive function, in trial 2 inhibition ($P = 0.004$); Stroop, trial 4 inhibition switching ($P = 0.003$); California Verbal Learning Test (CVLT)-II, total trials 1–5 ($P = 0.003$); CVLT-II, long delay free recall ($P = 0.006$). Improved sleep and fewer post-traumatic stress disorder (PTSD) symptoms, if present beforehand, were observed after treatment. Participants and family members also reported better social function and a better ability to perform interpersonal and occupational activities. Although these results were significant, further placebo-controlled studies will be needed to ensure the reliability of this these data [131].

Henderson and Morries [132] used a high-power NIR laser (10–15 W at 810 and 980 nm) applied to the head to treat a patient with moderate TBI. The patient received 20 NIR applications over a 2-month period. They carried out anatomical magnetic resonance imaging (MRI) and perfusion single-photon emission computed tomography (SPECT). The patient showed decreased depression, anxiety, headache and insomnia, whereas cognition and quality of life improved, accompanied by changes in the SPECT imaging.

PBM AND PAIN

PBM is often used clinically to treat pain. Very often this is pain resulting from some orthopedic disorder such as tendonitis, arthritis, traumatic joint injuries etc. [133].

LOCAL INFLAMMATORY PAIN

Several animal models have been used to test PBM for inflammatory pain. For instance injection of Complete Freund's Adjuvant (CFA) into the footpad of mice caused hyperalgesia to mechanical stimulus and heat. Application of PBM using 950 nm LEDs inhibited both types of hyperalgesia and increased the levels of IL-10. PBM abrogated the increase in TBARS and increased levels of both catalase (CAT) and superoxide dismutase (SOD). Pre-administration of naloxone or fucoidin prevented the analgesic effect of PBM [134].

Another application of PBM for inflammatory pain is concerned with the treatment of snake evenomation. A bite from a *Bothrops moojeni* viper causes systemic coagulopathy, severe local tissue damage including edema, hemorrhage, intense pain, and myonecrosis. A study in mice [135] tested PBM using a 685 nm laser (combined or not with antivenom) on the local pathological alterations induced by *B. moojeni* snake venom. PBM improved the pain as measured by the time (in seconds) spent in licking and biting the injected paw. Inflammatory infiltration was reduced histologically, phagocytosis was stimulated, myoblast proliferation and regeneration of muscle fibers was increased. Another study showed similar results with *B. moojeni* venom injected into the mouse gastrocnemius muscle and treated with 904 nm laser [136].

LOCAL NEUROPATHIC PAIN

A systematic review [137] analyzed 44 studies. In 13 of 18 human studies, pulsed or CW visible and CW NIR PBM slowed conduction velocity (CV) and/or reduced the amplitude of compound action potentials (CAPs). In 26 animal experiments, NIR PBM suppressed electrically and noxiously evoked action potentials including pro-inflammatory mediators. Disruption of microtubule arrays and fast axonal flow may underpin neural inhibition. In chronic pain, spinal cord changes induced by PBM may result in long-term depression of pain.

Anders and colleagues used a rat model of "spared nerve injury" (SNI) to test PBM [138]. The SNI model recapitulates peripheral neuropathic pain by partial denervation of the sciatic nerve by lesioning the tibial and common peroneal nerve branches, leaving the remaining sural nerve intact [139]. PBM (980 nm) was applied to the affected hind paw (output power 1 W, 20 s, 41 cm above skin, power density 43 mW/cm^2, dose 20 J), dorsal root ganglia and spinal cord regions every other day from day 7 to 30 post-operatively. The untreated but injured groups demonstrated mechanical hypersensitivity 1 to 30 days post-operatively. PBM-treated animals began to recover after two treatments, and at day 26, mechanical sensitivity returned to baseline.

Clinically, PBM has been used to treat diabetic-related polyneuropathy related pain [140], postherpetic neuralgia [141], neck pain (cervical radiculopathy) [142] and trigeminal neuralgia [143].

CENTRAL PAIN

Although there has not been a lot of clinical work on central pain sensitization, the ability of PBM to increase neuroplasticity suggests that it may have beneficial effects. de Sousa et al. [144] carried out a study of PBM on pain sensitivity in mice measured by stimulation of the footpad by von Frey filaments. They found that not only did delivering NIR light to the footpad decrease the sensitivity to pain, but also that applying the light to the lower back (dorsal root ganglion), the neck or the head was also effective. The maximum effect was found at 3 hours post-PBM. Hence it was proposed that PBM applied to the head can alter the pain pathways in the CNS and the brain.

PBM IN ORTHOPEDICS

ARTHRITIS

One in every two persons in US will experience some form of osteoarthritis in their lifetime and the incidence is 80 % in those over 75 [145]. Treatment is with analgesics (acetaminophen), non-steroidal anti-inflammatory drugs (NSAIDS, ibuprofen and diclofenac) and COX2 inhibitors (Celebrex), but these therapies have significant risks of adverse effects such as gastrointestinal bleeding with NSAIDs, and myocardial infarction with COX2 inhibitors [146]. PBM has been used clinically in osteoarthritis for many years but is still considered controversial. Although a Cochrane review [147] reported mixed and conflicting results, a subsequent analysis conducted by Bjordal et al. [148] concluded: "The Cochrane review conclusion was neither robust nor valid. Further sensitivity analyses with inclusion of valid non-included trials, performance of missing follow-up, and subgroup analyses revealed consistent and highly significant results in favor of active PBM for osteoarthritis." This disagreement existing in the literature suggests that much more work comprising animal studies, clinical trials and systematic reviews will need to be done before PBM becomes accepted as a valid therapy for arthritis.

Alves et al. [149] used a clinically relevant model of osteoarthritis in which the proteolytic enzyme papain is injected into the rat knee joint where it degrades the cartilage thus causing inflammation. The knees received a single application of 4J of energy from a 808 nm laser to the medial and lateral aspects of the knee delivered either at 50 mW or 100 mW and the rats were sacrificed after 24 hours. They found a significant reduction in inflammatory cells in fluid from synovial washing with both power levels but a bigger reduction in macrophages at the 50 mW power level. Reductions in interleukin (IL)-1beta and IL6 mRNA were found with 50 mW being better than

100 mW, while a bigger reduction in TNF alpha was seen with 100 mW. The authors hypothesized that the twice longer illumination time needed to deliver the same energy at half the power may have been responsible for the better effect of the 50 mW laser application, which agrees with a previous study that examined zymosan-induced arthritis in the rat knee [150] and found that a longer illumination time was more effective. Previous work from this group [151] had also shown that PBM in the same model increased angiogenesis and the amount of squamous epithelium while decreasing fibrosis in the joint. These results provide additional justification for the use of PBM (especially near-infrared laser that has the good penetration into tissue required for joints) as a treatment for osteoarthritis. Nevertheless, it should be pointed out that the study was only an animal model, not a clinical study in human disease and further studies will be necessary to define the benefits of PBM in osteoarthritis. In addition to the demonstrated anti-inflammatory effects, PBM may have additional benefits provided by its ability to act on nerves by reducing pain transmission and activating endogenous opioid receptors [152].

Lower Back Pain

Lower back pain (LBP) is a common disorder involving the muscles, nerves and bones of the back. The sensation can vary from a dull constant ache to a sudden sharp pain. LBP can be classified by its duration into: acute (pain lasting less than 6 weeks), sub-chronic (6 to 12 weeks) or chronic (more than 12 weeks). LBP may be further classified according to the underlying cause as either, mechanical, non-mechanical or referred pain. In most episodes of LBP, a specific underlying cause is not identified or even looked for, with the pain believed to be due to mechanical problems such as muscle or joint strain. The symptoms of LBP usually improve within a few weeks from the time they start, with 40–90 % of people completely recovered by 6 weeks. Despite this sufferers from chronic LBP are often desperate for relief having failed to find it with paracetamol NSAIDs and muscle relaxants.

PBM has been investigated for chronic LBP [153]. Glazov et al. published a systematic review of 15 studies including 1,039 participants. There was an overall significant reduction in pain with a weighted mean difference −1.40 cm (95 % CI −1.91 to −0.88 cm) in favor of PBM when patients with baseline pain < 30 months treated with at least 3 Joules (J) per point. Global assessment showed a risk ratio of 2.16 (95 % CI 1.61–2.90) in favor of PBM in the same groups at immediate follow-up. Another systematic review [154] by Huang et al. looked at 221 studies including seven RCTs (one triple-blind, four double-blind, one single-blind, one not mentioning blinding, totaling 394 patients) met the criteria for inclusion. Based on five studies, the WMD in visual analog scale (VAS) pain outcome score after treatment was significantly lower in the PBM group compared with placebo (WMD = −13.57 [95 % CI = −17.42, −9.72], I(2) = 0 %). No significant treatment effect was identified for disability scores or spinal range of motion outcomes.

Tendonitis

Bjordal et al. in Norway carried out a randomized, placebo-controlled trial of PBM (904 nm, 5.4 J per point, 20 mW/cm^2) for activated Achilles tendinitis [155]. In addition to clinical assessment, they used microdialysis measurement of peritendinous prostaglandin E2 concentrations. Doppler ultrasonography measurements at baseline showed minor inflammation shown by increased intratendinous blood flow and a measurable resistive index. PGE2 concentrations were significantly reduced with PBM vs. placebo. The pressure pain threshold also increased significantly. A systematic review by Nogueira [156] analyzed three studies and concluded that the use of PBM, compared to placebo, was consistently effective in treatment of tendinopathy.

Muscles

PBM for muscles aims to benefit athletic performance and training, to reduce delayed onset muscle soreness (DOMS), as well as to ameliorate signs of muscle damage (creatine kinase) after intense or prolonged exercise. Moreover, PBM can also be used to treat frank muscle damage caused by muscle strains or trauma. The International Olympic Committee and the World Anti-Doping Agency cannot ban light therapy for athletes considering (1) the intensity is similar to sunlight, and (2) there is no forensic test for light exposure. There have been several clinical trials carried out in Brazil in athletes such as elite runners [81], volleyball players [82] and rugby players [157]. Ferraresi et al. conducted a case-controlled study in a pair of identical twins [158]. They used a flexible LED array (850 nm, 75J, 15 sec) applied to both quadriceps femoris muscles (real to one twin and sham to the other) immediately after each strength training session (3 times/week for 12 weeks) consisting of leg press and leg extension exercises with load of 80 % and 50 % of the one-repetition maximum test, respectively. PBM increased the maximal load in exercise and reduced fatigue, creatine kinase and visual analog scale (DOMS) compared to sham. Muscle biopsies were taken before and after the training program and showed that PBM decreased inflammatory markers such as interleukin 1β and muscle atrophy (myostatin). Protein synthesis (mammalian target of rapamycin) and oxidative stress defense (SOD2, mitochondrial superoxide dismutase) were upregulated.

BONES

Due to the long-standing ability of PBM to improve wound healing, it has been used to treat problems with bones. The ability of PBM to stimulate mesenchymal stem cells, and in particular the osteogenic differentiation with upregulation of osteogenic markers [77]. These conditions have included bone defects that have been repaired with various kinds of bone graft and composite materials such as biosilicate [159, 160] and non-healing fractures [161]. Dentists and oral surgeons have often used PBM in applications such as: for orthodontic tooth movement into bone-grafted alveolar defects [162], new bone formation around implants [163] and bone consolidation in the period following mandibular distraction osteogenesis [164].

ELBOW

Lateral epicondylitis (LE, commonly known as tennis elbow) is a condition in which the forearm muscles and tendons become damaged from repetitive overuse. This leads to pain and tenderness on the outside of the elbow. Emanet et al. conducted a randomized trial of PBM (904 nm laser) with 49 patients (50 elbows) with 25 elbows receiving real and 25 getting placebo PBM 5 days/week for 3 weeks [165]. Although there was no difference between the groups immediately after the course of treatment, at 12 weeks the PBM group had significant improvements in visual analog scale, tenderness, Disability of the Arm Shoulder and Hand (DASH) questionnaire, the Patient-Related Lateral Epicondylitis Evaluation (PRTEE) test, pain-free grip strength and the Nottingham Health Profile (NHP) questionnaire.

Lam and Cheing also carried out a trial [166] of PBM using 904-nm laser in 39 patients with LE with an energy dose of 0.275 J per tender point (laser group) or sham irradiation (placebo group) for a total of 9 sessions. Significantly improvements were shown in all outcome measures with the laser group than with the placebo group ($P < 0.0125$), except in the two subsections of DASH.

SHOULDER

The effect of PBM on shoulder myofascial pain syndrome was tested in a randomized trial conducted by Rayegani et al. [167]. Sixty-three patients (46 females, 17 males; age range: 17–55 years old) were divided into groups receiving laser therapy, ultrasound and sham laser. PBM was effective in improving VAS pain scores during activity (54 %), at night (51 %) and at rest (51 %) and also improved Neck Disability Index (NDI) scores (73 %). Ultrasound was also effective, but PBM resulted in a higher NDI score and improvements in algometric assessment compared to ultrasound ($P < 0.05$).

Subacromial impingement syndrome is another shoulder disorder where the effects of PBM and ultrasound were compared by Yavuz et al. [168]. Thirty-one patients were randomly assigned to PBM ($n = 16$) and ultrasound ($n = 15$). Study participants received 10 treatment sessions over a consecutive period of 2 weeks (5 days per week). Outcome measures (visual analogue pain scale, Shoulder Pain and Disability Index, SPADI, patient's satisfaction level and sleep interference score) were assessed before treatment and at the first and third months after treatment. All patients were analyzed using the intent-to-treat principle. Mean reduction in VAS pain, SPADI disability and sleep interference scores from baseline to after 1 month and 3 months of treatment was statistically significant in both groups ($P < 0.05$). However, there was no significant difference in the mean change in VAS pain, SPADI disability and sleep interference scores between the two groups ($P > 0.05$). The mean level of patient satisfaction in group 1 at the first and third months after treatment was 72.45 ± 23.45 mm and 71.50 ± 16.54 mm, respectively. The mean level of patient satisfaction in group 2 at the first and third months after treatment was 70.38 ± 21.52 mm and 72.09 ± 13.42 mm, respectively. There was no significant difference in the mean level of patient satisfaction between the two groups ($P > 0.05$).

Ip and Fu studied elderly patients with painful adhesive capsulitis of the shoulder [169]. Thirty-five unselected elderly patients with mean age of 65 years were treated with PBM. All patients in this prospective cohort study had documentation of the diagnosis by contrast-enhanced magnetic resonance imaging before study entry and had failed to respond to a combination of conventional physical therapy and nonsteroidal anti-inflammatory medications. PBM used an 810 nm GaAIAs laser with 5.4 J per point at 20 mW/cm², on six predetermined anatomic points and two acupuncture points at 3× per week for 8 consecutive weeks. A total of 50 painful shoulder joints were treated, and all but four joints showed significant improvement in Constant-Murley shoulder score at the end of 8 weeks. The improvement was maintained at 1- and 2-year follow-up.

CONCLUSIONS AND FUTURE DIRECTIONS

The knowledge and acceptance of PBM by both the medical profession and the general public has been steadily increasing over the last 10 years. One development that may accelerate this transition into more general acceptance is the rise of popularity of LED devices.

Historically safety and expense limited PBM use. Originally PBM was largely practiced with lasers in keeping with its origins. This involved practitioners such as physical therapists or chiropractors treating a patient with a number of "points" in the area of the injury or other pathology. Safety issues and particularly concerns about eye safety restricted the practice of LLLT to qualified professionals who has undergone a "laser safety training course". Many of the lasers commonly used by these practitioners were, by anybody's calculation, rather expensive. Thousands of US dollars and even over $10,000 was not an unusual price to pay. By contrast with lasers, LED devices are relative inexpensive and considered almost completely safe. With power densities even as high as 100 mW/cm², the intensity of the light is no more than that of sunlight at noon on the equator. The production of commercial LEDs in the Far East has progressed to where these simple semiconductors are considered a commodity. The only challenge to manufacturing a highly effective device with optical power output in the tens of Watts spread over a large surface area of tissue is the dissipation of heat from the diodes. Some more powerful devices are fitted with small silent fans to keep them cool, while others rely on heat sinks to remove the heat. So with LED arrays the era of highly effective home-use devices has finally arrived. All that remains is the implementation of effective educational messages and marketing campaigns to convince the public to buy them. Most devices these days have rechargeable batteries, and many of them have been designed to be wearable for extra ease of use and consumer friendliness.

REFERENCES

1. Hamblin, M.R., M.V. de Sousa, and T. Agrawal, *Handbook of Low Level Laser Therapy.* 2016, Singapore: Pan-Stanford Publishing.
2. McGuff, P.E., R.A. Deterling, Jr., and L.S. Gottlieb, Tumoricidal effect of laser energy on experimental and human malignant tumors. *N Engl J Med*, 1965. 273(9): p. 490–492.
3. McGuff, P.E., et al., The laser treatment of experimental malignant tumours. *Can Med Assoc J*, 1964. 91: p. 1089–1095.
4. Mester, E., T. Spiry, and B. Szende, Effect of laser rays on wound healing. *Bull Soc Int Chir*, 1973. 32(2): p. 169–173.
5. Mester, E., B. Szende, and P. Gartner, The effect of laser beams on the growth of hair in mice. *Radiobiol Radiother (Berl)*, 1968. 9(5): p. 621–626.
6. Hode, L., The importance of the coherency. *Photomed Laser Surg*, 2005. 23(4): p. 431–434.
7. Mester, A., Laser biostimulation. *Photomed Laser Surg*, 2013. 31(6): p. 237–239.
8. Kim, W.S. and R.G. Calderhead, Is light-emitting diode phototherapy (LED-LLLT) really effective? *Laser Ther*, 2011. 20(3): p. 205–215.
9. Anders, J.J., R.J. Lanzafame, and P.R. Arany, Low-level light/laser therapy versus photobiomodulation therapy. *Photomed Laser Surg*, 2015. 33(4): p. 183–184.
10. Huang, Y.Y., et al., Biphasic dose response in low level light therapy. *Dose Response*, 2009. 7(4): p. 358–383.
11. Huang, Y.Y., et al., Biphasic dose response in low level light therapy – an update. *Dose Response*, 2011. 9(4): p. 602–618.
12. Sommer, A.P., et al., Biostimulatory windows in low-intensity laser activation: Lasers, scanners, and NASA's light-emitting diode array system. *J Clin Laser Med Surg*, 2001. 19(1): p. 29–33.
13. Calabrese, E.J., I. Iavicoli, and V. Calabrese, Hormesis: Its impact on medicine and health. *Hum Exp Toxicol*, 2013. 32(2): p. 120–152.
14. Agrawal, T., et al., Pre-conditioning with low-level laser (light) therapy: Light before the storm. *Dose Response*, 2014. 12(4): p. 619–649.
15. Passarella, S. and T. Karu, Absorption of monochromatic and narrow band radiation in the visible and near IR by both mitochondrial and non-mitochondrial photoacceptors results in photobiomodulation. *J Photochem Photobiol B*, 2014. 140: p. 344–358.
16. Beauvoit, B., T. Kitai, and B. Chance, Contribution of the mitochondrial compartment to the optical properties of the rat liver: A theoretical and practical approach. *Biophys J*, 1994. 67(6): p. 2501–2510.
17. Pastore, D., M. Greco, and S. Passarella, Specific helium-neon laser sensitivity of the purified cytochrome c oxidase. *Int J Radiat Biol*, 2000. 76(6): p. 863–870.
18. Karu, T.I. and S.F. Kolyakov, Exact action spectra for cellular responses relevant to phototherapy. *Photomed Laser Surg*, 2005. 23(4): p. 355–361.
19. Wong-Riley, M.T., et al., Photobiomodulation directly benefits primary neurons functionally inactivated by toxins: Role of cytochrome c oxidase. *J Biol Chem*, 2005. 280(6): p. 4761–4771.
20. Sarti, P., et al., Cytochrome c oxidase and nitric oxide in action: Molecular mechanisms and pathophysiological implications. *Biochim Biophys Acta*, 2012. 1817(4): p. 610–619.
21. Lane, N., Cell biology: Power games. *Nature*, 2006. 443(7114): p. 901–903.
22. Minke, B., The history of the Drosophila TRP channel: The birth of a new channel superfamily. *J Neurogenet*, 2010. 24(4): p. 216–233.
23. Hille, B., et al., Phosphoinositides regulate ion channels. *Biochim Biophys Acta*, 2015. 1851(6): p. 844–856.
24. Kim, C., Transient receptor potential ion channels and animal sensation: Lessons from Drosophila functional research. *J Biochem Mol Biol*, 2004. 37(1): p. 114–121.
25. Caterina, M.J. and Z. Pang, TRP channels in skin biology and pathophysiology. *Pharmaceuticals (Basel)*, 2016. 9(4): p. 77. https://doi.org/10.3390/ph9040077.
26. Montell, C., The history of TRP channels, a commentary and reflection. Pflugers Arch, 2011. 461(5): p. 499–506.
27. Ogawa, N., T. Kurokawa, and Y. Mori, Sensing of redox status by TRP channels. *Cell Calcium*, 2016. 60(2): p. 115–122.
28. Smani, T., et al., Functional and physiopathological implications of TRP channels. *Biochim Biophys Acta*, 2015. 1853(8): p. 1772–1782.
29. Cronin, M.A., M.H. Lieu, and S. Tsunoda, Two stages of light-dependent TRPL-channel translocation in Drosophila photoreceptors. *J Cell Sci*, 2006. 119 (Pt 14): p. 2935–2944.

30. Diani-Moore, S., et al., Sunlight generates multiple tryptophan photoproducts eliciting high efficacy CYP1A induction in chick hepatocytes and in vivo. *Toxicol Sci*, 2006. 90(1): p. 96–110.

31. Smirnova, A., et al., Evidence for new light-independent pathways for generation of the endogenous Aryl Hydrocarbon Receptor Agonist FICZ. *Chem Res Toxicol*, 2016. 29(1): p. 75–86.

32. Ulaszewski, S., et al., Light effects in yeast: Evidence for participation of cytochromes in photoinhibition of growth and transport in Saccharomyces cerevisiae cultured at low temperatures. *J Bacteriol*, 1979. 138(2): p. 523–529.

33. Hoang, N., et al., Human and Drosophila cryptochromes are light activated by flavin photoreduction in living cells. *PLoS Biol*, 2008. 6(7): p. e160.

34. Yang, Z., et al., Cryptochromes orchestrate transcription regulation of diverse blue light responses in plants. *Photochem Photobiol*, 2016. 93: p. 112–127.

35. Emery, P., et al., Drosophila CRY is a deep brain circadian photoreceptor. *Neuron*, 2000. 26(2): p. 493–504.

36. Yoshii, T., M. Ahmad, and C. Helfrich-Forster, Cryptochrome mediates light-dependent magnetosensitivity of Drosophila's circadian clock. *PLoS Biol*, 2009. 7(4): p. e1000086.

37. Liu, N. and E.E. Zhang, Phosphorylation regulating the ratio of intracellular CRY1 protein determines the circadian period. *Front Neurol*, 2016. 7: p. 159.

38. Chiou, Y.Y., et al., Mammalian period represses and de-represses transcription by displacing CLOCK-BMAL1 from promoters in a cryptochrome-dependent manner. *Proc Natl Acad Sci U S A*, 2016. 113(41): p. E6072–E6079.

39. Bailes, H.J. and R.J. Lucas, Human melanopsin forms a pigment maximally sensitive to blue light (lambdamax approximately 479 nm) supporting activation of G(q/11) and G(i/o) signalling cascades. *Proc Biol Sci*, 2013. 280(1759): p. 20122987.

40. Poletini, M.O., et al., TRP channels: A missing bond in the entrainment mechanism of peripheral clocks throughout evolution. *Temperature (Austin)*, 2015. 2(4): p. 522–534.

41. Koyanagi, M. and A. Terakita, Diversity of animal opsin-based pigments and their optogenetic potential. *Biochim Biophys Acta*, 2014. 1837(5): p. 710–716.

42. Mainster, M.A., Violet and blue light blocking intraocular lenses: Photoprotection versus photoreception. *Br J Ophthalmol*, 2006. 90(6): p. 784–792.

43. Chen, A.C.-H., et al., Role of reactive oxygen species in low level light therapy. *Proc. SPIE*, 2009. 7165: p. 716502-1.

44. Chen, A.C., et al., Low-level laser therapy activates NF-kB via generation of reactive oxygen species in mouse embryonic fibroblasts. *PLoS ONE*, 2011. 6(7): p. e22453.

45. Murphy, M.P., How mitochondria produce reactive oxygen species. *Biochem J*, 2009. 417(1): p. 1–13.

46. Candas, D. and J.J. Li, MnSOD in oxidative stress response-potential regulation via mitochondrial protein influx. *Antioxid Redox Signal*, 2014. 20(10): p. 1599–1617.

47. Suski, J.M., et al., Relation between mitochondrial membrane potential and ROS formation. *Methods Mol Biol*, 2012. 810: p. 183–205.

48. Zorov, D.B., M. Juhaszova, and S.J. Sollott, Mitochondrial reactive oxygen species (ROS) and ROS-induced ROS release. *Physiol Rev*, 2014. 94(3): p. 909–950.

49. Zorov, D.B., et al., Reactive oxygen species (ROS)-induced ROS release: A new phenomenon accompanying induction of the mitochondrial permeability transition in cardiac myocytes. *J Exp Med*, 2000. 192(7): p. 1001–1014.

50. Zorov, D.B., M. Juhaszova, and S.J. Sollott, Mitochondrial ROS-induced ROS release: An update and review. *Biochim Biophys Acta*, 2006. 1757(5–6): p. 509–517.

51. Storz, P. and A. Toker, Protein kinase D mediates a stress-induced NF-kappaB activation and survival pathway. *EMBO J*, 2003. 22(1): p. 109–120.

52. Sharma, S.K., et al., Dose response effects of 810 nm laser light on mouse primary cortical neurons. *Lasers Surg Med*, 2011. 43(8): p. 851–859.

53. Huang, Y.Y., et al., Low-level laser therapy (LLLT) reduces oxidative stress in primary cortical neurons in vitro. *J Biophotonics*, 2012.

54. Stone, J.R. and S. Yang, Hydrogen peroxide: A signaling messenger. *Antioxid Redox Signal*, 2006. 8(3–4): p. 243–270.

55. Sies, H., Hydrogen peroxide as a central redox signaling molecule in physiological oxidative stress: Oxidative eustress. *Redox Biol*, 2017. 11: p. 613–619.

56. Fukui, M., H.J. Choi, and B.T. Zhu, Rapid generation of mitochondrial superoxide induces mitochondrion-dependent but caspase-independent cell death in hippocampal neuronal cells that morphologically resembles necroptosis. *Toxicol Appl Pharmacol*, 2012. 262(2): p. 156–166.

57. Vasilenko, T., et al., The effect of equal daily dose achieved by different power densities of low-level laser therapy at 635 and 670 nm on wound tensile strength in rats: A short report. *Photomed Laser Surg*, 2010. 28(2): p. 281–283.

58. Oron, U., et al., Attenuation of infarct size in rats and dogs after myocardial infarction by low-energy laser irradiation. *Lasers Surg Med*, 2001. 28(3): p. 204–211.

59. Lanzafame, R.J., et al., Reciprocity of exposure time and irradiance on energy density during photoradiation on wound healing in a murine pressure ulcer model. *Lasers Surg Med*, 2007. 39(6): p. 534–542.

60. Ristow, M., et al., Antioxidants prevent health-promoting effects of physical exercise in humans. *Proc Natl Acad Sci U S A*, 2009. 106(21): p. 8665–8670.

61. Guaraldo, S.A., et al., The effect of low-level laser therapy on oxidative stress and functional fitness in aged rats subjected to swimming: An aerobic exercise. *Lasers Med Sci*, 2016. 31(5): p. 833–840.

62. Valero, T., Mitochondrial biogenesis: Pharmacological approaches. *Curr Pharm Des*, 2014. 20(35): p. 5507–5509.

63. Wei, Y., et al., The role of mitochondria in mTOR-regulated longevity. *Biol Rev Camb Philos Soc*, 2015. 90(1): p. 167–181.

64. Hood, D.A., et al., Unravelling the mechanisms regulating muscle mitochondrial biogenesis. *Biochem J*, 2016. 473(15): p. 2295–2314.

65. Li, S. and I. Laher, Exercise mimetics: Running without a road map. *Clin Pharmacol Ther*, 2017. 101(2): p. 188–190.

66. Wu, Z. and O. Boss, Targeting PGC-1 alpha to control energy homeostasis. *Expert Opin Ther Targets*, 2007. 11(10): p. 1329–1338.

67. Mormeneo, E., et al., PGC-1alpha induces mitochondrial and myokine transcriptional programs and lipid droplet and glycogen accumulation in cultured human skeletal muscle cells. *PLoS One*, 2012. 7(1): p. e29985.

68. Vaughan, R.A., et al., Dietary stimulators of the PGC-1 superfamily and mitochondrial biosynthesis in skeletal muscle. A mini-review. *J Physiol Biochem*, 2014. 70(1): p. 271–284.

69. Narkar, V.A., et al., AMPK and PPARdelta agonists are exercise mimetics. *Cell*, 2008. 134(3): p. 405–415.

70. Merrill, G.F., et al., AICA riboside increases AMP-activated protein kinase, fatty acid oxidation, and glucose uptake in rat muscle. *Am J Physiol*, 1997. 273(6 Pt 1): p. E1107–E1112.

71. Marin, T.L., et al., AMPK promotes mitochondrial biogenesis and function by phosphorylating the epigenetic factors DNMT1, RBBP7, and HAT1. *Sci Signal*, 2017. 10(464): pii: eaaf7478.

72. Zhang, Q., et al., Noninvasive low-level laser therapy for thrombocytopenia. *Sci Transl Med*, 2016. 8(349): p. 349ra101.

73. Luo, Z., et al., TRPV1 activation improves exercise endurance and energy metabolism through PGC-1alpha upregulation in mice. *Cell Res*, 2012. 22(3): p. 551–564.

74. Kida, R., et al., Direct action of capsaicin in brown adipogenesis and activation of brown adipocytes. *Cell Biochem Funct*, 2016. 34(1): p. 34–41.

75. Hsu, Y.J., et al., Capsaicin supplementation reduces physical fatigue and improves exercise performance in mice. *Nutrients*, 2016. 8(10): pii: E648.

76. Wang, Y., et al., Photobiomodulation of human adipose-derived stem cells using 810 nm and 980 nm lasers operates via different mechanisms of action. *Biochim Biophys Acta*, 2016. 1861: p. 441–449.

77. Wang, Y., et al., Photobiomodulation (blue and green light) encourages osteoblastic-differentiation of human adipose-derived stem cells: Role of intracellular calcium and light-gated ion channels. *Sci Rep*, 2016. 6: p. 33719.

78. Aquino, A.E., Jr., et al., Low-level laser therapy (LLLT) combined with swimming training improved the lipid profile in rats fed with high-fat diet. *Lasers Med Sci*, 2013. 28(5): p. 1271–1280.

79. Ferraresi, C., M.R. Hamblin, and N.A. Parizotto, Low-level laser (light) therapy (LLLT) on muscle tissue: Performance, fatigue and repair benefited by the power of light. *Photonics Lasers Med*, 2012. 1(4): p. 267–286.

80. Ferraresi, C., Y.Y. Huang, and M.R. Hamblin, Photobiomodulation in human muscle tissue: An advantage in sports performance? *J Biophotonics*, 2016. 9: p. 1273–1299.

81. Ferraresi, C., et al., Muscular pre-conditioning using light-emitting diode therapy (LEDT) for high-intensity exercise: A randomized double-blind placebo-controlled trial with a single elite runner. *Physiother Theory Pract*, 2015. 31(5): p. 354–61.

82. Ferraresi, C., et al., Light-emitting diode therapy (LEDT) before matches prevents increase in creatine kinase with a light dose response in volleyball players. *Lasers Med Sci*, 2015. 30: p. 1281–1287.

83. Johnstone, D.M., et al., Turning on lights to stop neurodegeneration: The potential of near infrared light therapy in Alzheimer's and Parkinson's disease. *Front Neurosci*, 2015. 9: p. 500.

84. Johnstone, D.M., et al., Indirect application of near infrared light induces neuroprotection in a mouse model of parkinsonism - an abscopal neuroprotective effect. *Neuroscience*, 2014. 274: p. 93–101.

85. Hopkins, J.T., et al., Low-level laser therapy facilitates superficial wound healing in humans: A triple-blind, sham-controlled study. *J Athl Train*, 2004. 39(3): p. 223–229.

86. Kazemikhoo, N., et al., Modifying effect of intravenous laser therapy on the protein expression of arginase and epidermal growth factor receptor in type 2 diabetic patients. *Lasers Med Sci*, 2016. 31(8): p. 1537–1545.

87. Momenzadeh, S., et al., The intravenous laser blood irradiation in chronic pain and fibromyalgia. *J Lasers Med Sci*, 2015. 6(1): p. 6–9.

88. Powers, S.K., E.E. Talbert, and P.J. Adhihetty, Reactive oxygen and nitrogen species as intracellular signals in skeletal muscle. *J Physiol*, 2011. 589(Pt 9): p. 2129–2138.

89. Buresh, R. and K. Berg, A tutorial on oxidative stress and redox signaling with application to exercise and sedentariness. *Sports Med Open*, 2015. 1(1): p. 3.

90. Ginani, F., et al., Effect of low-level laser therapy on mesenchymal stem cell proliferation: A systematic review. *Lasers Med Sci*, 2015. 30(8): p. 2189–2194.

91. Blatt, A., et al., Low-level laser therapy to the bone marrow reduces scarring and improves heart function post-acute myocardial infarction in the pig. *Photomed Laser Surg*, 2016. 34(11): p. 516–524.

92. Oron, U., et al., Autologous bone-marrow stem cells stimulation reverses post-ischemic-reperfusion kidney injury in rats. *Am J Nephrol*, 2014. 40(5): p. 425–433.

93. Oron, A. and U. Oron, Low-level laser therapy to the bone marrow ameliorates neurodegenerative disease progression in a mouse model of Alzheimer's disease: A minireview. *Photomed Laser Surg*, 2016. 34(12): p. 627–630.

94. Yang, J., et al., Low-level light treatment ameliorates immune thrombocytopenia. *Sci Rep*, 2016. 6: p. 38238.

95. Chen, A.C., et al., Effects of 810-nm laser on murine bone-marrow-derived dendritic cells. *Photomed Laser Surg*, 2011. 29(6): p. 383–389.

96. Yamaura, M., et al., Low level light effects on inflammatory cytokine production by rheumatoid arthritis synoviocytes. *Lasers Surg Med*, 2009. 41(4): p. 282–290.

97. Hwang, M.H., et al., Low level light therapy modulates inflammatory mediators secreted by human annulus fibrosus cells during intervertebral disc degeneration in vitro. *Photochem Photobiol*, 2015. 91(2): p. 403–410.

98. Imaoka, A., et al., Reduction of IL-20 expression in rheumatoid arthritis by linear polarized infrared light irradiation. *Laser Ther*, 2014. 23(2): p. 109–114.

99. Lim, W., et al., Anti-inflammatory effect of 635 nm irradiations on in vitro direct/indirect irradiation model. *J Oral Pathol Med*, 2015. 44(2): p. 94–102.

100. Choi, H., et al., Inflammatory cytokines are suppressed by light-emitting diode irradiation of P. gingivalis LPS-treated human gingival fibroblasts: Inflammatory cytokine changes by LED irradiation. *Lasers Med Sci*, 2012. 27(2): p. 459–467.

101. Sakurai, Y., M. Yamaguchi, and Y. Abiko, Inhibitory effect of low-level laser irradiation on LPS-stimulated prostaglandin E2 production and cyclooxygenase-2 in human gingival fibroblasts. *Eur J Oral Sci*, 2000. 108(1): p. 29–34.

102. Nomura, K., M. Yamaguchi, and Y. Abiko, Inhibition of interleukin-1beta production and gene expression in human gingival fibroblasts by low-energy laser irradiation. *Lasers Med Sci*, 2001. 16(3): p. 218–223.

103. Briken, V. and D.M. Mosser, Editorial: Switching on arginase in M2 macrophages. *J Leukoc Biol*, 2011. 90(5): p. 839–841.

104. Whyte, C.S., et al., Suppressor of cytokine signaling (SOCS)1 is a key determinant of differential macrophage activation and function. *J Leukoc Biol*, 2011. 90(5): p. 845–854.

105. Xu, H., et al., The polarization states of microglia in TBI: A new paradigm for pharmacological intervention. *Neural Plast*, 2017. 2017: p. 5405104.

106. Lu, J., et al., PTEN/PI3k/AKT regulates macrophage polarization in emphysematous mice. *Scand J Immunol*, 2017. 85: p. 395–405.

107. Saha, B., K. Kodys, and G. Szabo, Hepatitis C virus-induced monocyte differentiation into polarized M2 macrophages promotes stellate cell activation via TGF-beta. *Cell Mol Gastroenterol Hepatol*, 2016. 2(3): p. 302–316 e8.

108. Fernandes, K.P., et al., Photobiomodulation with 660-nm and 780-nm laser on activated J774 macrophage-like cells: Effect on M1 inflammatory markers. *J Photochem Photobiol B*, 2015. 153: p. 344–351.

109. Silva, I.H., et al., Increase in the nitric oxide release without changes in cell viability of macrophages after laser therapy with 660 and 808 nm lasers. *Lasers Med Sci*, 2016. 31(9): p. 1855–1862.

110. von Leden, R.E., et al., 808 nm wavelength light induces a dose-dependent alteration in microglial polarization and resultant microglial induced neurite growth. *Lasers Surg Med*, 2013. 45(4): p. 253–263.

111. Muili, K.A., et al., Photobiomodulation induced by 670 nm light ameliorates MOG35-55 induced EAE in female C57BL/6 mice: A role for remediation of nitrosative stress. *PLoS One*, 2013. 8(6): p. e67358.

112. Hofling, D.B., et al., Low-level laser therapy in chronic autoimmune thyroiditis: A pilot study. *Lasers Surg Med*, 2010. 42(6): p. 589–596.

113. Hofling, D.B., et al., Low-level laser in the treatment of patients with hypothyroidism induced by chronic autoimmune thyroiditis: A randomized, placebo-controlled clinical trial. *Lasers Med Sci*, 2013. 28(3): p. 743–753.

114. Hofling, D.B., et al., Assessment of the effects of low-level laser therapy on the thyroid vascularization of patients with autoimmune hypothyroidism by color Doppler ultrasound. *ISRN Endocrinol*, 2012. 2012: p. 126720.

115. Hofling, D.B., et al., Effects of low-level laser therapy on the serum TGF-beta1 concentrations in individuals with autoimmune thyroiditis. *Photomed Laser Surg*, 2014. 32(8): p. 444–449.

116. Oron, A., et al., low-level laser therapy applied transcranially to mice following traumatic brain injury significantly reduces long-term neurological deficits. *J Neurotrauma*, 2007. 24(4): p. 651–656.

117. Wu, Q., et al., Low-level laser therapy for closed-head traumatic brain injury in mice: Effect of different wavelengths. *Lasers Surg Med*, 2012. 44(3): p. 218–226.

118. Ando, T., et al., Comparison of therapeutic effects between pulsed and continuous wave 810-nm wavelength laser irradiation for traumatic brain injury in mice. *PLoS One*, 2011. 6(10): p. e26212.

119. Karu, T.I., L.V. Pyatibrat, and N.I. Afanasyeva, Cellular effects of low power laser therapy can be mediated by nitric oxide. *Lasers Surg Med*, 2005. 36(4): p. 307–314.

120. Xuan, W., et al., Transcranial low-level laser therapy improves neurological performance in traumatic brain injury in mice: Effect of treatment repetition regimen. *PLoS ONE*, 2013. 8(1): p. e53454.

121. Xuan, W., et al., Low-level laser therapy for traumatic brain injury in mice increases brain derived neurotrophic factor (BDNF) and synaptogenesis. *J Biophotonics*, 2015. 8(6): p. 502–511.

122. Xuan, W., et al., Transcranial low-level laser therapy enhances learning, memory, and neuroprogenitor cells after traumatic brain injury in mice. *J Biomed Opt*, 2014. 19(10): p. 108003.

123. Khuman, J., et al., Low-level laser light therapy improves cognitive deficits and inhibits microglial activation after controlled cortical impact in mice. *J Neurotrauma*, 2012. 29(2): p. 408–417.

124. Quirk, B.J., et al., Near-infrared photobiomodulation in an animal model of traumatic brain injury: Improvements at the behavioral and biochemical levels. *Photomed Laser Surg*, 2012. 30(9): p. 523–529.

125. Zhang, Q., et al., Low-level laser therapy effectively prevents secondary brain injury induced by immediate early responsive gene X-1 deficiency. *J Cereb Blood Flow Metab*, 2014. Aug, 34(8): p. 1391–1401.

126. Dong, T., et al., Low-level light in combination with metabolic modulators for effective therapy of injured brain. *J Cereb Blood Flow Metab*, 2015. Sep, 35(9): p. 1435–1444.

127. Naeser, M.A. and M.R. Hamblin, Traumatic brain injury: A major medical problem that could be treated using transcranial, red/near-infrared LED photobiomodulation. *Photomed Laser Surg*, 2015. Sep, 33(9): p. 443–446.

128. McClure, J., The role of causal attributions in public misconceptions about brain injury. *Rehabil Psychol*, 2011. 56(2): p. 85–93.

129. Naeser, M.A., et al., Improved cognitive function after transcranial, light-emitting diode treatments in chronic, traumatic brain injury: Two case reports. *Photomed Laser Surg*, 2011. 29(5): p. 351–358.

130. Naeser, M.A., et al., Improved language in a chronic nonfluent aphasia patient after treatment with CPAP and TMS. *Cogn Behav Neurol*, 2010. 23(1): p. 29–38.

131. Naeser, M.A., et al., Significant improvements in cognitive performance post-transcranial, red/near-infrared light-emitting diode treatments in chronic, mild traumatic brain injury: Open-protocol study. *J Neurotrauma*, 2014. 31(11): p. 1008–1017.

132. Henderson, T.A. and L.D. Morries, SPECT perfusion imaging demonstrates improvement of traumatic brain injury with transcranial near-infrared laser phototherapy. *Adv Mind Body Med*, 2015. 29(4): p. 27–33.

133. Clijsen, R., et al., Effects of low-level laser therapy on pain in patients with musculoskeletal disorders. A systemic review and meta-analysis. *Eur J Phys Rehabil Med*, 2017. 53(4): p. 603–610.

134. Martins, D.F., et al., Light-emitting diode therapy reduces persistent inflammatory pain: Role of interleukin 10 and antioxidant enzymes. *Neuroscience*, 2016. 324: p. 485–495.

135. Nadur-Andrade, N., et al., Effects of photobiostimulation on edema and hemorrhage induced by Bothrops moojeni venom. *Lasers Med Sci*, 2012. 27(1): p. 65–70.

136. Dourado, D.M., et al., Effects of the Ga-As laser irradiation on myonecrosis caused by Bothrops Moojeni snake venom. *Lasers Surg Med*, 2003. 33(5): p. 352–357.

137. Chow, R., et al., Inhibitory effects of laser irradiation on peripheral mammalian nerves and relevance to analgesic effects: A systematic review. *Photomed Laser Surg*, 2011. 29(6): p. 365–381.

138. Kobiela Ketz, A., et al., Characterization of macrophage/microglial activation and effect of photobiomodulation in the spared nerve injury model of neuropathic pain. *Pain Med*, 2017. 18(5): p. 932–946.

139. Richner, M., et al., The spared nerve injury (SNI) model of induced mechanical allodynia in mice. *J Vis Exp*, 2011(54), pii: 3092.

140. Bashiri, H., Evaluation of low level laser therapy in reducing diabetic polyneuropathy related pain and sensorimotor disorders. *Acta Med Iran*, 2013. 51(8): p. 543–547.

141. Knapp, D.J., Postherpetic neuralgia: Case study of class 4 laser therapy intervention. *Clin J Pain*, 2013. 29(10): p. e6–e9.

142. Chow, R.T., et al., Efficacy of low-level laser therapy in the management of neck pain: A systematic review and meta-analysis of randomised placebo or active-treatment controlled trials. *Lancet*, 2009. 374(9705): p. 1897–1908.

143. Falaki, F., A.H. Nejat, and Z. Dalirsani, The effect of low-level laser therapy on trigeminal neuralgia: A review of literature. *J Dent Res Dent Clin Dent Prospects*, 2014. 8(1): p. 1–5.

144. Pires de Sousa, M.V., et al., Transcranial low-level laser therapy (810 nm) temporarily inhibits peripheral nociception: Photoneuromodulation of glutamate receptors, prostatic acid phosphatase, and adenosine triphosphate., *Neurophotonics*, 2016. 3(1): p. 015003.

145. Arden, N. and M.C. Nevitt, Osteoarthritis: Epidemiology. *Best Pract Res Clin Rheumatol*, 2006. 20(1): p. 3–25.

146. Cheng, D.S. and C.J. Visco, Pharmaceutical therapy for osteoarthritis. *PM R*, 2012. 4(5 Suppl): p. S82–S88.

147. Brosseau, L., et al., Low level laser therapy (classes I, II and III) for treating osteoarthritis. *Cochrane Database Syst Rev*, 2004(3): p. CD002046.

148. Bjordal, J.M., et al., Can cochrane reviews in controversial areas be biased? A sensitivity analysis based on the protocol of a systematic cochrane review on low-level laser therapy in osteoarthritis. *Photomed Laser Surg*, 2005. 23(5): p. 453–458.

149. Alves, A.C., et al., Effect of low level laser therapy on the expression of inflammatory mediators and on neutrophils and macrophages in acute joint inflammation. *Arthritis Res Treat*, 2013. 15(5): R116.

150. Castano, A.P., et al., Low-level laser therapy for zymosan-induced arthritis in rats: Importance of illumination time. *Lasers Surg Med*, 2007. 39(6): p. 543–550.

151. da Rosa, A.S., et al., Effects of low-level laser therapy at wavelengths of 660 and 808 nm in experimental model of osteoarthritis. *Photochem Photobiol*, 2012. 88(1): p. 161–166.

152. Cidral-Filho, F.J., et al., Light-emitting diode therapy induces analgesia in a mouse model of postoperative pain through activation of peripheral opioid receptors and the L-arginine/nitric oxide pathway. *Lasers Med Sci*, 2013. 29(2): p. 695–702.

153. Glazov, G., M. Yelland, and J. Emery, Low-level laser therapy for chronic non-specific low back pain: A meta-analysis of randomised controlled trials. *Acupunct Med*, 2016. 34(5): p. 328–341.

154. Huang, Z., et al., The effectiveness of low-level laser therapy for nonspecific chronic low back pain: A systematic review and meta-analysis. *Arthritis Res Ther*, 2015. 17: p. 360.

155. Bjordal, J.M., R.A. Lopes-Martins, and V.V. Iversen, A randomised, placebo controlled trial of low level laser therapy for activated Achilles tendinitis with microdialysis measurement of peritendinous prostaglandin E2 concentrations. *Br J Sports Med*, 2006. 40(1): p. 76–80; discussion 76–80.

156. Nogueira, A.C., Jr. and J. Junior Mde, The effects of laser treatment in tendinopathy: A systematic review. *Acta Ortop Bras*, 2015. 23(1): p. 47–49.

157. Pinto, H.D., et al., Photobiomodulation therapy improves performance and accelerates recovery of high-level rugby players in field test: A randomized, crossover, double-blind, placebo-controlled clinical study. *J Strength Cond Res*, 2016. 30(12): p. 3329–3338.

158. Ferraresi, C., et al., Effects of light-emitting diode therapy on muscle hypertrophy, gene expression, performance, damage, and delayed-onset muscle soreness: Case-control study with a pair of identical twins. *Am J Phys Med Rehabil*, 2016. 95(10): p. 746–757.

159. Fangel, R., et al., Biomechanical properties: Effects of low-level laser therapy and Biosilicate(R) on tibial bone defects in osteopenic rats. *J Appl Biomater Funct Mater*, 2014. 12(3): p. 271–277.

160. Fangel, R., et al., Low-level laser therapy, at 60 J/cm^2 associated with a Biosilicate((R)) increase in bone deposition and indentation biomechanical properties of callus in osteopenic rats. *J Biomed Opt*, 2011. 16(7): p. 078001.
161. Briteno-Vazquez, M., et al., Low power laser stimulation of the bone consolidation in tibial fractures of rats: A radiologic and histopathological analysis. *Lasers Med Sci*, 2015. 30(1): p. 333–338.
162. Kim, K.A., et al., Effect of low-level laser therapy on orthodontic tooth movement into bone-grafted alveolar defects. *Am J Orthod Dentofacial Orthop*, 2015. 148(4): p. 608–617.
163. Soares, L.G., et al., New bone formation around implants inserted on autologous and xenografts irradiated or not with IR laser light: A histomorphometric study in rabbits. *Braz Dent J*, 2013. 24(3): p. 218–223.
164. Abd-Elaal, A.Z., et al., Evaluation of the effect of low-level diode laser therapy applied during the bone consolidation period following mandibular distraction osteogenesis in the human. *Int J Oral Maxillofac Surg*, 2015. 44(8): p. 989–997.
165. Emanet, S.K., L.I. Altan, and M. Yurtkuran, Investigation of the effect of GaAs laser therapy on lateral epicondylitis. *Photomed Laser Surg*, 2010. 28(3): p. 397–403.
166. Lam, L.K. and G.L. Cheing, Effects of 904-nm low-level laser therapy in the management of lateral epicondylitis: A randomized controlled trial. *Photomed Laser Surg*, 2007. 25(2): p. 65–71.
167. Rayegani, S., et al., Comparison of the effects of low energy laser and ultrasound in treatment of shoulder myofascial pain syndrome: A randomized single-blinded clinical trial. *Eur J Phys Rehabil Med*, 2011. 47(3): p. 381–389.
168. Yavuz, F., et al., Low-level laser therapy versus ultrasound therapy in the treatment of subacromial impingement syndrome: A randomized clinical trial. *J Back Musculoskelet Rehabil*, 2014. 27(3): p. 315–320.
169. Ip, D. and N.Y. Fu, Two-year follow-up of low-level laser therapy for elderly with painful adhesive capsulitis of the shoulder. *J Pain Res*, 2015. 8: p. 247–252.
170. Wu, Q., et al., Low-level laser therapy for closed-head traumatic brain injury in mice: Effect of different wavelengths. *Lasers Surg Med*, 2012. 44: p. 218–226.
171. Ando, T., et al., Comparison of therapeutic effects between pulsed and continuous wave 810-nm wavelength laser irradiation for traumatic brain injury in mice. *PLoS ONE*, 2011. 6(10): p. e26212–26220.

Section II

Clinical Approaches to Preventing and Treating Metabolic Dysfunction

7 Safeguarding Musculoskeletal Structures from Food Technology's Untoward Metabolic Effects

Ingrid Kohlstadt, MD, MPH

OVERVIEW

Medical advances give new tools to physicians and new hope to patients. Most health questions can now be answered with more treatment options. For one question, however, there are fewer options today. The question is, "Doc, what's good for me to eat?"

In the recent past, it may have been sufficient to advise patients to simply avoid junk food and fast food. Now the farm-to-fork changes in the food supply are complex and far-reaching. These changes affect whole foods, good-for-you foods, dietary supplements, and even oral hygiene products. Common foods that we keep in the refrigerator and the pantry shelf are grown, packaged, and prepared differently. These cumulative changes affect the musculoskeletal system.

This chapter explains the advantages the food industry derives from selected food technologies. This is concerning because for many food technologies biologic science demonstrates possible disadvantages for human health. Technologies impose departures from ancient metabolic pathways, digestion, absorption, satiety signaling, and the microbiome.

Since maintaining the musculoskeletal system is evolutionarily of low priority, long-term exposures to technologically changed foods may affect the musculoskeletal system disproportionately. Proactively identifying and avoiding foods associated with metabolic disturbance has been shown to improve outcomes in some situations. While these technologies are uniformly disadvantageous, patients vary in their risk for clinical symptoms.

Equipping our patients with answers to the question "Doc, what's good for me to eat?" is complex. It is sometimes difficult and left untried. That is why this chapter innovates how doctors can address the metabolic effects of food technology in clinical practice.

The impact of equipping our patients to restore metabolic and microbial normalcy may be far-reaching, based on the following lines of reasoning:

- Reducing *trans* fats has shown clinical impact [1]. Conversely, the adverse effects linger in societies that can't afford the pricy clean-up costs [2]. Several of the technologies presented in this chapter demonstrate the potential to be *trans* fat *déjà vu*.
- Further documentation comes from functional foods, those with evidence asserting health benefits beyond basic nutritional value. The broadening number of foods with scientific support to qualify them as functional foods is evidence of the converse. For example, if enriching a food with oat bran provides functional health benefits, then removing bran by refining oats could be considered dysfunctional. The FDA applied this logic to a warning letter to General Mills [3].
- According to The Centers for Disease Control and Prevention's health statistics, life expectancy in the U.S. is lower for the second year in a row [4]. Life expectancy is possibly the

best marker for the vibrant health of a society. In the setting of great advances in medical technologies, this national statistic reflects a failure. The analysis of a failure includes evaluating what is not being done, for example, addressing the metabolic underpinnings of disease.

- The USA is reputed to be the country with the cheapest food and most costly health care. This is not a coincidence but cost-shifting. In 2017 four former FDA commissioners jointly denounced the importation of cheaper drugs using the same rationale [5], that price does not equal cost.
- Science is under industry pressure. Scientific presentation of the risks of food technology has been derailed, and this forestall the public discourse [6].

The following sections detail the biologic rationale by which emerging food technologies may contribute to musculoskeletal disorders, including practical ways to avoid and mitigate the dietary exposures.

EMULSIFIERS

Food which is clumpy, separated, or in need of stirring rapidly loses its market share. Emulsifiers enable oil and water to mix. So, adding emulsifiers enables the food industry to provide consumers with foods that are smooth, creamy, thick, rich, and frothy.

Adding emulsifiers also makes food better able to permeate biologic structures. During digestion the rate and manner in which oil and water mix are carefully calibrated. Increasing the permeability of the intestinal lining is associated with symptoms sometimes referred to as "leaky gut."

The food industry's use of emulsifiers was challenged in March 2015 when *Nature* published the murine research of scientists Andrew Gewirtz and Benoit Chassaing from Georgia State University [7]. Mice exposed to the emulsifying agents developed metabolic syndrome faster than those unexposed. Differences were detected at levels one-tenth that permitted by the FDA. The authors and other scientists have since conducted human studies with the same finding [8]. Evidence mounted when removing exposure to emulsifiers demonstrated health benefits. A recent randomized study demonstrated that prescribing a no-carrageenan diet can extend remission of inflammatory bowel disease [9].

Emulsifiers affect the musculoskeletal system by promoting system-wide inflammation which includes joint disease and fasciitis. Metabolic syndrome represents a shift in body composition caused by muscle atrophy and fat acquisition.

As clinicians, we can raise our patients' awareness of emulsifiers and the preliminary findings above. The following information will help.

1. Emulsifiers have an absence of evidence but not evidence of absence. Our patients with musculoskeletal conditions draw their own conclusions. Emulsifiers have not been shown to be carcinogenic or toxic. By these standards, regulatory agencies consider emulsifiers safe. These safety criteria are outdated, not taking into account the physiological effects on the microbiome and intestinal permeability. Data fundamental to safety research is not being collected. For example, the U.S. population's exposure to emulsifiers is unknown, and this number is the "N" for epidemiologic study. In August 2017, more than 2 years after the *Nature* study which raised a safety concern, the following was published "Because no published dietary exposure estimates for commonly used emulsifiers exist for the U.S. population [10]."

2. Avoiding select emulsifiers may be adequate. While all emulsifiers act to enhance permeability, those that exist naturally in the diet don't raise as much concern as others. For example, lecithin is an emulsifier found in food naturally and is considered a safer additive than carrageenan and carboxymethyl cellulose. While carrageenan is "natural" because it is extracted from red seaweed, it is not a customary component of food and is not "natural"

to the human diet. Carboxymethyl cellulose is also "natural" because it's derived from cellulose which is made water-soluble through chemical reactions, but cellulose is not naturally digestible by humans. Synthetically-derived emulsifiers include polysorbates, currently used in medicines and vaccines with rising debate. I share the sentiments of Dr. George Lundberg voiced in his Medscape editorial [11].

3. Eliminating junk food does little to reduce emulsifier exposure. "Good-for-you" foods such as organic nut milks and kosher yogurt consumed for musculoskeletal health contain emulsifiers (Figure 7.1), as do some liquid medications, sports performance supplements, and everyday consumer health products such as tooth paste and mouth wash (Figure 7.2).

INTERESTERIFICATION OF FATS

In the first edition of this book, I coauthored a chapter on dietary fats with biochemist Dr. Mary Enig. Her life's work contrasted the untoward effects of *trans* fats with the benefits of saturated plant fats. From her perspective replacing *trans* fats with interesterified (IE) fats was exchanging one problematic food technology for another. Table 7.1 addresses terminology used for dietary fats.

Interesterification allows the food industry to achieve the desired melting point and texture of food. *Trans* and IE fats make this possible because the chemical structures of the fatty acids change the physical properties. Figure 7.3 depicts fatty acid molecules. The double lines represent double bonds, the location of fatty acid oxidation. The more *cis* (opposite of *trans*) double bonds, the more bends in the carbon structure. The more rigid the shape, the more solid the fat becomes. Interesterification doesn't change the fatty acid bonds *per se* but selects the fatty acids and their placement on the glycerol molecule. Fatty acids with fewer *cis* double bonds give oils the properties of animal fat.

NUTRITION   SPECIAL DIETS

INGREDIENTS

ROASTED HAZELNUT BASE (WATER,
GROUND ROASTED HAZELNUTS),
BROWN RICE SWEETENER (WATER,
BROWN RICE), TRICALCIUM
PHOSPHATE, GELLAN GUM, SEA SALT,
CARRAGEENAN, RIBOFLAVIN (B2),
VITAMIN A PALMITATE, VITAMIN D2

CONTAINS: HAZELNUTS

SOURCE

Nutrition Facts

Serving Size 1 cup (8 fl.oz.) 240 mL
Servings Per Container 4

Amount Per Serving

Calories 110	Calories from Fat 30

	% Daily Value*
Total Fat 3.5g	5%
Saturated Fat 0g	0%
Trans Fat 0g	
Cholesterol 0mg	0%
Sodium 120mg	5%
Potassium 75mg	2%
Total Carbohydrate 19g	6%
Dietary Fiber 1g	4%
Sugars 14g	
Protein 2g	

Vitamin A 10%	•	Vitamin C 0%
Calcium 30%	•	Iron 2%
Vitamin D 25%	•	Vitamin E 10%
Riboflavin 30%		

*Percent Daily Values are based on a 2,000 calorie diet.

FIGURE 7.1 The emulsifier carrageenan appears in the nutrition ingredients of a nut milk.

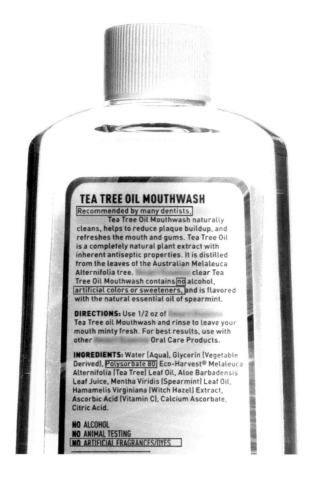

FIGURE 7.2 The artificial emulsifier polysorbate 80 is the third ingredient in this mouth wash, which correctly claims to contain no artificial colors, sweeteners, fragrances, or dyes.

The fatty acids from food form the lipid tails of bilipid membranes surrounding cells and cellular structures such as the mitochondria where ATP is synthesized. Similar to the way fatty acids change the physical properties of food, they alter the physical properties of the cell membranes (Figure 7.4), potentially making them more rigid.

A second distinct concern about interesterification is that the process disables and removes antioxidants. Without antioxidants, foods go rancid or change color, so antioxidants are added back in a process called enrichment. Enriched foods contain antioxidants sufficient for shelf life but not necessarily the type and amount required for healthy metabolism. Antioxidants are metabolic fire marshals, protecting against the potential damages of fatty acid oxidation. The absence and delay of metabolically requisite antioxidants yield system-wide inflammation.

Antioxidants chaperone the highly dynamic processing of the omega 3 and omega 6 fats presented in Figure 7.5. Substrate availability regulates the throughput of the pathways. IE fats include fewer omega 3 and omega 6 fats which have a high number of double bonds. This too contributes to inflammation.

Balance among the fatty acids is important for all musculoskeletal structures. Efficient utilization of dietary fats can reduce athletic performance. The laboratory tests which point to metabolic syndrome and include elevated triglycerides, low HDL cholesterol, and elevated glucose raise clinical suspicion of fatty acid imbalances. Dietary supplementation with omega-3 fats are sometimes

TABLE 7.1

Glossary of Terms Used in Labeling Oils

Term	Significance
Cold pressed	Solvents were not used to extract oil from seeds or nuts
Expeller pressed	Solvents were not used to extract oil from seeds or nuts
Extra virgin	The first oil to be extracted
Natural	No significance
Organic	Meets federally established criteria for organic, which has been shown to contain less pesticide contamination
Partially hydrogenated oil	Contains *trans* fats; another way to suspect the presence of *trans* fats is when the sum of saturated, monounsaturated, and polyunsaturated fat content is less than the total fats
Toasted	Safe; seeds and nuts are roasted before extracting; this makes the oils taste more flavorful
Genetically modified organism (GMO)	GMO is not universally labeled; GMO may impose health risk depending on what was modified; GMO may reduce pesticide content
Unrefined	Unprocessed to help retain nutrients
Pesticide content	Not labeled, although organic has been shown to have less contamination with persistent organic pollutants
Oxidized material	Not labeled; polyunsaturated oils should be refrigerated upon opening and the expiration date observed to avoid oxidation after purchase
Interesterification	A newer method of making plant oils, not yet indicated on the label
Fat free	Of course, cooking oil is fat; the label means that the portion size is small enough that the total fat falls below labeling criteria
Expiration date	Unsaturated oils should have a clearly marked expiration date; Rancidity occurs from oxidized fats and generally smells like stale potato chips

Note: The glossary is intended to help patients in selecting healthy oils.

consumed to help offset the effects of processed dietary fats, but can lead to further imbalances in the metabolic pathways depicted in Figure 7.5.

Avoiding IE fats in addition to avoiding *trans* fats may have added benefits, in terms of sports performance and the change in body composition from metabolic syndrome. Avoiding processed fats to the greatest extent possible may be the most effective way to avoid IE fats, since IE fats do not have the labeling requirements that *trans* fats and emulsifiers do. Prevalence data in food is also not collected; however, a 2012 U.S. estimate is that 3% of energy intake is IE, based on its use to replace *trans* fats [12].

FOOD COLORINGS

Food colorings are among the chemical additives with known effects on the central nervous system [13]. Consumption of the food colorings sunset yellow FCF, quinoline yellow, carmoisine, allura red, tartrazine, and ponceau aggravates attention deficit hyperactivity disorder (ADHD). The preservative sodium benzoate has similar effects. Conversely, removing the additives from diet ameliorates ADHD symptoms. The science has compelled Europe to take regulatory action [13].

Musculoskeletal benefits to avoiding the food additives for patients with ADHD include reduced need for treatment with medications such as first-line therapy methylphenidate. The FDA mandated drug label for the extended release of dexmethylphenidate hydrochloride includes warnings for cardiac muscle damage and long-term suppression of growth. Post-marketing surveillance identified

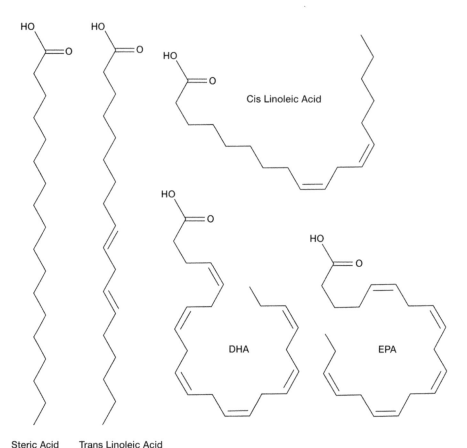

FIGURE 7.3 The chemical structure of fatty acids found in triglycerides confer structure and physical properties. The *trans* conformation of linoleic acid resembles a saturated fatty acid, whereas the *cis* conformation has some honeycombing of the highly unsaturated fatty acids DHA and EPA. (Reproduced with permission from Olmstead, S and Meiss, D. Chapter 8. Cardiac Arrhythmias. In Kohlstadt, I (ed), *Advancing Medicine with Food and Nutrients, Second Edition*. CRC Press. Boca Raton, FL. Jan 2013.)

an increased risk of rhabdomyolysis. The FDA does not require the study or reporting of long-term effects of discontinuation of ADHD medication [14]. Weight gain and obesity have been observed with discontinuation.

SWEETENERS: NEW FINDINGS

The food colorings and preservatives identified in the previous section are by far not the only neuroactive food additives. Because the mechanisms by which the chemicals exert drug-like effects on the brain are poorly understood, there is currently no efficient method for screening chemicals prior to introducing them into the food supply.

For the food industry, additives sometimes have dual roles. In addition to the labeled role as coloring agents, thickeners, preservatives, and so on, they may be intended to promote brand loyalty. Sugar, salt, colors, and caffeine are well understood to enhance brand loyalty.

It would be naïve to overlook that neuroactive food additives act on the craving and taste centers of the brain, including the parts of the brain which signal withdrawal. Chemicals which have been demonstrated to create drug-like effects on the brain may exert chemical dependence. Chemical dependence can make it more difficult for patients to choose healthful diets.

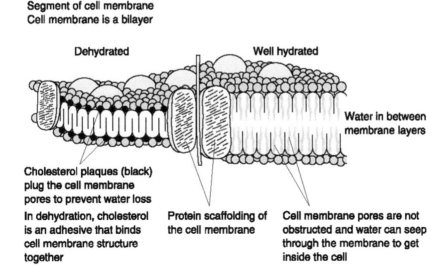

Segment of cell membrane
Cell membrane is a bilayer

Dehydrated   Well hydrated

Water in between
membrane layers

Cholesterol plaques (black)
plug the cell membrane
pores to prevent water loss

In dehydration, cholesterol   Protein scaffolding of   Cell membrane pores are not
is an adhesive that binds   the cell membrane   obstructed and water can seep
cell membrane structure   through the membrane to get
together   inside the cell

FIGURE 7.4 The bilayer membrane in two different states, hydrated and dehydrates, demonstrating the separation of the two layers. Water establishes a lateral diffusion pressure that helps in the enzyme-substrate actions. In a dehydrated state this ability is compromised. The physical properties of the hydrophobic fatty acid tails influence hydration status.

One example of food additives impairing healthful food selection is how high-intensity non-caloric artificial sweeteners (NAS) override taste. NAS are up to 10,000 times sweeter than natural bulk sweeteners such as sugar, honey, and maple syrup. Those accustomed to sweet tastes which are orders of magnitude more intense than natural sweetness find whole foods lacking in taste. It might be loosely compared to the way food tastes bland without chipotle and curry to those accustomed to spices.

Late-breaking research has elucidated a mechanism by which NAS alter satiety signaling [15]. A first-in-human study conducted by Dr. Richard Young of Adelaide School of Medicine elucidated this mechanism. In the presence of artificial sweeteners, less glucose may reach the distal portions of the intestine that release glucagon-like peptide 1 (GLP-1). GLP-1 is an incretin hormone that is protective against the metabolic syndrome.

The field of nutrigenomics detailed in Chapter 2 provides emerging evidence. A newly discovered association with *OTOP1* gene links sour taste with a sense of balance [16]. When sour taste is stimulated a protein known for preserving balance is synthesized in the vestibular system. Scientists are intrigued about why this gene association is highly conserved [16]. I hypothesize it is because sour and bitter tastes are located in the back of the tongue where they are stimulated not only by food but also by stomach acid. Imagine a lactating primate holding on to its mom who is fleeing predators in the arboreal canopy. In such a scenario if stomach acid could help command the lactating primate's ability to hold on there would indeed be a survival advantage. Nutrigenomics helps generate new hypotheses. For example, if sour taste is linked to balance, could the disproportionate sweet taste of NAS impair balance?

NAS are dehydrating. They impair neurologic signaling through dehydrating effects in the gut lumen, well-studied in the development of oral rehydration solution. In 1978 the British journal *The Lancet* expounded the importance for the public health of: "The discovery that sodium transport and glucose transport are coupled in the small intestine so that glucose accelerates absorption of solute and water (is) potentially the most important medical advance this century [17]." NAS are not glucose, and some NAS cause diarrhea, which is additionally dehydrating. Thirst mechanisms

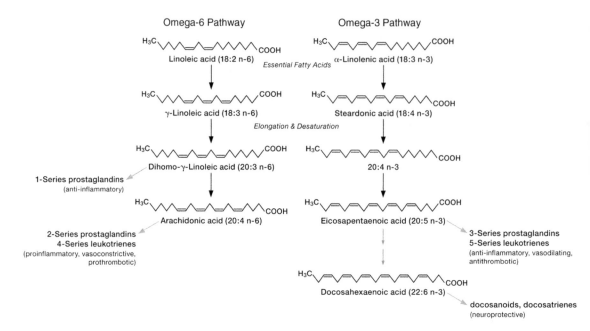

FIGURE 7.5 The metabolic pathways for essential fatty acids. (Reproduced with permission from Olmstead, S and Meiss, D. Chapter 8. Cardiac Arrhythmias. In Kohlstadt, I (ed), *Advancing Medicine with Food and Nutrients, Second Edition*. CRC Press. Boca Raton, FL. Jan 2013.)

override taste. Dehydration impairs musculoskeletal structures as elaborated in this book's first edition and illustrated in Figure 7.6.

In sum, taste has an important role in nutrient acquisition. It's a neurologic roadmap updated as metabolic needs change [18]. In this way, dulled taste challenges nutrient acquisition. As the primary reservoir for most nutrients, the musculoskeletal system is adversely affected.

ULTRA-PASTEURIZATION AND EMERGING DAIRY TECHNOLOGIES

Ultra-pasteurization and ultra-heat treatment (UHT) technologies extend milk's shelf life and reduce pathogen risk further than pasteurization alone. Before the technologies were widely adopted, nutrition studies were conducted to evaluate the safety of these new technologies for risk comparison studies.

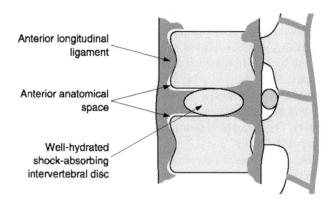

FIGURE 7.6 The anatomical design of the vertebral column highlighting the anatomical space and its relationship to the intervertebral disc in the vertebral column.

TABLE 7.2
Comparing Ultra-pasteurization and Aseptic (Ultra-high Temperature) Methods for Treating Milk to Pasteurization

Parameters	Pasteurization	Ultra-Pasteurization	Ultra-High Temperature
Heat treatment	161F for 15 seconds	280 F for 2 seconds	280 F for 2 seconds+
Bacterial kill	Some survival	Nearly "sterile"	Nearly "sterile"
Package treatment	Untreated	Treated with H_2O_2	Sterilized
Product storage	Refrigerated	Refrigerated	Shelf-stable
Shelf life	10–21 days	30–90 days	6 months+

As Table 7.2 details, nutrient values are comparable to pasteurized milk [19, 20]. However, the safety studies conducted in the 1980s did not consider the bioavailability of the nutrients or the impact on the human microbiome, since these affects were less understood at that time. Reanalysis of the original safety research in light of current knowledge has not been addressed in published literature. There are gaps in the safety literature and potential untoward metabolic effects are supported in the literature.

If microbes from livestock, the microbes that make yogurt, and microbes in the refrigerator are unable to digest milk due to these technologies, why would microbes in the human gastrointestinal tract be able to digest milk? If lactose in milk is not partially metabolized by microbial lactase, it is less bioavailable. When proteins are not digested in the upper gastrointestinal tract they engage more with GALT (gut-associated lymphoid tissue), which is why they are sometimes considered more immunogenic.

The intestinal microbiome is a competitive ecosystem where microbes that are fed flourish. Diet is the primary food of microbes. If *Lactobacilli* are unable to digest the lactose they are at a survival disadvantage. UHT and ultra-pasteurization would, therefore, be understood to reduce the presence of beneficial *Lactobacilli*.

UHT and ultra-pasteurization therefore likely impair musculoskeletal metabolism in the following ways. Symptoms of indigestion may cause patients to incorrectly conclude that they are lactose intolerant and therefore stop eating dairy products. If dairy products were previously part of their diet, they would have difficulty achieving adequate protein for muscle maintenance and adequate minerals for healthy bones. Diet-induced shifts in the microbiome and immune response are associated with inflammation involving the musculoskeletal structures.

Recently, one medical practice questioning the potential effects of UHT and ultra-pasteurization conducted a clinical trial. They demonstrated that homemade yogurt can resolve irritable bowel syndrome when prescribed in a clinical setting [21]. At a time that many patients have been instructed to avoid all dairy products in the setting of irritable bowel syndrome, the study findings attracted wide attention.

Making yogurt at home avoids the need for several food technologies, which may be problematic for digestion. Milk purchased to make yogurt can be pasteurized, but generally ultra-pasteurized and UHT milk aren't sufficiently digestible to the microorganisms known as live active yogurt cultures, and consequently don't culture.

Homemade yogurt avoids the need for microbiostatic additives such as natamycin, nanoparticles, excessive sugar, NAS, gluten-containing thickeners, and emulsifiers. There are several reasons such food technologies exacerbate irritable bowel syndrome. Thickeners such as food starch may contain gluten, which may be overlooked by consumers with sensitivies. Nanoparticle technology is sometimes considered part of the packaging and therefore not required to be labeled. Antimicrobials such as natamycin counteract the desired probiotic effect of yogurt. Emulsifiers reduce the microbial counts as well. The food technologies incorporated into yogurt understandably contribute to the variability in study results and conclusions about the health benefits of yogurt [22].

In summary, cultured dairy foods are an ancient and widely accessible source of musculoskeletal nutrients. Recent foods technologies have decreased the ability of some of these nutrients to be absorbed. Dairy has become allergenic and associated with gastrointestinal intolerances which cause people to instead select foods of lesser nutritional value.

GMO ENABLES GLYPHOSATES

Genetically modified organisms (GMOs) are a technology with enormous potential to help solve societal problems. GMOs have been used as an approach to reduce nutrient deficiencies and to promote drought-resistant resistant crops. Despite the tremendous advances GMOs could confer, the widest GMO application is herbicide resistance which has been proven detrimental to human health.

With glyphosate herbicides, the primary concern is not the GMO grains *per se* but the glyphosate residues on those grains. Glyphosates are newly synthetized. The glyphosate exposure appears to be ubiquitous. Presently most everyone has lab-detectable blood levels of glyphosate. A major route of exposure is food and not a single point source. Because human populations have not yet undergone natural selection to this new exposure, symptoms manifest differently among people and threshold doses vary. In sum, the epidemiology is exceedingly complex, and safety data is lacking.

The lack of safety data is accompanied by evidence that glyphosates harm the human musculoskeletal system. For example, glyphosates deplete manganese (Mn). Chondroitin sulfate synthesis depends on Mn, and its deficiency leads to osteoporosis and osteomalacia [23]. Glyphosates contribute to the rapid rise in celiac disease, an established risk factor for osteoporosis and muscle atrophy [24].

The human intestine is a garden and glyphosates are herbicides. As anticipated, glyphosates kill some microbes and thereby enable the growth of others. One pathogen which glyphosates enable is *Salmonella* [25]. Since livestock feed contains glyphosate residues, *Salmonella* would be increasingly common in milk, eggs, and meat. The increased risk might then require irradiating and ultra-pasteurizing food.

Musculoskeletal health relates to physical activity. Application of glyphosates limits outdoor physical activity. At a minimum, the pesticide warning signs at local parks make the grounds inaccessible for a few days [26]. Glyphosates are respiratory irritants, requiring those with sensitivities to stop their recreation immediately and remain indoors. Glyphosates are combined with adjuvants to help penetrate the plants, and adjuvants impose additional chemical toxicity.

IRRADIATION

Irradiation can protect food against foodborne illness such as *Salmonella* and *E. coli* poisoning. Foreign imported fruits are irradiated to prevent the spread of insects which could potentially spread to domestic crops. Irradiation extends the shelf life of food dramatically. Low doses of radiation preserve food and delay ripening and sprouting, while higher doses sterilize food, extending the shelf life by years.

Radioactivity is not retained in the food. Decades ago the U.S. government assessed the safety of food irradiation with the science available. At that time they concluded that the benefits outweigh the risks and took steps to reduce the perceived risks (Figure 7.7). The FDA's website emphasizes that sterilized foods make space travel safer [27]. Ironically another government website details the detrimental musculoskeletal effects of space travel [28]. These are attributed to the microgravity environment, but may also be mediated in part by the radiation exposures of space travel which may include the irradiated food products.

Microbiome research gives us reasons to reconsider irradiation's benefit-risk ratio. While radiation itself is not retained, there is minimal safety data on the breakdown products of radiation which do remain in food. Mineral content of irradiated food may not change but their bioavailability does, and irradiation's impact on digestibility of food has not been assessed.

In sum, irradiation makes food safe from transmitting infections but it diminishes the food quality. Byproducts of irradiation remain in the food, toxins formed prior to radiation remain in the food, and the food becomes less digestible. Nutrient levels may remain the same but the

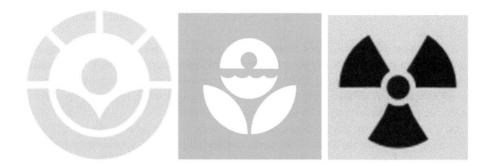

FIGURE 7.7 The food irradiation symbol Radura (left) is compared and contrasted to the symbol for the U.S. Environmental Protection Agency (center) and the radiation Tri-foil warning symbol (right).

body's ability to make use of these nutrients decreases and some nutrients alter their properties. In addition, transporting food to designated facilities for irradiation can extend the transit time from farm to fork.

Identifying food which has been irradiated is not straightforward. The Radura symbol is not uniformly required [29]. The process called cold pasteurization uses irradiation, which might not be inferred from the name. One may look closely at the foods which may be irradiated. These include meat, poultry, crustaceans, imported fresh fruits and vegetables, leaf vegetables, seeds for sprouting, shellfish, and seasonings. Currently, irradiated foods may not use the USDA organic label. Therefore choosing foods with the organic designation can help avoid exposure to irradiated food.

NANOPARTICLES

Nanotechnology is expanding what is possible in medical therapies. Scientists agree that there is much we have yet to learn about nanotechnology. This is an especially exciting field rich in potential for medical therapies. The new possibilities include delivery systems of medications and surgical materials. Future applications are anticipated to reduce exposure to toxic medications, improve uptake of bioactive substances, and provide more durable and less immunogenic orthopedic implants. The benefits of the medical applications of nanotechnology are anticipated to outweigh the potential harms of this new technology.

The food and cosmetic industries are also engaged in applying nanotechnology. There is specific interest in titanium dioxide nanoparticles. Titanium dioxide whitens various foods, adds texture to yogurt and cosmetics, serves as a mild abrasive and whitener in toothpaste, inhibits the growth of food pathogens, and blocks light especially in the UVB spectrum.

Sunscreens using nanoparticles of titanium oxide have been shown to be associated with lung cancer when they are applied by spraying. This is because the nanoparticles penetrate deeper into lung tissue than was realized [30]. Sunscreens travel deeper into the skin sometimes, too. There they can remain active for days, long beyond their needed protection for a swim at the beach. The longer-than-intended action is understood to not only prevent sunburn but also the vitamin D synthesizing action of ultraviolet light.

Nanoparticles, given their small size, are difficult to detect. For example, the food additive titanium dioxide (E171) is micronized, yet a fraction of this is nanoparticles [31]. Some food industry leaders have stopped adding titanium dioxide for this reason. But, not all titanium dioxide uses are labeled. Nanoparticles used in food production and handling are not labeled. For example, they can be applied to the packaging material and in this way wouldn't be considered part of the food, although it is understood that the nanoparticles enter the food.

To anticipate health effects of nanoparticles, it's not enough to think about quantity. Saying that "only" a fraction of titanium dioxide is nanoparticles lacks scientific credibility. For some metabolic purposes, what cellular structures a metal can penetrate is more important than the quantity consumed. Think *location*.

Once the immune system becomes sensitized to a metal, only a minute amount that penetrates the immune system barriers can trigger a significant inflammatory response. Could titanium-containing nanoparticles found in food and cosmetics be contributing to hypersensitivity reactions to titanium alloy dental and orthopedic implants? The answer is unknown. However, abductive reasoning and the Socratic method lead to "Yes."

The risks associated with titanium nanoparticles may be similar whether they are used for coating biomaterials, shielding the body from toxic medication, smooth application of sunscreen, or whitening a bag of Jordan almonds. The benefits from these applications, however, are not similar. Public discussion on weighing the risks and benefits would seem important, yet appears to be absent. Another way the public customarily "voices" their opinion is through purchasing power. However, without labeling requirements for nanoparticles in most foods and cosmetics, this avenue is also unavailable.

Clinicians can caution patients where applicable. To the extent possible avoiding food and cosmetic exposure to nanoparticles may benefit patients at risk for metal sensitivities and those with titanium alloy orthopedic implants. When there is a concern for low vitamin D levels such as in obesity, advanced age, and osteoporosis, avoiding nanotech sunscreens may provide benefits. Noting that a patient has metal sensitivity prior to elective orthopedic surgery may be helpful to select the best implant type as detailed in Chapter 1.

ACIDIFYING FOODS

Maintaining pH in the 7.35–7.45 range is crucial to human survival. Food is the primary substrate for the metabolic processes involved in maintaining pH. Lung and kidney physiology further assist in equilibration.

Equilibrating the pH equation involves adding more hydrogen ions or bicarbonate ions. When food technologies are combined in an individual's diet, they collectively pose a shortfall in bicarbonate. For example, salt, white vinegar, bleached flour, and white fat contribute less bicarbonate to the pH equation than spices, apple cider vinegar, whole grain, and unrefined oils. Processed foods are sometimes called acidifying.

Acidifying differs from acidic. Acidic is a term for pH where acidifying is a biochemical term for net H^+ production. These are not one and the same.

Citrus fruits, for example, are acidic with a low pH but they contribute citrate to the citric acid cycle (Kreb's cycle) as the name suggests. Citrus-derived products such as lemon water and the dietary supplement calcium citrate offer a double metabolic benefit. Because citrus is acidic, it assists in maintaining a low gastric pH allowing absorption of minerals and protein. One of the merits of citrus being alkalinizing is that it provides bicarbonate for blood pH.

In contrast to citrus, processed foods tend to create a double metabolic disadvantage. Processed foods have been shown to contribute to symptoms of dyspepsia, managed with H_2 blockers and proton pump inhibitors to neutralize stomach acid. The same processed foods then contribute H^+ which must be neutralized, either by diet, lungs, and kidneys or by the bicarbonate stored in bones.

Patients can monitor their pH as a way to measure their progress in diet modification. This is detailed in Chapter 3 (see Figure 3.9). The advantage of avoiding an acidifying diet is that muscle and bone will not be broken down to maintain pH, which is a physiologic priority over structural integrity.

ALLERGENIC FOODS

Processing food by various methods removes the food's natural components which modulate the human immune system. When nutrients are uncoupled, a type of inflammation called immune reactivity occurs. Immune reactivity is a summary biomarker for allergenicity.

A rise in allergenicity imposes on the musculoskeletal system. Food allergies contribute to sleep apnea with the impact on body composition described in Chapter 5. Sojourns at high elevation can compound the loss of muscle from hypoxia [32]. Food allergies are treated with medications known to decrease absorption of protein (Chapter 12). Treatment involves avoidance of reactive foods. In practical terms, removing otherwise healthful foods from the diet makes achieving a nutritious diet more difficult.

Diagnosing food allergies and intolerances can be difficult for both the health care provider and the patient. Chapter 3 explains how the lymphocyte response assay is one way to diagnose and monitor food allergies.

THE CLINICAL COSTS OF FOOD TECHNOLOGY AND INNOVATIONS TO ADDRESS THEM

Food technology keeps the price of food low. The costs of food technology, however, are high. This chapter stands shoulder to shoulder with the book's author team in concluding that we as physicians are disproportionately tasked with absorbing the societal costs.

- Physicians work through and around the stigma our patients understandably feel. They read diagnostic codes such as "dietary indiscretion" and "morbid obesity from excessive intake of calories" on their medical chart and wonder the same thing I do. "Where does the well-documented role of the food industry factor into these stigmatizing labels?"
- Physician services are "volunteered." When someone reaches for a vitamin supplement to help mitigate the damages of food technology the label advises "See your doctor." The direct-to-consumer prescription medication ads do the same, "Indigestion? Ask your doctor about…"
- In regards to food-as-medicine, physicians perform double duty. They write food prescriptions and are also the "pharmacists" guiding patients to take as directed.
- Physicians are sometimes wedged between the expectations of their patients and the expectations of management. One example is when patients determined to identify causes of their musculoskeletal symptoms order their own diagnostic tests including direct-to-consumer genetic test results. Increasingly, patients bring doctors nutrigenomic and metabolomic findings intended to guide food selection. Yet medical charts don't customarily handle potentially sensitive genetic information.

In context, patients come to their doctors when they feel "stuck." They've tried diet and exercise and were unable to reverse the tide of ill health. They feel pain or are too tired to sustain exercise. They experience food cravings that interfere with their livelihood. Their health goals seem a distant reach. The last thing such a patient would want to hear is that they should "do more." That is, unless that "do more" can help them succeed and break the cycle of ill health. And that is why physicians are choosing food as medicine.

Innovations are now available to enable practitioners to help their patients reunite food and medicine, and in this way treat musculoskeletal conditions. The following are innovative tools.

CHARTING THE NEWLY CONNECTED DATA POINTS

New diagnostic tests on the genome, epigenetics, adverse drug effects, environmental exposures, epigenetics, and concurrent medical conditions provide insights on underlying metabolic processes. These test results enable physicians to chart and code underlying causes, which have been known for some time [33]. Table 7.3 specifies diagnoses associated with some common musculoskeletal conditions. It puts metabolic diagnoses and therapies in code-able terms. Table 7.3 is developed primarily from my professional experience in reviewing medical charts and is intended as a practical tool.

TABLE 7.3

The Biologic Basis for Assigning Medical Diagnostic Codes to Clinical Recommendations Regarding Food Technologies

Musculoskeletal Condition	Underlying Biologic Mechanism Related to Food Technologies	ICD-10 Diagnosis Codes Which may Apply to Some Patients
Sarcopenia	Malabsorption of protein and minerals following Roux en Y bariatric surgery necessitated by obesogenic diet Acidifying diets Avoidance of dietary protein sources due to allergenicity necessitated by various food technologies Reduced absorption of irradiated protein sources Decreased bioavailability of muscle-building minerals and further reduction in mineral absorption due to inflammatory processes in the intestine Alterations in glucose signaling due to dietary sweeteners	K9589 Other complications of other bariatric procedure K9089 Other intestinal malabsorption E46 Unspecified protein-calorie malnutrition E71448 Other secondary carnitine deficiency Z681 Body Mass Index 19.9 or less, adult
Osteoporosis	Decreased mineral content of food due to allergenic foods Decreased bioavailability of minerals from food processing Decreased absorption of minerals due to inflammation from gluten sensitivity, emulsifiers and sweeteners Increased demand for minerals from acidifying diets Glyphosate-mediated effects Nanoparticles impair vitamin D synthesis	E8889 Other specified metabolic disorder K9089 Other intestinal malabsorption
Peripheral edema	Magnesium removed from food during processing, contrasted with added sodium Compromised integrity of cellular membranes from manipulation of fatty acids in foods Myxedema can sometimes be linked to food goiterogenic foods and loss of iodine Third-spacing due to low intravascular albumin levels, compounding the above	E8889 Other specified metabolic disorder E870 Hyperosmolality and hypernatremia E032 Hypothyroidism due to exogenous substances N179 Acute kidney failure from prerenal azotemia
Arthritis	Mechanical wear of the joint due to dehydrating effects of processed foods Gastrointestinal inflammation associated with emulsifiers and possibly inflammatory byproducts of food irradiation Proinflammatory shifts in the microbiome induced by various food technologies	K521 Toxic gastroenteritis and colitis
Myositis and rhabdomyositis	Direct effects of foods and the effects of medications such as statins and colchicine sometimes necessitated due in part to food technologies	M6088 Other myositis, which can induce N179 Acute kidney failure

(Continued)

TABLE 7.3 (CONTINUED)

The Biologic Basis for Assigning Medical Diagnostic Codes to Clinical Recommendations Regarding Food Technologies

Musculoskeletal Condition	Underlying Biologic Mechanism Related to Food Technologies	ICD-10 Diagnosis Codes Which may Apply to Some Patients
Obesity	Fatty acid imbalances predisposition to metabolic syndrome	E662 Obesity-related alveolar hypoventilation, also known as Pickwickian Syndrome
	Non-caloric artificial sweeteners interfere with glucose metabolism	E71318 Other disorders of fatty acid metabolism
	Allergenic foods contribute to hypoventilation with resulting inadequate oxygenation of tissues	Z6841 Body Mass Index 40.0–44.9, adult
	Obesogenic foods and indirect effects of medications required due to diet such as diuretics and some diabetic medications	
	Diminished taste perception and altered circadian rhythms from neuroactive food additives	
Fractures	Nanoparticles impair vitamin D synthesis	E211 Secondary hyperparathyroidism
	Sensitivity to gluten impairs proprioception and increases fall risk	G3281 Gluten ataxia
	Various dietary factors in diminished bone strength (See osteoporosis)	
Postoperative pain	Withdrawal symptoms from chemical dependency on food additives	G9782 other postprocedural disorders of the nervous system
	Secondary carnitine deficiency may be possible	
	Food technologies can impair tissue healing in many ways, this may be most evidenced by recent fascia research	
Decreased sports performance	Inefficient use of fatty acids manipulated as food is processed	E161 Other hypoglycemia
	Impaired utilization of glucose from sweeteners	G3281 Gluten ataxia
	"Brain fog" from gluten sensitivity and emulsifiers intensified during the physical stress of sports competition	G92 Toxic (metabolic) encephalopathy

FOOD AS PRESCRIBED

Disease physiology holds medication and avoidance of food technologies on equal footing. Most musculoskeletal conditions better respond to both types of interventions applied at the same time. A one-word explanation is tachyphylaxis. Within three months of any metabolic intervention, the body's compensatory mechanisms have adjusted to the change and the treatment effect diminishes. Therapies which combine lifestyle modification, avoidance of problematic food technologies and medications are robust against tachyphylaxis.

FOOD AS MEDICAL TREATMENT

The current understanding of metabolism demonstrates that food technologies are medical treatments. However, allopathic medicine tends to categorize these interventions as lifestyle choice and prevention. They maintain that avoidance of the problematic food technologies is within our patients' control. To what extent does the premise hold true that prescribing willpower is enough to achieve the desired improvement in musculoskeletal conditions? This chapter provides evidence that willpower is seldom enough. Additional support comes from the field of bariatric medicine, where diagnosing and treating the underpinnings of sarcopenic obesity, such as endocrine conditions and sleep apnea, enables patients to then leverage motivation to get the desired musculoskeletal results [34].

GROUP CLINIC VISITS

Avoidance of problematic foods can be communicated effectively in group clinical visits. This is why most health insurances and CMS reimburse physicians for leading group visits. Groups are not well-leveraged, largely due to attrition. Insurers pay for who shows up, not for who signs up. Doctors now have access to more engaging materials and various internet technologies. Group sessions can be interactive and accompanied by online materials. I've been involved in developing one such program for youths aged 9–12 [35, 36].

COLLABORATION

Metabolism is cross-specialty and this text intends to spark cross-specialty collaboration as evidenced by the diversity of its authors. The practice divide between dentists and doctors is not a biologic construct. The oral cavity offers the best views of the musculoskeletal system for those of us who aren't surgeons [37]. Insurance networks have limited doctors' ability to choose the colleagues to whom they refer. However, telemedicine, blockchain communication technology, and advances in internet information sharing offer new routes of collaboration.

ARTIFICIAL INTELLIGENCE

According to Medscape's Eric Topol, MD, medicine's top technology advances include artificial intelligence (AI) technology [38]. How might future AI applications help doctors guide their patients in food selection?

CONCLUSION

The chapter goal is to raise awareness among health care practitioners of the subtle, musculoskeletal effects of food technologies. In that way, health care practitioners can equip patients to restore the ancient handshake between food and human metabolism.

The chapter doesn't recommend any trend diets such as Paleo, vegetarian, or Mediterranean. It explains how common foods such as bread, yogurt, nut milk, fruit juice, and meat have changed their nutrient content, and how the changing face of food imposes on human metabolism.

Food technologies protect against microbial pathogens, reduce food spoilage, and make fresh produce more readily available. Offsetting the food safety benefits are untoward changes in nutrition, metabolism, and the microbiome. Recent research identifies metabolic changes not adequately conveyed by terms such as Generally Regarded as Safe (GRAS).

Food technologies with metabolic effects are pervasive. They are not limited to processed foods as sometimes assumed. Health foods, dietary supplements, good-for-you foods, and oral hygiene products incorporate newer food technologies. The lifestyle approach of healthful eating, therefore, does not limit exposure to the potential metabolic effects of food technologies presented in this chapter.

Innovations make it simpler to choose foods in the setting of multiple, converging, food technologies. Forthcoming innovations include artificial intelligence, new opportunities for collaboration among healthcare providers, materials for clinical groups, causal evidence to support billing codes, and media tools for using the latest science as a way to distinguish one's clinical practice. Doctors can use these tools to help personalize recommendations for their patients. The net result is that patients for whom diet and exercise were once Everest-steep are now able to summit their fitness goals and reduce their musculoskeletal symptoms.

ACKNOWLEDGMENTS

My young children have taken on the role of detectives, savvy to food labels. They are protégé taste testers. When they grab hold of a grocery cart it transforms into a vehicle of social change. Thank you, Raeha and Emmanuel, for living the change and for inspiring this chapter! I thank Ellis Richman for his enduring support and for taking on unexpected tasks too numerous to count.

Dr. Mary Enig and Dr. Fereydoon Batmanghelidj were authors in this book's first edition. Their understanding of membrane physiology remains ahead of its time and is therefore included posthumously in this chapter.

REFERENCES

1. Dietz WH, Scanlon KS. Eliminating the use of partially hydrogenated oil in food production and preparation. *JAMA Internal Medicine* 2012;308:143–44.
2. Downs S, Thow AM, Leeder SR. The effectiveness of policies for reducing dietary trans fat: A systematic review of the evidence. *Bulletin of the World Health Organization* 2013;91:262–69.
3. Press A. FDA takes issue with Cheerios health claims: Box labela suggest cereal can lower cholesterol and treat heart disease. 2009: Available online at www.nbcnews.com/id/30701291/ns/health-heart_health/t/fda-takes-issue-cheerios-health-claims/#.WsfRw39G3Sc
4. Health U. S. 2016 - Individual Charts and Tables: Spreadsheet, PDF, and PowerPoint files. Centers for Disease Control and Prevention National Center for Health Statistics 2018: Available online at www.cdc.gov/nchs/hus/contents2016.htm#fig06
5. McGinley L. Four former FDA commissioners denounce drug importation, citing dangers to consumers. *Washington Post* 2017;March 17: Available online at www.washingtonpost.com/news/to-your-health/wp/2017/03/17/four-former-fda-commissioners-denounce-drug-importation-citing-dangers-to-consumers/?utm_term=.1015d08c3249
6. Shanker D. Emails Show How the Food Industry Uses 'Science' to Push Soda. A conversation between two former Coke executives reveals some of the tricks of the trade. *Bloomberg News* 2017; September 13: Available online at www.bloomberg.com/news/articles/2017-09-13/emails-show-how-the-food-industry-uses-science-to-push-soda
7. Chassaing B, Koren O, Goodrich JK, Poole AC, Srinivasan S, Ley RE, Gewirtz AT. Dietary emulsifiers impact the mouse gut microbiota promoting colitis and metabolic syndrome. *Nature* 2015;519(7541):92–6.
8. Chassaing B, Van de Wiele T, De Bodt J, Marzorati M, Gewirtz AT. Dietary emulsifiers directly alter human microbiota composition and gene expression ex vivo potentiating intestinal inflammation. *Gut* 2017;66(8):1414–27.
9. Bhattacharyy S, Shumard T, Xie H, Dodd A, Varady KA, Feferman L, Halline AG, Goldstein JL, Hanauer SB, Tobacmana JK. A randomized trial of the effects of the no-carrageenan diet on ulcerative colitis disease activity. *Nutr Healthy Aging* 2017;4(2):181–92.
10. Shah R, Kolanos R, DiNovi MJ, Mattia A, Kaneko KJ. Dietary exposures for the safety assessment of seven emulsifiers commonly added to foods in the United States and implications for safety. *Food Addit Contam Part A Chem Anal Control Expo Risk Assess* 2017;34(6):905–17.
11. Lundberg G. Demonizing processed food: It's the additives. Medscape 2017: Available online at www.medscape.com/viewarticle/884444
12. Lefevre M, Mensink RP, Kris-Etherton PM, Petersen B, Smith K, Flickinger BD. Predicted changes in fatty acid intakes, plasma lipids, and cardiovascular disease risk following replacement of trans fatty acid-containing soybean oil with application-appropriate alternatives. *Lipids* 2012;47:951–62.
13. Government U.K. Food colours and hyperactivity. Food Standards Agency 2012: Available online at www.food.gov.uk/science/additives/foodcolours
14. Kohlstadt I, Murphy D. Systematic review of drug labeling changes that inform pediatric weight gain. *J J Neur Neurosci* 2014;1(2):013.
15. Young R. Artificial sweeteners alter gut response to glucose (Abstract). European Association for the Study of Diabetes (EASD) 2017 Annual Meeting Lisbon, Portugal: Medscape Medical News, 2017.
16. Tu YH, Cooper AJ, Teng B, et al. An evolutionarily conserved gene family encodes proton-selective ion channels. *Science* 2018; 359(6379):1047–1050.

17. Goodall R. Rehydration Project 2014: Oral Rehydration Therapy: How it Works. Available online at http://rehydrate.org/ors/ort-how-it-works.htm
18. Kohlstadt I. Coming to our senses on education and nutrition. *Time* 2014;Nov 12: Available online at http://time.com/3582298/coming-to-our-senses-on-education-and-nutrition/
19. Cornell. Dairy Foods Science Notes. Cornell University Department of Food Science 2007;October 10.
20. Burton H. *UHT Processing of Milk and Milk Products*. London: Elsevier Applied Science, 1988.
21. Chandran MaWH. The World Congress of Gastroenterology at the ACG 2017: Abstract P1152. Homemade Yogurt Resolves Irritable Bowel Symptoms. Medscape Medical News 2017;https://www.medscape.com/viewarticle/889752
22. Adolfsson O, Meydani SN, Russell RM. Yogurt and gut function. *Am J Clin Nutr* 2004;80(2):245–56.
23. Samsel A, Seneff S. Glyphosate, pathways to modern diseases III: Manganese, neurological diseases, and associated pathologies. *Surg Neurol Int* 2015;6:45.
24. Samsel A, Seneff S. Glyphosate, pathways to modern diseases II: Celiac sprue and gluten intolerance. *Interdiscip Toxicol* 2013;6(4):159–84.
25. Katholm C. Effects of Roundup (glyphosate) on gut microorganisms of farm animals. Department of Animal Science. Research Centre Foulum, Aarhus University 2017: Available online at http://library.au.dk/fileadmin/www.bibliotek.au.dk/fagsider/jordbrug/Specialer/Master_Thesis_final.pdf
26. Henderson AM, Gervais JA, Luukinen B, Buhl K, Stone D. Glyphosate general fact sheet. National Pesticide Information Center 2010: Available online at http://npic.orst.edu/factsheets/glyphogen.html
27. Government U.S. Food irradiation: What you need to know. Food and Drug Administration 2018: Available online at www.fda.gov/food/resourcesforyou/consumers/ucm261680.htm (accessed 2018).
28. Government U.S. Bones in space. National Aeronautics and Space Administration 2004: Available online at www.nasa.gov/audience/foreducators/postsecondary/features/F_Bones_in_Space.html (accessed 2018).
29. DiLuglio B, Cline J. Electromagnetic hypersensitivity and implications for metabolism. In: Kohlstadt I, ed. *Advancing Medicine with Food and Nutrients*, 2nd Edition. Boca Raton, FL: CRC Press, 2013:799–820.
30. Smijs TG, Pavel S. Titanium dioxide and zinc oxide nanoparticles in sunscreens: Focus on their safety and effectiveness. *Nanotechnol Sci Appl* 2011;4:95–112.
31. RVIM. Health effects due to titanium nanoparticles in food and toothpaste cannot be excluded. Government of Netherlands 2016: Available online at www.rivm.nl/en/Documents_and_publications/Common_and_Present/Newsmessages/2016/Health_effects_due_to_titanium_nanoparticles_in_food_and_toothpaste_cannot_be_excluded
32. Pasiakos SM, Berryman CE, Carrigan CT, Young AJ, Carbone JW. Muscle protein turnover and the molecular regulation of muscle mass during hypoxia. *Med Sci Sports Exerc* 2017;49(7):1340–50. doi:10.1249/MSS.0000000000001228
33. Young RC, Blass JP. Iatrogenic nutritional deficiencies. *Annu Rev Nutr* 1982;2:201–27.
34. Kohlstadt I. Primary care approaches to weight reduction. In: Kohlstadt I, ed. *Advancing Medicine with Food and Nutrients*, 2nd Edition. Boca Raton, FL: CRC Press, 2013:349–72.
35. Kohlstadt I, Gittelsohn J, Fang Y. NutriBee intervention advances diet and psychosocial outcomes among early adolescents. *J Am College Nutr* 2015;35(5):443–451.
36. Kohlstadt IC, Steeves ET, Rice K, Gittelsohn J, Summerfield LM, Gadhoke P. Youth peers put the "invent" into NutriBee's online intervention. *Nutr J* 2015;14:60. doi:10.1186/s12937-015-0031-2
37. Kohlstadt I. "Ahh-portunity" in crossing the dental-medical divide. *Townsend Letter* April 2018: Issue #417 13-15.
38. Topol E. Eric Topol's Top 10 Tech Advances Shaping Medicine. Medscape 2018: Available online at www.medscape.com/viewarticle/890982?src=WNL_infoc_180120_MSCPEDIT_TEMP2&uac=1364AR&impID=1538231&faf=1

8 Inflammatory Responses Acquired Following Environmental Exposures Are Involved in Pathogenesis of Musculoskeletal Pain

Ritchie C. Shoemaker, MD and James C. Ryan, PhD

INTRODUCTION

At first, one might not associate environmental exposures with pain. Warm climate versus cold causing pain? Humid climate versus dry causing pain? Urban versus rural? Pain isn't the first response a physician might necessarily associate with environmental exposures.

Contrast that perspective to environmental exposures to low molecular weight biotoxins and/or inflammagens made by one-celled creatures. Inflammation from innate immune responses dominates the illnesses created by biotoxins. Innate immunity can heal, but can also become the overwhelming source of illness caused by exuberant host responses. Add to the level of concern when exposures are to water-damaged buildings (WDB; schools, workplaces and residences), a problem seen in 50% of US buildings (NIOSH) [1]; or fresh water bodies hosting blooms of cyanobacteria (for example, Lake Erie [2]; or even just exposure to tick habitat, an increasing problem now extending well beyond the Northeast of the US. In the cohort of affected, environmentally exposed patients, pain syndromes are found in over 85% (Table 8.1).

Inflammation from innate immune mediators does not quickly come to mind thinking about "wear and tear" arthritis or overuse syndromes like rotator cuff injuries or tennis elbow.

Curiously, the same inflammatory mediators involved in response to adverse environmental exposures also play major roles in musculoskeletal pain, as will be discussed.

What we can't say is that environmental exposures are the sources of worn and torn, painful hips, knees and lower back; but we can say that understanding how to correct the pathogenic inflammatory responses to environmental exposures to toxins and inflammagens now has become fertile ground for development of therapies, both proteomically and genomically active, that control innate immune responses.

While one might speculate if new therapies would have been developed for musculoskeletal pain without learning how to heal illness caused by environmental exposures, one simply can conclude that as we learn more about innate immune responses, and transcriptomic changes associated with the immune responses, we learn how to think differently about common sources of pain. Said another way, there are few activities defined that are exempt from immune participation.

As we understand and catalogue the unknown biotoxin exposures we frequently encounter, such as consumption of fish contaminated by algal neurotoxins, we understand more about the importance of recording diverse environmental exposures in assessment of pain. Ciguatera, caused by ingestion of reef fish contaminated by ciguatoxins, a potent voltage gated sodium channel activator,

TABLE 8.1
Symptoms in Various CIRS Conditions

Symptoms	Controls	Cyano	WDB-1	WDB-2	WDB-3	PEAS	Ciguatera	Lyme
N=	239	10	156	288	21	42	100	352
Fatigue	6	100	89	83	100	70	91	94
Weak	<5	80	75	70	84	—	83	89
Ache	8	90	77	68	95	43	77	81
Cramp	<5	80	66	56	63	14	68	77
Unusual pains	<5	50	62	51	42	—	82	86
Ice pick pain	<5	40	49	41	—	—	45	82
Headache	9	90	78	66	84	73	78	88
Light sensitivity	<5	90	71	66	89	68	67	85
Red eyes	<5	50	52	48	63	68	48	61
Blurred vision	<5	40	61	56	63	—	53	66
Tearing	<5	30	41	48	63	—	28	55
SOB	11	60	78	63	74	57	63	77
Cough	7	50	72	53	53	43	62	71
Sinus congestion	8	60	79	65	74	41	70	68
Abdominal pain	<5	60	61	39	37	41	79	42
Diarrhea	<5	50	48	39	21	57	72	51
Joint pain	11	70	75	53	84	—	62	88
Morning stiffness	6	70	72	44	—	—	59	80
Memory impairment	<5	80	83	66	68	84	81	80
Difficulty concentrating	<5	70	81	62	53	35	83	82
Confusion	<5	40	75	57	26	24	66	72
Decreased word finding	<5	80	81	66	11	—	80	84
Decreased assimilation	<5	80	72	65	37	—	78	88
Disorientation	<5	30	51	40	11	—	28	33
Mood swings	<5	20	69	65	—	—	42	65
Appetite swings	<5	50	58	58	—	—	61	77
Sweats (night)	<5	50	61	54	—	—	42	68
Difficulty reg. body temp	<5	50	63	60	—	—	67	72
Excessive thirst	<5	60	69	54	—	—	59	71
Increased urinary frequency	<5	60	66	58	—	—	66	75
Increased susceptibility to static shocks	<5	40	41	44	—	—	38	32
Numbness	<5	40	48	44	37	—	74	66
Tingling	<5	40	61	51	47	—	78	71
Vertigo	<5	40	39	48	42	16	29	37
Metallic taste	<5	40	45	36	47	—	46	38

was marked early on [3, 4] as a source of a reversal of hot/cold sensation called "cold allodynia." In recent investigations, additional sources of this curious pain syndrome have been identified in other environmental, exposure-related syndromes [5] as having abnormalities related to a variety of sensory neurons with transient potential receptor vanilloid-1 ([TPRV-1]; 6). This singular finding of the link from biotoxin exposure to chronic pain has opened a flood of academic papers that show promise in bringing new approaches to management of chronic pain. We will return to an in-depth discussion of TPRV-1 and its family of receptors in the section "CGRP, SP and VIP: Pain Regulators". Ciguatera didn't have a prominent reputation for teaching us about chronic pain; that lack of notoriety no longer applies.

The underlying basis of pain syndromes from these different types of exposures to environmental biotoxins/inflammagens can be summed up in one word: inflammation. Inflammation is a time-honored cause of pain. From the first day of pathology class in medical school, physicians are trained to recognize heat, redness, swelling, loss of function and pain as manifestations of inflammation. What we learned in the 1970s about inflammation, however, was just a proverbial "drop in the bucket." In a seminal lecture at Cold Spring Harbor in 1989 [7], Charles Janeway foretold the future of inflammation research and therapies to come. Innate immune responses were in their infancy then; now it is routine to pick up an immunology journal that has at least half of its "state-of-the-art" papers either on innate immunity or transcriptomics.

The expanding world of inflammation has been unveiled over the past thirty years, beginning with publications on cytokines, expanding to receptors, cell-based immunity and more. Our current era of research shows us the incredible diversity – and speed – of genomic responses to environmental stimuli. When inflammatory responses become chronic, as abnormalities in immunity often will become, those who suffer with pain will surely have pain that becomes chronic as well.

There are two areas that will be highlighted in this chapter regarding musculoskeletal pain and environmental stimuli. First are manifestations of chronic inflammatory response syndromes (CIRS) in exposed and subsequently affected patients. This actually is an incredibly large subset of patients; most aren't diagnosed. Second are the associated effects of individual elements of CIRS, like TGF beta-1, VIP and microRNA, for example (definitions to follow) that appear by routes other than those acquired following environmental exposures. For example, we know that certain HLA haplotypes are associated with increased relative risk for CIRS [8] and we know that certain HLA haplotypes are also associated with ankylosing spondyloarthropathies (HLA B27). We will not discuss mechanisms of HLA association with epidemiologic risk so much as to say that the established body of evidence demands that we know to look for these associations now that we know those associations are not random occurrences.

We will look in detail at the lessons learned from transcriptomics [9, 10]. The central dogma of molecular biology states that genes produce transcripts that are translated into protein, at which point the protein can perform the task required by the cell. The genome is the ultimately the director of all cellular activity What's important to understand is in addition to the presence of any given gene in the genome is the *differential expression* of that same gene. Single nucleotide polymorphisms (SNP), may tell us about protein function but nothing about actual gene expression. If an SNP causes a 5% decrease in protein function, but that protein is expressed at an amount 5% greater than normal, the system likely suffers no effect. But of greater importance than expression of a single gene is differential gene expression of entire molecular pathways, as well as transcription factors, receptors, clusters of differentiation (CDs), pseudogenes, microRNA and long noncoding RNA, among others.

A second facet of pathway analysis of illness causation is readily observed by looking at genes that are overexpressed. What other unexpected adverse health effects follow? Since transforming growth factor beta-1 (TGF beta-1) is overexpressed in CIRS-WDB [11], and since TGF beta-1 turns on the processes involved in fibrosis, will there be more fibrotic lung tissue in CIRS-WDB, for example? The data that say yes are easily found but are anecdotal. The data are far less clear on matrix metalloproteinase-9 (MMP-9), also seen routinely to be a problem in CIRS-WDB. Can we show that herniated nucleus pulposus (HNP), a process involved with MMP9 is more common in CIRS-WDB patients? Or are TGF beta-1 and MMP9 simply reflecting redundancy of biological regulation of gene expression?

The argument regarding multiple sources of stimuli will be revisited when we discuss VIP and degenerative arthritis.

As an aside, this chapter will not focus on the cellular basis of nociception, the sensation of pain, so much as we will attempt to show that the diversities of inflammatory responses, ones that potentially can affect every cell in our body, are part of the daily maintenance of life itself. We suggest that pain, as part of what can be called disease, is dynamic, involving all regulatory and effector arms of innate and adaptive immune defenses, though the role of adaptive immunity in pain will be covered in less detail.

We will begin by exploring CIRS and then return to musculoskeletal conditions beginning in the section "Herniated Nucleus Pulposus and Innate Immune Effectors".

WHAT IS PAIN?

Multiple attempts have been made to define pain. For the purposes of this chapter, the definition from the International Association of the Study of Pain is adopted (www.iasp-pain.org, accessed 7/2/2107). "Pain is the unpleasant sensory and emotional experience associated with actual or potential tissue damage."

The perception of pain, nociception, involves multiple layers in which inflammatory effects might be exerted: (1) signal transduction by sensory neuron receptors; (2) transmission of signal via neurons: (3) modulation in the dorsal horn of the spinal cord; (4) and perception in the thalamus (ref). Each of these main elements of the experience of pain will be investigated for possible association with CIRS and its innate immune effectors.

WHAT IS CIRS?

Chronic inflammatory response syndromes (CIRS) are multisystem, multi-symptom illnesses acquired following exposure to environmentally produced biotoxins [11–15].

CIRS has gone through an evolution of names over the years. Initially, in the 1990s, CIRS was called a neurotoxin-mediated illness [12, 13]. As more information developed, the term was changed to chronic biotoxin-associated illness (CBAI). The third change to CIRS occurred following development of a commercial assay for TGFβ1 in 2008, readily available for insurance, coverage then by the development of a commercial assay for acquired T regulatory cells in 2009. CIRS was confirmed to involve many arms of the immune response systems acting simultaneously and in combination.

CIRS itself is modeled after an acute systemic inflammatory response syndrome (SIRS), an acronym typically only used to describe an acute inflammatory illness, sepsis. In patients with sepsis there is simultaneous activation of Th1-, Th2- and Th17-immunity; coagulation factors; and complement in response to an overwhelming stimulus of infection and endotoxin present in the blood stream. In this regard illness becomes the host response as eloquently described by Thomas [16].

Survivors of sepsis have been well studied; they do not have the same immune reactivity after one month as they did before sepsis started. Survivors have a significant increase in interleukin 10 and go on to develop greater incidences of chronic fatiguing illnesses [17, 18].

If an ICD code is to be used for an affected survivor of sepsis, should we be calling their illness chronic sepsis survivor syndrome? We clearly would not be able to call the illness an acute systemic inflammatory response syndrome. What should we call it?

In 2008, followed by a publication in 2010 [19], members of the small "mold" medical community began using a jargon term, CIRS-WDB, to describe illness seen with the same activation of Th1, Th2, Th17, coagulation, complement activation and more. If the illness came from water-damaged buildings, we called it CIRS-WDB. If it came from Post Lyme Syndrome, we called it CIRS-PLS. If it came from ciguatera we called the syndrome CIRS-ciguatera. Theoretically, we could call the syndrome most anything; possibly the syndrome would be codified by a regulatory agency, much as the CDC changed the name, "Pfiesteria health illness syndrome (affecting) humans," PHISH, for acute and chronic illness caused by exposure to blooms of toxigenic, fish-killing dinoflagellates, including Pfiesteria, to "Possible estuarine-associated syndrome" (PEAS) [11].

CASE DEFINITION OF CIRS

In 2008, the US General Accountability Office (GAO) published an overview of publications from US agencies working on the problem of damp indoor buildings [20]. Fifty-four studies were noted, showing no coordination of efforts across agency lines. But for the first time, a Federal case definition for what has become CIRS-WDB was proposed.

1. There must be the potential for exposure to a damp indoor space.
2. There must be a multisystem, multi-symptom illness present with symptoms similar to those seen in peer-reviewed publications.
3. There must be laboratory testing results similar to those seen in peer-reviewed, published studies.
4. There must be documentation of response to therapy (symptoms correction alone wasn't enough).

This definition still is used even though there has been an explosion of publications in the CIRS community noting various objective parameters in wide clinical use now (SM consensus).

Symptoms are noted to be essentially identical in multiple sources of environmental exposures resulting in CIRS (see Table 8.1). Of interest is the appearance of clusters of symptoms among the 37 symptoms recorded in CIRS (Table 8.2). Presence of eight or more (of the 13) clusters is virtually diagnostic of an unspecified type of CIRS (US Patent #US 9,770,170 B2).

Returning to the multiple sources of TGF beta-1, and the association of TGF beta-1 with painful musculoskeletal syndromes, the clinician can use the case definition and cluster analysis to quickly rule out CIRS in initial evaluation of a patient with a painful shoulder or low back pain. If there is

---

TABLE 8.2
Cluster Analysis

Cluster Analysis of Symptoms

Individual categories:

- Fatigue
- Weakness, assimilation, aching, headache, light sensitivity
- Memory, word finding
- Concentration
- Joint, AM stiffness, cramps
- Unusual skin sensations, tingling
- Shortness of breath, sinus congestion
- Cough, thirst, confusion
- Appetite swings, body temperature regulation, urinary frequency
- Red eyes, blurred vision, sweats, mood swings, icepick pains
- Abdominal pain, diarrhea, numbness
- Tearing, disorientation, metallic taste
- Static shocks, vertigo

A positive cluster analysis for biotoxin illness is presence of eight or more of 13 clusters

When we use persistent health symptoms as a group of 37, recorded by a trained health care provider in a medical history (never use patient-completed checklists), we can collate individual symptoms into groups, called clusters. Statistically, these clusters of symptoms, 13 in number, yield a diagnostic capability to separate out CIRS from essentially all diseases. If you have eight or more clusters of symptoms, the likelihood of CIRS exceeds 95%.

When combined with VCS deficits, symptom clusters can yield an accuracy in diagnosis of 98.5% (that means the sum of false positives and false negatives is less than 2%).

---

no multisystem illness identified by a medical history taken by a licensed health professional (NB: patient-completed checklists have too much potential for reporting bias to be used), CIRS is not the problem. But if elements of CIRS are present in the absence of actual CIRS, they must be noted and treated to affect clinical outcome. Elevated levels of TGF beta-1 cannot be simply ignored in cases of neuropathic pain, for example.

In the experience of this author, most consultants looking at pain are surprised when a seemingly isolated problem, like a rotator cuff tear or an enthesopathy, like lateral epicondylitis, are present as a part of a constellation of twenty other symptoms! Who knew? The medical historian. If the "diffusely positive review of systems," is not recorded, CIRS will never be diagnosed.

SYMPTOMS OF PAIN IN CIRS

In a medical history, the physician is not using a check list. Symptoms questioning is perhaps better understood after observing how a skilled attorney will question a witness. Essentially, he will likely be asking for the same information from multiple different angles trying to have a clear idea of what the witness actually said or did. Similarly, a physician will follow the line of thought of a patient in discussing symptoms, but will circle back to pin down any possible vagaries that might be present. In this manner, a physician will learn to a reasonable degree of medical certainty, more likely than not, on a day-to-day basis, does a patient have muscle aching? Does a patient have muscle cramps? Are there unusual pains, sharp stabbing pains that seemingly come unexpectedly and lancinate in one area of the body only to disappear and reappear elsewhere the next day? This type of pain description is typical of what CIRS patients experience and is absolutely not confabulated-but will sound odd to the physician who is not used to recording unusual pain histories.

Ask about unusual posturing of fingers or toes, sometimes called "clawing." These involuntary spasms in small muscles of fingers and toes can be painful, can be quite unusual for those affected and are certainly unusual elements of history. Some patients will have their long and fourth finger split apart making a sign of a V as we saw so often from Mr. Spock in Star Trek. Sometimes there will be arching of the MCP and MTP joints as well. If you don't ask about clawing, you won't be told. Patients will recognize a careful historian who asks about unusual muscle spasm when they have clawing.

Muscle cramping is a common problem in athletes (and CIRS patients!). How many times have we seen a star basketball player clutching at his calves in the middle of the 3rd quarter of a heated basketball game? Cramps are disabling! He limps off the court; his team's fans hold their breath until he stretches the cramp out and returns to the 4th quarter to win the game.

The calf cramps CIRS patients often have are not related to heat or to exertion. They are far more commonly brought on by lying down in bed or arising from sleep. The cramp is a muscle spasm; CIRS patients quickly learn that the spasm experienced in the middle of the night can be severe, especially if they have been sleeping with their ankles extended. Simple dorsiflexion of the ankles, stretching, for example, is mandatory but sometimes the spasm is so severe the gastrocnemius muscle essentially twists into a knot, occasionally tearing. Just so you know, in the middle of the night, that pain is agonizing. If you don't ask about cramps like these you won't be told. Physicians just aren't taught to take CIRS spasm histories. The spasms are real.

Joint stiffness is what we see often in CIRS as well as in day-to-day musculoskeletal medical practice. Stretching upon arising is a common way to start the day for both types of patients. Shoulders, elbows, knees, low back, all will require some sort of attention. The rate of stiffening, however, with *cessation* of activity, called "gelling," is far faster in CIRS than it is for patients with wear and tear degenerative arthritis. If a patient tells you that he would prefer to stay standing after activity rather than sit down and rest that may be an indication of his awareness of his own rate of gelling.

Aching is perhaps the most common CIRS pain. Not from over-doing the work in the yard or trying to work out excessively, muscle aching can be vague until the aching occurs almost every day regardless of antecedent activity, but not in the same area and not with the same intensity. CIRS aching won't respond to most meds, including NSAID. The aching often comes from areas of muscle insertion on tendons, raising the concern regarding enthesopathies. The enthesium has reduced blood supply and reduced capillary perfusion to begin with; inflammatory responses in CIRS make capillary hypoperfusion worse. Pain will be enhanced in the face of hypoperfusion. If one sees an enthesopathy but doesn't find a convincing history of overuse, spend a few minutes exploring the rest of the CIRS symptom roster with the patient.

As we will discuss in the section on transcriptomics, downregulation of nuclear encoded mitochondrial genes can be profound. Instead of postulating *intrinsic* mitochondrial disorders leading to abnormal mitochondrial metabolism of glucose, leading to lactic acid accumulation, a better approach is to recognize that nuclear transcription factors exert direct effect on mitochondrial function. By recording nuclear encoded mitochondrial gene activation, using Next Generation Sequencing, the physician can understand reduced energy delivery is abnormal due to aberrant genomic control. Still, whatever causes lactic acid accumulation, excessive lactic acid in capillary beds is a source of muscle pain, including aching.

Understanding that mitochondrial research is ongoing [21] looking at mitochondrial stress responses, we feel that a delineation of mitochondrial gene expression be examined as an upstream regulator of stress responses.

Headaches are not necessarily a musculoskeletal problem but can overlap with any pain syndrome. With CIRS we look for intravascular volume depletion and reduced antidiuretic hormone (ADH) levels for a given osmolality. If patients are troubled with headaches, especially if they have "migraine that lasts for more than 24 hours," think of ADH/osmolality and not an actual migraine.

Symptom variability is notoriously present in large segments of patient populations. Use of a physician history is necessary, as patient-completed questionnaires are unreliable. If someone presents a checklist of their health symptoms, the healthcare provider is obligated to review those symptoms to be sure whether they are present to a reasonable degree of medical certainty. Having said that, if a busy orthopedist needs to see eight patients per hour, he may need to delegate symptom recording to a staff member.

THE BIOTOXIN PATHWAY

Please refer to Figure 8.1 for a schematic representation of the series of events routinely seen in cases of CIRS. For a more detailed assessment of the elements of the Biotoxin Pathway, the reader is recommended to review information found on www.survivingmold.com.

The proteomic lab tests we rely on might be new to readers. We note abnormalities of a set of proteomic variables and have used proteomics to (1) aid in diagnosis of CIRS; and to (2) document systematic improvement with therapy, as self-healing won't occur in CIRS like it might in simple overuse syndromes.

The approach used to stratify lab abnormalities seen in CIRS encompasses a number of basic principles. First, there is a relationship between cases and controls that involves immune gene alleles on chromosome 6 (*HLA*). This relationship, called relative risk, looks at the incidence in cases for a given parameter, in this case the incidence of HLA-DR alleles in CIRS, divided by the incidence of the same parameter in controls. We have a data base of an approximately 10,000 patients for whom HLA has been recorded. What we see is the "susceptible" haplotypes of HLA, those with increased relative risk greater than 2.0, found in 95% of CIRS-WDB cases, are comprised of (1) 11-3-52B; (2) 4-3-53; (3) 7-2-53; (4) 13-6-52C; (5) 14-5-52B; and (6) 17-2-52A. The incidence of these haplotypes in control populations is 24% [8]. Of note, the HLA nomenclature has evolved, in particular the numbers used for haplotypes. At one time, we had approximately twenty identified haplotypes; now there are over 54, with subtyping extending HLA-DR to literally hundreds of additional descriptors. In an effort to keep things simple, we have maintained our registry of HLA based on what was current in 2000. It may be of use to look at a roster of HLA haplotypes and susceptibility by illness found in the Rosetta Stone appendix published in *Mold Warriors* in 2005 and in *Surviving Mold* in 2010 (Table 8.3).

The Biotoxin Pathway

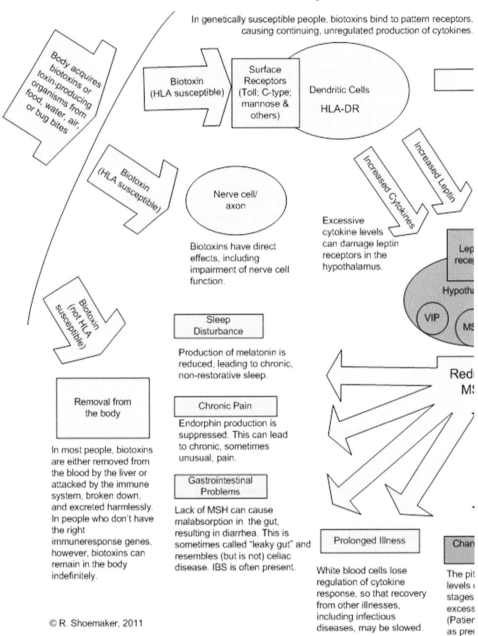

In genetically susceptible people, biotoxins bind to pattern receptors, causing continuing, unregulated production of cytokines.

Body acquires biotoxins or toxin-producing organisms from food, water, air, or bug bites

Biotoxin (HLA susceptible)

Surface Receptors (Toll: C-type; mannose & others)

Dendritic Cells
HLA-DR

Biotoxin (HLA susceptible)

Nerve cell/axon

Biotoxins have direct effects, including impairment of nerve cell function.

Increased Cytokines

Increased Leptin

Excessive cytokine levels can damage leptin receptors in the hypothalamus.

Lep rece

Hypotha

VIP   MS

Biotoxin (not HLA susceptible)

Sleep Disturbance

Production of melatonin is reduced, leading to chronic, non-restorative sleep.

Removal from the body

In most people, biotoxins are either removed from the blood by the liver or attacked by the immune system, broken down, and excreted harmlessly. In people who don't have the right immuneresponse genes, however, biotoxins can remain in the body indefinitely.

Chronic Pain

Endorphin production is suppressed. This can lead to chronic, sometimes unusual, pain.

Gastrointestinal Problems

Lack of MSH can cause malabsorption in the gut, resulting in diarrhea. This is sometimes called "leaky gut" and resembles (but is not) celiac disease. IBS is often present.

Red
M:

Prolonged Illness

White blood cells lose regulation of cytokine response, so that recovery from other illnesses, including infectious diseases, may be slowed.

Chan

The pit levels stages excess (Patier as prec levels

© R. Shoemaker, 2011

FIGURE 8.1   The biotoxin pathway

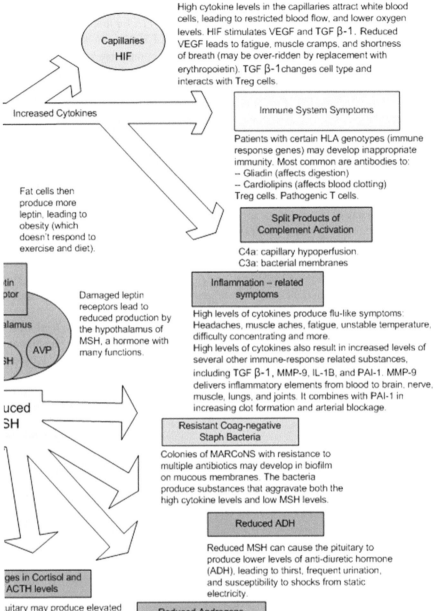

High cytokine levels in the capillaries attract white blood cells, leading to restricted blood flow, and lower oxygen levels. HIF stimulates VEGF and TGF β-1. Reduced VEGF leads to fatigue, muscle cramps, and shortness of breath (may be over-ridden by replacement with erythropoietin). TGF β-1 changes cell type and interacts with Treg cells.

Capillaries
HIF

Increased Cytokines

Immune System Symptoms

Patients with certain HLA genotypes (immune response genes) may develop inappropriate immunity. Most common are antibodies to:
-- Gliadin (affects digestion)
-- Cardiolipins (affects blood clotting)
Treg cells. Pathogenic T cells.

Fat cells then produce more leptin, leading to obesity (which doesn't respond to exercise and diet).

Split Products of
Complement Activation

C4a: capillary hypoperfusion.
C3a: bacterial membranes

Inflammation – related symptoms

tin
ptor

alamus

AVP

SH

Damaged leptin receptors lead to reduced production by the hypothalamus of MSH, a hormone with many functions.

High levels of cytokines produce flu-like symptoms: Headaches, muscle aches, fatigue, unstable temperature, difficulty concentrating and more.
High levels of cytokines also result in increased levels of several other immune-response related substances, including TGF β-1, MMP-9, IL-1B, and PAI-1. MMP-9 delivers inflammatory elements from blood to brain, nerve, muscle, lungs, and joints. It combines with PAI-1 in increasing clot formation and arterial blockage.

uced
SH

Resistant Coag-negative
Staph Bacteria

Colonies of MARCoNS with resistance to multiple antibiotics may develop in biofilm on mucous membranes. The bacteria produce substances that aggravate both the high cytokine levels and low MSH levels.

Reduced ADH

Reduced MSH can cause the pituitary to produce lower levels of anti-diuretic hormone (ADH), leading to thirst, frequent urination, and susceptibility to shocks from static electricity.

ges in Cortisol and
ACTH levels

uitary may produce elevated
of cortisol and ACTH in early
of illness, then drop to
ively low levels later.
ts should avoid steroids such
dnisone, which can lower
of ACTH.)

Reduced Androgens

Reduced MSH can cause the pituitary to lower its production of sex hormones.

Another cardinal feature seen in CIRS is reduction of levels of alpha melanocyte stimulating hormone (*MSH*) below 35 pg/ml. LabCorp has been the primary provider for this test. For unknown reasons, that lab changed the normal range of MSH in September of 2006 from where it had been placed correctly at 35–81 pg/ml to 0–40. Levels of MSH <1 are not compatible with life, so a level of -0- is not logically considered to be normal. Control testing published in several publications [11, 22] show that the newer normal range is not accurate; the older normal range is.

MSH is vitally important in regulation of inflammation, regulation of energy balance, regulation of circadian rhythm, regulation of limbic system parameters as well as regulation of keratinocytes, local mucus membrane defenses, immune defenses in blood and immune defenses in skin. It is a ubiquitously found regulatory neuropeptide [23]. With MSH deficiency we see enhanced development of CIRS following a priming inflammatory, cytokine event. Patients are borne with a given HLA, but HLA-based susceptibility to development of CIRS occurs only after an acute inflammatory event.

MSH is produced in a variety of tissues, especially in the hypothalamus and arcuate nucleus. The mechanism of production begins with activation of the leptin receptor, a primordial gp-130 cytokine receptor. Signaling from this receptor activates transcription of the gene for proopiomelanocortin (POMC). This parent molecule is split into MSH and beta endorphin, the natural opiate of the brain. In the presence of defective production of MSH, due to cytokine blockage of the leptin receptor, there will be MSH deficiency. Such a deficiency will be associated with decreased production of beta endorphin.

Deficiency of MSH can lead to chronic fatigue; blockade of leptin receptors leads to leptin resistance (the mechanism is similar to insulin receptor resistance [24]) and refractory weight gain; and deficiency of beta endorphin creates chronic pain. Here we have the basis for a devastating illness: chronic fatigue superimposed on chronic weight problems superimposed on chronic pain. When the clinician sees even one of this poisoned triad, think to add MSH deficiency and CIRS to the differential diagnosis.

TABLE 8.3

Human Leukocyte Antigen (HLA) Sequences Associated With Chronic Inflammatory Response Syndrome

	DRB1	DQ	DRB3	DRB4	DRB5
Multisusceptible	4	3		53	
	11/12	3	52B		
	14	5	52B		
Mold	7	2/3		53	
	13	6	52A, B, C		
	17	2	52A		
	18	4	52A		
Borrelia, post Lyme Syndrome	15	6			51
	16	5			51
Dinoflagellates	4	7/8		53	
Multi Antibiotic Resistant Staph epidermidis	11	7	52B		
Low MSH+melanocyte stimulating hormone	1	5			
No recognized significance	8	3,4,6			
Low-risk mold	7	9		53	
	12	7	52B		
	9	3/9		53	

Along with disruption of regulation of MSH production, (see discussion of beta-endorphins, below) are the influences of MSH on other hormone systems. For people with MSH deficiency, dysregulation of ACTH/cortisol is found in approximately 70% of patients; dysregulation of ADH/osmolality is found in 80% of patients; and dysregulation of gonadotrophins and androgens is found in approximately 40% of patients. Curiously, TSH and thyroid hormones are spared MSH regulation abnormalities.

MSH also exerts a damping effect on production of matrix metalloproteinase 9 (*MMP-9*), a protein made following cleavage of MMP-14, which is induced by the effects of cytokines in endothelial cells and white blood cells. We use MMP-9 because of the inability to accurately measure the total burden of Th1 and Th2 cytokines. The problem here is that cells that produce Th1/Th2 cytokines can bind given cytokines (autocrine effects) or cells nearby can also bind the cytokine (paracrine effects). When we measure IL1 beta or IL6 in the blood, the result is only the endocrine function of those cytokines. MMP-9 has additional important effects in chronic pain, namely delivery from inflammatory elements out of blood across cell membrane of endothelial cells through the basement membrane into the sub-intimal space. This delivery mechanism can create havoc in lung, brain, muscle, tendon and nerve [25].

The role of complement with generation of split products of activation, *C3a* and *C4a*, is also widespread in CIRS. These "built in" innate immune response agents are released quickly following cleavage of parent molecules, C3 and C4, respectively. When challenged by antigens, including infectious agents, C3a and C4a are vitally important to innate immune inflammatory responses.

TGF beta-1 remains a cytokine of great interest in musculoskeletal issues, specifically pain, as well as delayed healing in tendinous structures. We will return to TGF beta-1 in greater detail.

Of perhaps singular importance are levels of vasoactive intestinal polypeptide (*VIP*). VIP is a potent anti-inflammatory, neuroregulatory peptide, similar in function to MSH. It acts on three separate receptors, two of which, VIPR-1 and VIPR-2, are richly endowed on synovial cells as well as in joint tissue [26]. VIP is highly correlated with lack of inflammation, as we see in MSH, but it also has shown the ability to correct genomic abnormalities [10] as well as correct proteomics [11] and gray matter nuclear atrophy [27]. VIP replacement has revolutionized care of patients with CIRS. Given its important role in maintenance of joint integrity, one wonders how quickly use of this well-established anti-inflammatory neuropeptide will become standard practice. As new information on VIP comes to clinical trials, published data will lead the way.

An additional factor important to musculoskeletal problems, also present in CIRS, is vascular endothelial growth factor (VEGF). VEGF will stimulate enhanced delivery of oxygen in the capillary beds, especially important if there is enhanced reduction of capillary perfusion due to cytokine presence. Lack of oxygen delivery will compromise aerobic metabolism, particularly in muscle beds, creating reduced exercise tolerance, increased pain and absence of normal efficiency of electron transport chains in mitochondrial function.

These fundamental elements of CIRS also have importance for musculoskeletal pain and musculoskeletal injury, both as a whole and as individual effectors. The example of VIP in arthritic joints is one issue; similarly, enhanced entraining of TGF beta-1 into crosslinked collagen can increase susceptibility of those with hypermobility to the inflammation in fibromyalgia.

Two unanswered questions remain. First, if an inflammatory element is involved in musculoskeletal pain, and then that element is increased as part of CIRS, will the musculoskeletal pain increase? If so, will therapies known to be successful in CIRS cross over to be successful in musculoskeletal pain syndromes?

TRANSCRIPTOMICS

The most sophisticated research laboratory tool available today for testing physiology is performed using DNA sequencing. What this means is that scientists can now look at differential activation for all genes in the human genome using a Next Generation Sequencer. The Human Genome Project, completed in the early 2000s at the cost of billions of dollars, identified thousands of genes that code for proteins. What we saw then was the total genome structure, including duplicate copies called copy number variations (CNVs). Later, we learned that everyone had slight variations in most of their genes, called single nucleotide polymorphisms or SNPs. Many of these SNPs are now known to be important markers of disease because they can indicate a change in protein function or activity. However, these SNPs are fixed and do not change throughout your life. What may be the most impactful modulator of cellular activity is differential gene expression, since the amount of the gene expressed is ultimately in control of protein levels and cellular output. Based on current conditions, the genome will output a certain combination of genes, but when the conditions change, the gene output will change to best adapt to the new conditions or demands. This is generally what determines one's day-to-day, or even your morning-to-night, physiology.

What the first sequencing of human genome could not let us identify was this dynamic yet critical differential gene activity found over time.

We now know that the static genome is actively manipulated, constantly increasing production of some gene transcripts and decreasing others in response to its environment. Remarkably, environmental stimuli, and there are many, can cause gene activation in minutes, if not faster. Such rapid changes in gene activity provide incredibly precise adaptations of the host to a rapidly changing environment. Regulation is complex: nuclear transcription factors and newly discovered long noncoding RNAs, together with microRNAs and circular RNAs, as well as methylation and acetylation (don't forget demethylation and deacetylation!) can shut off and turn on gene function. If this sounds complicated, it is, though research into the interacting complexities of so many layers of regulation are only partially described.

We are at the dawn of a new era in science where we can use genomics and transcriptomics to our advantage in that we can find a distinct fingerprint for CIRS from water-damaged buildings, separating CIRS-WDB from ciguatera and from Post Lyme Syndrome. The application of genomics to complex human illness is in its early stages. Already, tremendous advances in medicine and science have resulted from transcriptomics.

HERNIATED NUCLEUS PULPOSUS AND INNATE IMMUNE EFFECTORS

Low back pain, discogenic back pain, slipped disc, ruptured disc, lumbar disc herniation, intervertebral disc degeneration/degradation are all names that basically imply pain and disability from back problems at some time in otherwise normal patients. The sufferers are many. Causes are relatively few, like repetitive microtrauma, overuse syndromes, improper ergonomics ("lift with your knees"), overweight, smoking, age ("time to use your brain, not your back"), malalignment, scoliosis, osteoporosis and more. Treatments are diverse but results are disheartening. Stretching, massage, physical therapy, disc injections and surgeries of all kinds are often recommended. Acupuncture, stress reduction and analgesics may have emerging roles.

What we rarely hear about is the benefits of reduction of inflammatory mediators in syndromes involving intervertebral discs [28]. Both disc cells and migrating macrophages release inflammatory cytokines in response to disc injury. We know that in injured discs, we see release of IL-1b, IL-6 and TNF as pro-inflammatory compounds and IL-8 as an anti-inflammatory compound, just like in CIRS. Enzymes that degrade extracellular matrix are induced by pro-inflammatory cytokines; matrix metalloproteinases worsen disc degeneration and pain [28].

Differential gene activation is observed in lumbar disc syndromes. From growth factors (VEGF and TGF beta-1, to platelet derived growth factors (PDGF)) the normal attempts to heal trauma include stimulation of new blood vessel growth to heal protruding discs; to intense pain from PDGF as part of the metabolic response to tissue healing [29]. If TGF beta-1 is activated, fibrosis won't be far behind.

It is possible that not all inflammatory effectors are going to cause pain in HNP. MMPs (there are many) and ADAM-4 ("a disintegrin and metalloproteinase with thrombospondin motifs") act synergistically and are associated with pain, but each may play a role in resorption of disc material after herniation is complete [30]. If we block MMP9 and ADAM-4, we might block pain acutely, but when do we stop as to not interfere with resorption of herniated fragments?

Perhaps transcriptomics can tell us [31] if we could see when tissue inhibitors of MMPs (TIMP) are activated. These effectors are increased in degenerated cells. Genetics plays a role, but so does the p38 mitogen-activated protein kinase pathway (MAP kinases), the same pathway turned on by exposure to trichothecene mycotoxins, especially deoxynivalenol [32]. For the 50% of the US work force (NIOSH) possibly employed in a WDB, do we know if their MAP kinases are actually helping them avoid ongoing pain?

To further confuse the issue of disc pain, look at comparisons of nucleus pulposus cells (NP) and articular chondrocytes in an animal model published by Ciu [33]. The cells look similar but gene profiling shows marked differences. Nucleus pulposus cells compared to chondrocytes are over-producers of MMP-2; MMP-14; ADAMS-1, -2, -17; as well as TIMP; but they are comparatively lower producers of MMP-1, -3, -7, -8, -10, -11, -13, -16, -19, -20, -21, -23, 24. 28; ADAMS-4, -5, -14, -18, -19; and TIMP-3. Chondrocytes expressed MMP-12 and MMP27, but NP cells did not. To confound these extraordinary results, we may ask what transcriptomic differences are created by being in cell culture instead of in vivo.

If genetics and activity, combined with overuse and obesity, remain underlying concerns about HNP, the same inflammatory mediators that we heard about in CIRS are supplying major loads of pain and disability. Does this mean that the salutary benefits from VIP apply to HNP independent of CIRS? Yes! (RCS, unpublished; 34).

OSTEOARTHRITIS AND VIP

The intriguing role of VIP in musculoskeletal pain is already well known [34]. Specific reasons for its benefits may simply relate to its presence in human synovial fibroblasts. Juarranz and colleagues report measurement of expression of VIP, VIP receptors, intracellular cAMP production and cell membrane adenylate cyclase [26]. VIP mRNA and VIP was detected in synoviocytes, with far less found in cells from patients with rheumatoid arthritis (RA) compared to cells from patients with osteoarthritis (OA). VIP receptor 1 (VIPR1/VPAC1) was more abundant on OA with VIP receptor 2 (VIPR2/VPAC2) in RA. Treatment of OA cells with tumor necrosis factor alpha (TNF) reproduced the findings of reduced VIP found in RA. VIP downregulated pro-inflammatory compounds IL-6, CCL2 and CXCL8 as did specific agonists of VPAC1 and VPAC2.

We can ask if the low VIP in RA was the result of pro-inflammatory compound generation, but we could also postulate either microRNA or long noncoding RNA blocking production of VIP. We know that in CIRS, VIP deficiency is associated with decreased production of Ikaros family transcription factors [10]. This transcriptomic work has not been done in RA to date.

Comparing VIP in human osteoarthritic cartilage to that of unaffected human controls was instructive. Jiang [35] published that VIP concentration in synovial cells from OA patients was much less than VIP from controls and that VIP was inversely correlated with progressive joint damage in OA.

In an excellent review article, Jang [34] notes the diversity of published benefits of VIP, though the correction of abnormal proteomics in CIRS by VIP is not referenced. VIP is downregulated in synovial fluid in OA; such downregulation leads to increases in pro-inflammatory cytokines. Moreover, VIP can prevent chronic joint cartilage damage and joint remodeling. Upregulation of VIP can counteract pro-inflammatory stimuli and *reduce pain*.

One must also consider the other sources of reduced pain from VIP. In mice lacking VIP, hypersensitivity apparently is mediated at a local mechanism in the spinal cord. This observation is complicated by the additional observation that VIP-deficient mice also had enhanced inflammatory and greater glial reactivity compared to controls [36].

Could VIP be (1) decreasing local generation of painful stimuli and (2) reducing dorsal cord hypersensitivity? Or is VIP affecting thalamus modulation of pain inputs?

CYTOKINES AND OSTEOARTHRITIS

A review looking at the literature of pro-inflammatory (and anti-inflammatory!) cytokines shows an evolution of thought from 1990 to the present. Myers [37], writing in 1990, suggests that while synovitis is common in advanced osteoarthritis (OA), prevalence and severity of synovial inflammation is uncertain in early cases with early changes in synovial thickening unimpressive. Biopsy studies found an association between synovial mononuclear cell infiltration and thickness of the synovial lining of only 12% of patients. The severity of cartilage lesions was unrelated to severity of synovitis. Contrast that work with that of Mathiessen [38] who writes in 2017 that modern imaging studies show significant changes even before visible cartilage degeneration has occurred. Imaging studies and tissue evaluation has confirmed a high prevalence of synovial inflammation in all stages of OA with multiple studies confirming synovitis is related to pain, poor function and possible progression of structural injury.

And yet, the middle ground in this timeline from Fernandes [39] published in 2002, acknowledges that activated synovial sites upregulate MMP gene expression. This finding is no different than what we have seen in CIRS. The thought of Fernandes was to block cytokines using antagonists to receptors for interleukin-1 to reduce experimental injury from cytokines such as TNF-alpha. They were able to show in experimental dogs and rabbits that in vivo intraarticular injections of IL-R antagonist genes can prevent progression of destructive changes.

In 2008, Ray [40] discusses the evidence for abundant expression of inflammation-responsive transcription factors paralleling what we look at in transcriptomics today. This transcription factor, called SAF-1 regulates increased synthesis of MMP-9 together with VEGF. We are accustomed to hearing those acronyms in arthritis as well as with CIRS. The implication from Ray's work is that more important than the MMP-9 effect on cartilage erosion are the factors that regulate MMP-9 reduction. Those factors, related to the genes of MMP-14, which are related to pro-inflammatory cytokine release. Pro-inflammatory cytokine release in turn is under regulatory control of a nuclear transcription agent.

Sandy [41] continues the approach looking at human genome-wide expression of inflammatory mediators in arthritis. This fascinating study looks at catabolic mediators in OA; discusses the prior focus of interleukin-1 beta; and shows that focus of interleukin-1 beta should be replaced by focus of soluble mediators such as IL17 or TGF beta-1 which are more likely to mimic disease in models of OA. Sandy concludes that early OA is related to the activity of soluble inflammatory mediators but late stage disease looks at the accumulation of biomechanical effects on the remaining cartilage.

The literature regarding cytokine inhibitors in arthritis is mixed. Calich [42] reviewed models of TNF neutralization through IL1Ra inhibitors in animals (NB: Sandy would substitute IL17 or/and TGF beta-1) but was not convinced there was adequate evidence that showed blocking TNF was beneficial in treatment of osteoarthritis in humans.

Kapoor [43] also reviewed the role of pro-inflammatory cytokines in the pathophysiology of osteoarthritis. The study defines osteoarthritis with its cartilage destruction, subchondral bone remodeling and inflammation of synovial membranes, and notes antecedent occurrences leading to degenerative changes. Kapoor also finds, (1) limited efficacy from blocking the effects of pro-inflammatory cytokines; and (2) little benefit in prevention of osteoarthritis in animal models.

It is likely that these studies looking at cytokines alone have overlooked the role of VIP and additional nuclear transcription factors, including Ikaros. Inflammatory mediators are invariably seen in a diverse group of pathologies with simultaneous activation of anti-inflammatory cytokines, Th-17 cells, neuroregulatory peptides and transcription-regulatory agents, making assessment of specific causation impossible.

TGF BETA-1 AND OSTEOARTHRITIS

Along with the progression of injury underlying the inflammatory bases of musculoskeletal pain is the increasing focus on transforming growth factor beta-1 (TGF beta-1) in osteoarthritis (OA). TGF beta-1 is defined as a "pleiotropic cytokine that is important in the regulation of joint homeostasis and disease." [44]. Of significance are both the direct effects of TGF beta-1 in immune signaling but also its indirect effects on differential gene transcription. Concentration of TGF beta-1 is normally low in healthy joints and high in osteoarthritic joints. This differential leads to enhanced activation of differential signaling pathways in joints themselves. There are indirect effects in TGF beta-1 including cartilage damage, osteophyte formation and synovial fibrosis as discussed earlier in this chapter but appear to be at least associated with, and possibly caused by, high levels of TGF beta-1. Interestingly, and consistent with the dual role of TGF beta-1, in younger patients, pathological changes are counteracted by TGF beta-1 but in joints of older patients those changes are enhanced. We know that TGF beta-1 acts in concert with T-regulatory cells, with those cells being anti-inflammatory in tissue, including joint, provided there is adequate presence of retinoic acid–related orphan receptor (ROR). In the absence of normal tissue levels ROR, TGF beta-1-driven T reg cells can be converted into T-effector cells, thereby enhancing tissue injury and releasing more TGF beta-1.

Although a significant literature on TGF beta-1 and OA has been published recently, there is reference to TGF beta overexpression contributing to experimental osteoarthritis as early as 2003 [45]. In experimental adenovirus transfection in an OA model in mice, TGF beta-1 had an important role in development of osteophytes in synovial thickening. These findings suggest that endogenous TGF beta-1 participates in pathogenesis of osteoarthritis.

Later work from 2006, [46] showed that lack of TGF beta-3 is associated with cartilage damage, suggesting loss of some protective effect and osteoarthritis progression.

Healthy cartilage is maintained by a dynamic balance of inflammatory effects on extracellular matrix and articular chondrocytes [47]. Cytokines and growth factors regulate the synthesis and degradation of extracellular matrix maintaining the stability and integrity of the joint. If the balance of synthesis/ degradation is disrupted, OA, a degenerative joint disorder characterized by destruction of articular cartilage, alterations of subchondral bone and synovial fibrosis, is likely to occur. According to Finnson, TGF beta-1 has emerged as an important regulator of osteoarthritis.

MICRORNA AND OSTEOARTHRITIS

Before leaving OA, one must return to the basic concepts of transcriptomics for added perspective. Our complement of protein-coding genes approximates 20,000. Many genes have been well-described and identified as part of discrete metabolic pathways. Another 30,000 genes are regulatory: they control gene transcription and translation. Not nearly enough is known about long noncoding RNA genes; this group of genes is a subject of intense research in 2017. Much more (though still not enough) is known about microRNA (miR). These small, regulatory RNA molecules fine-tune gene expression, participate in control of tissue development and homeostasis, with specific activities according to tissue and time [48]. In many instances, a single miR can influence multiple, different gene transcripts. Suffice to say, the layers of regulation exerted over mRNA translation are numerous and diverse.

As the reader has seen, we know OA is a dynamic interaction of cytokines, growth factors and regulatory neuropeptides and not just a wear and tear, degenerative process confined to overweight, inactive smokers. OA develops from aberrant regulatory control of effectors that act on synoviocytes, subchondral bone and inflammatory responses to the forces affecting abnormal control of synthesis and degradation. As one might expect, there is a developing literature on miR involvement with disruption of the normal process of joint surface healing.

Again, one might expect the literature on miR and OA is newer, but in 2008, Yamasaki [49] identified miR-146a as a participant in apparent protection of cartilage from injury. The highest levels of miR-146a were found in cartilage with the least injury (using Mankin scale). Expression of miR 146a was induced by IL-1b stimulation of chondrocytes.

In 2017, Zhang [50] extends this research, but as opposed to Yamasaki, this paper showed that mice without miR-146a had far less cartilage degeneration. This paper also showed that miR 146a "aggravated pro-inflammatory cytokines induced suppressing the expression of cartilage matrix-associated genes," especially targeting two specific genes, Camk2d and Ppp3r2. More importantly, miR-146a has a crucial role in cartilage homeostasis: inhibitors ameliorated OA.

In 2011, Li [51] found a multi-level effect of miR-146a; (i) high levels suppressed extracellular matrix-associated proteins and regulated inflammatory cytokines found in human knee joints; (ii) low levels are found both in dorsal root ganglia and dorsal horn of spinal column in rats experiencing experimental OA-induced pain. Further, miR-146a modulated pain related molecules in human glial cells.

In 2009, Miyaki et al. [52] demonstrated that a different compound, miR-140, was expressed normally in normal articular cartilage but much lower levels were found in OA tissue. IL-1beta suppressed miR-140.

IL-1beta also induces production of cyclooxygenase-2 (COX-2). COX-2 is an important contributor to chronic pain and inflammation in OA [53]. Normal human articular cartilage expresses miR-558, with lower levels seen in OA. IL-1beta induced suppression of miR-558 and induced MAP kinases, compounds also activated by trichothecene mycotoxins [32]. Finally, overexpression of miR-558 downregulated MMPs.

Meng published work [53] on regulation of MMPs in OA, finding an important regulatory role for miR-320. As seen with miR-558, IL-1beta suppressed miR-320 and upregulated MMP-13.

Another miR, Hsa-miR-148a expression is decreased in OA [54]. Overexpression inhibits hypertrophy; increases Type II collagen, which is accompanied by increased retention of proteoglycans.

Finally, both miR-29a and miR-140 protect chondrocytes against adverse effects induced by IL-1 beta [55].

With so many protective miR, one might wonder what is happening in our society that we see so much degenerative joint disease. This author submits that environmental exposure to toxigens and inflammagens are more common than suspected. Now that transcriptomics is readily available, we are likely to understand far more about sources of pro-inflammatory injury in OA, beginning with disruption of normal regulation of DNA transcription and regulation of miR.

TGF BETA-1, TENDON INJURY AND REPAIR

Musculoskeletal tissues are quite diverse in makeup and physiology. We have seen differences between nucleus pulposus cells, synoviocytes and muscle, for example. Two additional tissues where inflammatory mediators have important effects are tendon and enthesium. These next two sections are devoted to these tissues. Tendon is defined as a "uniaxial connective tissue component of the musculoskeletal system. Tendon is involved in forced transmission between the muscle and bone" [56]. While tendon is not avascular, it is poorly vascularized. It is largely composed of Type I collagen fibrils organized in parallel fashion along the long axis of the tissue. Injury to a tendon involves injury to production and assembly of Type 1 collagen. Tendons establish specific connections between muscles, enthesium and the skeleton by transferring contraction forces from muscle to bone allowing organized body motion. Because of the reduction of blood flow in tendon, it is not surprising that tendon injuries heal slowly; surgery cannot restore a damaged tendon to its normal structural integrity and mechanical strength [57].

Sakabe, in a review article, discusses the current status of tendon treatment as well as cell-based therapies in degenerative medicine approaches. As he writes in 2011, tissue engineering for tendon injury involves complex interactions among cellular sources, cytokines and gene delivery systems. This idea has arisen repeatedly in this area. Biological systems have limited means for diverse responses: the final common pathway of lab abnormalities in CIRS is paralleled by musculoskeletal tissue responses.

Nourissat and colleagues write in 2015 [59] that both growth factors and transcription factors involved in tenogenesis are emerging areas of focus in repair of tendon injury.

With this background in mind, one of the concerns in tendon injury is avoidance of development of TGF-mediated fibrosis. Indeed, downregulation of TGF beta-1 genes were studies by Chen [59] in 2009. This study looked at the role of four separate microRNA that could effectively impact TGF beta-1 expression in chickens *in vitro*. They found that delivery of microRNA to the tendons substantially downregulated expression TGF beta-1 but did not affect expression of the collagen 1 gene. This is an encouraging study showing that collagen 1 repair could possibly proceed without fibrosis; additionally, collagen 3 gene expression was reduced by over 50%.

Wu and colleagues write in 2016 [60] that microRNA, which specifically inhibits function of TGF beta-1, holds promise for prevention of adhesion formation during tendon healing, with reduction of adhesion formation and improvement of tendon gliding in digital flexor tendon injury was noted. Unfortunately, the strength of tendon healing was adversely affected. Reduction of adhesions in fibrosis is one arm of treatment approach to tendon surgery but additional work remains to be done.

Enhanced tendon healing, again in the chicken model, showed microRNA limiting adhesions around tendons. In this study [61] we have additional strength for a model in chickens to improve outcomes in tendon injury.

These investigations were continued [62] in 2017 by the same authors looking at the effects of VEGF genes delivered to enhance healing of tendons. Since VEGF can increase new blood vessel formation, improving oxygen delivery, perhaps this novel approach would show benefit. The results of this investigation showed that reduction of adhesion was accomplished and the strength of healing tendons was significantly increased. In this study, Type 3 collagen expression was not suppressed as it had been with microRNA affecting TGF beta-1. Type 3 collagen expression was increased.

Application of molecular processes remain desperately needed as shown by two studies on surgical interventions. In 2013 Roche [63] discussed Achilles tendon disorders, separating them by non-insertional and insertional conditions. Non-insertional injuries rarely require surgery and procedures are minimally invasive if indicated. Rehabilitation protocols have been shown to be of benefit. Still, surgery is not an option for Achilles tendon repair as discussed by Li [64] who calls for improvement in basic approaches to Achilles tendon injuries.

The same type of discussion applies to rotator cuff injures as discussed by Isaac [65]. Isaac summarizes more than 70 papers with a focus on original research. There are a number of therapies involving molecular approaches including, growth factors, stem cells and tissue engineering added to augment classical surgical approaches to rotator cuff repairs. This again is an emerging field of evaluation; preliminary studies are promising.

Another paper by Nixon [66] underscores the rapid advances in cell and gene-based approaches to tendon regeneration. Nixon suggests the ability to use RNA gene therapy to provide the ability for tendons to reduce matrix metalloproteinase injury in degradation.

In two 2017 papers [67, 68] additional importance is presented showing that upregulation of TGF beta-1 expression in stem cells of rabbits can actually improve tendon to bone healing after ACL reconstruction. The TGF-MAPK signaling pathway is underscored. Similarly, substance P increases connective tissue growth factors (CCN2) as an adjunct to TGF beta-1 in tissue repair and fibrosis. Substance P itself is linked to collagen production. In an *in vitro* study cells express proteins typically seen as made by tenocytes with evidence of increased proliferation following exposure to substance P and TGF beta-1. Substance P induced TGF-1 expression in tenocytes. Further approaches in tendon injury are focused not just on stem cells but discrete stimulation of substance P which can induce collagen Type 1, independent of the TGF beta-1 pathway. Taken together, the healing process is immediately involved with regulation of gene expression, controlled by microRNA and manipulation of TGF beta-1, VEGF and MMP-9. Understanding the importance of these inflammatory markers is vital to understanding excellent tendon healing and less than satisfactory tendon healing. Clearly, tendon injuries are an ongoing source of musculoskeletal pain.

ENTHESIUM

Between muscle and tendon lies tissue with its own unique construct, the enthesium. Here we see the emergence of increased amounts of Type 1 collagen suggestive of tendon structure intermingled with myocytes. As one looks closer to the tendon side of the enthesium, there is progressively less vascular supply and at the junction of the enthesium with tendons, the tissue becomes relatively avascular. As it so commonly happens in CIRS, there will be accumulation of inflammatory cells and mediators delivered to the end of capillary beds similar to what we see at the ends of fingers and at the ends of toes. There can also be accumulation of breakdown products of metabolism, including lactic acid. This combination of reduced blood flow and presence of inflammatory mediators from innate immune response leads to the increased incidence of extensor epicondylitis, patellar tendon pain and Achilles tendon pain at insertion sites together with plantar fascial pain. There are no reliable blood tests for inflammation of the enthesium. Fortunately, the painful syndrome of enthesitis usually responds to stretching and local heat. As opposed to classical overuse syndromes, in CIRS there is no therapeutic role for cessation of offending activity.

Of interest, is the appearance of psoriatic-related polyenthesitis and "classical" fibromyalgia. As noted previously, there are no reliable biomarkers for fibromyalgia. [69]

McGonagle [70] has looked in detail at psoriatic arthritis concluding that the arthritic pain in association with nail findings is actually clinically unrecognized enthesitis. He notes enthesitis is "associated with adjacent osteitis or bone and synovial inflammation." Normal insertion of tendons in McGonagle's view are associated with micro-damage and inflammatory change, strongly suggesting "that local tissue specific or what has been described as auto-inflammatory factors, may dictate disease expression."

In psoriatic arthritis, the diffuse inflammation involves the nail root and bed, but the nail itself is intimately related to entheses. McGonagle notes the extensor tendon of the DIP joint sends fibers from the bone that it envelopes the nail bed in an "interdigitation factor." His hypothesis is that "frequent micro-damage in tissue repair has resulted in a new model of pathogenesis which he calls auto-inflammation." Microtrauma leads to regional innate immune activation in persistent inflammation as an alternative to primary immunopathology driven by T and B cell abnormalities."

Similar findings are seen diabetes [71]. When studied by Ursini and his group, there was elevated prevalence of asymptomatic enthesopathic changes of the Achilles tendon insertions in Type 2 diabetes unrelated to peripheral neuropathy.

Approaches to treatment of enthesopathies have included conservative interventions as reviewed by the Cochrane Data Base [72]. The conclusion of this Cochrane Review, is that the available evidence from randomized trial is insufficient to advise on any specific conservative modality for treating exercise-related groin pain. Similarly, [73] Cochrane reviewers who looked at adhesive capsulitis or frozen shoulder, found that manual therapy and exercise were not convincingly shown to be of benefit. Further, injections of glucocorticoids provided short-term benefit. Finally, Page [74] looked at manual therapy and exercise from rotator cuff injury. Cochrane identified 60 studies but only one compared the combination of manual therapy and exercise to placebo. This study was judged to be high quality; no clinically important difference between groups were seen in any outcome. Cochrane calls for further trials of immunotherapy alone and exercise alone that would be needed to alter the opinions of the Cochrane Review. Compare that opinion to that of Moreno [75] who used intra-tissue electrolysis for enthesopathy of adductor longus in soccer players. These authors show that EPI (electro-pulse electrolysis) treatment together with physical therapy insured a greater more rapid reduction of pain in soccer players. The benefit lasts at least six months.

In another study looking at interventions for enthesopathy, ultrasound was felt to show benefit [76] in extensor epicondylitis.

While the hypothesis of capillary hypoperfusion remains of interest regarding pain in the enthesium, to date, there is no sustained opinion regarding interventions. Simply stated, if there is an enthesopathy, stretch, stretch, stretch. Based on academic reports presented in this chapter, this author suspects that when funding is made available for evaluating the transcriptomics and inflammatory mediators of enthesopathy, we will see the same group of compounds like VIP, TGF beta-1, MMPs, VEGF, miR and nuclear transcription regulators as we have seen in OA and tendons.

TGF BETA-1, SMAD 2, SMAD-3, FIBROSIS AND SCARS

A theme of this chapter has been the ubiquitous involvement of particular cytokines and regulators of inflammation, in all their various forms, in illnesses as seemingly diverse as CIRS-WDB and OA. Consistent with this theme is the idea that blood flow bringing these compounds to tissues will result in tissue-specific changes, but also in a *systemic illness*. The only tissues not affected by blood-borne inflammatory mediators are ones without blood flow.

Perhaps no biological function is a better example of the "final common pathway of inflammation," than fibrosis. When one says TGF beta-1 from the podium during an academic lecture, some listeners can immediately visualize TGF beta-1 interacting with its cell membrane receptor (TGF beta-1R), a member of the serine/threonine kinase family of receptors. Kinases put phosphoryl groups on compounds; in the case of TGF beta-1, what is phosphorylated are Smad 2 and Smad 3 [77]. These activated compounds migrate to the nucleus to regulate transcription of a complex series of genes.

Smad3 has a greater role acting on epithelial cells and fibroblasts [78] but also activates other transcription factors [79], including connective tissue growth factor (CTGF). CTGF is a major factor implicated in formation of fibrous tissues. Inhibition of TGF beta-1 can be accomplished. Such an effort will help illnesses as diverse as interstitial lung disease to scleroderma; and from cirrhosis to burn healing.

As one might expect, miRs influence TGF beta-1 signaling. In a revealing paper, Guo [80] shows the inhibitory effect of miR-29b in mice on scar formation. miR-29b is downregulated in thermal injury. Treatment with mir-29b suppressed collagen deposition and fibrotic gene transcription. Specifically, miR-29b inhibited the TGF beta-1/Smad/CTGF pathway.

Another approach [81] uses a cytoplasmic protein, TRAP-1, to regulate Smad expression by phosphorylating Smad3. By regulating phosphorylation, TRAP-1 can regulate collagen synthesis in fibroblasts, possibly avoiding initiation of pathologic scar formation.

Li published a provocative paper [82] showing efficacy of a plant-based treatment for uninhibited TGF beta-1/Smad signaling. Identification of a flavonoid polyphenol, kaempferol, downregulated Smad2/Smad3 phosphorylation in a dose-dependent manner. The mechanism apparently was selective binding of kaempferol to TGF beta-1R.

BETA ENDORPHINS AND PAIN

As discussed in the MSH section, deficiency of beta endorphins has long been associated with chronic pain. Hartwig writes in 1991 [83] that beta endorphin circulates in blood following production. Pain is blocked by inhibiting activation of peripheral somatosensory neurons. Unfortunately, exogenous opioids suppress production of beta endorphin. This 25-year-old concept has direct application to the explosion of opiate-related deaths currently afflicting the US. Even in 1991, beta endorphin deficiency was a recognized factor in multiple pain syndromes, including trigeminal neuralgia, migraines and rheumatoid arthritis (RA). The reader may be reminded of the occurrence of facial pain with MARCoNS; migraine diagnoses made in the face of ADH/osmolality dysregulation; and MSH deficiency as a typical finding in RA.

We can simply ask if pain perception from low back (for example) sources is worse in those with CIRS or MSH deficiency from another source. Bruehl [84] tells us that "endogenous opioid antinociceptive system dysfunction may contribute to elevated acute and chronic pain sensitivity among more disabled chronic pain patients."

By 2014, Bruehl added measurement of plasma beta endorphin to his approach [85]. Paradoxically, his group published that elevated resting levels of beta endorphins may be a biomarker for reduced analgesic capacity.

The disparity between reports that beta endorphin deficiency increased pain responses from one group and decreased pain responses from another suggests that additional mechanisms are involved. In 2011, we find reports of differential effects of mediators of chronic pain, namely neuropeptides substance P (SP), calcitonin gene-related peptide (CGRP) and VIP [86] in migraine. One may wonder if these neuropeptides have a role in pain from joint abnormalities as well.

CGRP, SP AND VIP: PAIN REGULATORS

Rapp [87] looked at differential effects of sensory neurons releasing SP and CGRP impacting cytokine release. Comparing fibroblasts in cell culture for patients with rheumatoid arthritis (RA) to those with osteoarthritis (OA), for example, RA fibroblasts increased release of IL-6 and IL-8 when treated with CGRP but not with SP. For OA fibroblasts, SP caused release of IL-8. When RA fibroblasts were treated with sympathetic nervous system mediators, adenosine and norepinephrine suppressed release of IL-6 and IL-8. The same treatment for OA caused release of both IL-6 and IL-8. Finally, Rapp presented evidenced that beta endorphin inhibited IL-8 secretion only at concentrations 1,000 times higher in RA compared to OA.

Moving from sensory neurons to dorsal root ganglia shows us more differential effects of SP, CGRP and VIP. Shadiack [88] showed that axotomy of superior cervical ganglia increased mRNA for VIP and SP. Axotomy of lumbar dorsal root ganglia increased mRNA for VIP but decreased mRNA for SP and CGRP. Use of an antiserum against nerve growth factor increased levels of VIP in cervical and lumbar dorsal root ganglia but decreased SP and CGRP when applied to sensory neurons.

Dallos [89] in 2006 provided some clarity by showing that neuropeptides SP, CGRP and VIP released from cutaneous nerves after an injury upregulated IL-1alpha and IL-8. The effects of SP, CGRP and VIP were to markedly increase release of nerve growth factor.

Two additional lines of inquiry support diversity of sources that affect pain in this complicated field. Dirmeier et al. published a paper [90] that possibly streamlines the understanding of SP and CGRP. Simply stated, SP is pro-inflammatory; CGRP is anti-inflammatory. Sensory nerve fibers carry both neuropeptides. OA had a greater density of CGRP nerve fibers; RA had more SP nerve fibers.

In a state-of-the-art paper from 2017, Grässel and Muschter [91] emphasize the crucial trophic effects from both sensory and sympathetic fibers required for normal growth of joint tissue and bone. The neurons are the source of neuropeptides including SP, CGRP and VIP. Given that neuropeptides are involved with inflammation in RA, it might be counter-intuitive to also see inflammation in OA controlled by neuropeptides. Given the massive role that OA plays in morbidity worldwide, therapies that enhance CGRP or VIP are likely to play important roles soon. As soon as clinicians have access to transcriptomic identification of abnormalities that are corrected by VIP, a shortcut to finding relief for OA sufferers may appear.

Finally, two papers from Lerner [92, 93] identify the role of SP, VIP and CGRP in regulation of bone formation and resorption. The working hypothesis is that the bone/joint link is regulated by neuropeptides. The burden of osteoporosis and arthritis, each a part of a system of tissues is due to systemic and local effects of neuropeptides. Therapies that address dysregulation of neuropeptides, at least as far as VIP is concerned, have a reasonable likelihood of benefit.

TRANSIENT RECEPTOR POTENTIAL RECEPTORS, INCLUDING TRPV1

At one time substance P was called capsaicin; its receptor TRPV1, is a nociceptive-specific ion channel [94]. This ion channel is activated by thermal injury and acidification as well. Other TRP ion channels are TRPV2, TRPV3, TRPV4, TRPM8 and TRPA1.Toxins [95] known to induce TRPV1 activation include scorpion venom, botulinum neurotoxin, spider toxin (NB: species not identified), ciguatoxin and brevetoxins. Vanillotoxins from a tarantula activate TRPV1 "via interaction with a region of TRPV1 that is homologous to voltage dependent ion channels."

Guilak and Liedtke [96] in 2010 suggests that TRPV4 is the "sixth sense," as it is activated by heat, cold, mechanical loading, osmolality, physical and chemical stimuli. TRPV4 is particularly relevant to musculoskeletal systems as it is expressed in articular cartilage and bone, reacting to osmotic stress. This paper suggests that TRPV4 exerts a regulatory role for a sensory channel in musculoskeletal tissues. Disruption of regulation by biotoxins is a recurrent theme in biotoxin medicine.

Liedtke, in 2016 [97], notes TRPV4 functions in peripheral neurons, and central nervous system cells (astrocytes and microglia) in physiologic and pathologic conditions. They are involved in pain and inflammation.

Cortright discusses TRP channels and pain in 2009 [98]. TRP channel inhibitors block pain by blocking receptors where pain signals are generated. Xu published a report [99] on benefits of an antagonist of TRPV1 (called SB-366791) that dramatically reduced abdominal pain. Similarly, Zhu also published [100] on correction of pancreatic pain in animals by blockade of nerve growth factor. In these animals, density of TRPV1 on pancreatic sensory neurons was reduced.

To no surprise, TGF beta-1increases pancreatic pain [101] in the same rat model presented earlier. This pain was associated with upregulation of TGF beta-1 receptors in dorsal root ganglion cells and was blocked by TGF beta-1 receptor 1 antagonist SB431542.

To add to the concept of an organized hierarchy of layers of pain perception, intrathecal injection of TGF beta-1 reproduced abdominal pain in rats. One can speculate regarding what is happening in unusual pain syndromes in CIRS where blood-brain barrier defenses against transport of TGF beta-1 are compromised.

The role of TRP in pain continues to be unveiled. Jardin [102] focuses on TRPV1, noting that the TRP super-family now has 28 known isoforms in mammals. TRPV1 is expressed in sensory neurons and dorsal root ganglion neurons.

Returning to the role of regulation of transcriptomics by miRNA, decreased expression of miR-199, found in irritable bowel disease [102] leads to enhanced expression of TRPV1 and greater abdominal pain.

CONCLUSIONS

Advances in molecular biological approaches to long-established medical problems have expanded diagnostics and therapeutics. CIRS is an example of state-of-the-art application of differential diagnosis, proteomics and transcriptomics to diagnosis and treatment of complex, chronic fatiguing illnesses acquired following exposure to biologically produced toxins and inflammagens. The disease entity is not just one abnormality; understanding the pathophysiology of CIRS comes from use of a systems or landscape approach. Treatment involves correction of abnormal regulation of inflammatory effectors, regulatory neuropeptides and multiple layers of control exerted on the results of gene transcription.

Applications of molecular methods to diagnosis have validated CIRS and shown the overlap of innate immune responses in musculoskeletal disorders, including pathogenesis of osteoarthritis (OA). Use of a systems approach to (1) innate immune activation and (2) dys-regulation of neuropeptide control of inflammation in OA and musculoskeletal pain opens a new window of treatment, one that is focused on the effects of inflammation on neuropeptide release by sensory neurons, differential regulation of activity of TRP channels and possibly dorsal root ganglia cells.

What we are missing at this time are reliable assays for transcriptomics of neural tissues involved in initiation of painful stimuli and propagation to the brain. It is unlikely that the whole blood analysis used successfully in defining abnormalities and successful correction of gene abnormalities in CIRS can be used without study of actual neural cell genomic function. Despite that need, now that we have data supporting regulatory roles for anti-inflammatory neuropeptides VIP and CGRP; and inflammatory roles for substance P, MMP9, VEGF, TGF beta-1 in generation of acute and chronic pain, we may be able to use methods used in delineation of the biological subtleties of CIRS to help unravel the complexities of chronic pain.

We are confident that increased use of transcriptomics and regulation of gene expression will enable us to understand pathophysiology of pain and disability in ways not seen before. Perhaps musculoskeletal pain will become a window on chronic pain syndromes. If so, innate immune inflammatory processes are likely to hold the keys to defeating pain.

REFERENCES

1. Park J and Cox-Ganser J. Mold exposure and respiratory health in damp indoor environments. *Front Biosci* 2011; E3: 757–771.
2. Wynne T, Davis T, Kelty R, Anderson A and Joshi J. NOAA forecasts and monitors blooms of toxic cyanobacteria in lake Erie. *Clear Waters* 2015 (summer); 21–23.
3. Litaker R, Vandersea M, Faust M, Kibler S, Nau A, Holland W, Chinain M, Holmes M and Tester P. Global distribution of ciguatera causing dinoflagellates in the genus Gambierdiscus. *Toxicon* 2010; 56: 711–730.
4. Bagnis R, Kuberski T, Laugier S. Clinical observation on 3,009 cases of ciguatera (fish poisoning) in the South Pacific. *Am J Trop Med Hyg* 1979; 28: 1067–1073.
5. Liu, D. *Handbook of Foodborne Diseases 2017.* Boca Raton, FL: CRC press *Ciguatera.*
6. Vetter I, Touska F, Hess A, Hinsbey R et al. Ciguatoxins activate specific cold pain pathways to elicit burning pain from cooling. *EMBO J* 2012; 31: 3795–3808.
7. Janeway, C. Approaching the asymptote? Evolution and revolution in immunology. *Cold Spring Harb Symp Quan Biol* 1989; 54: 1–13.
8. Shoemaker R, Rash J and Simon E. Sick building syndrome in water-damaged buildings: Generalization of the chronic biotoxin-associated illness paradigm to indoor toxigenic fungi; 5/2005; 66–77 in Johanning E. Editor, Bioaerosols, Fungi. Bacteria, Mycotoxins and Human Health.
9. Ryan J, Wu Q and Shoemaker R, Transcriptomic signatures in whole blood of patients who acquire a chronic inflammatory response syndrome (CIRS) following an exposure to the marine toxin ciguatoxin. *BMC Med Genomics* 2015 Apr 2; 8: 15. doi: 10.1186/s12920-015-0089-x.
10. Ryan, J and Shoemaker R. RNA-Seq on patients with chronic inflammatory response syndrome (CIRS) treated with vasoactive intestinal polypeptide (VIP) shows a shift in metabolic state and innate immune functions that coincide with healing. *Med Res Arch.* 2016; 4(7): 1–11.
11. Shoemaker R, House D and Ryan J. Vasoactive intestinal polypeptide (VIP) corrects chronic inflammatory response syndrome (CIRS) acquired following exposure to water-damaged buildings. *Health* 2013; 5(3): 396–401.
12. Shoemaker R. Possible estuary-associated syndrome, environmental health perspectives. *Grand Rounds Environ. Med.* 2001; 109(5): 539–545.
13. Shoemaker R. Residential and recreational acquisition of possible estuarine associated syndrome: A new approach to successful diagnosis and therapy, environmental health perspectives, *Special CDC Pfiesteria* Supplement, 2001; 109S5; 791–796.
14. Shoemaker R, House D and Ryan J. Defining the neurotoxin derived illness chronic ciguatera using markers of chronic systemic inflammatory disturbances: A case/control study. *Neurotoxicol Teratol* 2010 doi:10.1016/j.ntt.2010.05.07.

15. Shoemaker R and House D. Characterization of chronic human illness associated with exposure to cyanobacterial harmful algal blooms predominated by Microcystis. In *Cyanobacterial Harmful Algal Blooms: State of the Science and Research Needs*, edited by HK Hudnell, US Epa; ISOC Hab. Advances in Experimental Medicine and Biology. Volume 619 2/08. New York, NY: Springer Sciences. 653–654.

16. Thomas L. Notes of a biology-watcher. Germs. *NEJM* 1972; 287 (11): 553–555.

17. Griffith D, Lewis S, Rossi A., Rennie J, Salisbury L, Merriweather J, Templeton K and Walsh T, RECOVER Investigators. Systemic inflammation after critical illness: Relationship with physical recovery and exploration of potential mechanisms. *Thorax* 2016; 71: 820–829.

18. Grander W, Dunser M, Stollenwerk B, Siebert U, Dengg C, Koller B, Eller P and Tilg H. C-reactive protein levels and post-ICU mortality in nonsurgical intensive care patients. *Chest* 2010; 138: 856–862.

19. Berndtson, K, McMahon S, Ackerley M, Rapaport S, Gupta S and Shoemaker RC. Medically sound investigation and remediation of water-damaged buildings in cases of CIRS-WDB. Part 1.www.survivinmold.com; accessed 7/10/2017.

20. GAO. 2008; Report to the Chairman, HEAL, US Senate. Indoor Mold. Better coordination of research on health effects and more consistent guidance would improve Federal efforts.

21. Naviaux R, Naviaux J, Li K, Bright A et al. Metabolic features of chronic fatigue syndrome. *PNAS* 2016; 113(37): E5472–E5480.

22. Shoemaker R and House D. SBS and exposure to water damaged buildings: time series study, clinical trial and mechanisms; *Neurotoxicol Teratol* 2006; 28: 573–588.

23. Ichiyama T, Sato S. Okada K, Catania A and Lipton JM. The neuroimmunomodulatory peptide alpha-MSH. *Ann NY Acad Sci* 2000; 917: 221–226.

24. Mobbs C and Mizuno T. Leptin regulation of proopiomelanocortin. *Front Horm Res* 2000; 26: 25–70.

25. Shoemaker R and House D. A time-series of sick building syndrome; chronic, biotoxin-associated illness from exposure to water-damaged buildings. *Neurotoxicol. Teratol.* 2005; 27 (1) 29–46.

26. Juarranz Y, Gutierez-Canas I, Santiago B, Carrion M, Pablos J and Gomariz R. Differential expression of vasoactive intestinal peptide and its functional receptors in human osteoarthritic and rheumatoid synovial fibroblasts. *Arthritis Rheum* 2008; 58: 1086–1095.

27. Shoemaker RC, Katz D, Ackerley M, Rapaport S, McMahon S, Berndtson K and Intranasal RJ. VIP safely restores atrophic grey matter nuclei in patients with CIRS. *Internal Med Rev* 2017; 3 (4): 1–14.

28. Wuertz K and Haglund L. Inflammatory mediators in intervertebral disk degeneration and discogenic pain. *Global Spine* 2013; 3: 175–184.

29. Tsarouhas A, Soufla G, Tsarouhas K, Katonis P, Pasku D, Vakis A, Tsatsakis A and Spandidos D. Molecular profile of major growth factors in lumbar intervertebral disc herniation: Correlation with patient clinical and epidemiological characteristics. *Mol Med Rep* 2017; 15: 2195–2203.

30. Tsarouhas A, Soufla G, Katonis P, Pasku D, Vakis A and Spandidos D. Transcript levels of major MMPs and ADAMTS-4 in relation to the clinicopathological profile of patients with lumbar disc herniation. *Eur Spine J* 2011; 20: 781–790.

31. Vo N, Hartman R, Yurube T, Jacobs L, Sowa G and Kang J. Expression and regulation of metalloproteinases and their inhibitors in intervertebral disc aging and degeneration. *Spine J* 2013; 13: 331–341.

32. Petska J. Deoxynivalenol-induced pro-inflammatory gene expression: Mechanism and pathological sequelae. *Toxins* 2010; 2: 1300–1307.

33. Cui Y, Yu J, Urban J and Young D. Differential gene expression profiling of metalloproteinases and their inhibitors: A comparison between bovine intervertebral disc nucleus pulposus cells and articular cartilage. *Spine (Phila Pa 1976)* 2010; 35: 1101–1108.

34. Jang W and Li Juo W. Role of vasoactive intestinal peptide in osteoarthritis. *J Biomed Sci* 2016; 23: 63 doi:10.1186/s12929-016-0280-1.

35. Jiang W, Gao S, Chen X, Xu X, Xu M, Luo W, Zhang F, Zeng C and Leo G. Expression of synovial fluid and articular cartilage VIP in human osteoarthritic knee: A new indicator of disease severity? *Clin Biochem* 2012; 45: 1607–1612.

36. Gallo A, Leerink M, Michot B, Ahmed E, Forget P, Mouraux A, Hermans E and Deumens R. Bilateral tactile hypersensitivity and neuroimmune responses after spared nerve injury in mice lacking vasoactive intestinal peptide. *Exp Neurol* 2017; 3: 62–73.

37. Myers S, Brandt K, Ehlick J, Braunstein E, Shelbourne K, Heck D and Kalasinski L. Synovial inflammation in patients with early osteoarthritis of the knee. *J Rheumatol* 1990; 17: 1662–1669.

38. Mathiessen A and Conaghan P. Synovitis in osteoarthritis: Current understanding with therapeutic implications. *Arthritis Res Ther* 2017; 19: 18. doi:10.1186/s13075-017-1229-9.

39. Fernandes J, Martel-Pelletier J and Pelletier J. The role of cytokines in osteoarthritis pathophysiology. *Biorheology* 2002; 39: 237–246.

40. Ray A and Ray B. An inflammation-responsive transcription factor in the pathophysiology of osteoarthritis. *Biorheology* 2008; 45: 399–409.

41. Sandy J, Chan D, Trevino R, Wimmer M and Plaas A. Human genome-wide expression analysis reorients the study of inflammatory mediators and biomechanics in osteoarthritis. *Osteoarthritis Cartilage* 2015; 23: 1939–1945.

42. Calich A, Domiciano D and Fuller R. Osteoarthritis: Can anti-cytokine therapy play a role in treatment? *Clin Rheumatol* 2010; 29: 451–451.

43. Kapoor M, Martel-Pelletier J, Lajeunesse D, Pelletier J and Fahmi H. Role of proinflammatory cytokines in the pathophysiology of osteoarthritis. *Nat Rev Rheumatol* 2011; 7: 33–42.

44. Van der Kraan P. The changing role of TGFB in healthy, ageing and osteoarthritic joints. *Nat Rev Rheumatol* 2017; 13: 155–163.

45. Scharstuhl A, Vitters E, van der Kraan P and van den Berg W. Reduction of osteophyte formation and synovial thickening by adenoviral overexpression of transforming growth factor beta/bone morphogenetic protein inhibitors during experimental osteoarthritis. *Arthritis Rheum* 2003; 48: 3442–3451.

46. Blaney Davidson E, Vitters E, van der Kraan P and van den Berg W. Expression of transforming growth factor-beta (TGFbeta) and the TGFbeta signaling molecule SMAD-2P in spontaneous and instability-induced osteoarthritis: Role in cartilage degradation, chondrogenesis and osteophyte formation. *Ann Rheum Dis* 2006; 65: 1414–1421.

47. Finnson K, Chi Y, Bou-Gharios G, Leask A and Philip A. TGF-b signaling in cartilage homeostasis and osteoarthritis. *Front Biosci* 2012; 4: 251–268.

48. Miyaki S and Asahara H. Macro view of microRNA function in osteoarthritis. *Nat Rev Rheumatol* 2012; 8: 543–552.

49. Yamasaki K, Nakasa T, Miyaki S, Ishikawa M, Deie M, Adachi N, Yasunaga Y, Asahara H and Ochi M. Expression of MicroRNA-146a in osteoarthritis cartilage. *Arthritis Rheum* 2009; 60: 1034–1041.

50. Zhang X, Wang C, Zhao J, Xu J, Geng Y, Dai L, Huang Y, Fu S, Dai K and Zhang X. miR-146a facilitates osteoarthritis by regulating cartilage homeostasis via targeting Camk2d and Ppp3r2. *Cell Death Dis* 2017; 8: e2734.

51. Li X, Gibson G, Kim J, Kroin J, Xu S, van Wijnen A and Im H. MicroRNA 146a is linked to pain-related pathophysiology of osteoarthritis. *Gene* 2011; 480: 34–41.

52. Miyaki S, Nakasa T, Otsuki S, Grogan S, Higashiyama R, Inoue A, Kato Y, Sato T, Lotz M and Asahara H. MicroRNA-140 is expressed in differentiated human articular chondrocyte and modulates interleukin-2 responses. *Arthritis Rheum* 2009; 60: 2723–2730.

53. Park S, Cheon E and Kim H. MicroRNA-558 regulates the expression of cyclooxygenase-2 and IL-1B-induced catabolic effects in human articular chondrocytes. *Osteoarthritis Cartilage* 2013; 21: 981–989.

54. Vonk L, Kragten A, Dhert W, Saris D and Creemers L. Overexpression of has-miR-148a promotes cartilage production and inhibits cartilage degradation by osteoarthritic chondrocytes. *Osteoarthritis Cartilage* 2014; 22: 145–153.

55. Li X, Zhen Z, Tang G, Zheng C and Yang G. MiR-29a and MiR-140 protect chondrocytes against the anti-proliferation and cell matrix signaling changes by IL-1B. *Mol Cells* 2016; 39: 103–110.

56. Gaut L and Duprez D. Tendon development and diseases. *Wiley Interdiscip Rev Dev Biol* 2016; 5: 5–23.

57. Sakabe T. and Sakai T. Musculoskeletal diseases—tendon. *Br Med Bull* 2011; 99: 211–225.

58. Nourissat G, Berenbaum F and Duprez D. Tendon injury: From biology to tendon repair. *Nat Rev Rheumatol* 2015; 11: 223–233.

59. Chen C, Zhou Y, Wu Y, Cao Y, Cao J and Tang J. Effectiveness of microRNA in down-regulation of TG-beta gene expression in digital flexor tendons of chickens: In vitro and in vivo study. *J Hang Surg Am* 2009; 34: 1777–1784.

60. Wu Y, Mao W, Zhou Y, Wang X, Liu P and Tang J. Adeno-associated virus-2-mediated TGF-B1 microRNA transfection inhibits adhesion formation after digital flexor tendon injury. *Gene Ther* 2016; 23: 167–175.

61. Tang J, Zhou Y, Wu Y, Liu P and Wang X. Gene therapy strategies to improve strength and quality of flexor tendon healing. *Expert Opin Biol Ther* 2016; 16: 291–301.

62. Mao W, Wu Y, Yang Q, Zhou Y, Wang X, Liu P and Tang J. Modulation of digital flexor tendon healing by vascular endothelial growth factor gene transfection in a chicken model. *Gene Ther* 2017; 24: 234–240.

63. Roche A and Calder J. Achilles tendinopathy: A review of the current concepts of treatment. *Bone Joint* 2013; 95-B; 1299–1307.
64. Li H and Hua Y. Achilles tendinopathy: Current concepts about the basic science and clinical treatments. *Biomed Res Int* 2016; 2016: 6492597.
65. Isaac C, Gharaibeh B, Witt M, Wright V and Huard J. Biologic approaches to enhance rotator cuff healing after injury. *J Shoulder Elbow Surg* 2012; 21: 181–90.
66. Nixon A, Watts A and Schnabel L. Cell- and gene-based approaches to tendon regeneration. *J Shoulder Elbow Surg* 2012; 21: 278–294.
67. Frara N, Fisher P, Zhao Y, Tarr J, Amin M, Popoff S and Barbe M. Substance P increases CCN2 dependent on TGF-beta yet collagen type I via TGF-beta 1 dependent and independent pathways in tenocytes. *Connect Tissue Res* 2017; 1–15. doi:10.1080/03.
68. Wang R, Xu B and Xu H. Up-regulation of TGF-B promotes tendon-to-bone healing after anterior cruciate ligament reconstruction using bone marrow-derived mesenchymal stem cells through the TGF-B/MAPK signaling pathway in a New Zealand white rabbit model. *Cell Physiol Biochem* 2017; 41: 213–226.
69. De Marco, MAG, Merashli M, McKenna F, Tinazzi I, Marzo-Ortega H and McGonagle D. The problem in differentiation between psoriatic-related polyenthesitis and fibromyalgia. *Rheumatology* 2017; doi:10.1093/rheumatologh/kex079. (Epub ahead of print).
70. McGonagle D. Enthesitis: An autoinflammatory lesion linking nail and joint involvement in psoriatic disease. *J Eur Acad Dermatol Venereol* 2009; 23 Suppl 1: 9–13.
71. Ursini F, Arturi F, D'Angelo S, Amara L et al., High prevalence of Achilles tendon enthesopathic changes in patients with type 2 diabetes without peripheral neuropathy. *J Am Podiatr Med Assoc* 2017; 107: 99–105.
72. Almeida M, Silva B, Andriolo R, Atallah A and Peccin M. Conservative interventions for treating exercise-related musculotendinous, ligamentous and osseous groin pain. *Cochrane Database Syst Rev* 2013; 6: CD009565.
73. Page M, Green S, Kramer S, Johnston R, McBain B, Chau M and Buchbinder R. Manual therapy and exercise for adhesive capsulitis (frozen shoulder). *Cochrane Database Syst Rev* 2014; 26: CD011275.
74. Page M, Green S, McBain B, Surace S, Deitch J, Lyttle N, Mrocki M and Buchbinder R. Manual therapy and exercise for rotator cuff disease. *Cochrane Database Syst Rev* 2016; 10: CD012224.
75. Moreno C, Mattiussi G, Javier Nunez F, Messina G and Rejc E. Intratissue percutaneous electrolysis (EPI®) combined with active physical therapy for the treatment of adductor longus enthesopathy-related groin pain: A randomized trial. *J Sports Med Phys Fitness* 2017; doi:10.23736/S0022-4707.
76. Dones V 3rd, Grimmer K, Thoirs K, Suarez C and Luker J. The diagnostic validity of musculoskeletal ultrasound in lateral epicondylalgia: A systematic review. *BMC Med Imaging* 2014; 14: 10. doi: 10.1186/1471-2342-14-10.
77. Liu F. Receptor-regulated Smads in TGF-beta signaling. *Front Biosci* 2003; 8: S1280–S1303.
78. Brown K, Pietenpol J and Moses H. A tale of two proteins: Differential roles and regulation of Smad2 and Smad4 in TGF-beta signaling. *J Cell Biochem* 2007; 101: 9–33.
79. Denton C and Abraham D. Transforming growth factor-beta and connective tissue growth factor: Key cytokines in scleroderma pathogenesis. *Curr Opin Rheumatol* 2001; 13: 505–511.
80. Guo J, Lin Q, Shao Y, Rong L and Zhang D. miR-29b promotes skin wound healing and reduces excessive scar formation by inhibition of the TGF-B1/Smad/CTGF signaling pathway. *Can J Physiol Pharmacol* 2017; 95: 437–442.
81. Wang X, Qian Y, Jin R, Wo Y, Chen J, Wang C and Wang D. Effects of TRAP-1-like protein (TLP) gene on collagen synthesis induced by TGF-B/Smad signaling in human dermal fibroblasts. *PLoS One* 2013; e55899. doi:10.1371/journal.pone.0055899. (Epub ahead of print).
82. Li H, Yang L, Zhang Y and Gao Z. Kaempferol inhibits fibroblast collagen synthesis, proliferation and activation in hypertrophic scar via targeting TGF-B receptor type I. *Biomed Pharmacother* 2016; 83: 967–974.
83. Hartwig A. Peripheral beta-endorphin and pain modulation. *Anesth Prog* 1991; 38: 75–78.
84. Bruehl S, Chung O, Ward P and Johnson B. Endogenous opioids and chronic pain intensity: Interactions with level of disability. *Clin J Pain* 2004; 20: 283–292.
85. Bruehl S, Burns J, Chung O and Chont M. What do plasma beta-endorphin levels reveal about endogenous opioid analgesic function? *Eur J Pain* 2014; 16: 370–380.
86. Messlinger K, Fischer M and Lennerz J. Neuropeptide effects in the trigeminal system: Pathophysiology and clinical relevance in migraine. *Keio J Med* 2011; 60: 82–89.

87. Raap T, Justen H, Miller L, Cutolo M, Scholmerich J and Straub R. Neurotransmitter modulation of interleukin 6 (IL-6) and IL-8 secretion of synovial fibroblasts in patients with rheumatoid arthritis compared to osteoarthritis. *J Rheumatol* 2000; 27: 2558–2565.

88. Shadiack A, Sun Y and Zigmond R. Nerve growth factor antiserum induces axotomy-like changes in neuropeptide expression in intact sympathetic and sensory neurons. *J Neurosci* 2001; 21: 363–371.

89. Dallos A, Kiss M, Polyanka H, Dobozy A, Kemeny L and Husz S. Effects of the neuropeptides substance P, calcitonin gene-related peptide, vasoactive intestinal polypeptide and galanin on the production of nerve growth factor and inflammatory cytokines in cultured human keratinocytes. *Neuropeptides* 2006; 40: 251–263.

90. Dirmeier M, Capellino S, Schubert T, Angele P, Anders S and Straub R. Lower density of synovial nerve fibres positive for calcitonin gene-related peptide relative to substance P in rheumatoid arthritis but not in osteoarthritis. *Rheumatol (Oxford)* 2008; 47: 36–40.

91. Grassel S and Muschter D. Peripheral Nerve Fibers and their neurotransmitters in osteoarthritis pathology. *Int. J. Mol. Sci* 2017; 18: 1–23.

92. Lerner U. Deletions of genes encoding calcitonin/alpha-CGRP, amylin and calcitonin receptor have given new and unexpected insights into the function of calcitonin receptors and calcitonin receptor-like receptors in bone. *J Musculoskelet Neuronal Interact* 2006; 6: 87–95.

93. Lerner U and Persson E. Osteotropic effects by the neuropeptides calcitonin gene-related peptide, substance P and vasoactive intestinal peptide. *J Musculoskelet Neuronal Interact* 2008; 8: 154–165.

94. Numazaki M and Tominaga M. Nociception and TRP channels. *Curr Drug Targets CNS Neurol Disord* 2004; 3: 479–485.

95. Min J, Liu W, He H and Peng B. Different types of toxins targeting TRPV1 in pain. *Toxicon* 2013; 71: 66–75.

96. Guilak F, Leddy H. and Liedtke W. Transient receptor potential vanilloid 4: The sixth sense of the musculoskeletal system. *Ann N Y Acad Sci* 2010; 1192: 404–409.

97. Kanju P and Liedtke W. Pleiotropic function of TRPV4 ion channels in the central nervous system. *Exp Physiol* 2016; 101: 1472–1476.

98. Cortright D and Szallasi A. TRP channels and pain. *Curr Pharm Des* 2009; 15: 1736–1749.

99. Xu G, Winston J, Shenoy M, Yin H, Pendyala S and Pasricha P. Transient receptor potential vanilloid 1 mediates hyperalgesia and is up-regulated in rats with chronic pancreatitis. *Gastroenterology* 2007; 133: 1282–1292.

100. Zhu Y, Colak T, Shenoy M, Liu L, Pai R, Li C, Mehta K and Pasricha P. Nerve growth factor modulates TRPV1 expression and function and mediates pain in chronic pancreatitis. *Gastroenterology* 2011; 141: 370–377.

101. Zhang X, Zheng H, Zhu H, Hu S, Wang S, Jiang X and Xu G. Acute effects of transforming growth factor-B1 on neuronal excitability and involvement in the pain of rats with chronic pancreatitis. *J Neurogastroenterol Motil* 2016; 22: 333–343.

102. Jardin I, Lopez J, Diez R, Sanchez-Collado J et al. TRPs in pain sensation. *Front Physiol* 2017; 8: 392.

9 Periodontal Disease
Treatable, Nutrition-Related, and with Systemic Repercussions

David Kennedy, DDS

INTRODUCTION

Among orthopedic surgeons, it is common practice to note the integrity of soft tissue, muscle and bone in the operative report. Direct visualization of musculoskeletal structures is possible for all practitioners who examine the oral cavity. Noting findings in the patient medical record is also valuable for orthopedics since the integrity of tongue, teeth and gums correlates with the overall musculoskeletal system. Bleeding gums may increase clinical suspicion that vitamin C levels are inadequate for collagen synthesis. Noting an enlarged, "beefy" tongue in a patient with musculoskeletal injury from frequent falls could expedite the diagnosis of pernicious anemia. Similarly inflamed gums point to a biotoxin burden, which is amenable to treatment. Treatment of periodontal disease has been shown to reduce morbidity of inflammation-related systemic conditions.

Periodontal disease (PD) is an encompassing term for gingivitis and periodontitis. PD is the predominant underlying pathology of tooth loss. It is caused by various microorganisms and parasites. Host susceptibility, moderated by nutritional deficiencies, plays a significant role in the progress of the disease. Among the risk factors are diabetes, smoking, a diet characterized by refined carbohydrates and inadequate vitamin C.

PD has been called cyclical because it seems to come and go for reasons that are not totally clear. For example, when a woman is pregnant, her periodontal problems seem to accelerate. This is commonly called *pregnancy gingivitis*, and patients are often not counseled that PD is linked to the pregnancy outcome. The more severe the mother's periodontal condition, the more likely she is to have a low-birth-weight baby. In fact, periodontal pathogens have been isolated from the amniotic fluid [1, 2]. In addition, periodontal disease has been linked to systemic illness, including cancers, pneumonia, diabetes and cardiovascular disease [3–5].

EPIDEMIOLOGY

Research has confirmed through DNA testing a number of vectors for this infectious disease. The most common transmission pattern is from mother to child or caregiver to child, the pattern by which the gut microbiome is obtained [6]. Unlike the intestinal tract, which is colonized during the birth process, the organisms associated with periodontal disease need teeth to colonize, so they are typically not transferred until after the first teeth arrive.

Periodontal infections can also be transmitted to children from a father, siblings or playmates. In addition, a surprising development uncovered with DNA testing found transfer from dogs to humans.

Nutrition influences individual susceptibility, and changes in nutrient status and dietary patterns are thought to contribute to the cyclical pattern of PD progression. Other factors include personal hygiene, type of dentifrice, mercury/silver filling implants, smoking and stress [7]. Both fluoride-containing dentifrice and dental fluorosis have been linked to periodontal disease, probably through the mechanism of direct bone injury and/or increased inflammation [8]. Unsurprisingly, specific microbes, especially subgingival spirochetes and inflammatory crevicular leukocytes, are associated with PD progression [9].

PATHOPHYSIOLOGY

The pathophysiology of PD is the result of an inflammatory response resulting from the interaction between the pathogenic bacteria, the host's immune response, polymorph nuclear leukocytes (PMN) and heavy metal reactive oxygen species (ROS) production with depletion of glutathione [10–12]. The inflammation is induced either by direct action from bacterial invasion, like most infections, or by exotoxins released from colonizing bacteria.

Once the infection becomes established, amoebas that are secondary invaders play a significant role in the inflammatory process, producing large numbers of PMNs. Amoebas were identified in 1915 by the famous physician C. C. Bass as strongly implicated in periodontal disease [13]. He identified their presence by using a light microscope. They cannot be cultured and, as a result, are not picked up in most microbiological tests. Recently the presence of amoebas in PD sites and their absence where PD-related inflammation is not present has since been confirmed by polymerase chain reaction diagnostic techniques [14].

On microscopy, amoebas can be seen visibly attacking and consuming white blood cells, usually PMNs [15]. The damaged white blood cells then release histamine, which calls more PMNs to the area. The cycle produces enormous inflammation and accelerates the bone loss that is characteristic of the progressive destruction of the periodontal supporting structures. As the disease process advances, pockets form, and eventually, tooth mobility and abscess formation occurs.

The use of oral antibiotics such as metronidozole (Flagyl) alone for these parasites ultimately will fail to eradicate the oral infections, as the gingival crevicular fluid (GCF) generally carries very little antibiotic. A direct application of antiseptics to the sulcus followed by a direct application of metronidozole in ophthalmic solution to the sulcus, while at the same time providing oral systemic antibiotic coverage, has proven effective in eliminating this kind of infection. This method essentially treats all areas of infection simultaneously, and this way the amoeba is eradicated.

Heavy Metal Mercury in PD Pathophysiology

The dental profession has traditionally referred to a mixture of 50% elemental mercury and varying amounts of silver copper zinc and tin as a "silver" amalgam filling. As a result, most of the general public in a recent Zogby poll did not realize that mercury was even a component of a "silver" filling, much less the principal ingredient. A more appropriate term for such a filling in consideration of the patient's right to adequate informed consent would be a *mercury/silver* tooth filling.

Some dental organizations have claimed that the mercury forms a covalent bond with silver, a physical impossibility. It forms weak intermetallic bonds that are easily broken with heat or pressure and form microcurrents between the metals. Consequently, such fillings are now known to be the predominant source of in individual's exposure to mercury if present in the mouth [16].

In a series of elegant experiments at the University of Calgary School of Medicine, radioactively labeled mercury[203] fillings were installed in sheep and monkeys and the released mercury was imaged. In four weeks, the mercury had exited the fillings and accumulated in many distant organs including the kidney, liver and heart [17]. The deposits in the gut are likely particulate forms of amalgam that abrade during normal mastication. Human studies of stool have found high levels of mercury in amalgam bearers [18]. Although the absorption rate of inorganic mercury from the gut is low, the sheer volume of material was quite large. Absorption from the lung is very rapid, so approximately 80% of inhaled mercury is absorbed. The mercury deposited in the kidneys was first released as elemental mercury vapor from chewing absorbed from the lungs and then transported through the blood stream to the kidneys. The experiment with sheep was criticized by the American Dental Association as not reliable because sheep are ruminants, chewing more than humans. The authors of the research reported that a sheep was chosen precisely because the sheep is an exacerbated chewing model. However, the study was repeated a few months later in monkeys with similar results [19].

The sheep and monkey studies both revealed jawbone saturation with mercury. The mercury had rapidly migrated from the filling directly through the dental tissues into the bone. This appears to explain older research in humans that found bone loss surrounding teeth that have received "silver" fillings [20, 21]. Taken together, "silver" fillings are implicated in periodontal destruction. This is likely due to the production of ROS, depletion of GCF glutathione and inflammation.

In an interesting adaptation, exotoxin-producing bacteria which inhabit the oral cavity are able to couple mercury with their biological toxin to produce an even more toxic substance. This is particularly important in the case of root canals where dead roots are partially filled and retained in the jawbone. Research has confirmed that these root-filled teeth accumulate anaerobic bacteria in large numbers [22]. Wu reports that, "Histologic observation of root apices with surrounding bone removed from either patients or human cadavers has demonstrated that post-treatment apical periodontitis is associated with 50%–90% of root filled human teeth." [23] Apical periodontitis confirms that many root-filled teeth remain infected. The reaction of oral mercury with anaerobic toxicants can produce supertoxicants such as CH_3S-Hg^+ and $CH_3-S-Hg-S-CH_3$. Also, the excretion of mercury is variable, influenced by a diet containing milk or following an antibiotic by as much as 30 fold [24]. Since no dental research evaluates the systemic impact of root canal therapy, it falls upon the medical profession to identify this and rectify any injury from such misinformed dental treatments. It is likely that in a short amount of time, all nonvital or root-canaled teeth load with anaerobic organisms that release exotoxins. The impact of these diseased teeth on health have been reported for over 100 years, but until the development of the spiral CT scan, it was very difficult to verify the infection without first removing the tooth, since most apical lesions are not visible on standard dental X-rays.

PATIENT EVALUATION: REASONS TO NOTE PD IN A PHYSICAL EXAM

The classic method of diagnosing periodontal disease is based upon measurement of the gingival sulcus with a notched probe and clinically observing the presence of odor, pus, tooth mobility and/ or bleeding. Primarily anaerobic motile bacteria create inflammation and denude the crevicular epithelium to cause pocket formation.

Anaerobic culture is difficult to do in a clinical practice, and pocket measurement is an easy but very flawed approach. Even after the bacteria are eradicated, the pockets will remain as an artifact of the prior damage. Pus is not a consistent reliable feature of periodontal disease. Bleeding will occur in a healthy sulcus when sufficient pressure is applied to the probe. An undesirable consequence of probing an infected sulcus prior to disinfection the pathogenic organisms are seeded into deeper tissues. A much more accurate method of diagnosis is to visually assess the biological life and immune response in the gingival sulcus with a live wet slide using a microscope. Although this method is very easy in an office equipped with the necessary microscope, it is not typically found in most dental practices. The International Academy of Oral Medicine and Toxicology (IAOMT) strongly recommends this approach, but not all of its members provide the recommended level of examination. Less than 15% of the fees charged by dentists relate to periodontal disease, although an estimated 90% of adults have PD, pointing to a large disconnect between the problem and the treatment.

However, a physician during a routine exam may quickly screen for the presence of PD by assessing mouth odor, noting gingival color and asking pertinent questions regarding the stability of the teeth. A sure sign of advancing inflammation is seen when teeth begin to drift out of place and food impacts interproximally. Like most things in medicine, a careful diagnosis is going to lead to an appropriate treatment, but in the absence of a microscopic examination, there are steps that can easily be taken to avoid advancing disease.

Based on the pathophysiologic research presented above, noting "silver" fillings as a PD risk factor may not only be helpful for prevention and treatment of PD, but can also inform other systemic conditions associated with overburdened biopathways for toxin removal.

Noting the presence of PD in the chart is an inexpensive biomarker, described in the medical literature to be as strong a predictor of cardiovascular disease as is cholesterol [2]. PD can therefore contribute to clinical acumen in a diagnostic work-up.

PD can further guide clinical decision-making regarding compromised nutrient status and impaired digestion. Choice of antibiotics for a systemic illness may be appropriately influenced by the presence of PD, since responsive treatment regimens are better established than for some other conditions.

PD prevention is aligned with lifestyle medicine counseling. One of the most important steps in prevention is to promote daily oral irrigation as well as healthful nutrition, optimum hydration and the absence of negative oral habits like smoking or chewing tobacco.

PREVENTION

By far the simplest and most cost-effective approach to any dental disorder is prevention. Since almost all of the periodontal pathogens are anaerobic and highly motile organisms, the most efficacious approach in my opinion is daily application of antiseptics by oral irrigation. In the 19th century, physicians traditionally painted iodine on infected gums with a cotton swab. Applying a dilute solution with a pulsating water irrigator is the modern method, although some recent research into the prevention of baby-bottle tooth decay found the cotton swab with iodine is still an effective way to prevent decay [25].

Adequate saliva is vital to both preventing periodontal infections from advancing and to arresting tooth decay. Therefore, careful attention to the side effects of drugs is needed. Many medications can cause dry mouth. The most common ones are for blood pressure and psychiatric conditions. When such a medication is indicated, it should be accompanied with specific instructions on hydrating the mouth with sialogogue or another non-sugary method. Unfortunately, many people when faced with this condition reach for a sugary lozenge or beverage that will accelerate the problem of tooth decay. Sleep apnea and mouth breathing dehydrate the mucosa and can greatly accelerate PD if infectious organisms are present.

Various solutions for oral disinfection have been proposed, including ozone, colloidal silver and even salt water [26]. Early research found that water alone was more effective than nothing, and antimicrobial solutions enhanced the results [27]. Therefore, the actual solution is likely one of availability and preference rather than any hard dictates. It remains clear that the outer layers of plaque need to be disturbed mechanically first in order for the solution to penetrate sufficiently to flush out the periodontal pathogens. Simply put, stir it up and flush it out.

Fluoride irrigation solutions should not be applied as they have been shown to promote destruction of bone in the presence of preexisting PD [28]. The mouth has a thin mucosa, especially the floor of the mouth, and superb circulation; therefore, it can be used to supply nutrients such as vitamin B12 directly to the blood stream. By the same logic, a dentifrice that contains fluoride will give an unwanted systemic dose and impact the integrity of the jawbone. Inflammation is a known result of exposing soft tissues to fluoride. The patent application of a pharmaceutical company discloses that concentrations of fluorides from fluoridated toothpastes and mouthwashes activate G proteins in the oral cavity, thereby promoting PD and oral cancer. This is not surprising considering that research has linked fluoride to g protein activation [29].

In addition to the concerns about fluoride, two additional common toothpaste ingredients potentially exacerbate PD. (1) Sodium laurel sulfate is a soap derivative which will disrupt the oral mucosa and dramatically increase the frequency of oral aphthous or herpes outbreaks [30]. (2) Triclosan

(2,4,4' –trichloro-2'-hydroxydiphenyl ether) is a synthetic broad-spectrum antimicrobial agent first registered as a pesticide in 1969, and it is now under review at the FDA and EPA [31, 32]. Triclosan use is linked to discharges and impact on aquatic environments and possibly the development of antibiotic resistance. The association has a biologic basis. Triclosan may form dioxins in surface water, and its active ingredient is a polychloro phenoxy phenol [33].

Prevention is especially important during pregnancy. The hormone shift and immunosuppression during pregnancy can exacerbate existing periodontal conditions. Research has confirmed that a woman's oral health plays a significant role in her pregnancy outcome [34, 35]. Periodontal disease is associated with an elevated risk of undesirable pregnancy outcomes such as preterm birth and low-birth-weight infants [36]. Treatment of PD and tooth decay are difficult during pregnancy. For example, placing or removing a mercury/silver filling during pregnancy will significantly increase the maternal and cord-blood mercury. And while disinfection is beneficial, the trauma incurred during routine cleaning when PD is present will likely spread the organisms to the blood stream unless a pretreatment disinfection protocol is followed.

Bacteria living in the sulcus or in nonvital teeth exude short low-molecular-weight proteins that are more toxic than botulism. These exotoxins migrate to distant locations, and this is apparently how a septic site can exert its biotoxin in a remote area such as a heart or joint. Bacteria may also exert direct effects by getting into the placenta, an artery or inside the blood-brain barrier [37].

TREATMENT

Surgical periodontal therapy has been the standard of care for more than half a century, but more modern considerations now dictate an anti-infectious approach while enhancing host immunity to achieve a more predictable outcome. Some evidence now suggests that surgery can accelerate tooth loss [38]. This is because the target for such therapy was pocket reduction by excision of pocket tissue and bone remodeling and, occasionally, tissue grafts. Pathophysiology provides the rationale that treatment will fail unless the underlying causes of host susceptibility and specific microorganism or a group of specific microorganisms are addressed.

The IAOMT, after an extensive review of the literature and consultation with experts, concluded that the appropriate therapy for any periodontal condition starts with a careful analysis of the oral flora, followed by nonsurgical disinfection both in office and at home [39]. Frequent follow-up evaluations with a strong bias toward microbiological analysis provided the best avenue toward health. Mercury/silver fillings often play a significant role in the pathogenesis of PD, adding to the reasons to support the ban of mercury/silver fillings as the IAOMT first recommended in 1985. Daily mechanical hygiene coupled with irrigation with an antimicrobial agent is the most effective way to remove this common infection.

CLINICAL SUMMARY

PD is not limited to the oral cavity; it is systemically influenced and has systemic repercussions such as cardiovascular disease, low-birth-weight babies and cancers. It is an infectious process involving numerous forms of anaerobic bacteria and one-celled animals. Eradication of the amoebas or trichomonas should be considered a priority of any therapy. Control of PD is achieved by a combined approach of targeted oral hygiene with irrigation and antiseptics, mercury removal, optimizing nutrition and frequent monitoring of the oral flora to guard against recurrent infection.

REFERENCES

1. León, R. et al., Detection of porphyromonas gingivalis in the amniotic fluid in pregnant women with a diagnosis of threatened premature labor. *Journal of Periodontology*, 2007, 78(7): 1249–1255. (doi:10.1902/jop.2007.060368)

2. Xiaojing, L. I. et al., Systemic diseases caused by oral infections. *Clinical Microbiology Reviews*, 2000: 547–558.

3. Marques da Silva, R., Human atherosclerotic plaque contains viable invasive Actinobacillus actinomycetemcomitans and Porphyromonas gingivalis. *Journal of Vascular Surgery*, 2006, 44(5): 1055–1060.

4. Beck, J. D. et al., Periodontal disease and cardiovascular disease. *Journal of Periodontology*, 1996, 67: 1123–1137.

5. Paju, S. and Scannapieco, F. A., Oral biofilms, periodontitis, and pulmonary infections. *Oral Diseases*, 2007, 13(6): 508–512.

6. Li, Y. and Caufield, P. W., The fidelity of initial acquisition of mutans streptococci by infants from their mothers, *Journal of Dental Research*, 1995, 74(2): 681–685.

7. Chapple, I., Potential mechanisms underpinning the nutritional modulation of periodontal inflammation, *JADA*, 2009, 140(2): 178–184.

8. Vandana, K. L. and Sesha Reddy, M., Assessment of periodontal status in dental fluorosis subjects using community periodontal index of treatment needs. *Indiana Journal of Dental Research*, 2007, 18(2).

9. Keyes, P. H. and Rams, T. E., Subgingival microbial and inflammatory cell morphotypes associated with chronic periodontitis progression in treated adults. *Journal of the International Academy of Periodontology*, 2015, 17(2): 1–9.

10. Iwamoto, Y. et al., Antimicrobial periodontal treatment decreases serum C-reactive protein, tumor necrosis factor-alpha, but not adiponectin levels in patients with chronic periodontitis. *Journal of Periodontology*, 2003, 74(8): 1231–1236.

11. Salzberg, T. N., Overstreet, B. T., Rogers, J. D., Califano, J. V., Best, A. M., and Schenkein, H. A., C-reactive protein levels in patients with aggressive periodontitis. *Journal of Periodontology*, 2006, 77(6): 933–939.

12. Chapple, I. L. C., Role of free radicals and antioxidants in the pathogenesis of inflammatory periodontal diseases. *Clinical Molecular Pathology*, 1996, 49: 247–255.

13. Bass, C. C. and Johns, F. M., *Alveolodental Pyorrhea*, 1915. WB Saunders: Philadelphia.

14. Trim, R. D. et al., Use of PCR to detect Entamoeba gingivalis in diseased gingival pockets and demonstrate its absence in healthy gingival sites. *Parasitology Research*, 2011.

15. Author's personal observation

16. WHO Environmental Health Criteria 118, 1991, section 5.1. General population exposure, Table 2, http://www.inchem.org/documents/ehc/ehc/ehc118.htm

17. Hahn, L. J., Kloiber, R., Vimy, M. J., Takahashi, Y., and Lorscheider, F., Dental "silver" tooth fillings: A source of mercury exposure revealed by whole-body image scan and tissue analysis. *FASEB Journal*, 1989, 3: 2641–2646.

18. Skare, I. and Engqvist, A., Amalgam restorations – an important source of human exposure of mercury and silver. *Läkartidningen*, 1992, 15: 1299–1301.

19. Hahn, L. J., Kloiber, R., Leininger, R. W., Vimy, M. J., and Lorscheider, F. L., Whole-body imaging of the distribution of mercury released from dental fillings into monkey tissues. *FASEB*, 1990, 4: 3256–3260.

20. Fisher, D. et al., NIDR/ADA workshop. *Journal of Oral Rehabilitation*, 1984, 11: 399–405.

21. Ziff, M. F., Documented clinical side-effects to dental amalgam. *Advances in Dental Research*, 1992, 6: 131–134.

22. Shigetaka, N. et al., Bacterial invasion into dentinal tubules of human vital and nonvital teeth. *Journal of Endodontics*, 1995, 21(2): 70–73.

23. Wu, M. K. et al., Consequences of and strategies to deal with residual post-treatment root canal infections, *International Endodontic Journal*, 2006.

24. Rowland, Effects of diet on mercury metabolism and excretion in mice given methylmercury: Role of gut flora. *Archives of Environmental Health*, 1984, 39(6): 401–408.

25. Lopez, L., Berkowitz, R., Spiekerman, C., and Weinstein, P. Topical antimicrobial therapy in the prevention of early childhood caries: A follow-up report. *Paediatric Dentistry*, 2002, 24(3): 204–206.

26. Saini, R., Ozone therapy in dentistry: A strategic review. *Journal of Natural Science, Biology and Medicine*, 2011, 2(2): 151–153.

27. Roy Macaulay, W. J. and Newman, H. N., The effect on the composition of subgingival plaque of a simplified oral hygiene system including pulsating jet subgingival irrigation. *Journal of Periodontal Research*, 1986, 21(4): 375–385.

28. Sjostrom, S. and Kalfas, S., Tissue necrosis after subgingival irrigation with fluoride solution. *Journal of Clinical Periodontology*, 1999, 26(4): 257–260.

29. Strunecká, A. and Patočkab, J., Pharmacological and toxicological effects of aminofluoride complexes. *J. Fluoride*, 1999, 32: 4.

30. Herlofson, B. B. and Barkvoll, P., Sodium lauryl sulfate and recurrent aphthous ulcers. A preliminary study. *Acta Odontol Scand*, 1994, 52: 257–259.

31. Layton, L., FDA says studies on triclosan, used in sanitizers and soaps, raise concerns. *Washington Post* April 8, 2010.

32. http://www.epa.gov/oppsrrd1/REDs/factsheets/triclosan_fs.htm#summary

33. http://en.wikipedia.org/wiki/Polychloro_phenoxy_phenol

34. Offenbacher, S., Jared, H. L., O'Reilly, P. G., Wells, S. R., Salvi, G. E., Lawrence, H. P., Socransky, S. S., and Beck, J. D., Potential pathogenic mechanisms of periodontitis associated pregnancy complications. *Annals of Periodontology*, 1998, 3: 233–250.

35. León, R. et al., Detection of porphyromonas gingivalis in the amniotic fluid in pregnant women with a diagnosis of threatened premature labor. *Journal of Periodontology*, 2007, 78: 7.

36. Offenbacher, S., Beck, J. D., Lieff, S., and Slade, G., Role of periodontitis in systemic health: Spontaneous preterm birth. *Journal of Dental Education*, 1998, 62: 852–858.

37. Nicolson, G., Chronic bacterial and viral infections in neurodegenerative and neurobehavioral diseases. *Labmedicine*, 2008, 39, 5.

38. Ramfjord, S. P., Knowles, J. W., and Nissle, R. R., Longitudinal study of periodontal therapy. *Journal of Periodontology*, 1973, 44: 66.

39. Biocompatible Perio www.iaomt.org/articles/files/files188/biocompatible%20perio.pdf

10 Reduction in Orthopedic Conditions through Teledontic Treatment of Pharyngorofacial Disorders

Joseph Yousefian, DMD, MS and Michael N. Brown, DC, MD

AIMS:

A subspecialty of dentistry which is referenced hereinafter as teledontics, treats disorders involving the teeth, temporomandibular joint (TMJ) as well as the nasopharynx, oropharynx and maxillofacial structures, referred to as pharyngorofacial disorders (POFD). POFD correctly conveys that the dysfunction is not only in the TMJ and masticatory system but involves other oral, dental, nasopharyngeal, cervical, atlantooccipital and facial bone structures. POFD encompasses temporomandibular joint disorders (TMJD or TMD) as well as sleep breathing disorders such obstructive sleep apnea (OSA) and obstructive sleep apnea syndrome (OSAS). Dental clinicians specializing in treatment of POFD are increasingly being recognized for their contribution to regenerative orthopedics.[1] This chapter presents the biologic basis for why treating pharyngorofacial disorders (POFDs) is also clinically observed to alleviate musculoskeletal pain beyond the TMD, promote oxygenation to tissues, and make weight loss easier to achieve in response to standard lifestyle modifications.

This chapter is in three parts:

1. Pharyngorofacial disorders alter biomechanics of the face, oral cavity, airway and spine thereby predisposing to musculoskeletal pain.
2. Pharyngorofacial disorders alter metabolism, predisposing to musculoskeletal pain.
3. Correcting pharyngorofacial disorders restores structures to improve both biomechanical and metabolic function. Clinical cases demonstrate the resulting improvement in muscle preservation and fat reduction and pain management.

POFD AND THE BIOMECHANICS OF MUSCULOSKELETAL PAIN

The POF system is a complex biotensegrity unit, designed to carry out the tasks of breathing, chewing, swallowing, facial expression, and speech. These functions involve complex proprioceptive, mechanoreceptive and neuromuscular control mechanisms that allow for refined motor control. Perturbations in this system can lead to protective motor and sensory reflexes altering the kinematics of the POF complex leading to the development of POFDs (Figure 10.1).

POFDs represent a large group of disorders involving biomechanics and structural integrity of POF system impacting the growth and development of associated components. The site of dysfunction, structural damage and source of conceivable primary pain is located in the POF system.

During a normal function of the POF system, events as stressors of local or systemic origins may occur to influence the function (Table 10.1).

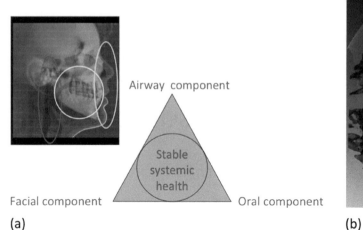

(a)

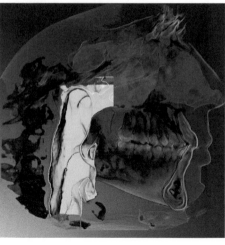

(b)

FIGURE 10.1   Structural and functional stability of pharyngorofacial triad and systemic health. Source: Diagrammatic representation of the pharyngorofacial triad components and systemic health.

TABLE 10.1

Proposed formula for the development of pharyngorofacial disorders (POFD)

				Host Adaptive		POF
Normal				Capacity		Structural remodeling
POF	+	Stressor	>	&	→	Dysfunction
Function				Psychosomatic		Symptoms
				Tolerance		

Local stressors leading to POF dysfunction include:

1. Placement of improperly occluding crown.
2. Local trauma such as injection response to local anesthesia.
3. Strain of opening the mouth too wide.
4. Unaccustomed use such as chewing gum for extended period of time.
5. Periodic episodes of bruxism
6. Effect of pain from surrounding tissues.

Systemic stressors leading to POF dysfunction include:

1. Emotional stress is one of the most common types of systemic alterations.
2. Elimination or reduction of REM sleep, which can lead to increased emotional stress and enhance generalized muscular tone of the body, head and neck leading to production of myofascial pain in the POF system (Figure 10.2).

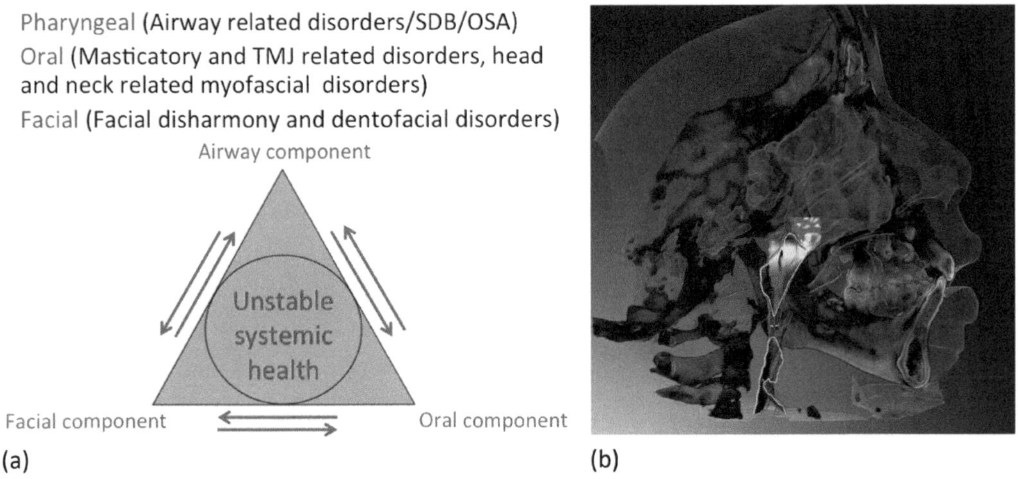

Pharyngeal (Airway related disorders/SDB/OSA)

Oral (Masticatory and TMJ related disorders, head and neck related myofascial disorders)

Facial (Facial disharmony and dentofacial disorders)

(a)   (b)

FIGURE 10.2   Pharyngorofacial disorders. SDB = sleep disordered breathing; OSA = obstructive sleep apnea; TMJ = temporomandibular joint Source: Remodeling of triad components of POFS and their vicious cycle as a major mechanism for decline of structural and functional integrity of the POF complex causing the development of POFD and their impact on the stability of systemic health.

METABOLIC DISTURBANCES ARISING FROM POFD

The change in biomechanics arising from POFD has many downstream metabolic effects associated with orthopedic conditions. Degeneration of POF musculoskeletal structures, obstructive sleep apnea (OSA) with metabolic syndrome, and musculoskeletal pain are presented here.

DEGENERATION OF POF MUSCULOSKELETAL STRUCTURES

Mandibular condylar cartilage was previously thought to be in the same category as the growth plate. However, it was later found that the condylar cartilage also possesses properties of epidphyseal cartilage.[2] Mandibular condylar cartilage as a hybrid of hyaline and fibrocartilage, has been categorized as chondroid bone, a tissue intermediate between bone and cartilage and thus functions as a growth site rather than a growth center.[2] Condylar cartilage is a secondary cartilage and therefore is subject to not only growth hormones, but local factors which can be modulated by mechanical stress modifying the amount of growth.[3] The authors have documented and appreciated abnormalities in the growth and development of the mandible in adolescence. This can result in various degrees of retrognathic mandible and thus can have long-term deleterious effects on the lumen of the airway and hence contributes to sleep disordered breathing (SDB) and OSA. This sets up a vicious cycle of desaturation and apneic events, chronic bruxism with further deterioration of the TMJ and condylar cartilage.

The authors have appreciated a high frequency of degenerative changes of the articular cartilage of the TMJ in both adult and adolescent patients with SDB and OSA. The integrity of the articular and soft tissue structures of TMJ can be caused by macro trauma or microtrauma to the TMJ and is influenced by bruxism, malocclusion and musculoskeletal instability of the masticatory system. It has been noted that prolonged concentric bruxism can cause functional overload of the TMJ.[4–6] The over loading of the joint causes, amongst various consequences, the collapse of lubricant in the join, which can result in degradation of hyaluronic acid by free radicals.[6] The regulation of hyaluronic acid production is controlled by various pro-inflammatory cytokines.[6] Excessive load to the mandibular condyle cause compression and narrowing of small vessels in the cancellous bone, which can cause injury to the articular cartilage and subchondral bone. This can lead to a chronic traumatic osteochondropathy (CTO) leading to degenerative changes of the TMJ, maxillary sutures and alveolar bone leading to maxillary and mandibular structural decline.

The progression of articular cartilage degenerative changes secondary to overload has unique effects on the POF structures. The mandibular condylar cartilage is somewhat unique in terms of several morphological, physiological and functional properties that are different from articular cartilage in long bones.[7] It has long been considered a critical growth site.[8] As mentioned previously, mandibular condylar cartilage previously thought to be the same as the growth plate has more

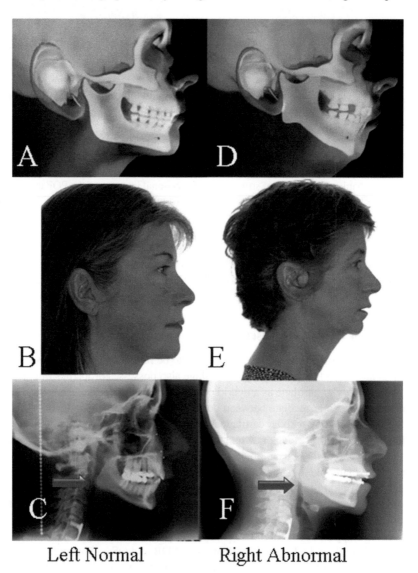

FIGURE 10.3 Degenerative changes in the TMJ causing remodeling in the POF structures. Source: *Left A, B, C: (A)* Schematic representation of normal facial skeletal and occlusal relationship. *(B)* Lateral facial photograph, representation of normal facial skeletal relationship. *(C)* Lateral cephalometric x-ray, representation of normal facial skeletal relationship and airway. Arrow pointing to the normal airway. *Right D, E, F: (D)* Schematic representation of abnormal facial skeletal and occlusal relationship, retrognathic jaw due to condylar remodeling. *(E)* Lateral facial photograph, representation of abnormal facial skeletal relationship including retrognathic jaw. *(F)* Lateral cephalometric X-ray, representation of adaptive facial skeletal as well as occlusal changes resulting constriction of the airway in response to condylar remodeling. Arrow pointing to the abnormal airway.

recently been found to possess properties of epiphyseal cartilage.[9] Thus, degenerative changes of the TMJ can alter growth and development of the mandible.

Patients with degenerative changes of the TMJ during the developmental years can develop a decrease in mandibular growth due to degenerative changes in the TMJ structures, resulting in decreased growth rate in the juvenile or progressive mandibular retrusion in the adult (Figure 10.3).[10,11] These patients also develop an anteroposterior retrusion of maxilla concomitant with a more retrusive position of the mandibular structures,[12] including the retropalatal, retroglossal and hypoglossal airway passages. As a result, the related airway passages may become more constricted.[13]

Schellhas, Gunson and Arnett showed that degenerative remodeling of the mandibular condyle and facial deformity occurs most often as a consequence of TMJ soft-tissue derangement with or without the presence of symptoms. At the initial clinical and radiographic examinations, they found externally visible chin displacement posteriorly (Figure 10.3). They also found a relatively high association between TMJ internal derangement and mandibular asymmetry, facial deformities and occlusal alterations.[14] Early onset of these structural deformities may impact the anteroposterior and vertical growth of the facial skeleton, including the maxillary structures.[12]

MRI studies performed by Tallents and colleagues on both symptomatic or asymptomatic female patients with a history of childhood bilateral degenerative joint disease showed that these patients had a moderate reduction of the anteroposterior dimension of the maxillary/mandibular (MM) structures, with a more pronounced overjet.[12] Due to these disharmonies, the related airway components may narrow, including retropalatal, retroglossal and hypoglossal areas. This constriction may contribute to the development of upper airway restriction during sleep causing SDB and OSA (Figure 10.3).[14,15]

Obstructive Sleep Apnea

OSA as one of more severe forms of SDB was once thought to be a disease of middle-age individuals, but it has become evident that individuals may experience apneic events at any age. OSA affects both genders and is encountered throughout the globe.

The data published by American Academy of Sleep Medicine on September 2014, estimated an increase in prevalence of OSA to 26% amongst adults between the ages of 30 and 70 years and gave much credit to the rising obesity epidemic.[16] Although Franklin et. al investigated 400 females from a population-based random sample of 10,000 Swedish females and found OSA (apnea-hypopnea index AHI $\geq$ 5) in 50% of females aged 20–70 years. Severe sleep apnea (AHI $\geq$ 30) was scored in

TABLE 10.2
The American Academy of Sleep Medicine (AASM) Task Force Classification of OSA[11]

Classification	AHI
Adults	
Mild	5–15/hr.
Moderate	15–30/hr.
Severe	>30/hr.
Children	
Mild	1–5/hr.
Moderate	5–10/hr.
Severe	>10/hr.

Note: The AHI is the number of apneas and hypopneas recorded during the study per hour of sleep. It is generally expressed as the number of events per hour.

14% of females aged 55–70 years with normal body mass index (BMI), and just in 31% of obese females with a BMI of >30 kg m^{-2}.[17] Asian men with severe OSAS have less tendency to be obese yet may present with significant posterior airway restriction leading to OSA.[18] Classification of OSA based on number of apnea events per hour is noted in Table 10.2.

The upper airway patency requires an interaction between structural and functional stability of POF anatomy and its related neuromuscular physiology.[13] Several studies of apnea patients and controls, found that the smallest airway luminal size was located at the level of the retropalatal (behind the soft palate) and retroglossal (behind the tongue).[19,20] Variables that affect the upper airway luminal size include the size of the jaw and tongue and the enlarging tonsillar bulk in children. POF abnormalities (*e.g.*, maxillary and mandibular retrognathia) also are associated with OSA.[21] Case reports correlate the development of OSA in individuals with various POF abnormalities. [22] Other risk factors include the size and position of the tongue, which are affected by the anteroposterior, transverse and vertical dimensions of the dental arches.[23]

It has been thought that the prevalence of OSA increases with age and weight gain.[24] Most often obesity as side effect of OSA initiated by POF structural and neuromuscular abnormalities as primary factors become secondary but a strong perpetuating element in development and severity of apneic events. As a result, the influence of obesity on airway anatomy was studied with controversial results. Some authors found that apneic subjects had extra fatty tissue deposition in the area of the upper airway when compared to weight-matched controls. Some studies more clearly relate OSA to potential changes in the POF complex and pharyngeal anatomy.[18,25]

POF structural and functional discrepancies create a vicious cycle of biomechanical and metabolic dysfunction. This is illustrated with the term metabolic syndrome. Metabolic syndrome and obesity were recognized by the late twentieth century as the major comorbidities of OSA and especially of OSAS in children[26] and adults, beyond just being sleepy.[27] Other major comorbidities of OSAS besides metabolic syndrome and obesity include; depression, 75% increased chance of motor vehicle accidents attributable to excessive daytime sleepiness, ADD & ADHD, Alzheimer's disease, sexual impotence, acid reflux, type II diabetes, High blood pressure, coronary artery disease, congestive heart failure, atrial fibrillation/cardiac arrhythmias, myocardial ischemia/infarction, heart attack, stroke (cerebral vascular accidents), 75% increased risk of development of cancer including breast and prostate in patients with moderate to severe OSAS and death.[28]

Sleep bruxism associated with SDB or OSA is an important phenomenon for physician to manage musculoskeletal disorders. Bruxism is the process of clenching the jaws and grinding teeth. Bruxism involves repetitive jaw muscle activity characterized by clenching or grinding of the teeth and/or by bracing or thrusting of the mandible.

Bruxism is classified into awake bruxism and sleep bruxism. Sleep bruxism is the most important for this discussion. Sleep bruxism (SB) has been found to be related to desaturation events and apneic events during sleep.[29–31] The TCR (Trigemino-cardiac reflex) is a powerful autonomic reflex that can reduce heart rate under challenging situations by acting as an oxygen conserving reflex.[32–34] Stimulation of the trigeminal nerve along its course can cause sympathetic withdrawal and parasympathetic overactivity through the vagus nerve resulting in bradycardia, apnea, bradypnea and hypotension. OSA occurs with frequent periods of collapse of the pharyngeal airway as we have addressed. This causes a reduction in oxygen saturation of blood leading to cortical and brainstem arousals.[35] It is reported that sudden micro-arousals (MA) occurring in the brain due to airway obstruction during sleep which cause a sudden tachycardia, which stimulates repetitive jaw movement and grinding that activates the TCR resulting in reflex bradycardia.[30,35] One of the key components of OSA is hypoxemia that itself acts as a potential risk factor for inciting the TCR.[35]

Several other risk factors are linked to SB. Psychological factors, such as stress, anxiety, and competitiveness, have been reported as exacerbators. In patients with OSA, 74% of episodes of SB are reported in the supine position.[36] Recent studies do not support the earlier findings that SB triggers sleep arousal; they suggest that SB is concomitant or secondary to cyclic alterations in the sleep patterns.[36]

An experimental model that could trigger arousals during the sleep without inducing awakenings has been developed.[36] Using it, the investigators were able to examine the mechanisms involved in the initiation of sudden SB. Using a brief vibrotactile stimulation, frequent sleep arousals were induced, followed by SB; teeth grinding occurred in 86% of the trials. The authors suggest that SB is one of the events that occur with physiologic activations associated with MAs.[36]

The authors describe a more exaggerated and continued EMG activity following apnea/hypopnea events in masseter/temporalis muscles of OSA patients with MD symptoms, eg, headaches and jaw pains upon awakening. Based on these observations, it is reasonable to suggest that SB is a multifactorial phenomenon. It may take place secondary to exaggerated transient motor and autonomic nervous system activation related to MAs following apnea/hypopnea events. This conclusion explains the phenomenon of MAs, concomitant with masticatory parafunctional activity, as the brain reacts to keep the constricted air passages open to prevent the choking that can develop following the episodes of apnea/hypopnea.

The authors suggest that there are also a number of clinical entities other than OSA that can lead activating the TCR causing bruxism without reduction in oxygen saturation levels. This would include upper airway resistant syndrome (UARS) and periodic leg movement (PLM) disorder, as we have discussed, that also lead to MAs and sleep bruxism. It has been appreciated that during CPAP titration at night most breathing abnormalities were eliminated and a complete eradication of SB events was also observed.[29]

MUSCULOSKELETAL PAIN

Pain initiated and felt in the POF system or in the related structures is defined as *primary pain*. Pain initiated from the adjacent head and neck structures and felt in POF system, known as *heterotopic* or referred pain. Pain regardless of the type, primary or heterotopic, often alters normal neuromuscular function by means of the central excitatory effects. This can lead to myofascial pain, headaches, maxillofacial pain syndromes, TMJ pain, intracapsular TMJ degenerative joint disease as well as postural abnormalities that can affect the cervical spine leading to neck pain and persistent myofascial pain extending through the whole upper trunk.[14]

Not all individuals respond to identical event(s) in the same manner. The variation depends primarily on the individual's physiologic and psychosomatic tolerance of certain stressors without feeling any adverse effects (Table 10.1). Under stable conditions, the POF complex including its cervical region and masticatory system is best able to tolerate the local and the systemic stressors. When orthopedic stability is compromised, relatively insignificant stressors may disrupt the normal function and initiate or aggravate clinical symptoms in the POF triad components.

The most orthopedically stable position of the POF complex is in natural head posture with mandible in centric occlusion and teeth in maximum intercuspation. The orthopedic instability may result from conditions that are related to the occlusion, the TM joints, the cervical region influenced by head and neck posture or combination. Other factors of instability include the genetic or epigenetic factors including developmental, or iatrogenic causes, arthritic condition, alterations in the normal anatomy of the TM joints, and disharmony between a stable intercuspal position (ICP) of the teeth and the musculoskeletal stable position of TM joints and cervical region. Spontaneous posturing of the head and neck or mandible including wear of unfitting oral appliances may also alter orthopedic stability of POF complex and cause dysfunction, symptoms, or in the long term, contribute to the development of POFD (Table 10.1).

The effectiveness of the physiologic pain modulation may also be altered by the systemic abnormalities associated with OSA, especially by fragmentation of the sleep stages and cycles. These changes may, in turn, alter the response of an individual to the local or systemic stressor(s). If the descending inhibitory system does not effectively modulate neuroreceptive input, the system becomes more vulnerable to encountered events. This condition may facilitate the development of local muscle disturbances, POFD-related symptoms including myofascial pain disorder, or fibromyalgia.

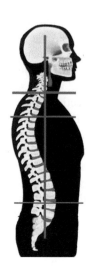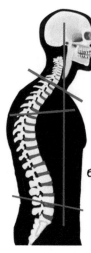

1. Forward head
   tilt shifting center
   of gravity.
2. Head thrust helps
   open the airway.
3. Upper body weight
   is shifted backward.
4. Hips are shifted
   forward.
5. Lumbar lordosis is
   increased.
6. Increased facet joint
   loading in upper
   cervical spine and
   cervicothroacic
   junction.

FIGURE 10.4 Postural compensations for narrowed airway. Source: The anterior head posture due to narrowed airway can lead to a number of postural aberrations.

The postural changes that begin with POFD often extend to the spine. A narrowed upper airway often leads to OSA. To reduce the obstruction postural compensation often occurs.[37] Most OSA patients will try to increase the airway patency by altering the posture of the head and neck during the daytime activities or sleep.[38] The anterior head carry position can lead to a number of postural aberrations that can lead to effects in the upper cervical spine, lower cervical spine, as well as lumbar spine and pelvis as noted in Figure 10.4 to the right.

In addition, some OSA patients, may develop masticatory dysfunction (MD) from nocturnal or diurnal anterior or lateral posturing of the mandible to increase the airway patency. MD may also result from anterior positioning by oral appliances, worn for management of snoring or OSA at bedtime.[39,40] The actual cause of the possible primary pain here is the compromised orthopedic stability of the TM joints and masticatory system causing MD and TMJD. This musculoskeletal instability may create primary pain and intracapsular dysfunction in the TMJ as well as other cervical spine joints including atlantooccipital complex. MD can also cause local myofascial pain in the masticatory, head, and neck musculature. The affected components can cause primary pain from the primary source of tissue change. The indirect effect of OSA on the development of POFD may be related to its impact on the orthopedic stability and altered function of the cervical facet joints, along with head and neck musculature. Overuse of the musculature in this condition may create myofascial pain in the cervical spine and craniofacial structures and may generate a source of heterotopic or referred pain to the other POF or head and neck regions.

The associated poor-quality sleep and hormonal changes are additional factors that may contribute to the development of joint degeneration, as well as functional damage to adjacent structures.[41,42] TMJs and other loadbearing joints can be equally affected by these perturbations. OSA patients have been known to have elevated inflammatory cytokines including tumor necrosis factor, IL-1, IL-6.[43] Among the inflammatory cytokines, tumor necrosis factor and interleukin-1 and-6, play a crucial role in the pathogenesis of osteoarthritis with regard to acceleration and progression of cartilage degeneration, as they promote bone restriction through osteoclastic differentiation and activation.[42]

There is emerging evidence that chronic recurrent hypoxia in OSA patients leads to activation of inflammatory pathways.[44–46] Levels of pro-inflammatory cytokines tumor necrosis factor alpha has been shown to correlate to severity of OSA and increase non-REM sleep and some authors suggest OSA to be a systemic inflammatory disease.[47] In addition, inflammatory markers such as C-reactive protein (CRP), interleukin-1b (IL-1b), IL-6, and IL-8 has also been identified in OSA patients.[45,46,48]

Pro-inflammatory cytokines IL-1b, IL-6 and TNF-α contributes to the regulation of sleep in the CNS hypothalamus and hippocampus.[49]

The intermittent hypoxia associated with OSA activates signaling cascades which can lead to production of reactive oxygen species (ROS), which include superoxide, and non-free radicals such as hydrogen peroxide and endogenous antioxidants defense mechanisms.[50] Reoxygenation (ischemic reperfusion) following a brief period of hypoxia in OSA in conjunction with periods of SB and overloading of the TM joints articular surfaces may predispose to cellular stress, possibly due to mitochondrial dysfunction thus promoting the activation of a pro-inflammatory response mediated by NF kappa B (NFκB), a major regulator of inflammatory gene expression. The effects of activation of this factor include increased expression of proatherogenic factors such as TNF-α, which may contribute to endothelial dysfunction and cardiovascular complications as well.[51] The ROS disrupts important signaling pathways in the arterial wall, promoting inflammatory and immune functions through the activation of NFκB.[52] Additionally, OSA in children have demonstrated abnormal levels of IL-17, an interleukin related to T helper 17 cells, a T helper cell involved in development of autoimmunity and inflammation.[53] With the complex interplay of OSA and an elevated pro-inflammatory state, there is no wonder that there is a higher risk of developing certain autoimmune diseases in OSA patients.[54] The co-existence of sleep apnea in rheumatic disease patients may influence the severity of patient-reported symptoms of pain and fatigue, as well as potentially impacting on levels of circulating inflammatory markers and mediators.[55-57]

It is important to note that upper-airway narrowing can occur in patients with rheumatoid arthritis (RA) when retrognathia develops secondary to TMJ destruction.[58,59] The authors opine that any condition causing destruction of mandibular condylar cartilage can lead to inadequate growth and development of the mandible and therefore causing varying degrees of retrognathia that can lead to the sequela of narrowed airway and OSA in children and adolescents. This can occur with any condition affecting the mandibular condylar cartilage which includes wear and tear and osteoarthritis. This phenomenon represents an example of an orthopedic condition that can lead to OSA and to all of the associated risks and comorbidities of OSA.

Systemic inflammation increasingly has been implicated in cardiovascular disease. Low-grade inflammation may be the "common ground" underlying the associations between OSA, metabolic syndrome and cardiovascular disease. Interleukin-6 is a proinflammatory cytokine, contributing to the synthesis of an acute phase reactant, C-reactive protein (CRP). Recent data suggest that CRP may predict an increased risk for diabetes, hypertension and metabolic syndrome.[60] Hypoxemia, occurring during the night in patients with OSA, together with sleep deprivation, causing an increase in cytokines, may induce a heightened state of systemic inflammation as evidenced by elevated CRP and serum amyloid A.[60] CRP levels are higher in OSA patients than in healthy individuals and may be associated with risk for hypertension. Along with OSA, sleep deprivation and obesity may induce an increase in cytokines and thereby contribute to the metabolic derangement.

Leptin, an adipocyte-derived hormone, exerts important effects on the cardiovascular system. Known as the central regulator of body fat mass, appetite and energy homeostasis, leptin also interacts with sleep. High serum leptin levels in obese patients is well documented and suggests the presence of leptin resistance.[61] Male patients with OSA have even higher levels of leptin than would be expected from obesity, which may have implications for weight gain in OSA patients.[62]

Other factors that contribute to the symptoms of metabolic syndrome due to OSA are sleep loss, daytime somnolence and decreased physical activity (Figure 10.5). Sleep deprivation may impair carbohydrate metabolism and endocrine function and lead to weight gain and insulin resistance, even in healthy subjects. Sleep deprivation for 60 hours elicits decreased insulin sensitivity.[63] Restricting sleep to four hours per night for six nights in young healthy individuals impairs glucose tolerance. Sleep deprivation results in increased plasma cortisol and resting blood pressure.[64] Sleep influences the nocturnal leptin profile and sleep deprivation disrupts this profile. Therefore, sleep is important in modulating metabolism and perhaps obesity.[64]

Insulin resistance is an independent risk factor in cardiovascular diseases, and its characteristics are present in patients with sleep apnea. Patients with OSA have significantly higher levels of fasting

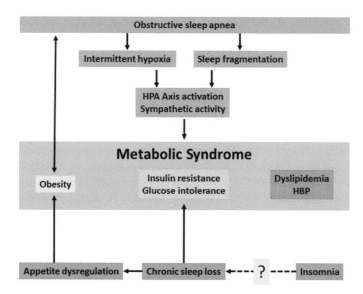

FIGURE 10.5 Chronic sleep loss and metabolic syndrome. Source: Diagrammatic pathway showing the effect of chronic sleep loss due to OSA, sleep deprivation or insomnia on the development of metabolic syndrome.

glucose and insulin resistance than non-OSA patients, independent of adiposity.[65] The severity of OSA is associated with increased insulin resistance through enhanced sympathetic activity, endothelial dysfunction and impairment of peripheral vasodilatation. The impairment of glucose tolerance is coupled with severity of nocturnal oxygen desaturation. Insulin resistance may contribute to development of metabolic syndrome.[65] In metabolic and neural hormonal changes in these patients also are shown to increase intake of high sugar-containing foods.[66]

Unrecognized POFD can lead to sleep disturbance and OSA, which is associated with neural hormonal, inflammatory, metabolic abnormalities, leading to obesity and the other comorbidities associated with sleep apnea. Weight gain and fatty deposits also alters the airway lumen further narrowing the upper airway, contributing to the development of OSA. The weight gain has profound effects on the spine and lower extremities. This eventually leads to progressive degenerative changes in the weightbearing joints. Pain and associated orthopedic disability leads to inactivity, which perpetuates obesity and metabolic disturbances and thus a vicious cycle is set up perpetuating orthopedic disability and shortening of patient's life span secondary to the comorbidities of OSA, which include obesity, coronary artery disease, hypercholesterolemia, and other metabolic disturbances.

In 2001, Warren and Bishara demonstrated a trend in North American children for more narrowed dental arch dimensions showing both maxillary and mandibular arch lengths in both sexes is significantly shorter over few generations.[67] The epigenetic factors like use of pacifiers, bottle feeding and change in quantity and quality of diet may play a role in this rapid change.[75]

The authors strongly believe that unrecognized POF abnormalities, leading to OSA and other sleep disturbances can lead to metabolic perturbations, obesity, neural hormonal effects, leading to a wide array of physiologic and anatomical disturbances. The combination of above factors including increased prevalence of POF structural discrepancies[67] are often exist as an underlying factor for development of OSA and its related comorbidities. OSA and its perpetuating factors including sleep loss, daytime somnolence, decreased activity and urge for consumption of high caloric intake may be contributing to the fact that 30% of American and Canadian children being obese.

Obesity and the associated metabolic abnormalities associated with obesity can lead to multiple musculoskeletal orthopedic difficulties. Despite the multifactorial nature of musculoskeletal disease, obesity consistently emerges as a key modifiable risk factor in the onset and progression of musculoskeletal conditions including spine and large joints.[68–70] Obesity has been associated with a greater risk of orthopedic and musculoskeletal pain and injury in both the military[71–73] as well as the general population.[70,74,75] Emerging evidence is now suggesting that with even the modest increase in weight-bearing activity in the obese patient can lead to pain and musculoskeletal difficulties.[76,77] For example, for every 5 kg weight gain, there is a commensurate 36% increased risk for developing osteoarthritis.[78] Obesity has been specifically implicated in disorders involving the back, hip, knee, ankle, and foot.[70,75,79–82] There is also a link to obesity and its profound effect on soft tissues, including tendons, fascia, and cartilage.[81,83,84] Patient with obesity are associated with more rapid progression of osteoarthritis, than their normal weight counterparts.[85] In a study of chronic pain complaints in a weight management service in patients with obesity, 91% of patients surveyed reported musculoskeletal pain.[86] In this population, 69% involved low back pain, 58%, knee pain, as well as a reported decrease in quality of life, decreased functional capacity and sleep.[86] The social economic impact of musculoskeletal conditions is staggering. One of the great fears of patients undergoing total joint arthroplasty for the knee is time to revision. Maintaining weight after a primary total knee arthroplasty (TKA) is protective against a later revision.[87] Failure to reduce weight after TKA is a risk factor for early revision for aseptic loosening, and osteolysis.[87] Orthopedic surgeons performing total joint arthroplasty procedures may recommend weight loss, but rarely recognize the complexity of POF abnormalities that can lead to sleep disorders and a metabolic perturbations that can cause obesity.

Obesity is a strong independent risk factor for pain. Adolescents with obesity were more likely to report musculoskeletal pain, including chronic regional pain, than their normal-weight peers. The disease nearly doubles the risk of chronic pain among the elderly—causing pain in soft-tissue structures such as tendons and ligaments, and worsening conditions such as fibromyalgia in individuals already living with constant pain in their muscles and joints.[88]

The odds of sustaining musculoskeletal injuries is 15% higher for persons who are overweight and 48% higher for people who are obese, compared to persons of normal weight.[88] In this way degeneration can occur secondarily from obesity-related injuries.

Osteoarthritis (OA) is a progressive "wear and tear" disease of the joints. Each pound of body weight places four to six pounds of pressure on each knee joint. Osteoarthritis of the knees is strongly associated with obesity.[88]

CLINICAL CONSIDERATIONS OF CHILDREN WITH POFD

POFD and OSA can also profoundly affect the pediatric population. The increased risk factor is especially true of those who have food or environmental allergies, chronic nasal congestion and mouth breathing. This phenomenon can be significantly magnified in children undergone certain orthodontic treatments causing constriction of the upper airway by severe retraction of front teeth and entrapment of the tongue in pharyngeal airway such as extraction of four bicuspids or extensive use of headgear and functional appliances. This can result in a phenomenon of "straight teeth – narrowed airway."

The sleep disorder occurring secondary to narrowed oral airway in children also lead to obesity in the pediatric population as well. Similar to the adult counterpart children also have adverse effects on the musculoskeletal system secondary to increasing weight gain.[89] This is also important because studies have demonstrated that overweight children are more than likely to become overweight adults compared to the normal weight peers.[90–92] Until recently, the majority of studies in children evaluated the association between orthopedic conditions such as slipped capital femoral epiphysis (SCFE) and Blount's disease with increased weight.[93,94] More recently, newer studies are showing that obesity affects the musculoskeletal system as a whole in the pediatric population and may impede the overall function of the individual.[95]

The biomechanics of the gait in an obese adolescent leads to a "fat thigh" gait which produces compressive forces on the medial aspect of the knee and may play a role in adolescent tibial varum.[96]

In addition, more recent studies have demonstrated an increased incidence in musculoskeletal pain associated with obesity when obese children were compared to other non-overweight counterparts. This is thought to be related to the compensatory biomechanical effects of the excess weight and misalignment on their joints as a factor for the increased incidence of pain in this population.[97,98] Although obese children have been noted to have better upper extremity strength their lower limb function are compromised.[99,100]

Detailed analysis of clinical symptoms is the first step for the diagnosis of OSA in children. Even when the clinical symptoms of OSA are evident, the cause(s) of breathing problems often remain undiagnosed for a long time. The long delay in diagnosis is the result of patients seeking treatment only when the complications, such as acute cardiorespiratory failure, already are severe. [101] The type and the frequency of clinical symptoms in children are different than those in adults. Excessive daytime sleepiness is infrequent in children.[101] There are three main nighttime symptoms of OSA in children and infants: snoring, difficulty in breathing with an inward movement of the upper part of the chest during inspiration, and apneas with noisy resumption of breathing.[102] Mouth breathing is common during wakefulness.[102] Drenching sweats, SB, restless sleep and frequent awakenings during the night are reported by parents. Nocturnal enuresis may be a symptom in older children.[102] Acute upper airway infections are common in younger children.[103] The severity of clinical symptoms increases during an infection and decreases with treatment.

Behavioral disorders (hyperactivity, aggressive behavior, ADD, and ADHD) and cognitive impairments have been reported in school children with OSA.[21] Recent studies have demonstrated that following appropriate treatment including tonsillectomy for treatment of OSA, behavioral and learning disorders can be alleviated in this group of patients.[21,102,104]

The mechanisms by which growth is stunted in some children remain a matter of debate. Some assumptions include an increase in the abnormally high oxygen consumption due to the overworking of the respiratory muscles during sleep.[105] Disturbance in the secretion of growth hormone, caused by disruptions in sleep cycles, is implicated as a cause for growth problems in children with OSA.[106] Children with mandibular retrognathia have an increased tendency to develop OSA, and the breathing problem becomes even worse when the seasonal allergies or repeated respiratory infections are increasing the risk of airway obstruction.

CORRECTING PHARYNGOROFACIAL DISORDERS

The most favorable care for patients with POFD suffering from SDB and OSA is treatment provided by an interdisciplinary team that includes members from the appropriate dental and medical disciplines.[15,107,108]

When dental treatment including orthodontic and orthognathic surgical procedures are used for the expansion and restoration of the POF complex for treatment of POFD including SDB and OSA, they are referred to as teledontics and telegnathic surgery.[15,107,108] This treatment protocol avoids the use of procedures and techniques, which can retract or constrict the jaws or dentition including; extraction of teeth, use of headgear or functional appliances or surgical set back of the jaws that in long run impacting the upper airway negatively.[109,110]

CASE STUDIES

Case #1

History

12 years old caucasian male patient with history of malocclusion and possible presence of OSA. The patient's parents reported presence of malocclusion, snoring and tooth grinding at bedtime. The patient was also noted to have depression, obesity, metabolic syndrome, fluctuating blood pressure, blood sugar, and hypercholesterolemia. He snored with restless sleep and his school performance

had significantly declined in the last few years and was becoming disruptive in class. He was unable to focus on his school work. Prozac and Adderall provided little benefit.

Exam

On exam patient was noted to have small jaws, narrow palate, cross bite with no evidence of tonsil or adenoid enlargement. Sleep study was obtained demonstrating severe OSA with AHI of 12. ENT consultant opined patient was not candidate for tonsillectomy and adenoidectomy.

Treatment

Intraoral appliances and braces as part of teledontic therapy were used to expand the palate, mandibular and maxillary dental arches which corrected his narrowed nasal cavity, pharyngeal airway. This also resolved the crowding avoiding the extraction of teeth. Following treatment patient had cessation of snoring and resolution of disrupted sleep. Post treatment sleep study confirmed resolution of OSA with AHI of 1. Patient was noted to have resolution of metabolic syndrome, obesity, with normalized blood pressure, cholesterol and blood sugar. Patient was noted to have improved performance in school with improved attentiveness and improved behavior in class. Patient was tapered off Adderall. Patient note to have improved nasal breathing rather than mouth breathing at night. Pre- and post-treatment images are presented in Figures 10.6 and 10.7.

NOTE: Diagnosis of probable OSA is easier in children who snore, have loud mouth breathing and/or bruxism. Inquiry should be made in these patients in regard to school performance and attention span.

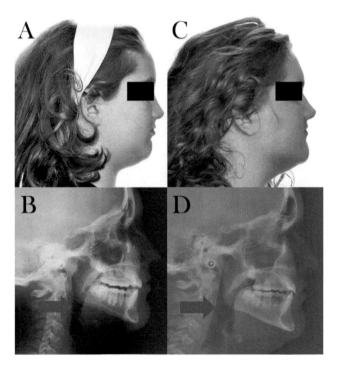

FIGURE 10.6 Case #1 Improvement of the facial growth and its impact on the enlargement of the jaws and airway. Source: (*A*) Lateral facial photograph (*B*) lateral cephalometric X-ray representation of abnormal facial skeletal relationship including retrognathic jaws and small airway in response to condylar remodeling. Arrow pointing to the abnormal airway. (*C*) Lateral facial photograph (*D*) lateral cephalometric X-ray representation of enhanced normal facial skeletal and airway as response to teledontic treatment. Arrow pointing to the normal airway.

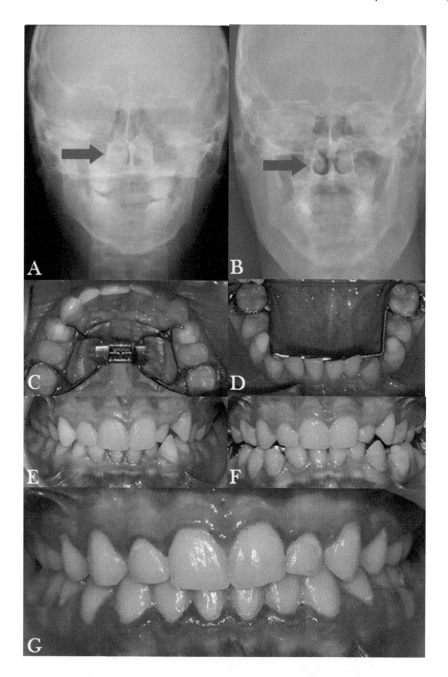

FIGURE 10.7 Case #1 Enlargement of the nasal cavity and oral cavity as response to the teledontic jaw expansion. Source: Pre-treatment *(A)*, post- treatment *(B)* frontal view cephalometric X-rays showing the significant enlargement of the nasal airway spaces as a favorable response to the teledontic expansion of palate. (arrows pointing to the nasal cavity). Intraoral photographs showing the significant expansion of the palate *(C)* and lower dental arch *(D)* for improvement of crowding to avoid four bicuspid extractions, also to create space for tongue to move forward out of the pharyngeal space to improve the airway. Intraoral photographs, pre-treatment *(E)* and post- treatment *(F)* showing the expansion of the dental arches for improvement of the crowding and tongue space. Post-treatment *(G)* intraoral photograph showing the ideal bite with expansion of the dental arches for improvement of the crowding and tongue space.

Case #2

History

A 46-year-old female presented with symptoms of POFD and MD including jaw pain, headaches, moderate OSA with AHI of 23, sleep efficiency of 82%, snoring, excessive daytime sleepiness, and fatigue. Patient was CPAP intolerant due to air leakage around her concave pre-oral area caused by four bicuspid extractions and severe retraction of her front teeth. Structurally she had deficient maxillary and mandibular dentition with protracted chin due to previous orthodontic treatment with an extended period of time using headgear and combined extraction of maxillary and mandibular first bicuspids. (Figure 10.8). Patient was obese with BMI of 55. Patient had history of failed multiple weight loss programs, including gastric bypass. Patient had previous arthroscopic meniscus debridement bilaterally with progressive worsening pain and functional disability secondary to advancing osteoarthritis of both knees with current recommendations from consulting orthopedist for a medial compartment hemiarthroplasty on the right. Conservative treatment directed to knees including viscoelastic supplement injections and PRP provided no benefit.

Diagnostic imaging

CBCT imaging of the TMJs revealed bilateral osteoarthrosis with flattening of the superior surfaces of the mandibular condyles, and loss of bony volume. The patient had a long history of tension and pain in the temporal areas and in front of the ears.

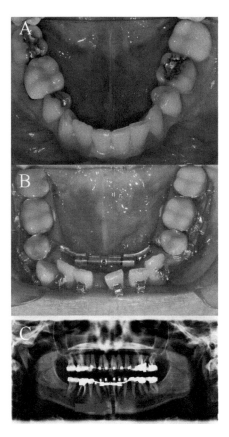

FIGURE 10.8   Case #2 Surgically assisted mandibular expansion "same" telegnathic technique for expansion of the lower jaw. Source: Intraoral photographs showing the before *(A)* and after *(B)* "same" telegnathic technique for expansion of the lower jaw. Panoramic X-ray *(C)* showing the "same" osteotomy site for expansion of mandible. Arrow pointing to the osteotomy site.

Treatment

The treatment began with management of her MD and OSA with pharyngorofacial stabilizing orthotic (PSO), combined with medication (Feldine, 20 mg) and home physical therapy for six months to stabilize the masticatory system and eliminate the masticatory and TMJ pain symptoms. Telegnathic surgery for correction of her OSA, included mandibular midline osteotomy followed by 8 mm teledontic expansion with surgically assisted mandibular expansion (SAME) utilizing author's technique[111] to resolve the crowding of the mandibular incisors and improvement of base of tongue constriction. Post-initial surgical intervention follow-up sleep study demonstrated AHI of 6 with reduction of EDS and snoring. Although functionally improved, patient opted for correction of maxillary and mandibular deficiencies causing aesthetic issues and mild OSA.

Patient proceeded with phase II-telegnathic procedure included an 8 mm maxillary expansion and an 8 mm maxillomandibular advancement (MMA). The postsurgical teledontic treatment was completed in 12 months. A remarkable increase in the retropalatal, retroglossal, and hypoglossal airway spaces was evident cephalometrically. Clinically patient reported absence of snoring, EDS and MD and TMJ symptoms. The post treatment sleep study showed improvement of AHI to 2.5, with sleep efficiency of 94%.

Patient was then able to complete a successful Medifast diet bringing her BMI to 27. Because of successful weight loss, patient reported marked improvement of lower back and knee complaints, which were then responsive to conservative treatment and opted to postpone her medial compartment hemiarthroplasty secondary to marked improvement of knee pain. Figure 10.8 and 10.9 demonstrate pre- and post-treatment images.

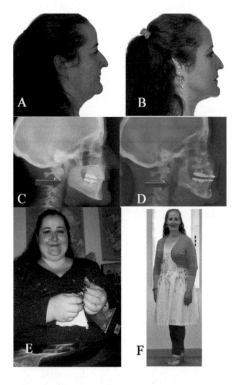

FIGURE 10.9   Case #2 Maxillomandibular advancement (MMA) telegnathic surgery for treatment of POFD and OSA. Source: Pre-treatment *(A)*, post- treatment *(B)* lateral view facial photographs showing the improvement of face by MMA telegnathic surgery. Pre-treatment *(C)*, post- treatment *(D)* lateral cephalometric X-ray showing the improvement of airway by "same and MMA" telegnathic surgery. Arrows pointing to the enlargement of the airway. Pre-treatment *(E)* and post-treatment *(F)* whole body photographs showing a favorable response to weight loss protocol due to resolved OSA.

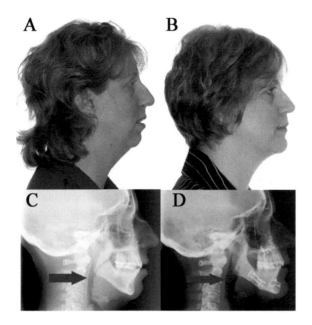

FIGURE 10.10   Case #3 Maxillomandibular advancement (MMA) telegnathic surgery for treatment of POFD and OSA. Source: Pre-treatment (A), post- treatment (B) lateral view facial photographs showing the improvement of face by CCR/MMA telegnathic surgery. Pre-treatment (C), post- treatment (D) lateral cepha-lometric X-ray showing the improvement of airway by "CCR/MMA" telegnathic surgery. Arrows pointing to the enlargement of the airway.

Case #3

History

39-year-old female presented with history of significant daytime somnolence, fatigue, long-standing history of TMJ and headache complaints, neck pain and low back pain, all non-responsive to conventional treatment. She described TMJ and temporal distribution of myofascial pain which was worse upon awakening and also aggravated by chewing. Patient was overweight with BMI of 31 and history of depression and hypertension.

Related past history

At age 15. Patient underwent orthodontic treatment with use of headgear and extraction of the 4 first premolar teeth in order to correct her overbite.

Examination

Sleep study demonstrated severe OSA with AHI of 68. The retrusive position of the maxillary and mandibular teeth was caused by excessive use of headgear and previous four bicuspid extractions.

Treatment intervention

The patient began treatment by wearing a PSO at bed time to manage the OSA and stabilize the masticatory system and reduce her frequent headaches and TMJ sensitivity.

The surgical procedures included pre-surgical teledontic preparation combined with 12 mm counterclockwise rotation advancement of maxillomandibular (CCR/MMA) structures. Total treatment time was 24 months. Patient noted interval resolution of TMJ pain, neck and back pain. Follow-up sleep study demonstrated AHI of 2.9, and sleep efficiency of 92%, demonstrating interval resolution of OSA. Patient's hypertension resolved and over a period time gradual improvement of mood and resolution of depression. An additional 2 years was required for behavioral modification to improve diet, lifestyle and exercise. Patient then was able to lose weight with BMI reduced to 27. Post-treatment facial photographs noted in Figure 10.10.

CONCLUSION

POFDs are at the "jaws" of chronic musculoskeletal pain, sleep disordered breathing and unintended weight gain. Advances in regenerative orthopedics have enabled dentists to improve treatment outcomes for POFDs especially in younger populations where a "teledontic" approach may be especially effective when uptake of CPAP has been poor. This involves use of oral appliances and sometimes oral surgery as described in the preceding cases. The dental profession has observed marked improvement not only in parameters of dental health, but parameters relevant to orthopedic medicine most of which are mediated by correction of sleep apnea. Outcomes include reduction in chronic musculoskeletal pain, success in patient-initiated diets, and reduction in risk factors of osteoarthritis.

REFERENCES

1. Yousefian J. Pharyngorofacial regenerative orthopedics, advances in understanding TMD. *34th American Association of Orthopedic Medicine Annual Conference and Scientific Seminar Seattle WA.* 2017.
2. Salo LA, Hoyland J, Ayad S. The expression of types X and VI collagen and fibrillin in rat mandibular-condylar cartilage. Response to mastication forces. *Acta Odontol Scand.* 1996;54(5):295–302.
3. Petrovic A, Stutzmann J. Growth hormone: Mode of action on different varieties of cartilage. *Pathol Biol (Paris).* 1980;28(1):43–58.
4. Mori H, Horiuchi S, Nishimura S, et al. Three dimensional finite element analysis of cartilaginous tissues in human temporomandibular joint during prolonged clenching. *Arch Oral Biol.* 2010;55:879–886.
5. Cairns B. Pathophysiology of TMD pain—basic mechanisms and their implications for pharmacotherapy. *J Oral Rehabil.* 2010;37:391–410.
6. Tanaka E, Detamore M, Mercuri L. Degenerative disorders of the temporomandibular joint: Etiology, diagnosis, and treatment. *J Dent Res.* 2008; 87:296–307.
7. Ren C, Yang Y. Mandibular condyle: Structure properties and growth regulation. *J Oral Sci Health.* 2014;1(1):1–6.
8. Sicher H. Growth of the mandible. *Am J Orthod.* 1947; 33(1):30–35.
9. Salo L, Hoyland J, Ayad S, et al. The expression of types X and VI collagen and fibrillin in rat mandibular condylar cartilage. Response to mastication forces. *Acta Odontol Scand.* 1996;54(5):295–302.
10. Arnett W, Milam S, Gottesman L. Progressive mandibular retrusion, Idiopathic condylar resorption. Part I. *Am J Orthod Dentofacial Orthop.* 1996;110(1):8–5.
11. Arnett W, Milam S, Gottesman L. Progressive mandibular retrusion, Idiopathic condylar resorption. Part II. *Am J Orthod Dentofacial Orthop.* 1996;110(2):117–127.
12. Gidarakou I, Tallents R, Kyrkanides S. Comparison of skeletal and dental morphology in asymptomatic volunteers and symptomatic patients with bilateral degenerative joint disease. *Angle Orthodontist.* 2003;73(1):71–78.
13. Yousefian J, Moghadam B. *The Role of Contemporary Orthodontics in the Diagnosis and Treatment of Sleep-disordered Breathing.* Vol 2. 2nd ed. USA: Roth Williams Legacy Foundation; 2015.
14. Gunson M, Arnett W. Oral contraceptive pill use and abnormal menstrual cycles in women with severe condylar resorption: A case for low serum 17β-estradiol as a major factor in progressive condylar resorption. *Am J Orthod Dentofacial Orthop,* 2009;136(6):772–779.
15. Yousefian J. Correction of severe obstructive sleep apnea syndrome with interdisciplinary medical and dental treatment planning. *J Dent Sleep Med.* 2016;3(3):1–3.
16. Medicine AAoS. 2014.
17. Franklin KA, Sahlin C, Stenlund H. Sleep apnoea is a common occurrence in females. *Eur Respir J.* 2013;41(3):619–615.
18. Li KK, Powell NB, Guilleminauilt C. Obstructive sleep apnea syndrome: A comparison between Far-East Asian and white men. *Laryngoscope.* 2000;110(10):1689–1693.

19. Davies R, Stradling J. The relationship between neck circumference, radiographic pharyngeal anatomy, and the obstructive sleep apnea syndrome. *Eur Respir J.* 1990;3(5):509–514.
20. Schwab R. Upper airway imaging. *Clin Chest Med.* 1998;19(1):33–54.
21. Gozal D. Sleep-disordered breathing and school performance in children. *Pediatrics.* 1998;102:616–620.
22. Cistulli P, Sullivan C. Sleep-disordered breathing in Marfan's syndrom. *Am Rev Respir Dis.* 1993;147:645–648.
23. Davidson T. The role of the dental profession in the diagnosis and treatment of sleep-disorders breathing. *Dentistry today.* 2005;24(9):1–3.
24. Burwell C. Extreme obesity associated with alveolar hypoventilation: A pickwickian syndrome. *Am J Med.* 1956;21:811–818.
25. Joosten SA, Hamilton GS, Naughton MT. Impact of weight loss management in OSA. *Chest.* 2017;3692(17):30157–30155.
26. Gozal D, Khalyfa A, Qiao Z. Angiopoietin-2 and soluble Tie-2 receptor plasma levels in children with obstructive sleep apnea and obesity. *Obesity.* 2017;25(6):1083–1090.
27. Cortese R, Zhang C, Gozal D. DNA methylation profiling of blood monocytes in patients with obesity hypoventilation syndrome: Effect of positive airway pressure treatment. *Chest.* 2016;150(1):91–101.
28. Jonas DE, Amick HR, Feltner C. Screening for obstructive sleep apnea in adults: Evidence report and systematic review for the US Preventive Services Task Force. *JAMA.* 2017;317(4):415–433.
29. Oksenberg A, Arons E. Sleep bruxism related to obstructive sleep apnea: The effect of continuous positive airway pressure. *Sleep Med.* 2002 Nov;3(6):513–515.
30. Kostrzewa-Janicka J, Jurkowski P, Zycinska K, Przybyłowska D, Mierzwińska-Nastalska E. Sleep-related breathing disorders and bruxism. *Adv Exp Med Biol.* 2015;873:9–14. doi:10.1007/5584_2015_151.
31. Jokubauskas L, Baltru A, Saityt E. Relationship between obstructive sleep apnoea syndrome and sleep bruxism: A systematic review. *J Oral Rehabil.* 2017;44:144–153.
32. Sandu N, Spiriev T, Lemaitre F, Filis A, Schaller B. Trigemino-Cardiac Reflex Examination Group (TCREG). New molecular knowledge towards the trigemino-cardiac reflex as a cerebral oxygen-conserving reflex. *Sci World J.* 2010;10:811–817.
33. Schaller B, Cornelius J, Sandu N, Ottaviani G, Perez-Pinzon M. Oxygen- conserving reflexes of the brain: The current molecular knowledge. *J Cell Mol Med.* 2009 13:644–647.
34. Sandu N, Cornelius J, Filis A, et al. Cerebral hemodynamic changes during the trigeminocardiac reflex: Description of a new animal model protocol. *Sci World J.* 2010;10:1416–1423.
35. Chowdhury T, Bindu B, Singh G, Scha B. Sleep disorders: Is the trigemino- cardiac reflex a missing link? *Front Neurol.* 2017;8(63):1–7.
36. Lavigne G, Mazini C, Kato T. Sleep bruxism. *Principales and practice of sleep medicine,* Kryger, roth *and* dement *editors.* 2005 (4 th Edition):946–959.
37. Piccin CF, Pozzebon D, Scapini F. Craniocervical posture in patients with obstructive sleep apnea. *Int Arch Otorhinolaryngol.* 2016;20(3):189–195.
38. Sokucu O, Oksayan R, Uyar M. Relationship between head posture and the severity of obstructive sleep apnea. *Am J Orthod Dentofacial Orthop.* 2016;150(6):945–949.
39. Yousefian J, Moghadam B. Orofacial complications associated with forward repositioning of the mandible in snore guard users. *J General Dentistry.* 2003;51(6).
40. Jones DE, Amick HR, Feltner C. Screening for obstructive sleep apnea in adults: Evidence report and systematic review for the US Preventive Services Task Force. *JAMA.* 2017;317(4):415–433.
41. Hoz-Aizpurua J, Diaz E, Latouche A, et al. Sleep bruxism. Conceptual review and update. *Med Oral Patol Oral Cir Bucal.* 2011;16:231–238.
42. Dias G, Bonato L, Guimarães J, et al. A study of the association between sleep bruxism, low quality of sleep, and degenerative changes of the temporomandibular joint. *J Craniofac Surg.* 2015 Nov;26(8): 2347–2350.
43. Nadeem R, Molnar J, Madbouly E, et al. Serum inflammatory markers in obstructive sleep apnea: A meta-analysis. *J Clin Sleep Med.* 2013;9(10):1003–1012.
44. McNicholas W. Obstructive sleep apnea and inflammation. *Prog Cardiovasc Dis.* 2009;51:392–399.
45. Wolf J, Lewicka J, Narkiewicz K. Obstructive sleep apnea: An update on mechanisms and cardiovascular consequences. *Nutr Metab Cardiovasc Dis.* 2007;17:233–240.
46. Gozal D. Sleep, sleep disorders and inflammation in children. *Sleep Med.* 2009;10(Suppl 1):S12–16.
47. Quercioli A, Mach F, Montecucco F. Inflammation accelerates atherosclerotic processes in obstructive sleep apnea syndrome (OSAS). *Sleep Breath Schlaf Atm.* 2010;14:261–269.
48. Garvey J, Taylor C, McNicholas W. Cardiovascular disease in obstructive sleep apnoea syndrome: The role of intermittent hypoxia and inflammation. *Eur Respir J.* 2009;33:1195–1205.

49. Kang W, Park H, Chung J-H, Kim J. REM sleep deprivation increases the expression of interleukin genes in mice hypothalamus. *Neurosci Lett.* 2013;556:73–78.
50. Lam S-Y, Liu Y, Ng K-M, et al. Chronic intermittent hypoxia induces local inflammation of the rat carotid body via functional upregulation of proinflammatory cytokine pathways. *Histochem Cell Biol.* 2012;137:303–317.
51. Ryan S, Taylor C, McNicholas W. Selective activation of inflammatory pathways by intermittent hypoxia in obstructive sleep apnea syndrome. *Circulation.* 2005;112:2660–2667.
52. Lavie L, Lavie P. CrossTalk opposing view: Most cardiovascular diseases in sleep apnoea are not caused by sympathetic activation. *J Physiol.* 2012;590:2817–2819.
53. Huang Y, Gulleminault C, Hwang F, et al. Inflammatory cytokines in pediatric obstructive sleep apnea. *Medicine.* 2016;95:41.
54. Kang J, Lin H. Obstructive sleep apnea and the risk of autoimmune diseases: A longitudinal population-based study. *Sleep Med.* 2012;13:583–588.
55. Lui M, Lam J, Mak H, et al. C-reactive protein is associated with obstructive sleep apnea independent of obesity. *Chest.* 2009;135:950–956.
56. de la Pena B, Serpero L, Barcelo A, et al. Inflammatory proteins in patients with obstructive sleep apnea with and without daytime sleepiness. *Sleep Breath.* 2007;11:177–185.
57. Taylor-Gjevre R, Nair B, Gjevre J. Obstructive sleep apnoea in relation to rheumatic disease. *Rheumatology.* 2013;52:15–21.
58. Alamoudi O. Sleep-disordered breathing in patients with acquired retrognathia secondary to rheumatoid arthritis. *Med Sci Monit.* 2006 Dec;12(12):CR530–534. Epub 2006 Nov 23.
59. Paul S, Simon S, Issac B, Kumar S. Management of severe sleep apnea secondary to juvenile arthritis with temporomandibular joint replacement and mandibular advancement. *J Pharm Bioallied Sci.* 2015 Aug;7(Suppl 2):S687–S690.
60. Laaksonen D, Niskanen I. C-reactive protein and the development of the metabolic syndrome and diabetes in middle-aged men. *Diabetologia.* 2004;108:1815–1821.
61. Considine R, Sinha M. Serum immunoreactive-leptin concentrations in normal-weight and obese humans. *N Engl J Med.* 1996;334:292–295.
62. Hirotsu C, Albuquerque RG, Nogueira H, et al. The relationship between sleep apnea, metabolic dysfunction and inflammation: The gender influence. *Brain Behav Immu.* 2017;59:211–218.
63. VanHelder T, Symons J, Radomski M. Effects of sleep deprivation and exercise on glucose tolerance. *Aviat Space Environ Med.* 1993;64:487–492.
64. Vgontzas A, Zoumakis M. Impaired nighttime sleep in healthy old versus young adults is associated with elevated plasma interleukin-6 and cortisol levels:physiologic and therapeutic implications. *I Clin Endocrinol Metab.* 2003;88:2087–2095.
65. Abate N. Obesity and cardiovascular disease. Pathogenetic role of the metabolic syndrome and therapeutic implications. *I Diabetes Complications.* 2000;14:154–174.
66. Rodriquez LA, Madsen KA, Cotterman C. Added sugar intake and metabolic syndrome in US adolescents: Cross-sectional analysis of the National Health and Nutrition Examination Survey 2005–2012. *Public Health Nutr.* 2016;19(13):2424–2434.
67. Warren JJ, Bishara SE. Comparison of dental arch measurements in the primary dentition between contemporary and historic samples. *Am J Orthod Dentofac Orthop.* 2001;119(3):211–215.
68. Wearing S, Henning E, Byrne N, Steele J, Hills A. Musculoskeletal disorders associated with obesity: A biomechanical perspective. *Proobesity Reviews.* 2006;7:239–250.
69. Frilander H, Solovieva S, Mutanen P, Pihlajamäki H, Heliövarra M, Viikari-Juntura E. Role of overweight and obesity in low back disorders among men: A longitudinal study with a life course approach. *BMJ Open.* 2015;5(8):e007805. doi:10.1136/bmjopen-2015-007805.
70. Peltonen M, Lindroos A, Torgerson J. Musculoskeletal pain in the obese: A comparison with a general population and long-term changes after conventional and surgical obesity treatment. *Pain.* 2003;104:549–557.
71. Jones BH, Bovee MW, Harris JM 3rd, Cowan DN. Intrinsic risk factors for exercise-related injuries among male and female army trainees. *Am J Sports Med.* 1993;21:705–710.
72. Heir T, Eide G. Age, body composition, aerobic fitness and health condition as risk factors for musculoskeletal injuries in conscripts. *Scand J Med Sci Sports.* 1996;6:222–227.
73. Ross J, Woodward A. Risk factors for injury during basic military training. Is there a social element to injury pathogenesis? *J Occup Med.* 1994;36:1120–1126.
74. Kortt M, Baldry J. The association between musculoskeletal disorders and obesity. *Aust Health Rev.* 2002;25:207–214.

75. Aoyagi K, Ross P, Okano K, et al. Association of body mass index with joint pain among community-dwelling women in Japan. *Aging Clin Exp Res.* 2002;14:378–381.
76. Mattsson E, Larsson U, Rössner S. Is walking for exercise too exhausting for obese women? *Int J Obes Relat Metab Disord.* 1997;21:380–386.
77. Hulens M, Vansant G, Claessens A, Lysens R, Muls E. Predictors of 6-minute walk test results in lean, obese and morbidly obese women. *Scand J Med Sci Sports.* 2003;13:98–105.
78. Lementowski P, Zelicof S. Obesity and osteoarthritis. *Am J Orthop (Belle Mead NJ).* 2008;37(3):148–151.
79. Hootman J, Macera C, Ainsworth B, Martin M, Addy C, Blair S. Association among physical activity level, cardiorespiratory fitness, and risk of musculoskeletal injury. *Am J Epidemiol.* 2001;154:251–258.
80. Tsuritani I, Honda R, Noborisaka Y, Ishida M, Ishizaki M, Yamada Y. Impact of obesity on musculoskeletal pain and difficultyof daily movements in Japanese middle-aged women. *Maturitas.* 2002;42:23–30.
81. Riddle D, Pulisic M, Pidcoe P, Johnson R. Risk factors for plantar fasciitis: A matched case-control study. *J Bone Joint Surg.* 2003;85A:872–877.
82. Andersen R, Crespo C, Bartlett S, Bathon J, Fontaine K. Relationship between body weight gain and significant knee, hip, and back pain in older Americans. *Obes Res.* 2003;11:1159–1162.
83. Wendelboe A, Hegmann K, Gren L, Alder S, White GJ, Lyon J. Associations between body-mass index and surgery for rotator cuff tendinitis. *J Bone Joint Surg Am.* 2004;86-A:743–747.
84. Ding C, Cicuttini F, Scott F, Cooley H, Jones G. Knee structural alteration and BMI: A cross-sectional study. *Obes Res.* 2005;13:350–361.
85. Nebel M, Sims E, Keefe F, et al. The relationship of self-reported pain and functional impairment to gait mechanics in overweight and obese persons with knee osteoarthritis. *Arch Phys Med Rehabil.* 2009;90(11):1874–1879.
86. MacLellan G, Dunlevy C, O'Malley E, et al. Musculoskeletal pain profile of obese individuals attending a multidisciplinary weight management service. PAIN prepublished review 2017.
87. Lim C, Goodman S, Huddleston III J, et al. Weight gain after primary total knee arthroplasty is associated with accelerated time to revision for aseptic loosening. *J Arthroplasty.* 2017;1–4.
88. Mihalko W, Bergin F, Kelly F, Canale SM. Obesity, orthopaedics, and outcomes. *J Am Acad Orthop Surg.* 2014;22(11):683–690. doi:10.5435/JAAOS-22-11-683.
89. Krul M, van der Wouden J, Schellevis F, Suijlekom-Smit L, Koes B. Musculoskeletal problems in overweight and obese children. *Ann Fam Med.* 2009;7:352–356. doi:10.1370/afm.1005.
90. Guo S, Wu W, Chumlea W, Roche AF. Predicting overweight and obesity in adulthood from body mass index values in childhood and adolescence. *Am J Clin Nutr.* 2002;76(3):653–658.
91. Whitaker R, Wright J, Pepe M, Seidel K, Dietz W. Predicting obesity in young adulthood from childhood and parental obesity. *N Engl J Med.* 1997;337(13):869–873.
92. Eriksson J, Forsén T, Osmond C, Barker D. Obesity from cradle to grave. *Int J Obes.* 2003;27(6):722–727.
93. Bhatia N, Pirpiris M, Otsuka N. Body mass index in patients with slipped capital femoral epiphysis. *J Pediatr Orthop.* 2006;26:197–199.
94. Pirpiris M, Jackson K, Farng E, et al. Body mass index and Blount disease. *J Pediatr Orthop.* 2006;26:659–663.
95. Chan G, Chen C. Musculoskeletal effects of obesity. *Curr Opin Pediatr.* 2009;21:65–70.
96. Davids J, Huskamp M, Bagley A. A dynamic biomechanical analysis of the etiology of adolescent tibia vara. *J Pediatr Orthop.* 1996;16:461–468.
97. Bell L, Byrne S, Thompson A, et al. Increasing body mass index z-score is continuously associated with complications of overweight in children, even in the healthy weight range. *J Clin Endocrinol Metab.* 2007;92:517–522.
98. Taylor E, Theim K, Mirch M, et al. Orthopedic complications of overweight in children and adolescents. *Pediatrics.* 2006;117:2167–2174.
99. Riddiford-Harland D, Steele J, Baur L. Upper and lower limb functionality: Are these compromised in obese children? *Int J Pediatr Obes.* 2006;1:42–49.
100. Haerens L, Deforche B, Maes L, et al. Physical activity and endurance in normal weight versus overweight boys and girls. *J Sports Med Phys Fitness.* 2007;47:344–350.
101. Carroll J, Loughlin G. Dianosis criteria for obstructive sleep apnea syndrome in children. *Pediatr Pulmonol.* 1992;14:71–74.
102. Wang R, Elkins T, Keech D. Accuracy of clinical evaluation in pediatric obstructive sleep apnea. *Otolaryngol Head Neck Surg.* 1998;118:69–73.
103. Brouillette R, Fernbach S, Hunt C. Obstructive sleep apnea in infants and children. *J Pediatr.* 1982;100(1):31–40.

104. Redline S, Amin S. The childhood adenotonsillectomy trial (chat): Rationale, design, and challenges of a randomized controlled trial evaluating a standard surgical procedure in a pediatric population. *Sleep.* 2011;34(11):1509–1517.
105. Marcus C, Koerner C, Pysik P. Determinants of growth failure in children with the obsructive sleep apnea syndrome. *J Pediatr.* 1994;125:556–562.
106. Goldstein S, Wu R, Thorpy M. Reversibility of deficient sleep entrained growth hormone sectrion in a boy with achondroplasia and obstructive sleep apnea. *Acta Endocrinol.* 1987;116:95–101.
107. Yousefian J, Trimble D, DePaso W. Correction of severe obstructive sleep apnea with interdisciplinary treatment. *Dentitry Today.* 2015;34(8):80–88.
108. Prinsell J. Telegnatic maxillomandibular advancement surgery for OSA. *Dental Sleep Pratice.* 2015 Fall(Fall):6–9.
109. Wang Q, Jia P, Anderson NK. Changes of pharyngeal airway size and hyoid bone position following orthodontic treatment of Class I bimaxillary protrusion. *Angle Orthodontist.* 2012;82(1):115–121.
110. Germec-Cakan D, Taner T, Akan S. Uvulo-glossopharyngeal dimensions in non-extraction, extraction with minimum anchorage, and extraction with maximum anchorage. *Eur J Orthod.* 2011 33(5):515–520.
111. Yousefian J. A simple technique for mandibular symphyseal distraction osteogenesis. *J Clin Orthod.* 2010 Dec;44(12):731–737.

11 Drug-Related Muscular Pain

Sahar Swidan, PharmD

INTRODUCTION

In order to facilitate prompt diagnosis and, where possible, avoidance, this chapter provides an overview of common perpetrators of drug-related muscle pain.

Skeletal muscle makes up a large portion of the body's mass and receives a large amount of blood supply.[1] Due to its metabolic activity, many drugs that enter the body's circulatory system are passed throughout skeletal muscles leading to various drug-induced disorders. Adverse drug effects on muscle include myalgias, myositis, and rhabdomyolysis.[1]

Myalgia is muscle pain that is characterized by diffuse muscle pain, tenderness, and cramps.[1] This can be associated with muscle weakness, but it is not always a characteristic. Myalgia is not accompanied by elevations in creatinine kinase, but symptoms of cramps and aches can be a precursor to more serious conditions such as rhabdomyalgia.[1]

Myositis is inflammation of voluntary muscle fibers and is associated with muscle symptoms that are similar to myalgia in addition to elevations in serum creatine kinase (CK).[1] Creatine kinase originates in the myocardium and skeletal muscle. Skeletal muscle accounts for around 94% of creatine kinase, and CK is a marker for muscle damage.[1] Myopathy, which is sometimes used interchangeably with myositis, is a general term for disease of the muscles. It can be either acquired or inherited; inherited forms can occur at birth or have an onset later in adult life.[1] There is a strong correlation between many drugs and the presence of myopathies associated with fatigue, generalized muscle pain, muscle tenderness, muscle weakness, significantly elevated CK > 10 times the upper limit of normal (ULN), nocturnal cramping, and tendon pain.[1]

Rhabdomyolysis usually presents as an acute event, but it can have an insidious onset over a period of weeks. Approximately 50% of cases present with pain, but most if not all cases present with muscle weakness, muscle swelling, myoglobinuria, and a marked elevation in serum CK (between 10 and 100 times ULN).[1] Myoglobinurias present as a tea or cola colored urine with elevated serum myoglobin levels that can result in secondary renal failure and result in the release of intracellular contents such as enzymes and myoglobin from damaged monocytes into circulation.[1] This can be toxic to the kidney. Rhabdomyolysis can also cause hyperkalemia, hypocalcemia, disseminated intravascular coagulation, cardiomyopathy, respiratory failure, and severe metabolic acidosis.[1] In order to resolve rhabdomyolysis, the offending agent must be discontinued and supportive care with IV fluids, correction of electrolyte imbalances, and alkalization of the urine.[1] Patients can recover fully if the syndrome is recognized early and treated appropriately.

MECHANISMS BY WHICH DRUGS CAN INDUCE MYOPATHIES

There are various drugs that cause myopathies. In order to facilitate easy referencing, they are listed in Table 11.1 by class, family, and drug example.

Table 11.2 explains the known mechanisms of myopathies of drugs that cause myopathies. Not all of the mechanisms for all drug-induced myopathies are known at this time, but Table 11.2 describes the known mechanisms of actions including examples of drugs that are not limited to the list below.

Coenzyme Q10 deficiency is the most common associated muscle defect. CoQ10 is an essential cofactor in mitochondrial respiration pathways in the electron transport chain.[1] Moreover,

TABLE 11.1

Common Drugs that Cause Myalgia and Myopathy

Class	Family	Examples
Antibiotics	Quinolones	Ciprofloxacin, norfloxacin, ofloxacin
	Miscellaneous	Clotrimazole, isoniazid, minocycline, piperacillin-tazobactam
Anti-neoplastic agents and related compounds	Anti-metabolites	Cladribine, cytarabine, methotrexate
	Miscellaneous	Docetaxel, paclitaxel, letrozole, leuprorelin, procarbazine, vincristine
Anti-ulcer agents	Histamine H2 receptor antagonists and proton pump inhibitors	Cimetidine, ranitidine, nizatidine, pantoprazole
Antiviral agents	Antiretroviral agents	Indinavir, lamivudine, ritonavir, saquinavir, stavudine, zidovudine
	Other	Ganciclovir
Corticosteroids		Steroids such as dexamethasone, betamethasone, and triamcinolone, but may be any steroid taken by injection, inhalation, or oral ingestion
Bisphosphonates		Alendronate, ibandronate, pamidronate, risedronate
Lipid-lowering drugs	Fibrates	Fenofibrate, gemfibrozil, nicotinic acid
	Statins	Atorvastatin, fluvastatin, pravastatin, simvastatin
Antifungal agents		Amphotericin B, terbinafine
Antithyroid drugs		Carbimazole, propylthiouracil
Immunosuppressants		Cyclosporine, mycophenolate mofetil, tacrolimus
Cardiovascular agents		Amiodarone, beta-blockers, bumetanide, captopril, diuretics, enalapril, eprosartan, lecranidipine, methyldopa
Miscellaneous		Baclofen, chloroquine, colchicine, ethanol, iloprost, isotretinoin, ivermectin, infliximab, mebeverin, mefloquine, metoclopramide, montelukast, nafarelin, naltrexone, penicillamine, phenytoin, salmeterol, sildenafil, somatropin, triazolam

Source: Table adapted from Lee A, ed., *Adverse Drug Reactions*, 2nd ed. Great Britain: Pharmaceutical Press, 2009; Bannwarth B. *Expert Opinion on Drug Safety*, 1(1), 69, 2002; and Holder K., *FP Essentials*, 420, 23–7, 2016.

TABLE 11.2

Proposed Mechanism of Drug-Induced Myalgias

Classification and Example Mechanism	Examples
Necrotizing myopathies: Reduced essential co-enzyme production, myocyte membrane changes, and increased oxidation	HMG CoA-reductase inhibtiors (Statins), fibrates, nicotinic acid
Corticosteroid myopathy: Disruption of RNA synthesis	Fluorinated steroids such as dexamethasone and triamcinolone
Mitochondrial myopathies: Inhibition of mitochondrial DNA polymerase	Zidovudine
Lysosomal storage myopathy: Increased lysosomal activity degrading muscle fibers	Hydroxychloroquine, amiodarone
Antimicrotubular myopathy: Accumulation of lysosomes and autophagic vacuoles	Colchicine, vincristine
Hypokalemic myopathy: Disruption of water and electrolyte homeostasis	Diuretics, oral contraceptives
Inflammatory myopathies: Activation of immune system, resembles autoimmune disease	D-penicillamine and interferon-alpha

carnitine palmityl transferase (CPT) II deficiency is a mitochondrial abnormality most likely acquired as a result of exposure to statins opposed to a genetic inheritance. CPT II is located in the mitochondrial membrane where it facilitates the transport of long-chain fatty acids into the mitochondrion.[1]

CORTICOSTEROIDS

Corticosteroid-induced myalgia is a result of the *chronic* use of oral corticosteroids that can cause proximal muscle weakness and atrophy of lower limbs. It does not result from acute use of corticosteroids. It is the most common cause of drug-induced toxic muscle disease.[1] The result of corticosteroid-induced myalgias are usually accompanied by other systemic side effects of corticosteroids such as hyperglycemia, increased risk of infections, weight gain, fluid retention, and hypertension. These myalgias are often dose related and occur with inhaled steroid doses of greater than 10 mg of prednisolone (or equivalent) daily for more than 30 days. Fluorinated steroids present a higher risk of these associated myalgias compared to non-fluorinated corticosteroids.[1] Risk factors that increase this associative risk of myalgia include accumulative doses, concomitant use of other myotoxic drugs, electrolyte disturbances that manifest as muscle weakness, and sepsis or multi-organ failure.[1] The disruption of RNA synthesis that occurs with corticosteroid-induced myopathies leads to type-II muscle fiber atrophy and muscle necrosis.[1]

Moreover, corticosteroids such as the glucocorticoids promote bone loss through other mechanisms that are directly related to hormonal regulation impacted by these medications: [2]

- Reduction of GI calcium absorption[2]
- Increased urinary calcium excretion[2]
- Induced secondary hyperparathyroidism[2]
- Decreased production of skeletal growth factors[2]
- Decreased responsiveness to luteinizing hormone to gonadotropin releasing hormone, which decreases gonadal hormone production[2]
- Suppression of corticotropin, which leads to suppression of the adrenal production of androstenedione, a substrate for both testosterone and estrone production[2]
- Decreased osteoblast-medicated bone formation[2]
- Increased bone resorption[2]

All the above mechanisms in some combination result in a disproportionate loss of cancellous or trabecular bone. Since trabecular bone has an inherently greater rate of turnover compared to cortical bone; this can lead to reduced turnover directly affecting trabecular bone.[2] Moreover, bone GLA protein, osteocalcin is inhibited with the use of glucocorticoids, which contributes to this disproportionate loss of trabecular bone.[2]

CHOLESTEROL-LOWERING AGENTS

Cholesterol-lowering agents such as fibrates, nicotinic acid derivatives, and statin are well known to be associated with myopathies.[1] The occurrence rate among statin users is about 1.5%–3% in some controlled clinical trials and up to 10%–13% in other prospective clinical trials.[1] If statins and other lipid-lowering drugs are used in combination, there is an increased risk of myopathy that can result in a more severe clinical presentation leading to rhabdomyolysis. The risk of rhabdomyolysis increases with advanced age, statin dose greater than 40 mg, concurrent cyclosporine, gemfibrozil, and diltiazem administration and diabetes. Fibrates inhibit phase 2 glucuronidation reaction in statin metabolism and may be a better option in combination with statins compared to gemfibrozil.[1] The mechanism of myopathy from cholesterol-lowering agents is not well understood, but is possibly due to the reduced synthesis of mevalonate. Mevalonate is a precursor to multiple critical components of the cell membrane as well as a precursor molecule for the steroid hormones, vitamin D, and bile acids.[1] The mechanism for statin-induced myopathy can be attributed to an increase in the fluidity of the myocyte membrane due to changes in cholesterol, impaired synthesis of compounds in the cholesterol pathway, and an increase in activity of carnitine palmityl transferase. Decreased synthesis of cholesterol pathway compounds, especially hemeA and CoQ10, results in mitochondrial dysfunction, reduced energy, and eventually cell death. Increased activity of CPT II leads to carnitine and fatty acid deficiency, and subsequently damage to muscle fibers.[1] The greater the lipophilicity of the statin, the greater the penetration into muscle tissue and greater risk for myopathies. Simvastatin is the most lipophilic agent, pravastatin is the most hydrophilic agent. It is recommended that a baseline creatinine kinase is measured before initiating lipid-lowering therapy, and if symptoms such as muscle weakness or pain are reported by the patient, a new creatinine kinase should be obtained to compare to the initial value upon starting therapy.[1]

ANTIPSYCHOTIC DRUG THERAPIES

Antipsychotic drug therapies such as aripiprazole, buspirone, amitriptyline, haloperidol, and atypicals (clozapine, olanzapine, quetiapine, risperidone, and ziprasidone) act on the 5-hydroxytryptamine (5-HT) receptor family. 5-HT receptors are a group of G protein-coupled receptors and ligand-gated ion channels that are found in the central and peripheral nervous systems. Drugs with potent 5-HT2A activity produced a larger increase in CK as compared to dopamine D2 neuroleptics. CK levels can increase in up to 10% of patients who are treated with clozapine, risperidone, olanzapine, or haloperidol. If any symptoms of muscle pain or weakness are reported among these patients, a CK should be obtained to determine the clinical implications of the myopathy.

QUINOLONE ANTIBIOTICS

Quinolone antibiotics such as levofloxacin, ciprofloxacin and moxifloxacin are broad spectrum antibiotics that are effective against both gram positive and gram negative bacteria. They are often used to treat urinary tract infections (UTIs). Other antibiotics such as sulfamethoxazole-trimethoprim, cephalexin, and nitrofurantoin monohydrate are also frequently used to treat UTIs. First generation quinolones and fluoroquinolones can produce cartilage lesions, especially in weight-bearing joints, that can in rare instances lead to tendinopathies such as tendonitis and tendon rupture.[3] Tendon rupture can occur even after a single dose of a quinolones with the risk beginning at 48 hours after starting treatment and lasting over several months after the completion of treatment. Tendinopathies due to quinolones are especially a concern in sports medicine where patients may exert themselves more and increase their risk of tendon rupture after taking a quinolone antibiotic. There have been reports of non-erosive arthropathies that are involved with the lower extremities and often occur in patients with cystic fibrosis. Articular symptoms generally appear within the first two weeks of the initiation of therapy, though late onset is possible and does not need to start within two weeks of beginning the antibiotic therapy.[3] These effects often occur in younger patients; therefore, fluoroquinolones are contraindicated in children and adolescents. This drug class is also contraindicated during pregnancy and lactation due to risk of the mother passing the drug through the placenta.[3]

NON-STEROIDAL ANTI-INFLAMMATORY DRUGS (NSAIDS)

NSAIDs increase the risk of developing osteoporosis of the hip and knee. The mechanism associated with this musculoskeletal drug-induced occurrence results from affecting cartilage metabolism that may occur. NSAIDs can stimulate or suppress the synthesis of cartilage glycosaminoglycan synthesis.[4] This is mainly associated with long-term use, and is especially seen with diclofenac and less commonly in ibuprofen, naproxen, and piroxicam.[3] Moreover, this is more likely to occur in patients that already have osteoporosis. In the normal joint, there is a balance between the continuous process of cartilage matrix degradation and repair. However, in osteoarthritis there is a disruption in this homeostatic balance of the catabolic process of chondrocytes.[4]

DRUGS USED IN HORMONE-DEPENDENT CANCERS

Hormone-dependent cancers requiring therapy have been associated with an increased risk of musculoskeletal disorders. Androgen deprivation therapy with the use of GnRH analogues is used in the treatment of prostate cancer.[3] It is also used in women who have endocrine-responsive breast cancer and other sex-hormone dependents disorders. GnRH analogues lead to a decrease in estradiol levels in premenopausal women, with decreases comparable to that of postmenopausal women.[3] Testosterone levels also fall using GnRH analogues resembling castration values in men. This results in hypogonadism which then leads to increased bone turnover, bone loss, and risk of bone fractures.[3] Up to 19.4% of men who survive 5 years after diagnosis of prostate cancer experience a bone fracture after treatment with androgen deprivation therapy as compared to 12.6% seen in control patients.[3]

Third generation aromatase inhibitors such as letrozole, anastrozole, and exemestane are used in breast cancer. Peripheral aromatase activity is the major source of estrogens in postmenopausal women, so aromatase inhibitors decrease estrogen levels to starve the tumor of its primary growth factor.[3] Lowered estrogen also effects the bone, leading to an increase in bone loss and increased risk of bone fractures, especially at the spine and wrist.[5] Aromatase inhibitors are associated with an incidence of arthralgia in 25% of patients, with more than half of these patients already having an existing joint disease that was exacerbated by the aromatase inhibitor therapy. Symptoms appear within the first two years of therapy, with a peak incidence of 6 months. In 75% of patients, the arthralgia resolves within 18 months.[6] Stiffness, aching, or pain in the hands, arms, knees, feet, pelvic, hip bones, and back has been described. The pain is usually symmetrical and can be associated with mild soft-tissue thickening that can be observed by clinicians.[6] While the pathogenic features of aromatase inhibitor-associated arthralgia have not been clearly defined, these symptoms spontaneously resolve.

Moreover, aside from drugs directly causing arthralgia, the actual hormone-dependent cancers themselves may cause joint pain. This is due to the increase in nerve growth factor, which is associated with inflammatory and painful conditions leading to synovial fluid in inflammatory joint disease.[7] Chronic nerve growth factor exposure leads to an increase in the expression of TRPV1 receptors in sensory neurons, which increases ASIC expression and bradykinin receptor binding. Both contribute heavily to cancer pain.[7]

THYROID REPLACEMENT DRUGS

Drugs used to treat thyroid disorders such as levothyroxine for hypothyroidism may be associated with decreased bone mineral density.[8] This has been found to be of particular importance when using doses that exceed 150 mcg/day. The elderly population is at greater risk for this effect, as well as patients who have already been diagnosed with osteoporosis.[8] The risk of decreased bone mineral density has also been shown in postmenopausal women; therefore, it is important to monitor elderly women that use high doses of levothyroxine.

Moreover, not only can treatment with levothyroxine cause drug-induced musculoskeletal pain, but the under-treatment of hypothyroidism itself can lead to a myxedema coma.[9] A myxedema coma is a life-threatening clinical manifestation that occurs due to long-standing untreated or severe hypothyroidism. It leads to a significant alteration in mental status, hypothermia, and severe weakness of muscles that can result in respiratory muscle dysfunction. There is a 40% change of mortality, so early recognition is crucial.[9]

DIURETICS

Diuretic medications such as furosemide are commonly used to treat fluid retention and swelling in heart failure, and can be associated with reduced bone mineral density.[5] These medications work by increasing urination and promoting calcium excretion from the kidneys, resulting in a decreased amount of calcium reabsorption.[5] The subsequent reduction in bone mineral density is thought to be due to a bone-sparing effect that is thought to occur through the blockage of renal sodium chloride cotransporter leading to a decrease in urinary calcium excretion.

Additionally, diuretic therapy with thiazides and loop diuretics can lead to hypokalemia, which is often associated with muscle weakness and severe cases of muscle cramps and pain.[10] These effects can often be seen during exercise when there is a disruption of the skeletal muscle cells and potassium is being released from the muscle. Lack of potassium in muscle prevents adequate widening of blood vessels which results in decreased muscle blood flow, cramps, and the destruction of skeletal muscle.[10]

Effects are mostly seen in the first week of diuretic therapy. The first week is associated with an increased risk of falls, particularly in older adults.

DRUGS WHICH ALTER METABOLISM OF VITAMIN D

Vitamin D is a fat-soluble vitamin that is essential strong bones and for calcium homeostasis.[11] *In vivo* vitamin D is metabolized to 25(OH)D and then subsequently to the active form of vitamin D 1,25(OH)$_2$D. Low vitamin D levels are common in the general population and lead to decreased amounts of calcium absorption.[11] This triggers the release of parathyroid hormone, which promotes skeletal calcium resorption and consequently bone loss. Vitamin D deficiency is defined as a serum 25(OH)D concentration of <25–37 nmol (<10–15 ng/mL). Optimal fracture protection occurs in patients whose doses exceed 700 IU/day and are 80% compliant with their vitamin D supplement.

Hypovitaminosis D causes sarcopenia, muscle weakness, and contributes to the risk of falls among older adults. It can also cause pain in the bone marrow which has a clinical presentation similar to myalgias. Vitamin D-deficiency associated myopathies are due to type II fiber atrophy leading to a decrease in muscle strength.[11] Administration of vitamin D and calcium leads to an increase in muscle strength and decreases the risk of falls. This occurs by increasing the number of myocytes and type II muscle fibers.[11] While the serum level of vitamin D needed to obtain optimal muscle strength is unknown, improvement is based more on functional improvement rather than laboratory testing. Reversal of secondary hyperparathyroidism can also be an indicator of improvement.[11]

Several classes of medications alter vitamin D synthesis, not necessarily resulting in hypovitaminosis D. Alterations in synthesis can lead to levels of active vitamin D outside of the therapeutic range.

SYNTHETIC PTH- FORTEO

Forteo (teriparatide) is an anabolic agent that is used for the treatment of osteoporosis. It is a synthetic parathyroid hormone that stimulates new bone formation on the trabecular and cortical bone surfaces by preferential stimulation of osteoblastic over osteoclastic activity.[12] This treatment for osteoporosis can lead to hypercalcemia which presents clinically with profound myalgias (stones, bones, groans). Myalgia is one of the most common side effects of Forteo. Routine calcium-level monitoring is recommended with the use of the drug to help prevent myalgias.[12]

MEDICATIONS THAT RELAX THE AIRWAY

Any medications that relax the airway would increase the risk of myalgias from hypoxia. We see this clinically in patients with pre-existing OSA that becomes more severe with a pain medication for example.

THE INFLUENZA VACCINATION

By itself, immunization against influenza does not lead to myalgia. However, studies show that it can do so with concomitant use of a myotoxic medication. Specifically, the medical literature mentions myalgias post-influenza vaccination in patients taking statins.[13] This is explained by an immunologically mediated response to the vaccination interacting with a statin. There is usually no report of prior muscle pain in these patients on a statin, but this rhabdomyolysis that can result is attributed to the influenza vaccine-statin combination. This can be a higher risk in patients with existing renal dysfunction.[13]

MANAGEMENT OF DRUG-INDUCED MUSCULOSKELETAL DISORDERS

Ensuring safe living environments and eliminating drugs that can increase the risk of fall are two ways to decrease the likelihood of muscle pain and injury.[14] With adverse drug effects, clinical decision-making begins with awareness of the interactions. Treatments vary based on the adverse drug effect, the availability of substitutes and support options. Treatment options include discontinuing a medication, substituting a medication for another with a more favorable risk-benefit profile, adjusting the dose, or modifying the treatment regimens. Sometimes adding supporting nutrients and maintaining sufficient hydration are sufficient.

CONCLUSION

The musculoskeletal system is highly perfused tissue that has vast exposure to the circulatory system, which leaves it susceptible to many drug-induced adverse effects. Drug exposure within skeletal muscle can cause myalgias, myositis, and rhabdomyolysis. There are various drugs that have an increased risk for muscle-related effects including corticosteroids, cholesterol-lowering agents, antipsychotics, antibiotics, NSAIDs, and hormone therapies, among others. These drug-related adverse effects can be debilitating and limit the use of current and future therapies for patient conditions. The most important way to manage drug-induced musculoskeletal disorders is to first withdraw the drug if symptoms occur. Some musculoskeletal disorders may involve supportive care options such as nutrients and hydration as supplemental management techniques. Healthcare professionals are equipped to help manage drug-related musculoskeletal disorders.

REFERENCES

1. Smithson J. Drug induced muscle disorders. *Pharmacist.* 2009;28(12):1056–62.
2. Medscape. Osteoporosis in Solid Organ Transplantation Overview of Treatment. http://emedicine.medscape.com/article/128108-overview?pa=sDFLakkr8Hd7%2BCPequ5JfTQN61Bz68bbK4eK9QC6n0LZQXRjvv0W4XVs2A9yBos%2B0AJj%2B91DQx08bi5u979cV8Edx1ifJJK66DE1LVU1RZo%3D#a1 (accessed 2 August 2017).
3. Bannwarth B. Drug-induced musculoskeletal disorders. *Drug Safety.* 2007;30(1):27–46.
4. Hauser RA. The acceleration of articular cartilage degradation in osteoporosis by nonsteroidal anti-inflammatory drugs. *Journal of Prolotherapy.* 2010;1:305–22.
5. Osteoporosis Canada. Medications that can Cause Bone Loss, Falls and/or Fractures. http://www.osteoporosis.ca/osteoporosis-and-you/secondary-osteoporosis/medications-that-can-cause-bone-loss-falls-and-or-fractures/ (accessed 2 August 2017).
6. Thorne C. Management of arthralgias associated with aromatase inhibitor therapy. *Current Oncology* 2007;14(Supp 1):S11–19.
7. Schmitdt BL, Hamamoto DT, Simon DA, et al. Mechanism of cancer pain. Molecular Interactions. 2010;10(3):164–78.
8. Ko YJ, Kim JY, Lee J, et al. Levothyroxine dose and fracture risk according to the osteoporosis status in elderly women. Journal *of Preventive* Medicine *and* Public Health. 2014;47:36–46.
9. Chaker L, Bianco AC, Jonklaas J, et al. Hypothyroidism. *Lancet.* 2017.

10. National Organizations for Rare Disorders. Hypokalemia. https://rarediseases.org/rare-diseases/hypo-kalemia/ (accessed 11 September 2017).
11. Wolff AE, Jones AN, and Hansen KE. Vitamin D and musculoskeletal health. *Nature*. 2008;4(11):580–88.
12. Mulgund M, Beattle KA, Wong AKO, et al. Assessing adherence to teriparatide therapy, causes of nonadherence and effect of adherence on bone mineral density measurements in osteoporotic patients at high risk for fracture. *Therapeutic Advances in* Musculoskeletal *Disease*. 2009;11(1):5–11.
13. Raman KS, Chandrasekar T, Reeve RS, et al. Influenza vaccine-induced rhabdomyolysis leading to acute renal transplant dysfunction. *Nephrology Dialysis Transplantation*. 2006;21:530–1.
14. American Colleges of Clinical Pharmacy. Bowles SK. Drug-Induced Osteoporosis. https://www.accp.com/docs/bookstore/psap/p7b03.sample04.pdf (accessed 2 August 2017).
15. Velloso CP. Regulation of muscle mass by growth hormone and IGF-1. *British Journal of Pharmacology*. 2008;154:557–68.
16. ACE. 8 Hormones Involved in Exercise. https://www.acefitness.org/blog/5593/8-hormones-involved-in-exercise (accessed 2 July 2017).
17. Dimitriadis G, Mitrou P, Lambadiari V, et al. Insulin effects in muscle and adipose tissue. *Diabetes Research and Clinical Practice*. 2011;93S:S52–9.
18. Rooyackers OE and Nair KS. Hormonal regulation of human muscle protein metabolism. *Annual Review of Nutrition Darby* 1997;17:457–85.
19. Izquierdo M, Hakkinen K, Anton A, et al. Maximal strength and power, endurance performance, and serum hormones in middle-aged and elderly men. *Medicine and Science in Sports Exercise*. 2001;33(9):1577–87.
20. Hormone Health Network. What Does Testosterone Do? http://www.hormone.org/hormones-and-health/what-do-hormones-do/testosterone (accessed 5 July 2017).
21. West DW and Phillips SM. Anabolic processes in human skeletal muscle: Restoring the identities of growth hormone and testosterone. *Physician and Sportsmedicine*. 2010;38(3):97–104.
22. Lowe DA, Baltgalvis KA, and Greising SM. Mechanisms behind estrogens' beneficial effect on muscle strength in females. *Exercise and Sport Sciences Reviews Journal*. 2010;38(2):61–7.
23. Tiidus PM. Benefits of estrogen replacement for skeletal muscle mass and function in post-menopausal females: Evidence from human and animal studies. *EAJM*. 2011;43:109–14.
24. Machida S and Booth FW. Insulin-like growth factor 1 and muscle growth: Implication for satellite cell proliferation. *Proceedings of the Nutrition Society*. 2004;63:337–40.
25. Salvatore D, Simonides WS, Dentice M, et al. Thyroid hormones and skeletal muscle—new insights and potential implications. *Nature*. 2014;10:206–14.
26. Rejnmark L. Effects of vitamin D on muscle function and performance: A review of evidence from randomized controlled trials. *Therapeutic Advances in* Chronic Disease. 2011;2(1):25–37.
27. Livestrong. Role of Calcium in the Skeletal System. http://www.livestrong.com/article/274233-role-of-calcium-in-the-skeletal-system/ (accessed 11 July 2017).
28. Khazai N, Judd SE, and Tangpricha V. Calcium and vitamin D: Skeletal and extraskeletal health. Current Rheumatology *Reports*. 2008;10(2):110–17.
29. U.S. Food & Drug Administration. FDA Drug Safety Communication: FDA revises label of diabetes drug canagliflozin (invokana, Invokamet) to include updates on bone fracture risk and new information on decreased bone mineral density. https://www.fda.gov/Drugs/DrugSafety/ucm461449.htm (accessed 2 August 2017).
30. Taylor SI, Blau JE, and Rother KI. SGLT2-inhibitors trigger downstream mechanisms that may exert adverse effects upon bone. Lancet Diabetes *and* Endocrinology. 2015;3(1):8–10.
31. Holder K. Myalgias and myopathies: Drug-induced myalgias and myopathies. *FP Essentials*. 2016;420:23–7.

12 Metabolic Interventions for Sarcopenic Obesity

Gabrielle Lyon, D.O. and Jamie I. Baum, PhD

INTRODUCTION

As obesity increases in the population, the amount of dieting also increases. Most dieting strategies lead to combined loss of fat and muscle. The weight that is regained is mostly fat. Therefore, over time the ratio of fat to muscle changes. Loss of muscle becomes sarcopenia and when it is accompanied by obesity it is more difficult to treat. This chapter presents methods for early detection of sarcopenia and treatment strategies for preserving muscle during weight loss.

BACKGROUND

The loss in muscle mass observed with aging is often accompanied by an increase in fat mass [1], which can happen even in the absence of changes in body mass index (BMI) [2]. The loss of muscle mass results in a decrease in basal metabolic rate (BMR), or the amount of caloric energy we use while at rest [3]. Loss of muscle mass induces a 2%–3% decrease in BMR per decade after the age of 20, and a 4% decline in BMR per decade after the age of 50 [3, 4]. Muscle loss and subsequent reduction in metabolic rate contribute to obesity that accompanies the aging process.

Sarcopenia is the term for age-associated loss of muscle mass and function [2]. The loss of muscle function associated with sarcopenia is often referred to as dynapenia [5]. A loss or reduction in skeletal muscle function often leads to increased morbidity and mortality either directly, or indirectly, via the development of secondary diseases such as diabetes, obesity, and cardiovascular disease [2, 6]. The causes of sarcopenia include poor nutrition, diminished responsiveness to anabolic hormones and/or nutrients, and a sedentary lifestyle. The etiology of sarcopenia includes malnutrition, increased inflammatory cytokine production, oxidative stress, hormone reduction (e.g. growth hormone and testosterone), and decreased physical activity [7, 8]. Maintaining skeletal muscle function throughout the lifespan into old age is essential for independent living and good health. The efficient activation of the mechanistic processes that regulate muscle development, growth, regeneration, and metabolism is required for skeletal muscle to function at optimal levels [2, 9].

Obesity is another important risk factor associated with aging [1, 10, 11]. Obesity rates increase over the age of 65, and like sarcopenia, obesity has been consistently associated with several negative health outcomes such as chronic disease, disabilities, falls, and mobility limitations [11]. However, in older adults over 65 years of age, it has been found that a body mass index (BMI) in the overweight range is not associated with an increased risk of mortality [12–14]. It has been observed that obese older patients with cardiovascular disease have demonstrated better survival rates compared with non-obese older patients [1, 15]. However, even if mortality rates decrease with obesity in older adults, the problem remains that the negative effects of obesity on function may lead to disability with age [11].

Both sarcopenia and obesity are potential health risks for older adults and it has been shown that when both sarcopenia and obesity exist, they synergistically increase the risk of negative health outcomes and earlier onset of disability [11, 16, 17]. This combination of sarcopenia and obesity is commonly referred to as sarcopenic obesity [11] or obesogenic sarcopenia (Figure 12.1). The prevalence of sarcopenic obesity is estimated to be 18% in women and 43% in men and is predicted to increase with increasing age [18, 19].

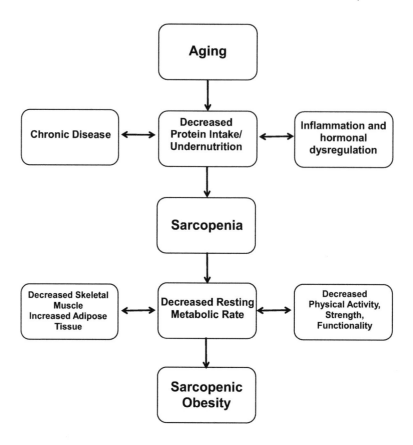

FIGURE 12.1 Sarcopenic obesity: determinants and associated factors. This figure shows the contributors to the development of sarcopenic obesity.

CLINICAL DIAGNOSIS

STRUCTURAL ASSESSMENT

Measuring skeletal muscle mass and strength is important for diagnosing older adults at risk for developing sarcopenia. The clinical definition of sarcopenia can be found in Table 12.1. Muscle mass can be measured using different methods that are available for both clinical and research purposes. However, these methods vary in cost, complexity, and availability [5]. Approaches for measuring muscle mass include anthropometry, urinary metabolites, ultrasound, bioimpedence analysis, imaging [5], and new technology using stable isotopes [20] or measuring total body water [21]. These methods, their advantages and disadvantages, and applicability in a clinical setting are summarized in Table 12.2. Obesity makes sarcopenia difficult to diagnose. Therefore, diagnosing sarcopenic obesity also needs to include measurements such as BMI and total body fat (if available).

METABOLIC ASSESSMENT

Plasma or serum assessments are also available [22]. Aging is associated with changes in the endocrine system characterized by a natural reduction in secretion of growth hormone (GH), testosterone, and insulin-like growth factor 1 (IGF-1), which are all closely associated with protein metabolism and rates of muscle excitation and contraction [22]. Aging can also be characterized by a low-grade

TABLE 12.1

Clinical Definition of Sarcopenia

Organization	Diagnostic Criteria and Cut-Points for Sarcopenia				
	Physical Function (Gait Speed)	Or	Muscle Strength (Handgrip Strength)	And	Muscle Mass (DXA, ALM/height^2; BIA, SMM/height^2)
European Working Group on Sarcopenia in Older People (2010)	<0.8 m/s		Men: <30 kg Women: <20 kg		DXA, ALM/height^2 Men: <7.23 kg/m^2 Women: <5.67 kg/m^2 BIA – Asians, SMM/height^2 Men: <8.87 kg/m^2 Women: <6.42 kg/m^2 BIA – Caucasians, SMM/height^2 Men: <10.76 kg/m^2 Women: <6.76 kg/m^2
Asian Working Group for Sarcopenia (2014)	<0.8 m/s		Men: <26 kg Women: <18 kg		DXA, ALM/height^2 Men: <7.0 kg/m^2 Women: <5.4 kg/m^2 BIA, ALM/height^2 Men: <7.0 kg/m^2 Women: <5.7 kg/m^2
Foundation for the NIH Sarcopenia Project (2014)	<0.8 m/s		Men: <26 kg Women: <16 kg		DXA, ALM/BMI Men: <0.789 Women: <0.512

Source: Adapted from Lee, D.C., et al., *Future Sci OA*, 2(3), FSO127, 2016 and Afilalo, J., et al., *J Am Coll Cardiol*, 56(20), 1668–1676, 2010.

ALM, appendicular lean mass (arms and legs); BIA, bioelectrical impedance analysis; BMI, body mass index; DXA, dual-energy x-ray absorptiometry; SMM, skeletal muscle mass (whole-body).

inflammatory state. Inflammatory molecules such as TNFα and IL-6 have catabolic effects on muscle mass and are involved in sarcopenia and are often elevated with obesity and aging [1].

Obesity is also associated with low-grade inflammation and endocrine changes. Endocrine changes related to obesity in older adults include decreased estrogen levels (females), decreased total testosterone (females and males), decreased testosterone (males), decreased sex hormone binding globulin (SHBG), decreased dihydroepiandrosterone (DHEA) levels, increased prolactin, increased cortisol, changes in thyroid hormones (increased free T4 and reversed T3 and decreased T3 levels), and secondary hyperparathyroidism in the presence of low vitamin D levels. Decreased GH, IGF-1, leptin and insulin resistance, and downregulation of ghrelin are also present [1, 23]. These changes that occur with normal aging seem to be exacerbated in the presence of abdominal obesity [23].

FUNCTIONAL ASSESSMENT

Muscle strength and physical function are also important tools for identifying sarcopenia. Handgrip strength has widely been used as a measurement of muscle strength because it is inexpensive, easy to use in a clinical setting by using a handheld dynamometer, and is well correlated with most relevant health outcomes such as mortality [24]. However, leg strength is more related to physical functions such as gait, chair standing, and stair climbing, leg strength tests have also been used, especially in research [25]. Common leg strength tests include knee flexion and extension and various velocities

TABLE 12.2

Skeletal Muscle Mass Measurement Methods

Method	Measurements	Advantages	Disadvantages
Anthropometry	• Skinfold thickness • Waist circumference • Body Mass Index (BMI) • Height • Weight	• Noninvasive • Cost-effective • Safe • Easy to implement in clinical setting	• Training required • Poor precision in obese people • Skinfold difficult with aging due to loss of skin elasticity and muscle tone
Urinary metabolites	• 24-hour creatinine • 3-methyl histidine	• Noninvasive • Relatively inexpensive • Safe • Reflects muscle cell mass	• Requires several 24-hour urine samples while ingesting a meat-free diet
Ultrasound	• Muscle width and area	• Noninvasive • Safe • Widely available • Useful for longitudinal monitoring	• Requires training/technical skill • Requires identification of reproducible measurement sites • Important to control for exercise • Muscle needs to be in a relaxed state
Bioimpedance	• Segmental impedance • Resistance and reactance • Phase angle	• Cost is variable • Safe • Equipment potentially portable • Useful for long-term monitoring	• Measurements sensitive to individual conditions such as hydration and physical activity • Instrument predictions may be population specific
Computed Topography (CT) Imaging	• Cross-sectional muscle area • Muscle attenuation	• High resolution • 3-dimensional reconstruction • Regional and whole-body measures	• Cost • Radiation exposure • Individual size limitations
Dual-Energy X-ray Absorptiometry (DXA) Imaging	• Lean soft tissue • Fat content • Bone content • Bone quality	• Wide availability • High precision • Low radiation • Regional and whole-body measures	• Modest cost • Size (height and weight) limitations • Cannot measure skeletal muscle mass and quality
Magnetic Resonance Imaging (MRI)	• Cross-sectional muscle area	• High resolution • 3-dimensional reconstruction • Multiple measures of muscle quality	• Relatively high cost • Individual size limitations
Labeled Creatine	• Indicator of skeletal muscle mass	• Noninvasive • Safe • Useful for long-term monitoring	• Labeled creatine not widely available • Requires special equipment for analysis which could be expensive • Training needed

Source: Adapted from Heymsfield, S.B., et al., *Proc Nutr Soc*, 74(4), 355–366, 2015 and Hellerstein, M. and W. Evans, *Curr Opin Clin Nutr Metab Care*, 20(3), 191–200, 2017.

TABLE 12.3

Classification of Overweight and Obesity by BMI, Waist Circumference, and Associated Disease Risks

	BMI (kg/m²)	Obesity Class	Disease Risk[a] Relative to Normal Weight and Waist Circumference[b]	
			Men 102 cm (40 in) or less Women 88 cm (35 in) or less	Men > 102 cm (40 in) Women > 88 cm (35 in)
Underweight	<18.5		—	—
Normal weight	18.5–24.9		—	—
Overweight	25.0–29.9		Increased	High
Obesity	30.0–34.9	I	High	Very high
	35.0–39.9	II	Very high	Very high
Extreme obesity	40+	III	Extremely high	Extremely high

Source: Adapted from NIH. Classification of overweight and obesity by BMI, waist circumference, and associated disease risks https://www.nhlbi.nih.gov/health/educational/lose_wt/BMI/bmi_dis.htm [84].

BMI, Body Mass Index.

[a] Disease risk for type 2 diabetes, hypertension, and CVD.

[b] Increased waist circumference can also be a marker for increased risk, even in normal weight individuals.

using isokinetic equipment, which can also measure muscle power [25]. Measuring muscle power is important in sarcopenia because it could be a better predictor of functional capacity since muscle power is lost faster than strength during aging [25]. There are several physical function tests that are easier to implement in a clinical setting, including gait speed, 6 minute or 400 m walk tests, timed get-up-and-go test, and chair stand tests [25]. Measuring gait speed is the most popular physical function test because it is simple, fast, and easy to measure as a predictor of mobility limitations and mortality [25–28].

RATIO OF MUSCLE TO FAT

BMI is one method that can be used to determine obesity (Table 12.3). Body mass index, which correlates with body fat in most young and middle-aged adults, can either underestimate the degree of adiposity in older adults due to changes in body composition (e.g. muscle loss and fat gain) or overestimate BMI due to loss of height from vertebral compression [1]. This means that the relationship between BMI and disease risk is weaker in older adults than in younger adults. In older adults, in the presence of certain diseases, a higher BMI has even been found to be protective, a phenomenon which is referred to as the obesity paradox [29, 30]. Fat distribution also changes with aging, resulting in an increase in visceral fat, which is more pronounced in women versus men. There is also increased fat deposition in the muscle and liver, thereby increasing the risk of developing chronic diseases such as insulin resistance [1].

Waist circumference, which has a high correlation with total fat mass and intra-abdominal fat, might be a better predictor of adverse health effects of obesity in the elderly and is easy to implement in a clinical setting; however, more work is needed to define the cut-off values for the elderly [1].

THERAPIES

OVERVIEW

Interventions for treating and preventing sarcopenic obesity that are presented in this chapter include specifics on dietary protein, concurrent weight loss, and exercise. Interventions targeting sarcopenia and sarcopenic obesity should focus on maintaining or building skeletal muscle mass and targeting fat mass to prevent the onset or worsening of functional decline with age [31]. Dietary, weight loss and exercise intervention have all been associated with positive effects on muscle mass, muscle health, and adiposity. However, since the objective in treating sarcopenic obesity needs to address gaining of muscle mass while losing fat mass, the changes in sarcopenic obesity cannot be measured by change in body weight alone, but need to also measure changes in body composition and/or functional parameters [11], as described above.

Protein

Nutrition is important for health and function in older adults. Inadequate nutrition can contribute to the development of sarcopenia and obesity [6, 8]. As life expectancy continues to rise, it is important to consider optimal nutritional recommendations that will improve health outcomes, quality of life, and physical independence in older adults [32].

The current protein intake guidelines for aging adults is discussed here. Several studies identify protein as a key nutrient for aging adults [6, 8]. Low protein intake is linked to a decrease in physical ability in aging adults [33]. However, protein intake greater than the dietary guidelines (Table 12.4) may prevent sarcopenia [34], help maintain BMR [35], improve bone health [36–39], and improve cardiovascular function [40–42]. These benefits of increasing protein in the diet may improve function and quality of life in healthy older adults, as well as improve the ability older patients to recover from disease and trauma [6].

The current dietary recommendations for protein intake include the dietary reference intakes (DRI) for macronutrients, which include an estimated average requirement (EAR), a recommended dietary allowance (RDA), and an acceptable macronutrient distribution range (AMDR) [43]. In the case of daily protein intake, the EAR for dietary protein is 0.66 g/kg/day and the RDA is 0.8 g/kg/day for all adults over 18 years of age, including elderly adults over the age of 65 [6, 8]. This can become confusing when trying to make recommendations for patients. Even the Food and Nutrition Board recognizes a difference between what is recommended with the RDA and the level of protein intake needed for optimal health. Therefore, there is a third recommendation for protein called the AMDR. The AMDR includes a range of optimal protein intakes in the context of a complete diet ranging from 10 to 35% of daily energy or calorie intake coming from protein [43], which makes the AMDR easier to use when developing dietary recommendations (Table 12.4) [6].

Experts in the field of protein and aging recommend a protein intake between 1.2 and 2.0 g/kg/day or higher for elderly adults [6, 8, 44]. The RDA of 0.8 g/kg/day is well below these recommendations and reflects a value at the lowest end of the AMDR. It is estimated that 38% of adult men and 41% of adult women have dietary protein intakes below the RDA [45, 46]. For a sample diet plan, refer to Table 12.5.

TABLE 12.4
Dietary Protein Intake Recommendations

	Gram protein/kg body weight/day
EAR	0.66
RDA	0.8
AMDR	1.05–3.67

Source: Adapted from Baum, J.I. and R.R. Wolfe, *Healthcare (Basel)*, 3(3), 529–543, 2015.

EAR, Estimated Average Requirement; RDA, Recommended Dietary Allowance; AMDR, Acceptable Macronutrient Distribution Range.

TABLE 12.5
Sample Diet Plan[a]

	Non-Vegetarian	Lacto-Ovo Vegetarian
Meal 1[b]	• 4–6 oz ground chicken, beef, or turkey OR lean ground breakfast sausage • 1 cup of dark green vegetables sautéed with 1 T olive oil • 1 slice of whole-grain toast	• 1 egg • 5 egg whites • 1 scoop of branched-chain amino acids scrambled into eggs • 1 cup of dark green vegetables sautéed with 1 T olive oil • 1 slice of whole-grain toast
Snack	10 almonds	10 almonds
Meal 2	• 1.5 scoops of whey protein • ½ cup of berries • 1 cup of milk (almond or dairy)	• 1 scoop of pea protein • 1 scoop of branched-chain amino acids • ½ cup of berries • 1 cup of milk (almond or dairy)
5-hour break		
Meal 3[2]	• 4–6 oz lean beef, chicken, or fish • 40 g of carbohydrate • 1 T healthy fat (avocado, olive oil, etc.), if desired	• 4 oz Temeh • 1 scoop of branched-chain amino acids • 40 g of carbohydrate • 1 T healthy fat (avocado, olive oil, etc.), if desired

[a] Target approximately 30 g of protein per meal.
[b] Keep protein and carbohydrates in 1:1 ratio.

PROTEIN QUALITY

Both protein amount and source, whether the protein comes from animal or plant sources, are important to consider when recommending protein intake to older adults [2, 47]. There are three important aspects to take into consideration when recommending a protein source: (1) the characteristics of the specific protein, such as the amount of essential amino acids (EAA), (2) the food matrix in which the protein is consumed, for example, as part of a beverage or a complete meal; and (3) the characteristics of the individuals consuming the food, including health status, physiological status, and energy balance [47].

Essential amino acids, especially the branched-chain amino acids (BCAA), are strong stimulators of muscle protein synthesis [48–50]. Several studies demonstrate that maximal stimulation of muscle protein synthesis is possible with only 15 g of EAA [51]. This translates to ~35 g of high-quality protein (e.g. animal source or whey protein supplement). A larger amount of lower quality protein (e.g. plant sources of protein), which contains a lower content of EAA, would be required to achieve the same health benefits.

In addition, the difference in digestibility and bioavailability of a protein can impact the quantity of protein that needs to be ingested to meet metabolic needs, this is especially important in older adults since gastric motility and nutrient absorption decrease with age. The speed of protein digestion and absorption of amino acids from the gut can influence whole-body protein building [52]. Proteins with differing amino acid profiles exhibit different digestion and absorption rates [52–55]. Amino acid availability depends directly on both the quality and quantity of the dietary protein [53].

For example, the digestion and absorption rates of fast (e.g. whey) versus slow (e.g. casein) proteins need to be taken into consideration when developing protein recommendations. When young, healthy subjects were provided with either a whey protein meal (30 g) or a casein meal (43 g), both containing the same amount of leucine, a BCAA, and whole-body protein building was measured, the subjects consuming the whey (fast) protein meal had a high, rapid, increase in plasma amino acids, while subjects consuming the casein (slow) protein meal had a prolonged plateau of essential amino acids [56]. In addition, consumption of whey protein stimulated postprandial protein synthesis by 68%, while consumption of casein only stimulated protein synthesis by 31%. However, ingestion of casein inhibited whole-body protein breakdown by 34%, while whey protein had no effect [56]. These results indicate that slow proteins, when adjusted for leucine content, may promote postprandial protein deposition by an inhibition of protein breakdown. When the influence of protein digestion rate on protein turnover was tested in older subjects, the opposite occurs [55]. When older men consumed 20 g of either whey (2.5 g leucine), casein (1.7 g leucine) or casein hydrolysate (1.7 g leucine), the whey protein stimulated postprandial protein accretion more effectively than either casein or casein hydrolysate [55]. These results demonstrate that older and younger individuals respond differently to protein source and dose and highlight the need for separate protein recommendations for young and older adults.

Whether or not the amino acid source is whole protein or a mixture of free amino acids can also influence the rate of muscle protein synthesis [57]. For example, when older subjects were given either an EAA mixture (15 g) or a whey protein supplement (13.6 g) after an overnight fast, subjects consuming the EAA mixture had higher mixed muscle fractional synthetic rate [57], which is associated with increases in muscle mass. The differing responses could be due to differing leucine content between the supplements (EAA; 2.8 g leucine and whey; 1.8 g leucine) or because the EAA supplement was composed of individual amino acids while the whey protein supplement was intact protein. This could influence the rate of appearance of the amino acids into circulation and the protein synthetic response. Another example is form or texture of the protein itself, such as ground beef versus a beef steak [58]. When older men consumed 135 g as ground beef or as a beef steak, the amino acids from the ground beef appeared more rapidly in the circulation than the amino acids from the beef steak. Whole-body protein balance was higher after consumption of the ground beef versus the beef steak. However, six hours after the beef meals, muscle protein synthesis was not different [58]. However, these data support that the form of protein we eat impacts digestion, absorption and rate of appearance of amino acids into circulation [2].

It is well established that eating more than 30 g of protein at a meal does result in a further stimulation of muscle protein synthesis. This suggests that there is a protein threshold of ~25–30 g of protein per meal [59, 60]. However, with increasing age it may become more difficult to consume 30 g of protein per meal. There are several risk factors for reduced protein intake in adults including reduced energy needs, difficulty acquiring and preparing food, overall reduction in energy and protein intake due to changes in appetite, changes in food preference, and/or food insecurity [44]. Therefore, when incorporating protein into the diet of older adults it is important to consider protein density, the grams of protein provided per calorie of protein food source [46]. It is especially important to consider protein density when designing diets for older adults with sarcopenic obesity, to ensure that the calories consumed count towards maintaining muscle mass. Estimated protein density per protein source can be found in Figure 12.2. In addition, a list of specific food sources and the quantity needed to maximize muscle protein synthesis can be found in Table 12.6. Since consuming 30 g of protein from whole-food sources may be difficult for some older adults, supplementation with EAAs could be an alternative strategy.

Timing of Protein Intake

Another issue related to defining the optimal protein recommendations for older adults is defining the optimal timing of protein intake throughout the day. Dietary protein provides substrates for newly (*de novo*) synthesized proteins and the EAA derived from dietary protein also act as signaling molecules to stimulate the muscle protein synthetic response [61]. However, the muscle protein synthetic response is short-lived and lasts for 4–5 hours post protein ingestion [62]. Therefore, the consumption of protein in regular intervals throughout the course of the day becomes necessary to maximize muscle protein building [61]. Older adults typically consume the majority of their protein (and energy) intake at dinner [45, 63, 64], 38 g versus 13 g of protein at breakfast (Figure 12.3). Current research demonstrates that

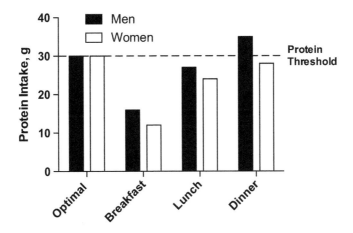

FIGURE 12.2 Protein density of animal protein foods, dairy protein foods, and plant protein foods. Data expressed as an average of foods containing at least 1% animal protein, dairy protein, or plant protein as calculated in [46]. (Adapted from Pasiakos, S.M., et al., *Nutrients*, 7(8), 7058–7069, 2015.).

TABLE 12.6
Amount of Dietary Protein Needed to Maximize Muscle Protein Synthesis[a]

Protein Source	Amount Needed to be Ingested per Meal to Match Leucine Value Found in whey Protein (g)	Amount of Protein per Meal to Reach ~3 g of Leucine (g)
Animal Sources		
Whey	27	23
Milk	876	28
Casein	35	30
Beef	164	35
Egg	5 eggs	36
Cod	211	38
Plant Sources		
Maize	264	25
Black Bean	167	36
Soy	104	28
Rice	500	37
Pea	180	39
Wheat	299	45
Potato	2891	58

Source: Adapted from van Vliet, S. et al., *J Nutr*, 145(9), 1981–1991, 2015.

[a] Amount of protein source to be ingested to maximize post-exercise muscle protein synthesis rates in response to feeding in young subjects. A higher leucine content suggests that a lower amount of dietary protein from a given source is needed to maximize postprandial muscle protein synthesis response rates.

even distribution of protein intake throughout the day is more effective at stimulating 24-hour protein synthesis compared to an uneven distribution [65, 66]. This is supported by data from a longitudinal study on nutrition and aging, which found that even distribution of daily protein intake across meals is independently associated with greater muscle strength and higher muscle mass in older adults, but is not associated with loss in muscle mass [64] or mobility [63] over 2–3 years.

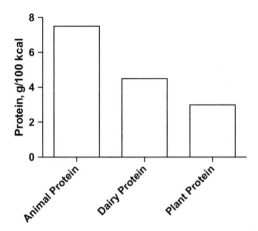

FIGURE 12.3 Meal distribution of protein intake in older men (74.2 + 4.1 years) and women (74.5 + 4.2 years) compared to the optimal protein intake per meal. (Adapted from Farsijani, S., et al., *Am J Clin Nutr*, 106(1), 113–124, 2017 and Phillips, S.M., et al., *Appl Physiol Nutr Metab*, 41(5), 565–572, 2016.

However, there are some studies that fail to confirm the importance of spreading protein intake out over the course of the day [67, 68]. Additional studies have compared pulse feeding (72% of daily protein at lunch) versus protein being evenly distributed over four daily mails in hospitalized older patients for 6 weeks [69, 70]. These studies found that pulse feeding of protein increased postprandial amino acid bioavailability [69] and increased lean mass [70] compared to spreading protein intake throughout the day. Taken together, the optimal timing and distribution of protein intake in older adults still needs to be determined.

WEIGHT LOSS

Diet-induced weight loss results in a decrease in both fat mass and lean body mass [1, 71], which could worsen age-related muscle loss, increase sarcopenia, and further impair physical function. Several population-based studies have evaluated the effect of weight loss on mortality in middle-age to older age groups [71–75]. The data for these studies indicate that weight loss in older adults is associated with increased, rather than decreased, mortality. However, it is important to note that these are purely observational-based studies and not randomized, controlled trials. Several studies, primarily conducted in middle-aged adults, found that intentional weight loss is associated with reduced mortality rates in people with diabetes, impaired glucose tolerance, and other health conditions [71]. Specifically, weight loss diets higher in protein (>30% of energy intake) and lower in carbohydrate have been shown to promote weight loss, improve body composition (i.e. decrease fat mass and increase lean mass), and regulate glycemic response [76–80]. However, it is important to note that the meal and/or diet recommendations for increased protein consumption are based on studies including animal-based, high-quality protein sources. The reason for focusing on animal sources of protein in weight loss studies is because lean animal sources of protein allow for the highest protein content with the fewest calories (refer to Figure 12.2) [81]. In addition, increasing evidence suggests that animal proteins, particularly whey protein, promote gains in lean mass through increased skeletal muscle protein synthesis [61, 81].

EXERCISE

Sarcopenic obesity has been attributed, in part, to an age-related decline in physical activity. However, data show that regular physical activity, including aerobic and resistance exercise, is important for the prevention and treatment of obesity and/or sarcopenia in older adults [25]. Exercise has been shown to increase muscle protein synthesis, increase intramuscular IGF-1, and restore insulin sensitivity [19]. One research group recommends working towards an exercise intervention incorporating progressive resistance training (PRT), with three approximately 90 minutes sessions per week consisting of 15 minutes of flexibility, 30 minutes of low-impact aerobic exercise, 30 minutes of high-intensity PRT, and 15 minutes of balance training [19, 82]. This is supported by the recommendation from the American College of Sports Medicine consisting of a multi-component training program composed of strength, endurance, balance, and flexibility [83]. There are barriers and perceived constraints for older adults when it comes to participating in exercise. These include poor health, pain, diseases, tiredness, fear, and negative experiences, which tend to be more frequent among the severely obese [1].

The most effective intervention for treatment of sarcopenic obesity includes both a weight loss diet and regular exercise. The combination of these interventions acts synergistically to improve muscle mass and reduce frailty more than either diet or exercise alone [1, 19].

CLINICAL CASE

CASE PRESENTATION

History of Present Illness:
Joan is a 65-year-old woman who presented to my integrative medicine consulting service with the twin goals of weight loss and improved strength and energy.

Past Medical History:
Untreated hypothyroidism and a binge eating disorder which recurs intermittently. In her 20s she had anorexia and bulimia. Low energy and increasing body fat mass over the last 5 years have been accompanied by a 5-pound annual weight gain. Her highest adult weight was 215 pounds at age 45; lowest adult weight was 160 pounds. Her dieting history is positive for yo-yo dieting since the age of 19. Growing up she was very physically active and in high school she played softball competitively. After high school, her physical activity shifted to more cardio-type activities.

Family History:
Both parents having obesity and type II diabetes.

Exercise:
Her physical activity includes walking 10,000 steps daily and Pilates twice a week. Data was collected from a cronometer iPhone app.

Diet:
Currently, her dietary habits are largely vegan. Macronutrients are as follows: 250 g of carbohydrates, 30 g of plant-based protein, and 50 g of fat per day. Macronutrient pattern per meal is 62.5 g of carbohydrates, 7.5 g of protein, and fat 12.5 g per meal. Total caloric intake is 1570 calories.

Diagnostics:
Total cholesterol 235, HDL 40, LDL 174, VLDL 35, TG 180, ferritin 19, vitamin D 45, hemoglobin 12.6, hematocrit 36.8, TSH 5.4, Free T3 1.0, Free T4 0.76, with a reverse T3 of 35. Complete metabolic panel was within normal limits, with a homocysteine of 6.0, CRP 0.5, ESR 20, Omega Index of 4.5, fasting insulin 10, fasting leptin level 35, and a fasting blood glucose 93. HbA1c is 5.7. She declined having her hormones tested as she said she was not interested in addressing this part of her health.

Physical exam:
Waist-to-hip ratio of 0.90 and a BMI of 30. She presents with a weight of 186 pounds and her height is 5'6. Skeletal muscle mass as measured by inBody 570 is 62.8 pounds, with a body fat mass of 69.9, a percent body fat of 38.1, and visceral body fat level of 15.

Vitals:

Blood pressure 130/80, heart rate of 70, and an otherwise unremarkable physical exam. Supplements include 5,000 international units (IU) of vitamin D3 and a multivitamin.

Initial intervention:

Macronutrients were adjusted to the following: 150 g of carbohydrates, 125 g of protein (non-plant based), and 50 g of fat. Total caloric intake 1550. Macronutrients were divided into four meals with the following breakdown: 37.5 g of carbohydrates, 31.25 g of protein, and 12.5 g of fat. The meals consisted of either 4–5 oz of ground chicken, beef, turkey, or bison, or the option to supplement with a whey protein shake. Carbohydrates were largely green vegetables or complex carbohydrates with sugar limited to 20 g a day. Fat was derived from sources naturally occurring in the above-mentioned foods–none was to be added.

Medications and supplemental nutrients:

Thyroid medication was recommended but the patient declined this therapy. Vitamin D was continued at the previous dose. Omega-3 fatty acids, 2 grams twice a day, was initiated.

Exercise:

Three days a week of resistance exercise (one hour-long sessions) were added to Joan's current activity. This included seated rows, chest presses, leg extensions, hamstring curls, leg presses, and shoulder presses. These exercises were chosen due to their safety as well as the incorporation of large muscle groups. The training started with a 10-minute warm up followed by three sets of high-volume training, roughly 25 repetitions, or until muscular exhaustion. The weight training routine was calculated at 30-50% of her one "rep" maximum. This training strategy was chosen based on the emerging data that it is not the heaviness of the load that generates muscular and metabolic change but rather the effort. Thus, fatigability of the muscle is key and can be accomplished with heavy or light loads. The training ended with a 5-minute cool down. The exercise program was developed by certified trainers and a physiotherapist–training sessions were also supervised by certified trainers. Immediately after exercise sessions, Joan consumed a whey protein shake of 30–40 g.

Four week follow-up:

Joan lost a total of 4 pounds of fat and gained 2 pounds of muscle. Her BMI decreases to 29.7, skeletal muscle mass increased to 66.8, body fat mass decreased to 65.9, percent body fat decreased to 35.1 (a reduction of 3%). All strength exercises increased. In addition, she reported that her binge eating had reduced by 50%. Her lab values were largely unchanged except for fasting insulin which decreased to 6μ/ml.

CASE DISCUSSION

Joan had little exercise prior to her treatment. We sometimes refer to this as being untrained. Untrained individuals tend to show the greatest improvement.

The type and timing of protein is important. Joan's diet was largely devoid of branched-chain amino acids in amounts sufficient enough to stimulate protein synthesis. Her nutrition protocol was designed to optimize muscle protein synthesis with at least 2.5 g of leucine per meal. By designing her intake to include a carbohydrate to protein ratio of roughly 1:1, this minimized fat storage.

In subsequent visits, Joan became more willing to address her elevated levels of reverse T3, her low free T3 as well as her leptin resistance. Research demonstrates that the laboratory-guided medical treatment of hypothyroidism could be anticipated to help Joan continue to achieve her goals of weight reduction and an increase in strength and energy.

Clinical suspicion for sleep apnea and sex hormone imbalances were high at the initial visit. They were not measured initially and are anticipated to improve with improvement in body composition.

CONCLUSIONS

Early detection of sarcopenia in the setting of obesity allows for early intervention. Treatment should begin with exercise, especially resistance training. Exercise should not exceed the patient's metabolic wherewithal. The metabolic processes of muscle preservation during weight reduction depend on protein. The quality of the protein and the nature of the amino acid composition influence how well the body can utilize the protein for rebuilding muscle and other body structures. The timing of protein intake is also important, with morning and post-exercise being common times of protein shortfall. The clinical setting provides an opportunity to further optimize metabolic processes to achieve the twin goals of fat reduction and energy increase.

REFERENCES

1. Mathus-Vliegen, E.M. and Obesity Management Task Force of the European Association for the Study of Obesity, Prevalence, pathophysiology, health consequences and treatment options of obesity in the elderly: A guideline. *Obes Facts*, 2012. 5(3): p. 460–483.
2. Baum, J.I. and R.R. Wolfe, The link between dietary protein intake, skeletal muscle function and health in older adults. *Healthcare (Basel)*, 2015. 3(3): p. 529–543.
3. Buch, A., et al., Muscle function and fat content in relation to sarcopenia, obesity and frailty of old age–An overview. *Exp Gerontol*, 2016. 76: p. 25–32.
4. Kim, T.N., et al., Impact of visceral fat on skeletal muscle mass and vice versa in a prospective cohort study: The Korean Sarcopenic Obesity Study (KSOS). *PLoS One*, 2014. 9(12): p. e115407.
5. Heymsfield, S.B., et al., Skeletal muscle mass and quality: Evolution of modern measurement concepts in the context of sarcopenia. *Proc Nutr Soc*, 2015. 74(4): p. 355–366.
6. Wolfe, R.R., The role of dietary protein in optimizing muscle mass, function and health outcomes in older individuals. *Br J Nutr*, 2012. 108 (Suppl 2): p. S88–S93.
7. Kim, T.N. and K.M. Choi, Sarcopenia: Definition, epidemiology, and pathophysiology. *J Bone Metab*, 2013. 20(1): p. 1–10.
8. Wolfe, R.R., S.L. Miller, and K.B. Miller, Optimal protein intake in the elderly. *Clin Nutr*, 2008. 27(5): p. 675–684.
9. Guller, I. and A.P. Russell, MicroRNAs in skeletal muscle: Their role and regulation in development, disease and function. *J Physiol*, 2010. 588(Pt 21): p. 4075–4087.
10. Finucane, M.M., et al., National, regional, and global trends in body-mass index since 1980: Systematic analysis of health examination surveys and epidemiological studies with 960 country-years and 9.1 million participants. *Lancet*, 2011. 377(9765): p. 557–567.
11. Goisser, S., et al., Sarcopenic obesity and complex interventions with nutrition and exercise in community-dwelling older persons–a narrative review. *Clin Interv Aging*, 2015. 10: p. 1267–1282.
12. Graf, C.E., et al., Impact of body composition changes on risk of all-cause mortality in older adults. *Clin Nutr*, 2016. 35(6): p. 1499–1505.
13. Heiat, A., V. Vaccarino, and H.M. Krumholz, An evidence-based assessment of federal guidelines for overweight and obesity as they apply to elderly persons. *Arch Intern Med*, 2001. 161(9): p. 1194–1203.
14. Janssen, I. and A.E. Mark, Elevated body mass index and mortality risk in the elderly. *Obes Rev*, 2007. 8(1): p. 41–59.
15. Dorner, T.E. and A. Rieder, Obesity paradox in elderly patients with cardiovascular diseases. *Int J Cardiol*, 2012. 155(1): p. 56–65.
16. Baumgartner, R.N., et al., Sarcopenic obesity predicts instrumental activities of daily living disability in the elderly. *Obes Res*, 2004. 12(12): p. 1995–2004.
17. Rolland, Y., et al., Difficulties with physical function associated with obesity, sarcopenia, and sarcopenic-obesity in community-dwelling elderly women: The EPIDOS (EPIDemiologie de l'OSteoporose) Study. *Am J Clin Nutr*, 2009. 89(6): p. 1895–1900.
18. Batsis, J.A., et al., Sarcopenia, sarcopenic obesity and mortality in older adults: Results from the National Health and Nutrition Examination Survey III. *Eur J Clin Nutr*, 2014. 68(9): p. 1001–1007.
19. Bouchonville, M.F. and D.T. Villareal, Sarcopenic obesity: How do we treat it? *Curr Opin Endocrinol Diabetes Obes*, 2013. 20(5): p. 412–419.

20. Hellerstein, M. and W. Evans, Recent advances for measurement of protein synthesis rates, use of the 'Virtual Biopsy' approach, and measurement of muscle mass. *Curr Opin Clin Nutr Metab Care*, 2017. 20(3): p. 191–200.

21. Schoeller, D.A., Changes in total body water with age. *Am J Clin Nutr*, 1989. 50(5 Suppl): p. 1176–1181; discussion 1231-5.

22. Ribeiro, S.M. and J.J. Kehayias, Sarcopenia and the analysis of body composition. *Adv Nutr*, 2014. 5(3): p. 260–267.

23. Kennedy, R.L., K. Chokkalingham, and R. Srinivasan, Obesity in the elderly: Who should we be treating, and why, and how? *Curr Opin Clin Nutr Metab Care*, 2004. 7(1): p. 3–9.

24. Leong, D.P., et al., Prognostic value of grip strength: Findings from the Prospective Urban Rural Epidemiology (PURE) study. *Lancet*, 2015. 386(9990): p. 266–273.

25. Lee, D.C., et al., Physical activity and sarcopenic obesity: Definition, assessment, prevalence and mechanism. *Future Sci OA*, 2016. 2(3): p. FSO127.

26. Afilalo, J., et al., Gait speed as an incremental predictor of mortality and major morbidity in elderly patients undergoing cardiac surgery. *J Am Coll Cardiol*, 2010. 56(20): p. 1668–1676.

27. Guralnik, J.M., et al., Lower-extremity function in persons over the age of 70 years as a predictor of subsequent disability. *N Engl J Med*, 1995. 332(9): p. 556–561.

28. Toots, A., et al., Usual gait speed independently predicts mortality in very old people: A population-based study. *J Am Med Dir Assoc*, 2013. 14(7): p. 529 e1–e6.

29. Oreopoulos, A., et al., The obesity paradox in the elderly: Potential mechanisms and clinical implications. *Clin Geriatr Med*, 2009. 25(4): p. 643–659, viii.

30. Chapman, I.M., Obesity paradox during aging. *Interdiscip Top Gerontol*, 2010. 37: p. 20–36.

31. Schaap, L.A., A. Koster, and M. Visser, Adiposity, muscle mass, and muscle strength in relation to functional decline in older persons. *Epidemiol Rev*, 2013. 35: p. 51–65.

32. Prevention, C.f.D.C.a., *The State of Aging and Health in America 2013*, U.D.o.H.a.H.S. Centers for Disease Control and Prevention, Editor. 2013: Atlanta, GA.

33. Welch, A.A., Nutritional influences on age-related skeletal muscle loss. *Proc Nutr Soc*, 2014. 73(1): p. 16–33.

34. Morais, J.A., S. Chevalier, and R. Gougeon, Protein turnover and requirements in the healthy and frail elderly. *J Nutr Health Aging*, 2006. 10(4): p. 272–283.

35. Wilson, M.M., R. Purushothaman, and J.E. Morley, Effect of liquid dietary supplements on energy intake in the elderly. *Am J Clin Nutr*, 2002. 75(5): p. 944–947.

36. Dawson-Hughes, B., Calcium and protein in bone health. *Proc Nutr Soc*, 2003. 62(2): p. 505–509.

37. Dawson-Hughes, B., Interaction of dietary calcium and protein in bone health in humans. *J Nutr*, 2003. 133(3): p. 852S–854S.

38. Thorpe, M.P., et al., A diet high in protein, dairy, and calcium attenuates bone loss over twelve months of weight loss and maintenance relative to a conventional high-carbohydrate diet in adults. *J Nutr*, 2008. 138(6): p. 1096–1100.

39. Heaney, R.P. and D.K. Layman, Amount and type of protein influences bone health. *Am J Clin Nutr*, 2008. 87(5): p. 1567S–1570S.

40. Hu, F.B., et al., Dietary protein and risk of ischemic heart disease in women. *Am J Clin Nutr*, 1999. 70(2): p. 221–227.

41. Obarzanek, E., P.A. Velletri, and J.A. Cutler, Dietary protein and blood pressure. *JAMA*, 1996. 275(20): p. 1598–1603.

42. Stamler, J., et al., Inverse relation of dietary protein markers with blood pressure. Findings for 10,020 men and women in the INTERSALT Study. INTERSALT Cooperative Research Group. INTERnational study of SALT and blood pressure. *Circulation*, 1996. 94(7): p. 1629–1634.

43. Institute of Medicine, *Dietary Reference Intakes for Energy, Carbohydrate, Fiber, Fat, Fatty Acids, Cholesterol, Protein and Amino Acids*. 2005, National Academy Press: Washington, D.C.

44. Volpi, E., et al., Is the optimal level of protein intake for older adults greater than the recommended dietary allowance? *J Gerontol A Biol Sci Med Sci*, 2013. 68(6): p. 677–681.

45. Fulgoni, V.L., 3rd, Current protein intake in America: analysis of the National Health and Nutrition Examination Survey, 2003–2004. *Am J Clin Nutr*, 2008. 87(5): p. 1554S–1557S.

46. Pasiakos, S.M., et al., Sources and amounts of animal, dairy, and plant protein intake of US adults in 2007–2010. *Nutrients*, 2015. 7(8): p. 7058–7069.

47. Millward, D.J., et al., Protein quality assessment: Impact of expanding understanding of protein and amino acid needs for optimal health. *Am J Clin Nutr*, 2008. 87(5): p. 1576S–1581S.

48. Anthony, J.C., et al., Orally administered leucine stimulates protein synthesis in skeletal muscle of postabsorptive rats in association with increased eIF4F formation. *J Nutr*, 2000. 130(2): p. 139–145.
49. Anthony, J.C., et al., Leucine stimulates translation initiation in skeletal muscle of postabsorptive rats via a rapamycin-sensitive pathway. *J Nutr*, 2000. 130(10): p. 2413–2419.
50. Gordon, B.S., A.R. Kelleher, and S.R. Kimball, Regulation of muscle protein synthesis and the effects of catabolic states. *Int J Biochem Cell Biol*, 2013. 45(10): p. 2147–2157.
51. Wolfe, R.R., Regulation of muscle protein by amino acids. *J Nutr*, 2002. 132(10): p. 3219S–3224S.
52. Boirie, Y., et al., Slow and fast dietary proteins differently modulate postprandial protein accretion. *Proc Natl Acad Sci U S A*, 1997. 94(26): p. 14930–14935.
53. Dangin, M., et al., The digestion rate of protein is an independent regulating factor of postprandial protein retention. *Am J Physiol Endocrinol Metab*, 2001. 280(2): p. E340–E348.
54. Dangin, M., et al., Influence of the protein digestion rate on protein turnover in young and elderly subjects. *J Nutr*, 2002. 132(10): p. 3228S–3233S.
55. Pennings, B., et al., Whey protein stimulates postprandial muscle protein accretion more effectively than do casein and casein hydrolysate in older men. *Am J Clin Nutr*, 2011. 93(5): p. 997–1005.
56. Boirie, Y., P. Gachon, and B. Beaufrere, Splanchnic and whole-body leucine kinetics in young and elderly men. *Am J Clin Nutr*, 1997. 65(2): p. 489–495.
57. Paddon-Jones, D., et al., Differential stimulation of muscle protein synthesis in elderly humans following isocaloric ingestion of amino acids or whey protein. *Exp Gerontol*, 2006. 41(2): p. 215–219.
58. Pennings, B., et al., Minced beef is more rapidly digested and absorbed than beef steak, resulting in greater postprandial protein retention in older men. *Am J Clin Nutr*, 2013. 98(1): p. 121–128.
59. Symons, T.B., et al., A moderate serving of high-quality protein maximally stimulates skeletal muscle protein synthesis in young and elderly subjects. *J Am Diet Assoc*, 2009. 109(9): p. 1582–1586.
60. Paddon-Jones, D. and B.B. Rasmussen, Dietary protein recommendations and the prevention of sarcopenia. *Curr Opin Clin Nutr Metab Care*, 2009. 12(1): p. 86–90.
61. van Vliet, S., N.A. Burd, and L.J. van Loon, The skeletal muscle anabolic response to plant- versus animal-based protein consumption. *J Nutr*, 2015. 145(9): p. 1981–1991.
62. Moore, D.R., et al., Differential stimulation of myofibrillar and sarcoplasmic protein synthesis with protein ingestion at rest and after resistance exercise. *J Physiol*, 2009. 587(Pt 4): p. 897–904.
63. Farsijani, S., et al., Even mealtime distribution of protein intake is associated with greater muscle strength, but not with 3-y physical function decline, in free-living older adults: The Quebec longitudinal study on Nutrition as a Determinant of Successful Aging (NuAge study). *Am J Clin Nutr*, 2017. 106(1): p. 113–124.
64. Farsijani, S., et al., Relation between mealtime distribution of protein intake and lean mass loss in free-living older adults of the NuAge study. *Am J Clin Nutr*, 2016. 104(3): p. 694–703.
65. Mamerow, M.M., et al., Dietary protein distribution positively influences 24-h muscle protein synthesis in healthy adults. *J Nutr*, 2014. 144(6): p. 876–880.
66. Murphy, C.H., et al., Hypoenergetic diet-induced reductions in myofibrillar protein synthesis are restored with resistance training and balanced daily protein ingestion in older men. *Am J Physiol Endocrinol Metab*, 2015. 308(9): p. E734–E743.
67. Kim, I.Y., et al., Quantity of dietary protein intake, but not pattern of intake, affects net protein balance primarily through differences in protein synthesis in older adults. *Am J Physiol Endocrinol Metab*, 2015. 308(1): p. E21–E28.
68. Arnal, M.A., et al., Protein pulse feeding improves protein retention in elderly women. *Am J Clin Nutr*, 1999. 69(6): p. 1202–1208.
69. Bouillanne, O., et al., Long-lasting improved amino acid bioavailability associated with protein pulse feeding in hospitalized elderly patients: A randomized controlled trial. *Nutrition*, 2014. 30(5): p. 544–550.
70. Bouillanne, O., et al., Impact of protein pulse feeding on lean mass in malnourished and at-risk hospitalized elderly patients: A randomized controlled trial. *Clin Nutr*, 2013. 32(2): p. 186–192.
71. Villareal, D.T., et al., Obesity in older adults: Technical review and position statement of the American Society for Nutrition and NAASO, The Obesity Society. *Obes Res*, 2005. 13(11): p. 1849–1863.
72. Andres, R., D.C. Muller, and J.D. Sorkin, Long-term effects of change in body weight on all-cause mortality. A review. *Ann Intern Med*, 1993. 119 (7 Pt 2): p. 737–743.
73. Williamson, D.F. and E.R. Pamuk, The association between weight loss and increased longevity. A review of the evidence. *Ann Intern Med*, 1993. 119(7 Pt 2): p. 731–736.
74. Lissner, L., et al., Variability of body weight and health outcomes in the Framingham population. *N Engl J Med*, 1991. 324(26): p. 1839–1844.

75. Blair, S.N., et al., Body weight change, all-cause mortality, and cause-specific mortality in the multiple risk factor intervention trial. *Ann Intern Med*, 1993. 119(7 Pt 2): p. 749–757.

76. Farnsworth, E., et al., Effect of a high-protein, energy-restricted diet on body composition, glycemic control, and lipid concentrations in overweight and obese hyperinsulinemic men and women. *Am J Clin Nutr*, 2003. 78(1): p. 31–39.

77. Gannon, M.C., et al., An increase in dietary protein improves the blood glucose response in persons with type 2 diabetes. *Am J Clin Nutr*, 2003. 78(4): p. 734–741.

78. Layman, D.K., et al., Increased dietary protein modifies glucose and insulin homeostasis in adult women during weight loss. *J Nutr*, 2003. 133(2): p. 405–410.

79. Layman, D.K., et al., A reduced ratio of dietary carbohydrate to protein improves body composition and blood lipid profiles during weight loss in adult women. *J Nutr*, 2003. 133(2): p. 411–417.

80. Baum, J.I., M. Gray, and A. Binns, Breakfasts higher in protein increase postprandial energy expenditure, increase fat oxidation, and reduce hunger in overweight children from 8 to 12 years of age. *J Nutr*, 2015. 145(10): p. 2229–2235.

81. Phillips, S.M., S. Chevalier, and H.J. Leidy, Protein "requirements" beyond the RDA: Implications for optimizing health. *Appl Physiol Nutr Metab*, 2016. 41(5): p. 565–572.

82. Frimel, T.N., D.R. Sinacore, and D.T. Villareal, Exercise attenuates the weight-loss-induced reduction in muscle mass in frail obese older adults. *Med Sci Sports Exerc*, 2008. 40(7): p. 1213–1219.

83. Haskell, W.L., et al., Physical activity and public health: Updated recommendation for adults from the American College of Sports Medicine and the American Heart Association. *Med Sci Sports Exerc*, 2007. 39(8): p. 1423–1434.

84. National Heart, Lung, and Blood Institute. Classification of overweight and obesity by BMI, waist circumference, and associated disease risks. [cited 2017 July 31]; Available from: https://www.nhlbi.nih.gov/health/educational/lose_wt/BMI/bmi_dis.htm.

13 Drug-Related Sarcopenia

Sahar Swidan, PharmD

Physical exercise with resistance training is considered the most effective treatment for sarcopenia. Resistance changes metabolic signaling to effectively maintain muscle mass, but only 15% of United States adults achieve recommended levels of physical activity. Concordantly sarcopenia is common and clinically manifest in most adults over 75 years of age. Sarcopenia is a significant contributor to orthopedic conditions among the elderly, particularly hip fractures. Once deconditioning and sarcopenia manifest the requisite resistance exercise is difficult to achieve and the metabolic milieu is unlikely to be conducive to muscle reacquisition. Therefore prevention and early identification for risk modification are important for orthopedic outcomes on population and patient levels.

This chapter details pharmacologic strategies for sarcopenia risk reduction and management. Currently medication is not considered a primary therapy. However, medications exert both favorable and unfavorable effects on muscle metabolism. Clinicians aware of these well-studied mechanisms can select medications, hormone therapies, and nutrients to minimize adverse effects and potentially preserve muscle mass in patients at risk for sarcopenia.

EPIDEMIOLOGY

Sarcopenia is the loss of muscle mass and strength, associated with aging.[1] It affects balance and gait, decreases mobility, reduces muscle endurance, and impairs overall ability to perform tasks of daily living.[2] The degree of muscle mass and strength alteration is most commonly due to inactivity, but can also affect those that have been physically active throughout their lives.[1] All elderly women and men experience some amount of muscle loss with aging. The prevalence of clinically significant sarcopenia is estimated to be 13% to 24% among men and women aged 65–70 years. More than 50% of adults over 75 have sarcopenia, with higher prevalence among men.

DIAGNOSIS

Sarcopenia is sometimes considered a silent disease, often unrecognized until its clinical manifestations are many. Diagnosis is therefore very important.

Few diagnostic tests are as famous as the first test for sarcopenia. Archimedes is renowed for shouting "eureka!" when he stepped into the bath. At that moment he realized that he was able to measure his body's volume by measuring the rise in water level. Since muscle is denser than fat, underwater weighing was used for centuries to estimate body composition. Given the difficulty in feasibility of the method, underwater weighing has been "displaced".

Current diagnostic tools are broken into two categories: muscle size and physical performance.[2] Muscle size is assessed using a dual-energy X-ray absorptiometry (DXA), bioelectrical impedance analysis (BIA), CT scan, or MRI scan. For physical performance, a short physical performance battery (SPPB) is used to assess sarcopenia.[2] Table 13.1 shows the reliability of the tests and measurements assessed using these techniques.

A consensus on a standard of diagnosis has not been established for sarcopenia. Studies have evaluated each of the listed diagnostic measurements in Table 13.1, but have not established a gold standard for diagnosis since the disease state itself is still not completely understood and well-developed in terms of definition, cause, and treatment protocol.

TABLE 13.1

Measuring Techniques for Sarcopenia[2]

Parameters	Techniques	Measurements	Comments
Muscle Size	DXA scan	Total skeletal muscle mass	Reliable, low radiation exposure
	BIA	Tissue conductivity	Less reliable
	CT scan	Muscle cross-sectional area	Radiation exposure, expensive
	MRI scan	Muscle cross-sectional area	Expensive, less available
Physical performance	SPPB	Lower extremity function	Validated tool for older adults

Abbreviations: CT, computed tomography; MRI, magnetic resonance imaging; BIA, bioelectric impedance analysis; DXA, dual-energy X-ray absorptiometry; SPPB, short physical performance battery.

The above techniques are used in clinical practice. They are also used for research purposes to determine the effects of various drugs on body composition. Lack of a single blood test or biomarker is a limitation in research and may be a reason pharmacology is less often considered in the management of sarcopenia than in other chronic conditions.

PATHOPHYSIOLOGY

The pathophysiology of sarcopenia provides a roadmap by which to understand the direct and many indirect effects of medications on sarcopenia. Figure 13.1 identifies the established pathways.

There are two types of fibers that compose skeletal muscle: type I and type II fibers. Type I are slow fibers that are known as "fatigue-resistant fibers" because they have a higher density of mitochondria, capillaries, and myoglobin content.[2] Most muscle fiber are type I fibers. Type II fibers are fast fibers that exhibit higher glycolytic potential, lower oxidative capacity, and faster response.[2]

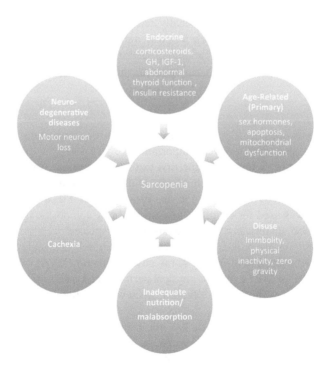

FIGURE 13.1   Pathophysiologic mechanisms of sarcopenia.[2]

Sarcopenia has been proposed to be a neurodegenerative process that leads to anabolic hormone production or sensitivity, dysregulation of cytokine secretions, and modification in the inflammatory state as outlined in Figure 13.1.[2]

Neurodegenerative process is a progressive, irreversible process that results in neuron loss as age increases. Neuron loss can be related to the effects of muscles as they age leading to alterations in the motor cortex, spinal cord, peripheral neurons, and the neuromuscular junction.[2] Age-related change also occurs for hormone levels and hormone sensitivity. There is a decrease in growth hormone, insulin-like growth factor-1 (IGF-1), corticosteroids, androgens, estrogens, and insulin.[2] Each of these hormones are involved in the anabolic and catabolic state for the regulation of muscle protein metabolism. The decrease in these hormone levels as people age directly relate to the decrease in muscle mass that is observed in the elderly population. Moreover, age-related changes in inflammatory factors and cytokines can contribute to protein-energy wasting associated with obese patients. While not a drug-induced factor it, is a contributing factor that must be considered in older adults with sarcopenia.[2]

Skeletal muscle is an endocrine organ that secretes hormone-like factors which influence the metabolism in tissues and organs throughout the body. Myokines are muscle-derived proteins that oppose adipokines and cytokines.

RISK FACTORS

There are various risk factors associated with sarcopenia including genetic influence, diet, body composition, pharmacological therapy, intrinsic factors, and lifestyle habits.[3,4] Similar to the pathophysiology, risk factors provide insights into effects of medications.

Obesity is a risk factor; it increases muscle wasting through pathophysiologic mechanisms. Studies have shown that diagnosis of sarcopenia occurs more often in advanced obesity patients than in lower-weight individuals.

Cigarette smoking has direct dose-related effects on muscle mass, but the mechanisms have not been fully elucidated. The oxidative damage resulting from the cigarette smoke is one factor. According to various studies, metabolites of smoking may be important in this process such as aldehydes, reactive oxygen species, and reactive nitrogen species. These components enter the bloodstream, reach the skeletal muscles, and accelerate muscle loss.[5–7]

Heavy alcohol consumption can influence muscle mass due to many factors. Heavy intake of alcohol displaces protein from the diet and creates micronutrient and mineral deficiencies. Moderate alcohol consumption does not seem to be associated with sarcopenia.[3] A study by Thapalia et al. indicates that patients with alcoholic cirrhosis and hepatitis have severe muscle loss. Ethanol impairs skeletal muscle protein synthesis but does not increase ubiquitin proteasome-mediated proteolysis. Therefore, autophagy is increased by alcohol exposure and contributes to sarcopenia.[8]

Lack of physical activity is an important contributor to the loss of muscle mass and strength.[4] Physical activity is protective against the development of sarcopenia, but *it also depends on* the type of activity that is pursued. Aerobic activities such as walking, running, cycling, or swimming increases maximal oxygen consumption and improves muscle quality, neuromuscular adaptation, and muscle function. Resistance training is advantageous because it increases myofibrillar protein synthesis, muscle mass, and strength even in older adults.[4] Currently, it is not known whether resistance or aerobic training is preferred to prevent sarcopenia, so both training modalities are recommended for the improvement of muscle mass and strength among individuals.[4]

There is a neurological component to sarcopenia that results in the loss of alpha motor-neuron axons. This decreases the electro-physical nerve velocity, which reduces intermodal length and segmental demyelization that occurs throughout the aging process.[4] The role of demyelization in sarcopenia seems minor, but the progressive demyelization and renervation process that is observed throughout aging and resulting fiber type grouping is the primary mechanism that is involved in the development of sarcopenia among patients.[4] The loss of alpha motor neurons leads to an effect in the types of neurons in the lower extremities, which can lead to less coordinated muscle action and a reduction in muscle strength.[4] This is related to the loss of type II fast fibers throughout aging.

Alterations in endocrine function, apart from those natural to the aging process, are risk factors. Even in the setting of the aging process, when these factors are treated, function improves. Insulin, estrogens, androgens, growth hormone, prolactin, thyroid hormones, catecholamines, and cortico-steroids are involved in the etiology and pathogenesis of sarcopenia and have a role and effect on skeletal muscle throughout the aging process.

Insulin resistance increases with age, leading to an increase in intramyocellular fat mass, which is a risk factor for the development of obesity-induced sarcopenia. Insulin selectively stimulates skeletal muscle mitochondrial protein synthesis, so decreased sensitivity of insulin on muscle synthesis can be a contributing factor to sarcopenia.[4]

Decrease in estrogen throughout aging leads to a decrease in muscle mass since estrogens are protective of muscle mass. Decrease in estrogens lead to an increase in pro-inflammatory cytokines that causes apoptosis. Hormone replacement therapy may be beneficial combat this decrease in muscle mass that is seen once estrogens decrease, but data is controversial.[4]

Reduction in growth hormone and IGF-1 contribute to sarcopenia. Growth hormone lowers fat mass, increases lean body mass, and improves blood lipid profile. IGF-1 activates satellite cell pro-liferation and differentiation, and increases protein synthesis in existing fibers. However, as people age the levels of these hormones decrease and lead to decreased muscle strength.[4]

Testosterone reduction over the aging process is associated with a decrease in muscle mass, strength, and function. Hormone replacement therapy with testosterone is controversial due to its adverse effects, but it does have a dose-dependent response to an increase in muscle mass, muscle strength, and protein synthesis.[4] Dehydroepiandrostedione (DHEA) also decreases over time, leading to an effect on muscle size, strength, and function. However, the effect of DHEA is understudied and needs more data to fully understand its implications on sarcopenia development within men and women.[4]

Vitamin D and parathyroid hormone (PTH) levels correlate to muscle mass, muscle strength, balance and the risk of falls among older adults. Low levels of vitamin D that occur with aging is correlated to an increased PTH level. High PTH occurs independently of sarcopenia, but is associ-ated with an increased risk of falling, which can be a greater risk factor among patients with low vitamin D and low muscle mass and strength.[4] Therefore, vitamin D as well as PTH levels should be monitored and considered in relation to modulation of muscle tissue functioning. Moreover, vitamin D replacement helps with increasing intracellular calcium, which is crucial for the mainte-nance of strong bones.[4]

Genetic factors contribute highly to variability in muscle strength and provide a strong risk fac-tor for the development of sarcopenia among older adults.[4] Studies have shown that genes growth/differentiation factor 8 (GDF8), cyclin-dependent kinase inhibitor 1A (CDKN1A), and myogenic differentiation antigen 1 (MYOD1) are possible candidate genes that affect lower extremity muscle strength.[4] In regards to the myostatin pathway, cyclin-dependent kinase 2 (CKD2), retinoblastoma (RB1), and IGF01 are correlative to muscle strength.[4] Moreover, polymorphisms in the vitamin D receptor (VDR) are also associated with muscle strength, because vitamin D has an effect on both smooth and striated muscle. Genetic research is anticipated to facilitate sarcopenia diagnosis and guide therapies.

DRUG-RELATED SARCOPENIA

Here we consider the convergence of factors. Sarcopenia of clinical significance is common among the elderly. Prevention is more effective than treatment. Knowledge of the pathophysiology and risk factors are tools clinicians can use to detect elevated risk of sarcopenia. These same tools can guide which medications could potentially worsen or improve sarcopenia.

A recent review considered not only one drug class, but provided a broad overview of medica-tions that are helpful or harmful to muscle. Campins et al., defined oral drugs that are associated with muscle function and categorized them as harmful or beneficial. Drugs that were found to be beneficial to muscle function include ACE inhibitors, ARBs, biguanides, thiazolidinediones, incretins, allopurinol, formoterol, and vitamin D. Statins, sulfonylureas, and glinides (meglitinide) were found to be harmful to muscle function.[9] The following sections will expand on these and other drug-related effects.

Selecting Antihypertensive Medications: Angiotensin Converting Enzyme Inhibitors and Diuretics

In a double-blind, randomized controlled trial, patients received an angiotensin converting enzyme (ACE) inhibitor or a placebo. It was shown that the patients receiving the ACE inhibitor had an improvement in their mean six-minute walking distance compared to the placebo group.[9] Therefore, it is postulated that ACE inhibitors may improve muscle strength and walking speed and have a protective effect on the risk of sarcopenia.[9] Similar to ACE inhibitors, angiotensin receptor blockers (ARBs) may have the same beneficial effect on skeletal muscle since they work by a similar mechanism.[9] It has been shown that a decrease in the inflammatory cytokine IL-6 associated with ARB therapy and the blockade of the angiotensin 1 receptor has beneficial effects on skeletal muscle remodeling associated with sarcopenia. This occurs by modulating the transforming growth factor-β, which is known to inhibit skeletal muscle regeneration.[9]

A study conducted by Mandai et al. showed that bumetanide and furosemide impair myoblast fusion into myogenic multinucleate myotubes, which is a crucial step in skeletal myogenesis that is associated with muscle generation, regeneration, and hypertrophy.[10] These two medications decrease Ca^{2+} transients that are triggered by KCl-induced depolarization in differentiated myotube, which is seen in smooth muscle cells.[10] Since Ca^{2+} is a component involved in skeletal myogenesis, the use of loop diuretics can inhibit muscle hypertrophy.[10] In conclusion, NKCC1 expression is increased in differentiating C2C12 cells and in mouse skeletal muscle after exercise training, and NKCC1 inhibition with bumetanide or furosemide impairs myogenic differentiation and exercise-induced muscle hypertrophy. Loop diuretics that are commonly administered to patients with heart failure or kidney failure may be involved in the pathogenesis of sarcopenia in these populations.

Selecting Oral Antidiabetic Drugs

Oral antidiabetic drugs can be either beneficial or harmful to the prevention of sarcopenia. Diabetes itself as a disease state has been associated with the loss of muscle mass and strength. Metformin, a biguanide, has data to support its ability to prevent the development of sarcopenia in older adults with prediabetes by reducing pro-inflammatory cytokines independent of glucose.[9] Also, metformin induces the atrophic gene MurF1, which is located in muscle and causes autophagic cell death. AMPK activation that occurs as part of the mechanism of metformin to potentiate the actions of insulin leads to this autophagic stimulus.[11]

The oral antidiabetic family of thiazolidinediones are PPAR receptor agonists that increases insulin sensitivity and anabolic effects.[9] Rosiglitazone has been shown in studies to decrease the breakdown of proteins and decrease muscle atrophy. This family as a whole could be protective of sarcopenia, but more research needs to be conducted to further examine its effects on bone mass and strength.[9] In regards to pioglitazone in non-diabetic patients who are obese, treatment along with resistance training did decrease visceral fat loss, but did not improve muscle loss.[11]

Incretins are oral antidiabetic drugs that inhibit the enzyme dipeptidyl peptidase IV, which is responsible for the degradation of endogenous incretin.[9] They have a hypertrophic and anti-apoptotic effect in addition to a positive effect on insulin resistance sensitivity and muscle oxygen intake. As a result, it is speculated that these drugs may be protective against sarcopenia and the muscular atrophy that results from the age-progressive disease.[9] Moreover, GLP-1 agonists may facilitate neuroprotective effects. A study found that four weeks of administration of a GLP-1 lead to nerve regeneration.[11]

Sodium glucose co-transport (SGLT2) inhibitors are a newer class of medications used in the treatment of diabetes mellitus type II. This class of medications reduces hyperglycemia and body weight by inhibiting the renal SGLT2 co-transport without significantly affecting the GLUT1 transport in skeletal muscle.[11] There is speculation that the reduction of plasma glucose with SGLT2 may have an indirect effect of muscle insulin sensitivity. There is currently no evidence of these medications' effect on muscle, so more studies need to be explored to better understand the class effect on muscle mass, strength, and function.[11]

Sulfonylureas are a class of anti-diabetic drugs that may increase the risk of sarcopenia.[9] Sulfonylureas block potassium channels and produce a secretagogue effect on insulin. Studies have shown that sulfonylureas may induce cell apoptosis, leading to atrophy. Glinides have a similar mechanism of action to that of sulfonylureas but with a shorter half-life that may also cause atrophy of muscles.[9] Both the sulfonylureas and glinides may induce atrophy in pancreatic beta cells as well as skeletal muscle. Glimepiride is less of an atrophic agent as compared to repaglinide, which was shown in studies to have the most potent atrophic effect. These effects are due to the blockade of KATP channels in muscle.[11]

ALLOPURINOL IN THE MANAGEMENT OF GOUT

Allopurinol is a drug that is used to prevent reoccurring gout in patients. This particular medication works by reducing plasma levels of uric acids by inhibiting xanthine oxidase.[9] Xanthine oxidase has been shown to increase oxidative stress, resulting in decreased muscle mass and strength. Therefore, by inhibiting xanthine oxidase, oxidative stress is reduced and muscle mass can be maintained.[9] As a result, it has been postulated that allopurinol may prevent muscle atrophy and sarcopenia. A ten-year analysis showed that allopurinol-treated patients had better overall function compared to those that were not on allopurinol.[9]

FORMOTEROL IN THE MANAGEMENT OF ASTHMA

Formoterol, which is a potent β2-adrenoceptor-selective agonist, is traditionally used to treat asthma.[9] This medication can cause an increase in protein synthesis, which decreases apoptosis and can increase muscle regeneration.[12] Other β2 adrenergic agonists have not been investigated regarding possible positive effects on preventing sarcopenia, so this medication family needs to be further investigated.[9]

HMG-CoA REDUCTASE INHIBITORS

Statin medications are another class of medications that can have a negative effect on the development of sarcopenia.[9] Statins are cholesterol-lowering medications that inhibit HMG-CoA reductase to reduce cardiovascular risk.[9] These drugs are well known for their propensity to cause muscular-related side effects that can occur in up to 29% of patients. These adverse drug effects are the most common reason for discontinuing statin medication.[9] The muscle toxicity is dose-dependent and usually resolves after decreasing the dose or discontinuing treatment. Toxicity is associated with decreased coenzyme Q-10 which is essential for the mitochondrial respiratory chain. However, it has also been proposed that its effect on statins may also be related to cell apoptosis and dysfunction in glucose oxidation.[9] The overall effects patients notice are decrease in muscle strength, pain in their leg muscles, and an increased risk of falls.[9] Patients taking statins should have their CPK levels monitored to assess their risk for myopathies and sarcopenia.

CORTICOSTEROIDS

Corticosteroids are associated with sarcopenia:[13] glucocorticoid-associated atrophy is seen in type II or phasic muscle fibers.[14] The mechanism of this type of muscle atrophy occurs by the upregulation of myostatin and glutamine synthetase. Glucocorticoids inhibit the physiological action of GH, and appear to induce IGF-1 activity in target organs. These changes in steroid-induced glutamine synthetase represent dose-dependent inhibition of the enzyme.[14] Moreover, glucocorticoids induce leucine resistance to muscle protein synthesis leading to protein degradation.[14] Glucocorticoids produce oxidative stress in multiple tissues, including the bone, nervous tissue, and possibly muscle.[15] The body reacts by upregulating antioxidant transcription factors in the forkhead box O family (FOXO). These may be partially responsible for the conditions of hypodynamic and adynamic bone and muscle atrophy.[15] FOXO upregulation may be responsible for the biphasic response of bone inflammation and stress with initial high bone turnover followed by hypodynamic bone.[15]

PROTON PUMP INHIBITORS

Proton pump inhibitors such as pantoprazole, esomeprazole, and omeprazole contribute to sarcopenia as an adverse effect of long-term use.[16] These drugs are known for their use in treating acid-related disorders such as reflux, heartburn, and ulcers. Long-term use of these medications, particularly at higher doses, is a well-established contributor to hip fractures in older adults.[17] Less known is the association with sarcopenia which may be from the same mechanism. Lowering pH in the gastrointestinal tract reduces calcium absorption leading to osteoporosis risk. Lowering pH also changes the microbiome to a likely more proinflammatory milieu. Impaired absorption of protein is critical for sarcopenia. Dietary intake of protein is emphasized, but this is only part of the process; the protein must also be absorbed. It is broken down in the stomach to facilitate absorption in the small intestine, but insufficient stomach acid results in a net reduction in protein intake.

PSYCHOTROPIC MEDICATIONS

Sarcopenia can result from mitochondrial damage, which can be exacerbated by various psychotropic medications. Mechanisms of mitochondrial damage and tissues are different among different medications.[18] Medications can directly inhibit mtDNA transcription of electron transport chain (ETC) complexes and inhibit enzymes required for steps of glycolysis and beta oxidation.[19] Medications can also indirectly damage mitochondria by producing free radicals through the reduction of endogenous antioxidants such as glutathione, and by depleting nutrients in the body that are required for construction and function of mitochondrial enzymes or ETC complexes.[18]

Barbiturates inhibit mitochondrial respiration by inhibiting NADH dehydrogenase. NADH dehydrogenase is a part of complex I of the ETC.[18] Drugs and some endogenous compounds sequester CoA (aspirin, divalproex), inhibit mitochondrial β-oxidation enzymes (tetracyclines, 2-arylpropionate anti-inflammatory drugs), or inhibit both mitochondrial β-oxidation and oxphos (bile acids, amiodarone). Valproic acid depleted carnitine and decreases β-oxidations in the liver inducing mitochondrial damage.[18] Moreover, many psychotropic medications also cause mitochondrial dysfunction, including antidepressants, antipsychotics, dementia medications, seizure medications, mood stabilizers, benzodiazepines, and Parkinson's Disease medications. There are many other drugs that can induce mitochondrial damage. Understanding the mechanism of how these drugs cause mitochondrial damage is important to develop ways to protect patients.[18]

TREATMENT

There are currently no approved medications for the treatment of sarcopenia. None of the pharmacological or behavioral interventions currently considered for the reversal of sarcopenia have been proven to be as efficacious as resistance training. Therefore, it is the basis of all recommendations for patients with sarcopenia.[4] According to the American College of Sport Medicine and the American Heart Association, resistance training should be pursued on two or more consecutive days per week to produce a gain in muscle size and strength, even in frail elderly patients. While disuse of resistance training can result in rapid detraining, it can be maintained by a minimum of one exercise per week.[4] Currently, only 12% of the United States older adult population performs strength training at least twice a week, so this is an important intervention that can be made to prevent and treat sarcopenia in this patient population.[20]

While there are no approved medications to treat sarcopenia, β-hydroxy β-methylbutyrate (HMB), which is a metabolite of the amino acid leucine, has been shown to have efficacy as a dietary supplement in preventing the loss of muscle mass in individuals who have sarcopenia.[21,22] It has been noted to help preserve lean muscle mass in older adults.[22] HMB has shown efficacy in reducing, or even reversing, the loss of muscle mass, muscle function, and muscle strength in hypercatabolic disease states.[22,23] Overall recommendations as of June 2016 for treating sarcopenia include supplementation with HMB, regular resistance exercise, and consumption of a high-protein diet.[22,23]

Supplementation with DHEA and growth hormone has shown little to no effect on the treatment or prevention of sarcopenia. While growth hormone may increase muscle protein synthesis and muscle mass, it has not been shown to result in an increase in strength and function.[23] Testosterone as well as other anabolic steroids have also been investigated for the treatment of sarcopenia, and may have some positive effects on muscle strength and mass[24,25]

Myostatin is a natural inhibitor of muscle growth and mutations in the myostatin gene result in muscle hypertrophy. Therefore, antagonism of myostatin enhances muscle tissue regeneration by increasing satellite cell proliferation.[4] Myostatin antagonists have a potential therapeutic impact on sarcopenia, but more studies need to be conducted to further investigate its use. Recombinant human antibodies to myostatin have been studied in regards to muscular dystrophy, and may be a treatment approach for sarcopenia in the future.[4]

Vitamin D supplementation with a dose of 800 IU per day can help to reduce hip fractures in the older adult population.[4] Vitamin D leads to increased muscle strength as a result of preventing type II fibers from undergoing muscle atrophy.[4] It is unknown if vitamin D can prevent sarcopenia, but this is an area of research that should be further explored to better identify the effects of vitamin D and calcium supplementation on sarcopenia and the development of muscle mass and function among older adults.[4] Vitamin D has been known to protect bones in bone mineral density disorders. Low vitamin D levels are common, especially among older adults, where the deficiency has a prevalence of around 50%. Prolonged deficiency in vitamin D can lead to muscle weakness and loss of muscle mass and strength.[9] Changes in muscle morphology due to atrophy of the type II fast muscle fibers has been seen. Moreover, low vitamin D levels have been seen to cause lower physical performance in walking speed, maintaining balance, and risk of falls among elderly patients.[9] A randomized controlled clinical trial showed that vitamin D supplementation for over four months resulted in a 10% increase in muscle fiber size among older women.[26] Other studies have also shown that vitamin D causes an increase in proximal strength of the lower extremities in those with vitamin D deficiency, but does not have a clinically significant effect on muscle strength in adults with baseline vitamin D levels >25 nmol/L.[27] The Society on Sarcopenia, Cachexia and Wasting Diseases recommends checking vitamin D levels and replacing levels if low in all sarcopenic patients.[12, 26] Apart from vitamin D, the drugs explained above would not be added as a prophylaxis for sarcopenia, but co-existing conditions requiring treatment using these drugs may be of benefit to patients with sarcopenia risk.

Carnitine is one of the most important amino acids in the body for fat transport and metabolism and as a mitochondrial energy source. Muscles store up to 95% of the body's total carnitine. Carnitine is critical for normal skeletal muscle bioenergetics, and skeletal muscle is greatly affected in states of carnitine deficiency.[28]

Some studies have shown that L-carnitine may present an important role in the treatment of the myopathy induced by several etiologies. Study of carnitine use in uremic patients with some degree of muscular atrophy, reports that 24-week treatment with l-carnitine (2 g IV at the end of

TABLE 13.2
Sarcopenia Treatment Option Summary[30]

Intervention		Effect	Comments
Exercise – Increased cardiovascular fitness with increased endurance	Aerobic	Increases mitochondrial volume and activity	• *Pros*: Overall beneficial effects of exercise to individual
	Resistance	Increased muscle mass and strength, increases skeletal muscle protein synthesis and muscle fiber size, improves physical performance	• *Cons*: Motivation to exercise remains low
Nutritional protein supplement		Varying evidence of increased muscle mass and strength	• *Pros*: Ensures good protein intake • *Cons*: May reduce natural food intake
β-hydroxy β-methylbutyric acid (HMB; a bioactive metabolite of leucine) supplementation with arginine or alone		HMB showed some effects on muscle mass and function in these high-quality studies, but sample sizes were small	• *Pros*: Good amino acid to enhance muscle fibers • *Cons*: Small sample size and short-term studies
Hormone therapy	Testosterone	Testosterone also can increase muscle bulk through an anabolic process to increase skeletal muscle	• *Cons*: Masculinization of women; increased risk of prostate cancer in men if they over artomatize to estrogens
	Estrogen	Poor evidence of increased muscle mass but not function	• *Cons*: Risk of breast cancer
	Growth hormone	Some evidence for increased muscle mass, varying evidence for increased muscle strength	• *Cons*: Side effects including fluid retention, orthostatic hypotension
Vitamin D		Variable evidence for increased muscle strength, reduced falls in nursing home residents	• *Pros*: Fracture reduction, possible cardiovascular benefits
ACE inhibitors		Some evidence for increased exercise capacity	• *Pros*: Other cardiovascular benefits • *Cons*: Renal function needs monitoring
Creatine – Creatine synthesis mainly occurs in the liver and kidneys. On average, 1 gram is produced by the body per day in young adults. Creatine is also obtained through the diet at a rate of about 1 g/d from diet		Variable evidence of increased muscle strength and endurance especially when combined with exercise	• *Cons*: Reports of nephritis • It also raises creatinine causing false positive lab tests in physical exams
Potential new treatments	Myostatin antagonists	No trials in older adults	
	Peroxisome proliferator-activated receptor (PPAR) agonist	No human trials	
	5-aminoimidazole-4-carboxamide-1β-4-ribofuranoside	No human trials	

hemodialysis, or in dialysis solution, or oral twice daily) leads to an increase of about 7% in the diameter of type I and type IIa fibers, as well as a reduction in atrophic fibers. No remarkable changes were documented in type IIb fibers. These results along with other results in patients with cancer cachexia indicate possible utilization in the treatment of sarcopenia.[29]

It is known that cancer and other conditions that create chronic systemic inflammation triggered and sustained by cytokines as well as increased oxidative stress, contribute to the pathogenesis of cachexia. Recent findings indicate that muscle-specific genes (i.e., myosin heavy chain) and their products must be targeted to initiate muscle wasting]. Muscle atrophy occurs at different levels, starting from repressed gene expression and ending with accelerated protein degradation. Furthermore, the studies show that, besides myofibrilar protein loss, apoptosis is also present in skeletal muscle of cachectic tumor-bearing animals and human patients with cancer cachexia (Table 13.2). [31,32]

CONCLUSION

It is estimated that 5–13% of elderly people aged 60–70 years are affected by sarcopenia. The numbers increase to 11–50% for those aged 80 or above. Sarcopenia may lead to frailty, but not all patients with sarcopenia are frail and sarcopenia is about twice as common as frailty. Several studies have shown that the risk of falls is significantly elevated in subjects with reduced muscle strength. Treatment of sarcopenia remains challenging and we do not have many options with strong clinical efficacy. However, more research is being done and progress is being made. Most promising treatments have been found with exercise and resistance training, and hormone replacement therapy that includes testosterone, estrogens, and growth hormone. Vitamin D has always been a critical player in the prevention of disease including osteoporosis and sarcopenia. Other agents such as angiotensin-converting enzyme inhibitors and nutritional supplements such HMB show promise in the treatment of sarcopenia. We are all excited to see the new and progressive research on PPAR agonists and AICAR.

REFERENCES

1. International Osteoporosis Foundation. What is sarcopenia? https://www.iofbonehealth.org/what-sarcopenia (accessed 27 June 2017).
2. Kim TN and Choi KM. Sarcopenia: Definition, epidemiology, and pathophysiology. *J Bone Metab.* 2013; 20: 1–10.
3. Dennison EM, Sayer AA, and Cooper C. Epidemiology of sarcopenia and insight into possible therapeutic targets. *Nature.* 2017; 13: 340–347.
4. Rolland Y, Czerwinski S, Van Kan GA, et al. Sarcopenia: Its assessment, etiology, pathogenesis, consequences and future directions. *J Nutr Health Aging.* 2008; 12(7): 433–450.
5. Lee JSW, Auyeung T-W, Kwok T, Lau EMC, Leung P-C and Woo J. Associated factors and health impact of sarcopenia in older Chinese men and women: A cross-sectional study. *Gerontology.* 2007; 53: 166–172.
6. Rom O, Kaisari S, Aizenbud D, and Reznick AZ. Sarcopenia and smoking: A possible cellular model of cigarette smoke effects on muscle protein breakdown. *Ann N Y Acad Sci* 2012; 1259: 47–53.
7. Rom O, Kaisari S, Aizenbud D, and Reznick AZ. The effects of acetaldehyde and acrolein on muscle catabolism in C2 myotubes. *Free Radic Biol Med.* 2013; 65C: 190–200.
8. Thapaliya S, Runkana A, Megan R et al. Alcohol-induced autophagy contributes to loss in skeletal muscle mass. *Autophagy* 2014; 10: 4, 677–690.
9. Campins, L, Camps M, Riera A, et al. Oral drugs related with muscle wasting and sarcopenia: A review. *Pharmacology.* 2017; 99: 1–8.
10. Mandai S, Furukawa S, Kodaka M, et al. Loop diuretics affect skeletal myoblast differentiation and exercise-induced muscle hypertrophy. *Sci Rep.* 2017; 7: 46369.
11. Cetrone M, Mele A and Tricarico D. Effects of the antidiabetic drugs on the age-related atrophy and sarcopenia associated with diabetes type II. *Curr Diabetes Rev.* 2014; 10: 231–237.
12. Morley JE, Argiles JM, Evans F, et al. Society for sarcopenia, cachexia, and wasting disease: Nutritional recommendations for the management of sarcopenia. *J Am Med Dir Assoc.* 2010; 11: 391–396.

13. Umegaki H. Sarcopenia and diabetes: Hyperglycemia is a risk factor for age-associated muscle mass and functional reduction. *J Diabetes Investig.* 2015; 6(6): 623–624.
14. Sakuma K and Yamaguchi A. Sarcopenia and age-related endocrine function. *Int J Endocrinol.* 2012.
15. Klein GL. The effect of glucocorticoids on bone and muscle. *Osteoporosis Sarcopenia.* 2015; 1: 39–45.
16. Steves CJ, Bird S, Williams FMK, et al. The microbiome and musculoskeletal conditions of aging: A review of evidence for impact and potential therapeutics. *J Bone Mineral Res.* 2016; 21(2): 261–269.
17. Osteoprosis Canada. Medications that can cause bone loss, falls and/or fractures. http://www.osteo-porosis.ca/osteoporosis-and-you/secondary-osteoporosis/medications-that-can-cause-bone-loss-falls-and-or-fractures/ (accessed 2 August 2017).
18. Neystadt J and Pieczenik SR. Medication-induced mitochondrial damage and disease. *Mol Nutr Food Res.* 2008; 52: 780–788.
19. Busquets S, Figueras MT, Fuster G, et al. Anticachectic effects of formoterol: A drug for potential treatment of muscle wasting. *Cancer Res.* 2004; 64: 6725–6731.
20. MMWR. US Department of Health and Human Services. 2004. Strength training among adults aged 65 years - United States 2001; 25–28.
21. Brioche T, Pagano AF, Py G, et al. Muscle wasting and aging. Experimental models, fatty infiltrations, and prevention. *Mol Aspects Med.* 2016; 5: 56–87.
22. Wu H, Xia Y, Jiang J, et al. Effect of beta-hydroxy-beta-methylbutyrate supplementation on muscle loss in older adults: A systematic review and meta-analysis. *Archives of Gerontology and Geriatrics.* 2015; 61: 168–175.
23. Argiles JM, Campos N, Lopez-Pedrosa JM, et al. Skeletal muscle regulates metabolism via interogan crosstalk: Roles in health and disease. *JAMDA.* 2016; 17: 789–796.
24. Sakuma K and Yamaguchi A. Sarcopenia and age-related endocrine function. *Int J Endocrinol.* 2012.
25. Wakabayashi H and Sakuma K. Comprehensive approach to sarcopenia treatment. *Curr Clin Pharmacol.* 2014; 9(2): 171–180.
26. Ceglia L, Niramitmahapanya S, da Silva Morais M, et al: A randomized study on the effect of vitamin D3 supplementation on skeletal muscle morphology and vitamin D receptor concentration in older women. *J Clin Endocrinol Metab* 2013; 98: E1927–E1935.
27. Stockton KA, Mengersen K, Paratz JD, et al. Effect of vitamin D supplementation on muscle strength: A systematic review and meta-analysis. *Osteoporos Int.* 2011; 22: 859–871.
28. EP Brass.Supplemental carnitine and exercise. *Am J Clin Nutr.* 2000; 72: 618S–623S.
29. Spagnoli LG, Palmieri G, Mauriello A, Vacha GM, D'Iddio S, and Giorcelli G. Morphometric evidence of the trophic effect of L-carnitine on human skeletal muscle. *Nephron.* 1990; 55: 16–23, 10.1159/000185912.
30. Burton LA and Sumukadas D. Optimal management of sarcopenia. *Clin Interventions.* 2010; 5: 217–228.
31. Li Y-P and Schwartz RJ. TNF-α regulates early differentiation of C2C12 myoblasts in an autocrine fashion. *FASEB J.* 2001; 15: 1413–1415.
32. Busquets, S, Deans C, Figueras M, Moore-Carrasco R, López-Soriano FJ, and Fearon KC. Apoptosis is present in skeletal muscle of cachectic gastro-intestinal cancer patients. *Clin Nutr.* 2007; 26: 614–618, 10.1016/j.clnu.2007.06.005.

14 Sex Hormones and Their Impact on Sarcopenia and Osteoporosis

Pamela W. Smith, MD, MPH, MS

This chapter addresses the changes in sex hormones that occur with aging in both men and women. It provides a health care practitioner's synthesis of the medical literature on the role of sex hormones in preserving muscle mass and bone strength during aging.

INTRODUCTION

Men experience andropause, which is defined as an absolute or relative insufficiency of testosterone or its metabolites in relation to the needs of that individual at that time in his life [1]. Studies have shown that half of healthy men between the ages of 50 and 70 years will have a testosterone level below the lowest level seen in healthy men who are 20–40 years of age and that 30%–60% of men in their 70s are hypogonadal [2–3]. These numbers may actually be under reported. Testosterone has many functions in the male [4–12]. Key functions are listed in Table 14.1.

Women experience a decline in estrogen, progesterone, and testosterone during menopause and throughout the aging process. Testosterone production is equally as important for women as it is for men. For women, testosterone has the functions outlined in Table 14.1 [13–18]. In women, estrogen has 400 functions in the body, including those outlined in Table 14.2 [19–31]. Progesterone also has many functions in a woman's body including stimulating the production of new bone [31]. This and other key functions of progesterone in women are listed in Table 14.2 [32–36].

Men also make estrogen in the form of estrone, estradiol, and estriol. Estradiol has a protective effect on the brain structure in older males and has been shown to help maintain bone structure [37–39].

SARCOPENIA

Sarcopenia is a major contributing factor to fractures, weakness, disability, falls, and mortality [40]. Sarcopenia is common and it is becoming more common as patients live longer. Sarcopenia affects almost 20% of men aged 70–75 and 50% of men over the age of 80. In women, about 25% have sarcopenia between the ages of 70 and 75 years and 40% by the time they reach the age of 80 [41]. Another study has shown that after the age of 50, muscle mass declines at a yearly rate of about 1%–2% and that strength decreases about 1.5% yearly, which soars to 3% yearly after the patient is aged 60 [42]. These numbers, however, vary depending on the definition of sarcopenia that is used [43].

Muscle mass is regulated by the optimal balance between the synthesis and breakdown of muscle proteins. This mechanism is controlled by various hormones, two of which are testosterone and estrogen [44].

Beginning around age 35 years, testosterone levels in men decrease by 1%–3% per year [45]. The Massachusetts Male Aging Study showed a 30-year fall in total testosterone in men averaging 48% and a decline in free testosterone levels of 85% [46]. The decline that occurs with aging in skeletal muscle mass is greater in males than females [47]. Testosterone is the main anabolic steroid hormone produced by the body and optimal testosterone levels are needed for the maintenance of

TABLE 14.1

Key Functions of Testosterone in Men and Women

Men

Involved in the making of protein and muscle formation

Helps manufacture bone

Improves oxygen uptake throughout the body

Helps regulate blood sugar

Needed for normal sperm development

Regulates acute hypothalamic–pituitary–adrenal responses under dominance challenge

Helps regulate cholesterol production

Decreases the risk of heart disease

Helps protect the brain from cognitive decline

Aids in maintaining a powerful immune system

Aids in mental concentration

Regulates platelet aggregation indirectly by modifying thromboxane A2 receptor
  concentration on megakaryocytes and platelets

Decreases anxiety

Improves mood

Women

Increases sexual interest

Increases sense of emotional well-being

Increases muscle mass and strength

Helps maintain memory

Helps the skin from sagging

Decreases excess body fat

Helps maintain bone strength

Elevates norepinephrine in the brain having a tricyclic affect

muscle mass. Testosterone concentrations decline as the patient ages, suggesting that low testosterone levels should be considered one of the etiologies for loss of muscle mass and sarcopenia.

In young patients who are healthy, the skeletal muscle mass is almost 60% of the total body mass. After age 40, this percentage begins to decrease [48]. One medical trial revealed that when the value was adjusted for height, the testosterone that is bioavailable is responsible for 2.6% of the change in appendicular skeletal muscle mass, which is 75% of the total skeletal muscle mass [49]. Furthermore, studies have shown that low testosterone levels increase the risk of developing sarcopenia, since low testosterone in men results in lower protein synthesis and loss of muscle mass [50].

Several studies have shown that testosterone replacement increases muscle mass and muscle strength with a congruent increase in protein synthesis when given to men with low testosterone levels [51–56]. Another study showed that testosterone replacement increased lean body mass and lowered fat content compared to placebo but had no effect on muscle strength. Other studies indicated that testosterone replacement had an anabolic action that improved muscle strength and increased muscle size [57–59]. In addition, studies have shown that testosterone replacement increases fat-free mass, but the studies conflict as to whether the dimensions of muscle performance show improvement when the patient used testosterone replacement [60–65]. Furthermore, a recent study evaluated the possible mechanisms by which androgens alter protein balance with a suggestion that further studies need to be done that are controlled for diet and other confounding factors to better understand testosterone's effects on the building and breakdown of protein [66]. This may be partially due to the fact that previous medical trials have also shown that the effects of testosterone on muscles are mediated by a number of different factors such as the amount of exercise the patient participates

TABLE 14.2
Key Functions of Estrogen and Progesterone in Women

Estrogen

Maintains bone density

Stimulates the production of choline acetyltransferase, an enzyme that prevents Alzheimer's disease

Increases metabolic rate

Improves insulin sensitivity

Regulates body temperature

Helps prevent muscle damage

Helps maintain muscle

Improves sleep

Reduces risk of cataracts

Helps maintain the elasticity of arteries

Dilates small arteries

Increases blood flow

Inhibits platelet stickiness

Decreases the accumulation of plaque on arteries

Enhances magnesium uptake and utilization

Maintains the amount of collagen in the skin

Decreases blood pressure

Decreases low-density lipoprotein and prevents its oxidation

Helps maintain memory

Increases reasoning and new ideas

Helps with fine motor skills

Increases the water content of skin and is responsible for its thickness and softness

Enhances the production of nerve-growth factor

Increases high-density lipoprotein by 10%–15%

Reduces the overall risk of heart disease by 40%–50%

Decreases lipoprotein(a)

Acts as a natural calcium channel blocker to keep arteries open

Enhances energy

Improves mood

Increases concentration

Helps prevent glaucoma

Increases sexual interest

Reduces homocysteine

Decreases wrinkles

Protects against macular degeneration

Decreases risk of colon cancer

Helps prevent tooth loss

Aids in the formation of neurotransmitters in the brain such as serotonin, which decreases depression, irritability, anxiety, and pain sensitivity

Progesterone

Helps balance estrogen

Leaves the body quickly

Improves sleep

Has a natural calming effect

Lowers high blood pressure

Helps the body use and eliminate fats

(Continued)

TABLE 14.2 (CONTINUED)

Key Functions of Estrogen and Progesterone in Women

Lowers cholesterol

Increases scalp hair

Helps balance fluids in the cells

Increases the beneficial effects of estrogen on blood vessels

Increases metabolic rate

Natural diuretic

Natural antidepressant

Is anti-inflammatory

Enhances the action of thyroid hormones

Improves libido

Helps restore proper cell oxygen levels

Induces conversion of E1 to the inactive E1S form

Promotes Th2 immunity

Is neuroprotective, promoting myelination

in, the patient's nutritional status, the individual's genetic background, their level of growth hormone, whether the person has optimal thyroid function, and the patient's cytokine production [67].

Even though testosterone replacement in males produces an increase in lean body mass and strength, as the patient ages, the effect of testosterone on lean mass and strength is not as great as when he was younger. A meta-analysis showed a moderate increase in muscle strength in men on testosterone replacement [68]. In a single trial, testosterone replacement has been shown to reverse sarcopenia in aging patients through the regulation of the following signaling pathways: myostatin, Akt, c-Jun HN2-terminal kinase, and Notch [69].

Estrogen is also important when it comes to muscle since it functions as an anti-inflammatory in both men and women. Furthermore, elevated levels of estrogen in a male increase sex hormone binding globulin, which decreases the level of free testosterone, the amount that is available for the body to use.

In women, the postmenopausal decline in estrogen may have a catabolic effect on muscle. As the level of estrogen falls with age, the level of cytokines in the body escalates, which are inflammatory such as tumor necrosis factor alpha (TNF-alpha) and interleukin 6 (IL-6). Estrogen and testosterone inhibit IL-1 and IL-6 and may also have an indirect catabolic effect upon muscle [70, 71]. Additionally, studies report that estrogen aids in the prevention of muscle mass loss [72, 73]. Furthermore, lower levels of estrogen in women lead to declining muscle mass, which can contribute to decreased activity levels. This decline can be reversed with hormone replacement therapy [74].

For both men and women, testosterone replacement balanced with other sex hormone replacement can improve muscle mass by increasing protein anabolism and reducing protein catabolism in both sexes. Further studies will be helpful in quantifying the extent to which hormone replacement therapy will have a positive effect on sarcopenia in both men and women. Whatever therapeutic decisions are jointly made in the context of the doctor–patient relationship, treatment for sarcopenia should include resistance strength training whenever feasible since this has established effectiveness.

OSTEOPOROSIS

Primary osteoporosis is the result of bone loss related to the decline in gonadal function associated with aging. Secondary osteoporosis may result from chronic diseases, exposures, or nutritional deficiencies that adversely impact bone metabolism. This section will focus on primary osteoporosis.

In women, estradiol plays a major role in preserving skeletal integrity. Loss of bone mass occurs commonly with estrogen loss. Bone loss due to estrogen regression follows a foreseeable pattern. Initially, bone loss is rapid and affects trabecular bone first. After 10–15 years of estrogen deficiency, the rate of loss each year decreases to less than one-half of its level before menopause. Due to the fragility of the resulting bone, mild trauma can produce fractures of the wrist and spine. After another 10–15 years of bone loss, hip fractures become more common [75].

The beneficial effects of estrogen on bone structure are, to some extent, due to the ability of estrogen to decrease the development of osteoclastic cytokine production in T-cells and in osteoblasts. Estrogen has been shown to hasten the apoptotic death of osteoclasts as a method by which to suppress cytokine production. The main action of estrogen at the cellular level is to inhibit the osteoclast by increasing the levels of osteoprotegerin (OPG). OPG attaches to the receptor activator of NFkB and slows osteoclast differentiation and its activity [76, 77].

Other effects of estrogen on bone cells and bone remodeling have also been discussed at length in the medical literature. In healthy patients, bone is renewed on an endless basis by the reabsorption of old bone by osteoclasts and the formation of new bone by osteoblasts. The cells involved in this process of bone regeneration are called the bone remodeling units (BMU), where the bone is reabsorbed before new bone is formed [78]. In patients with estrogen loss, the numbers of BMU are increased, which results in an imbalance in the making of bone. This increase in osteoclasts and the consequent increase in bone resorption can be decreased by estrogen replacement. Likewise, studies have described that mRNA levels for IL-6 and IL-1 have been shown to be increased in trabecular bone in postmenopausal women with osteoporosis when compared to controls without this disease process who are the same age [79]. However, the levels of IL-6 and IL-1 in the serum are not affected by bone status [80]. This research supports the perception that estrogen has a direct effect on bone cells by altering the making and secretion of cytokines which act as paracrine factors in the proximate area around the bone. Furthermore, Winding and others discuss the positive effects that estrogen has on bone structure that are dependent on the number of estrogen receptors in the body.

In addition, studies have shown that estrogen functions in other ways to help build and maintain bone structure. Estrogen decreases bone resorption and diminishes lysosomal proteinase secretion [81,82]. Furthermore, findings have shown that osteoclast formation was suppressed by estrogen replacement [83, 84]. Estrogen replacement therapy has also been shown to increase type I collagen synthesis and secretion in osteoclasts [85]. Another study did not demonstrate this effect [86]. Other trials have revealed that estrogen positively affects the production of transforming growth factor beta (TGF-β) by intensifying its production [87]. Likewise, estrogen also has an anti-resorption influence through a direct consequence that is inhibitory on the osteoclasts. Recently, it has been suggested that reactive oxygen species (ROS) may play a role in postmenopausal bone loss by generating a more oxidized bone microenvironment [88, 89]. One of the roles of estrogen is as an antioxidant. Likewise, estrogen has an indirect effect by suppressing inflammatory cytokines IL-6, IL-1, and TNF-alpha release and the release of TGF-B by bone-derived stromal cells and osteoblasts [90–93].

Estrogen also has a positive effect on markers of bone remodeling. The rate of bone turnover in a patient can be evaluated indirectly by examining biochemical markers. The main part of the organic bone matrix is made of type I collagen. When bone is reabsorbed, collagen is broken down into breakdown products that are excreted in the urine. These breakdown products can be measured, including hydroxyproline, pyridinoline, and doxypyridinoline. These bone resorption markers are a good way to evaluate the effectiveness of therapies such as estrogen replacement [94]. Another study showed that the level of bone remodeling was reduced and the bone mass was increased with hormone replacement. The placebo group did not show any increase in bone mass [95]. Likewise, in clinical trials, estrogen has been shown to reverse bone loss in areas of trabecular and cortical bone due to postmenopausal hormone loss [96–98]. Both osteoblasts and osteoclasts have been shown to have estrogen receptor sites [99, 100]. As you have seen, studies have revealed that estrogen has positive direct effects on both the osteoblasts and osteoclasts and also helps prevent bone loss in postmenopausal women.

The greatest osteoporosis prevention benefit from hormone replacement therapy is obtained if it is begun shortly after menopause. However, the literature is clear that hormone replacement therapy prevents bone loss in patients who are postmenopausal no matter when the therapy is instituted [101, 102]. In addition, the positive effect of estrogen on bone structure lasts only as long as the patient is using estrogen and is lost if the patient discontinues the therapy.

Progesterone is a hormone that has been shown to benefit bone building. Progesterone loss after menopause can lead to bone loss. Clinical trials have shown that using a combination of estrogen and progesterone replacement prevents bone loss after menopause [103, 104]. Furthermore, the combination of estrogen and progesterone together has been shown to be even more effective than estrogen alone [105, 106].

Loss of estrogens and/or testosterone increases the rate of bone remodeling by removing the restraining effects on the making of osteoblasts and osteoclasts. Likewise, loss of androgens and estrogens also causes an imbalance between resorption and formation by extending the life of osteoclasts and decreasing the life of osteoblasts. Furthermore, endogenous androgens increase bone mineral density (BMD) in women of all ages. In fact, women with excess endogenous testosterone, such as women with polycystic ovary syndrome, have increased BMD when compared with women with normal testosterone levels [107]. Testosterone and estrogens maintain bone mass and integrity, regardless of the age of the patient or if they are male or female [108].

The Framingham Osteoporosis Study revealed that as men age, they lose BMD at a rate of 1% per year [109]. Other studies have shown that one in five men will suffer a fracture from osteoporosis during their lifetime [110,111]. One of the major causes of osteoporosis in men is hypogonadism, which is found in up to 20% of men with symptomatic vertebral fractures and 50% of older men with hip fractures, according to a recent trial [112]. In addition, osteoporotic fractures in men are associated with increased morbidity and greater mortality than in women. One-half of men who fall and break a hip die within a year [113]. Moreover, almost one in four men older than 60 years will have a fracture that is related to osteoporosis [114]. Furthermore, the rate of hip fracture is projected to increase by 310% in men and 240% in women by 2050. If a male reference range is used to evaluate bone loss: 3%–6% of men have osteoporosis and 28%–47% of men have osteopenia [115].

When the patient or the practitioner thinks of osteopenia or osteoporosis, they usually think of female patients. However, one-third of cases of osteoporosis in the United States are men [116].

Bone loss in hypogonadal men has been shown to be related to testosterone deficiency. One study showed that bone density decreased with declining total testosterone levels with a four- to five-fold greater decrease for each nanomole-per-liter decrease in total testosterone [117]. However, studies have shown that testosterone and estrogen are both key players in building and maintaining bone in males. Testosterone stimulates periosteal growth, whereas estrogen is important for the maintenance of trabecular bone mass and structure [118]. In addition, testosterone has a direct effect on osteoclasts and osteoblasts in males [119]. In fact, androgen receptors are located on osteoblasts [120]. Furthermore, testosterone modifies the effects induced by osteoblastic cells by affecting adhesion molecule expression, which is a major requirement for the development and function of osteoblasts [121]. Additionally, OPG secretin increases if the hypogonadal male is on testosterone replacement when he exercises. This affect does not occur due to exercise alone. OPG works as a decoy for the receptor activator of the nuclear factor kappa beta ligand, which is secreted by osteoblasts. It also provokes the formation of osteoclasts and stimulates their differentiation [122]. Likewise, testosterone inhibits the discarding of this ligand by osteoblasts [123]. Moreover, testosterone inhibits IL-6 gene expression [124]. It also inhibits IL-1 expression [125].

Testosterone has many other functions related to bone health. It reduces the number of bone remodeling cycles by changing the manufacturing of osteoclasts and osteoblasts from progenitor cells. Testosterone also has effects on the duration of mature bone cells and has a pro-apoptotic effect on osteoclasts and an opposite effect on osteoblasts and osteocytes. Furthermore, testosterone modulates the effects caused by other hormones and cytokines that are part of bone metabolism. For example, studies have revealed that calcitonin levels are lower in patients with low testosterone and the levels can be increased with testosterone replacement therapy [126]. Likewise, giving testosterone to males who have low levels can increase growth hormone secretion [127]. Growth hormone increases bone mass and density [128]. Furthermore, a medical trial showed that when testosterone was replaced in males with low levels, osteocalcin (a marker of osteoblastic activity) levels increased and bone breakdown products were decreased in the urine [129, 130].

Estrogen is also a key player in building and maintaining bone in males. Therefore, aromatization of testosterone into estradiol is paramount in bone metabolism. In fact, several studies have shown that low estradiol levels in males were associated with an increased risk of developing osteoporosis [131–135]. Estrogen is needed to suppress bone resorption, but both testosterone and estrogen are paramount for the formation of bone. Estrogen receptors are present on osteoblasts, osteoclasts, and osteocytes. Testosterone stimulates periosteal growth, whereas estrogen is important for the maintenance of trabecular bone mass and structure [136–140].

CONCLUSION

The physiologic roles of sex hormones include the maintenance of musculoskeletal structures. The effects of age-associated decline in gonadal function on muscle and bone can lead to osteoporosis and sarcopenia. This chapter is a resource to clinicians as they distinguish healthy aging from osteoporosis and sarcopenia in their patients.

Patients with osteoporosis and sarcopenia may benefit from referral to endocrinologists, geriatric specialists, and other health care providers practiced in hormone replacement therapy. An additional resource to referring practitioners is the drug labels of hormone replacement therapy, which outline the indications for the US Food and Drug Administration (FDA) approved use and adverse effects. An emerging adverse drug effect from topical hormone therapies is unintended secondary exposure via direct contact with skin. Drug labels can be accessed through FDA.gov and dailymed.nlm.nih.gov.

REFERENCES

1. Carruthers, M., The diagnosis of androgen deficiency, *Aging Male* 2002; 4:254.
2. Wang, C., et al., ISA, ISSAM, EAU, EAA, and ASA recommendations: Investigation, treatment and monitoring of late-onset hypogonadism in males, *Aging Male* 2009; 12:5–12.
3. Korenman, S., et al., Secondary hypogonadism in older men: Its relationship to impotence, *J Clin Endocrinol Metab* 1990; 71:963–69.
4. van den Beld, A., et al., Measures of bioavailable serum testosterone and estradiol and their relationships with muscle strength, bone density, and body composition in elderly men, *Jour Clin Endo & Met* 2000; 85(9):3276–82.
5. Harman, S., et al., Male menopause, myth or menace, *The Endocrinologist* 1994; 4(3):212–17.
6. Swerdloff, R., et al., Androgen deficiency and aging in men, *West J Med* 1993; 159(5):579–85.
7. Vermuelen, A., et al., Androgens in the aging male, *J Clin Endocrinol Metab* 1991; 73(2):221–24.
8. Menta, P., et al., The social endocrinology of dominance: Basal testosterone predicts cortisol changes and behavior following victory and defeat, *J Pers Soc Psychol* 2008; 94(6):1078–93.
9. Ajayi, A., et al., Testosterone increases human platelet thromboxane A-2 receptor density and aggregation responses, *Circulation* 1995; 91(11):2742–47.
10. English, K., et al., Low-dose transdermal testosterone therapy improves angina threshold in men with chronic stable angina, *Circulation* 2000; 120:1906–11.
11. Dardona, P., et al., Update: Hypogonadotropic hypogonadism in type 2 diabetes and obesity, *J Clin Endocrinol Metab* 2011; 96(9):2643–51.
12. Araujo, A., et al., Endogenous testosterone and mortality in men: A systematic review and meta-analysis, *J Clin Endocrinol Metab* 2011; 90:3007–19.
13. Bachmann, G., et al., Female androgen insufficiency: The Princeton consensus statement on deficiency, classification, and assessment, *Fertil Steril* 2002; 77(4):660–65.

14. Davis, S., et al., Testosterone influences libido and well-being in women, *Trends Endocrinol Metab* 2001; 2(1):33–37.
15. Ehrenreish, H., et al., Psychoendocrine sequelae of chronic testosterone deficiency, *J Psychiatr Res* 1999; 33(5):379–87.
16. Worboys, S., et al., Evidence that parenteral testosterone therapy may improve endothelium-dependent and -independent vasodilation in postmenopausal women already receiving estrogen, *J Clin Endocrinol Metab* 2001; 86(1):158–61.
17. Rohr, U., The impact of testosterone imbalance on depression and women's health, *Maturitas* 2002; 41(Suppl):S25–S46.
18. Jensen, M., Androgen effect on body composition and fat metabolism, *Mayo Clin Proc* 2000; 75(Suppl):S65–S68.
19. Weitzmann, M., et al., Estrogen deficiency and bone loss: An inflammatory role, *J Clin Invest* 2006; 116(5):1186–94.
20. Bush, T., et al., Preserving cardiovascular benefits of hormone replacement therapy, *J Reprod Med* 2000; 45(3 Suppl):259–73.
21. Chetkowski, R., et al., Biologic effects of transdermal estradiol, *NEJM* 1986; 314:1615–20.
22. Fink, G., et al., Estrogen control of central neurotransmission: Effect on mood, mental state, and memory, *Cell Mol Neurobiol* 1996; 16(3):325–44.
23. Duff, S., et al., A beneficial effect of estrogen on working memory in postmenopausal women taking hormone replacement therapy, *Horm Behav* 2000; 38(4):262–76.
24. Halbreich, U., Role of estrogen in postmenopausal depression, *Neurology* 1997; 48(5 Suppl 7): S16–S20.
25. Inukai, T., et al., Estrogen markedly increases LDL-receptor activity in hypercholesterolemia patients, *J Med* 2000; 32:247–61.
26. Nike, E. and Nakano, M., Estrogens as antioxidants, *Methods Enzymol* 1990; 186:330–33.
27. Pansini, F., et al., Control of carbohydrate metabolism in menopausal women receiving transdermal estrogen therapy, *Ann NY Acad Sci* 1990; 592:460–62.
28. Seely, E., et al., Estradiol with or without progesterone and ambulatory blood pressure in postmenopausal women, *Hypertension* 1999; 33(5):1190–94.
29. Rice, M., et al., Estrogen replacement therapy and cognitive function in postmenopausal women without dementia, *Am J Med* 1997; 103(3A):26S–35S.
30. Puder, J., et al., Estrogen modulates the hypothalamic-pituitary-adrenal and inflammatory cytokine responses to endotoxin in women, *J Clin Endocrinol Metab* 2001; 86(6):2403–8.
31. Steifert-Klauss, V., et al., Progesterone and bone: Actions promoting bone health in women, *J Osteoporos* 2010; 2010:845180.
32. Gruber, D., et al., Progesterone and neurology, *Gynecol Endocrinol* 1999; 13(Suppl 4):41–45.
33. Kalkoff, R., et al., Metabolic effects of progesterone, *J Obstet Gynecol* 1982; 142–46, 735–38.
34. Sumino, H., et al., Hormone replacement therapy decreased insulin resistance and lipoid metabolism in Japanese postmenopausal women with impaired and normal glucose tolerance, *Horm Res* 2003; 60(3):134–42.
35. Stein, D., The case for progesterone, *Ann NY Acad Sci* 2005; 1052:152–59.
36. Rosano, G., et al., Natural progesterone, but not medroxyprogesterone acetate, enhances the beneficial effect of estrogen on exercise-induced myocardial ischemia in post-menopausal women, *J Am Coll Cardiol* 2000; 36:2154–59.
37. Gibbs, R., et al., Estrogen and cognition: Applying preclinical findings to clinical perspectives, *J Neurosci Res* 2003; 74(5):637–43.
38. Hogervorst, E., et al., Serum total testosterone is lower in men with Alzheimer's disease, *Neuro Endocrinol Lett* 2001; 22(3):163–68.
39. Mosekilde, L., et al., The pathogenesis, treatment and prevention of osteoporosis in men, *Drugs* 2013; 73(1):15–29.
40. Ferrucci, L., et al., Designing randomized, controlled trials aimed at preventing or delaying functional decline and disability in fragile, older persons: A consensus report, *J Am Geriatr Soc* 2004; 52(4):625–34.
41. Vandervoort, A., Aging of the human neuromuscular system, *Muscle Nerve* 2002; 25(1):17–25.
42. Gallagher, D., et al., Appendicular skeletal muscle mass: Effects of age, gender, and ethnicity, *J Appl Physiol* 1997; 83(1):229–39.
43. Zinna, E., et al., Exercise treatment to counteract protein wasting of chronic diseases, *Curr Opin Clin Metab Care* 2003; 6(1):87–93.
44. Marcell, T., et al., Comparison of GH, IGF-I, and testosterone with mRNA of receptors and myostatin in skeletal muscle in older men, *Am J Physiol Endocrinol Metab* 2001; 281:E1159–64.

45. Horstman, A., et al., The role of androgens and estrogens on healthy aging and longevity, *J Gerontol A Biol Sci Med Sci* 2012; 67:1140–52.

46. Feldman, H., et al., Age trends in the level of serum testosterone and other hormones in middle-aged men: Longitudinal results from the Massachusetts Male Aging Study, *J Clin Endocrinol Metab* 2002; 87:589–98.

47. Janssen, I., et al., Estimation of skeletal muscle mass by bioelectrical impedance analysis, *J Appl Phys* 2000; 89:465–71.

48. Lexell, J., Distribution of different fiber types in human skeletal muscles: Effects of aging studied in whole muscle cross sections, *Muscle Nerve* 1983; 6:588–95.

49. Malmström, T., et al., Low appendicular skeletal muscle mass (ASM) with limited mobility and poor health outcomes in middle-aged African Americans, *J Cachexia Sarcopenia Muscle* 2013; 4(3):179–86.

50. Galvao, D., et al., Exercise can prevent and even reverse adverse effects of androgen suppression treatment in men with prostate cancer, *Prostate Cancer Prostatic Dis* 2007; 10(4):340–46.

51. Emmelot-Vonk, M., et al., Effect of testosterone supplementation on functional mobility, cognition, and other parameters in older men: A randomized controlled trial, *JAMA* 2008; 299(1):39–52.

52. Bhasin, S., et al., Testosterone effects on the skeletal muscle. In Nieschlag, E., Behre, N. (Eds.) *Testosterone: Action, Deficiency, Substitution*, 3rd Ed., pp. 191–206, Cambridge, UK: Cambridge University Press, 2004.

53. Bhasin, S., et al., Testosterone replacement increase fat-free mass and muscle size in hypogonadal men, *J Clin Endocrinol Metab* 1997; 82:407–13.

54. Brodsky, I., et al., Effects of testosterone replacement on muscle mass and muscle protein synthesis in hypogonadal men: A clinical research center study, *J Clin Endocrinol Metab* 81:3469–75.

55. Snyder, P., et al., Effects of testosterone replacement in hypogonadal men, *J Clin Endocrinol Metab* 2000; 85:2670–77.

56. Wang, C., et al., Transdermal testosterone gel improves sexual function, mood, muscle strength, and body composition parameters in hypogonadal men, *Testosterone Gel Study Group*, *J Clin Endocrinol Metab* 2000; 85:2839–53.

57. Borst, S., Interventions for sarcopenia and muscle weakness in older people, *Age Ageing* 2004; 33:548–55.

58. Mauras, N., et al., Testosterone deficiency in young men: Marked alterations in whole body protein kinetics, strength, and adiposity, *J Clin Endocrinol Metab* 1998; 83:1886–92.

59. Surampudi, P., et al., Hypogonadism in the aging male diagnosis, potential benefits, and risks of testosterone replacement therapy, *Int J Endocrinol* 2012; 2012:625434.

60. Urban, R., et al., Translational studies in older men using testosterone to treat sarcopenia, *Trans Am Clin Climatol Assoc* 2014; 125:27–44.

61. Storer, T., et al., Testosterone dose-dependently increases maximal voluntary strength and leg power, but does not affect fatigability or specific tension, *J Clin Endocrinol Metab* 2003; 88:1478–85.

62. Ferrando, A., et al., Testosterone administration to older men improves muscle function: Molecular and physiological mechanisms, *Am J Physiol Endocrinol Metab* 2002; 282:E601–7.

63. Blackman, M., et al., Growth hormone and sex steroid administration in healthy aged women and men: A randomized controlled trial, *JAMA* 2002; 288:2282–92.

64. Urban, R., et al., Testosterone administration to elderly men increases skeletal muscle strength and protein synthesis, *Am J Physiol* 1995; 269:E820–26.

65. Tenover, J., et al., Effects of testosterone supplementation in the aging male, *J Clin Endocrinol Metab* 1992; 75:1092–98.

66. Rossetti, M., et al., Androgen-mediated regulation of skeletal muscle protein balance, *Mol Cell Endocrinol* 2017; 447:35–49.

67. Fryburg, D., et al., Short-term modulation of the androgen milieu alters pulsatile, but not exercise- or growth hormone (GH)-releasing hormone-stimulated GH secretion in healthy men: Impact of gonadal steroid and GH secretory changes on metabolic outcomes, *J Clin Endocrinol Metab* 1997; 82:3710–19.

68. Ottenbacher, K., et al., Androgen treatment and muscle strength in elderly men: A meta-analysis, *J Am Geriatr Soc* 2006; 54(11):1666–73.

69. Kovacheva, E., et al., Testosterone supplementation reverses sarcopenia in aging through regulation of myostatin, c-Jun NH2-terminal kinase, Notch, and Akt signaling pathways, *Endocrinology* 2010; 151(2):628–38.

70. Roubenoff, R., et al., Sarcopenia current concepts, *J Gerontol A Biol Sci Med Sci* 2000; 55:M716–24.

71. Perry, H., et al., Testosterone and leptin in older African-American men: Relationship to age, strength, function and season, *Metabolism* 2000; 49:1085–91.

72. Rolland, Y., et al., Loss of appendicular muscle mass and loss of muscle strength in young postmenopausal women, *J Gerontol A Biol Sci Med Sci* 2007; 62(3):330–35.

73. Dionne, I., et al., Sarcopenia and muscle function during menopause and hormone-replacement therapy, *J Nutr Health Aging* 2000; 4(3):156–61.

74. Dillon, E., et al., Hormone treatment and muscle anabolism during aging: Androgens, *Clin Nutr* 2010; 29:697–700.

75. Ettinger, B., Prevention of osteoporosis: Treatment of estradiol deficiency, *Obstet Gynecol* 1998; 72(5 Suppl):12S–17S.

76. Fitzpatrick, L., Estrogen therapy for postmenopausal osteoporosis, *Arg Bras Endocrinol Metabol* 2006; 50(4):705–19.

77. Krum, S., et al., Unraveling estrogens action in osteoporosis, *Cell Cycle* 2008; 7(10):1348–52.

78. Winding, B., et al., Effect of estrogen and progesterone on bone. In Fraser, I. (Ed.) *Estrogens and Progestogens in Clinical Practice*, Chapter 18, New York: Churchill/Livingstone, 2000.

79. Ralston, S., Analysis of gene expression in human bone biopsies by polymerase chain reaction: Evidence for enhanced cytokine expression in postmenopausal osteoporosis, *J Bone Min Res* 1994; 9:883–90.

80. McKane W., et al., Circulating levels of cytokines that modulate bone resorption: Effect of age and menopause in women, *J Bone Min Res* 1994; 9:1313–18.

81. Oursler, M., et al., Estrogen modulation of avian osteoclast lysosomal gene expression, *Endocrinology* 1993; 132:1373–80.

82. Pederson, I., et al., Evidence of a correlation of estrogen receptor level and avian osteoclast estrogen responsiveness, *J Bone Min Res* 1997; 12:742–52.

83. Manolagas, S., et al., Estrogen, cytokines and the control of osteoclast formation and bone resorption in vitro and in vivo, *Osteoporos Int* 1993; 3:114–16.

84. Kaji, H., et al., Estrogen blocks parathyroid hormone (PTH)-stimulated osteoclast-like cell formation by selectively affecting PTH-responsive cyclic adenosine monophosphate pathway, *Endocrinology* 1996; 137:2217–24.

85. Benz, D., et al., Estrogen binding and estrogenic responses in normal human osteoblast-like cells, *J Bone Min Res* 1991; 6:531–41.

86. Verhaar, H., et al., A comparison of the action of progestins and estrogen on the growth and differentiation of normal adult human osteoblast-like cells in vitro, *Bone* 1994; 15:307–11.

87. Komm, B., et al., Estrogen binding, receptor mRNA and biologic response in osteoblast-like osteosarcoma cells, *Science* 1988; 241:8–4.

88. Basu, S., et al., Association between oxidative stress and bone mineral density, *Biochem Biophys Res Commun* 2001; 288:275–79.

89. Maggio, D., et al., Marked decrease in plasma antioxidants in aged osteoporotic women: Results of a cross-sectional study, *J Clin Endocrinol Metab* 2003; 88:1523–27.

90. Ibid., Girasole.

91. Ibid., Kassem.

92. Passeri, G., et al., Increased interleukin-6 production by murine bone marrow and bone cells after estrogen withdrawal, *Endocrinology* 1993; 133:822–28.

93. Jika, R., et al., Increased osteoclast development after estrogen loss, mediation by interleukin-6, *Science* 1992; 257:88–91.

94. Hassager, C., et al., Effect of the menopause and hormone replacement therapy on the carboxy-terminal pyridinoline cross-linked telopeptide of type I collagen, *Osteoporos Int* 1994; 4:349–52.

95. Bonde, M., et al., Applications of an enzyme immunoassay for a new marker of bone resorption (CrossLaps): Follow-up on hormone replacement therapy and osteoporosis risk assessment, *J Clin Endocrinol Metab* 1995; 80:864–68.

96. Christiansen, C. et al., Bone mass in postmenopausal women after withdrawal of oestrogen/gestagen replacement, *Lancet* 1981; 1:459–62.

97. Gotfredsen, A., Bone changes occurring spontaneously and caused by oestrogen in early postmenopausal women: A local or generalized phenomenon? *Br Med J* 1986; 292:1098–110.

98. Canderelli, R., et al., Benefits of hormone replacement therapy in postmenopausal women, *J Am Acad Nurse Pract* 2007; 119(12):635–41.

99. Oursler, M., et al., Avian osteoclasts as estrogen target cells, *Proc Natl Acad Sci USA* 1991; 88:6613–17.

100. Eriksen E., et al., Evidence of estrogen receptors in normal human osteoblast-like cells, *Science* 1988; 241:84–86.

101. Christiansen, C., Prevention and treatment of osteoporosis with hormone replacement therapy, *Menopausal Stud* 1993; 38(Suppl 1):45–54.

102. Wells, G., et al., Meta-analysis of the efficacy of hormone replacement therapy in treating and preventing osteoporosis in postmenopausal women, *Endocr Res* 2002; 23:529–39.
103. Christiansen, C., et al., Uncoupling of bone formation and resorption by combined oestrogen and progestogen therapy in postmenopausal osteoporosis, *Lancet* 1985; 2:800–1.
104. Gallagher, J., et al., Effects of oestrogen and progestogen therapy on calcium metabolism in postmenopausal women, *Front Horm Res* 1975; 3:150–76.
105. Scheven, B., et al., Stimulatory effects of estrogen and progesterone on proliferation and differentiation of normal human osteoblast-like cells in vitro, *Biochem Biophys Res Comm* 1992; 186(1):54–60.
106. Prior, J., Progesterone as a bone-trophic hormone, *Endocr Rev* 1990; 11(2):386–98.
107. Notelovitz, M., Androgen effects on bone and muscle, *Fertil Steril* 2007; 77(Suppl 4):S34–41.
108. Vanderschueren, D., et al., Androgens and bone, *Endocr Rev* 2004; 25(3):389–425.
109. Hannan, M., et al., Risk factors for longitudinal bone loss in elderly men and women: The Framingham Osteoporosis Study, *J Bone Min Res* 2000; 15(4):710–20.
110. Khosla, S., Update in male osteoporosis, *J Clin Endocrinol Metab* 2010; 95(1):3–10.
111. Melton, L., et al., Perspective. How many women have osteoporosis? *J Bone Min Res* 1992; 7(9):1005–10.
112. Tuck, S., et al., Testosterone, bone and osteoporosis, *Front Horm Res* 2009; 37:123–32.
113. Ducharme, N., Male osteoporosis, *Clin Geriatr Med* 2010; 26(2):301–9.
114. Gruntmanis U., Male osteoporosis: Deadly, but ignored, *Am J Med Sci* 2007; 333:85–92.
115. Drake, M., et al., Male osteoporosis, *Endocrinol Metab Clin North Am* 2012; 41(3):629–41.
116. Ibid., Eastell.
117. Zitzmann, M., et al., Monitoring bone density in hypogonadal men by quantitative phalangeal ultrasound, *Bone* 2002; 31:422–29.
118. Slemenda, C., et al., Sex steroids and bone mineral density in older women and men: The Rancho Bernardo Study, *J Bone Min Res* 1997; 12(11):1833–43.
119. Zitzmann, M., et al., Androgens and bone metabolism. In Nieschlag, E., Behre, N., (Eds.) *Testosterone: Action, Deficiency, Substitution*, 3rd Ed., Cambridge, UK: Cambridge University Press, 2004.
120. Colvard, D., et al., Identification of androgen receptors in normal human osteoblast-like cells, *Proc Natl Acad Sci USA* 1989; 86:854–57.
121. Liegibel, U., et al., Concerted action of androgens and mechanical strain shifts bone metabolism from high turnover into an osteoanabolic mode, *J Exp Med* 2002; 196:1387–92.
122. Khosla, S., Minireview: The OPG/RANKL/RANK system, *Endocrinology* 2001; 142:5050–55.
123. Huber, D., et al., Androgens suppress osteoclast formation induced by RANKL and macrophage-colony stimulating factor, *Endocrinology* 2001; 142:3800–8.
124. Hofbauer, L., et al., The anti-androgen hydroxyflutamide and androgens inhibit interleukin-6 production by an androgen-responsive human osteoblastic cell line, *J Bone Min Res* 1999; 14:1330–37.
125. Pilbeam, C., et al., Effects of androgens on parathyroid hormone and interleukin-1-stimulated prostaglandin production in cultured neonatal mouse calvariae, *J Bone Min Res* 1990; 5:1183–88.
126. Foresta, C., et al., Testosterone and calcitonin plasma levels in hypogonadal osteoporotic young men, *J Endocrinol Invest* 1985; 8:377–79.
127. Bondanelli, M., et al., Activation of the somatotropic axis by testosterone in adult men: Evidence for a role of hypothalamic growth hormone-releasing hormone, *Neuroendocrinology* 2003; 77:380–87.
128. Monson, J., Long-term experience with GH replacement therapy: Efficacy and safety, *Eur J Endocrinol* 2003; 148:S9–S14.
129. Wang, C., et al., Effects of transdermal testosterone gel on bone turnover markers and bone mineral density in hypogonadal men, *Clin Endocrinol (Oxf.)* 2001; 54:739–50.
130. Katznelson, L., et al., Increase in bone density and lean body mass during testosterone administration in men with acquired hypogonadism, *J Clin Endocrinol Metab* 1996; 81:4358–65.
131. Ibid., Slemanda.
132. Center, J., et al., Hormonal and biochemical parameters in the determination of osteoporosis in elderly men, *J Clin Endocrinol Metab* 1999; 84(1):3626–35.
133. Amin, S., et al., Association of hypogonadism and estradiol levels with bone mineral density in elderly men from the Framingham study, *Ann Inter Med* 2000; 133(12):951–63.
134. Szulc, P., et al., Bioavailable estradiol may be an important determinant of osteoporosis in men: The MINOS study, *J Clin Endocrinol Metab* 2001; 86(1):192–99.
135. Khosala, S., et al., Relationship of serum sex steroid levels to longitudinal changes in bone density in young versus elderly men, *J Clin Endocrinol Metab* 2001; (8698):3555–51.
136. Falahati-Nini, A., et al., Relative contributions of testosterone and estrogen in regulating bone resorption and formation in normal elderly men, *J Clin Invest* 2000; 106:1553–60.

137. Komm, B., et al., Estrogen binding receptor mRNA, and biologic response in osteoblast-like osteosarcoma cells, *Science* 1988; 241:81–84.

138. Oursler, M., et al., Human giant cell tumors of the bone (osteoclastomas) are estrogen target cells, *Proc Natl Acad Sci USA* 1994; 91:5227–31.

139. Braidman, I., et al., Preliminary evidence for impaired estrogen receptor-protein expression in osteoblasts and osteocytes from men with idiopathic osteoporosis, *Bone* 2000; 26:423–27.

140. Cetin, A., et al., Predictors of bone mineral density in healthy males, *Rheumatol Int* 2001; 21:85–88.

15 Treating the Dysmetabolism Underlying Osteoporosis

Xaviour Walker, MD, MPH, DTMH and Joseph Lamb, MD

INTRODUCTION

Osteoporosis, literally "porous bone," is defined as a reduction in the mass and quality of bone and/or the presence of a fragility fracture. Osteoporosis can be a clinically silent systemic skeletal disease characterized by compromised bone strength, predisposing to an increased risk of fracture. Osteoporosis is common, preventable when diagnosed early, and serious though treatable. This chapter presents the pathophysiology of osteoporosis to guide clinicians to early diagnosis and metabolic interventions.

Three lines of reasoning lend urgency to early diagnosis of osteoporosis in the setting of orthopedic medicine:

1. Patients with osteoporosis even in its early manifestations are more likely to have trauma or other conditions requiring orthopedic management. In such cases, the preexisting osteoporosis can forestall healing. In the setting of elective surgery, undiagnosed and untreated osteoporosis is a missed opportunity to optimize recovery.
2. Osteoporosis is increasingly recognized as a "lifestyle disease," preventable or ameliorated by appropriate lifestyle choices. As such, bone health needs to be understood in the context of a broad clinical picture involving frailty (sarcopenia and osteoporosis) and metabolic syndromes [1].
3. Understanding patients' pretest probability of having osteoporosis prior to screening with bone density testing is recommended [2]. It is becoming increasingly recognized that bone density is an imperfect and sometimes inadequate surrogate for bone strength. For example, heavy metals such as lead create dense bones which are weaker. Medications prescribed to make bones denser might not be adding to bone strength to the extent previously anticipated. These examples underscore the added importance of thoroughly assessing risk factors for inadequate bone strength presented in this chapter.

PHYSIOLOGY

Bone is a metabolically active endocrine organ with regulatory functions in calcium homeostasis, energy expenditure, and bone and muscle remodeling. The organic component of bone consists of a cellular component and the extracellular cartilage matrix that is the scaffolding for mineralization. The strength of bone is determined by both bone quality and bone density. Bone quality is a measure of the functional status of the organic matrix and is often a significant determinant of fracture risk [3]. Bone density is a function of the adequacy of mineralization.

Bone mineralization is regulated primarily by the activity of three cell types, osteoclasts with bone reabsorption, osteoblasts involved in bone formation, and osteocytes, which act as mechanosensors and orchestrators of the bone remodeling process. These processes are under both local (e.g. cytokines and growth factors) and systemic (e.g. estrogens and calcitonin) control, which work together for bone homeostasis. These bone cells respond to changing environmental stimuli such as nutrient availability, hormonal messaging, inflammation, and physiological demands. Mechanical loading is one such physiologic demand, modulated by the osteocyte through a complex array of cell signaling pathways. The mechanical message is transformed into altered gene expression resulting in proliferation and matrix synthesis. This message leads to upregulation of growth factors including insulin-like growth factor 1 (IGF-1), vascular endothelial growth factors, and bone morphogenetic proteins (BMP) 2 and 4 [4].

The bone remodeling cycle has three consecutive phases: reabsorption, where osteoclasts digest old bone, over two to four weeks; reversal, when mononuclear cells appear on the bone surface; and finally, formation, when over two to four months new bone is made by osteoblasts until the reabsorbed bone is replaced [5, 6]. Activated osteoclasts reabsorb bone and are regulated by several hormones, including parathyroid hormone (PTH), calcitonin from the thyroid, and growth factor interleukin 6. The activity of osteoclasts is also mediated by osteoprotegerin (OPG) and the receptor-activator of nuclear factor-κB ligand (RANKL) [5, 6]. RANKL, a member of the tumor necrosis (TNF) cytokine family, induces the formation of osteoclasts by binding the receptor-activator of NFKappaB (RANK) to osteoclast precursors. OPG, also a member of TNF cytokine family, can also bind to RANKL and inhibits the binding of RANK to RANKL and therefore the differentiation and reabsorption of osteoclasts [6].

A broad range of cell surface receptors and intercellular skeletal structures including those in the extracellular matrix and the cellular cytoskeleton (integrins, cadherins, and Ca^{+2} channels), intracellular signaling kinases, prostaglandins, and nitric oxide are intimately involved in the regulation of matrix secretion and mineralization [4]. Many of the messengers involved in mediating bone growth are intimately involved in inflammatory signaling pathways. The interplay of these messages is complex and bidirectional. Many growth factors influence osteoblast formation. Core binding Factor A1 (CBFA1) is a transcription factor expressed in osteoblast progenitors and stromal support cells that has been shown to be important in the control of osteoblast development. It regulates the expression of several osteoblast-specific genes including type 1 collagen, the receptor-activator of NFKappaB (RANK) ligand also called the osteoclast differentiation factor, osteocalcin, osteopontin, and bone sialoprotein.

In addition to the cell-mediated local control, several hormones provide system-wide oversight of bone metabolism. Both parathyroid hormone (PTH) and 1,25-dihydroxy-vitamin D_3 directly modulate osteoclastic activity to maintain appropriate serum calcium and phosphorus levels. Estrogen influences bone metabolism. Deficiency increases bone remodeling intensity, which exacerbates propensity to bone resorption in functionally challenged bone and contributes to the development of primary osteoporosis in peri-menopausal women. Testosterone deficiency has also been shown to be associated with osteoporosis [7]. Intervention trials have demonstrated that supplementation with estrogen in women, DHEA in men and women, and testosterone in hypogonadal men is effective.

The interaction of local cells, communicating by growth factors and cytokines and modulated by systemic hormones, and simultaneously modulating basic energy regulation and body composition, is the healthy norm of bone metabolism. Osteoporosis is the pathophysiologic disturbance of this process.

Nutrients obtained primarily in our diet are biology's building blocks to erect strong bone. Table 15.1 lists these nutrients and the required intake in the absence of disease.

PATHOPHYSIOLOGY

As we explore the pathophysiology of osteoporosis, we find that underlying mechanisms rather than broad organ system classifications may cast more light on the underlying causes of osteoporosis. These broad mechanistic categories include diminished achievement of peak bone mass, decreased mineral availability, decreased osteoblast activity, increased osteoclast activity, abnormal protein metabolism, and systemic inflammation.

Indeed, much research over the last decade has demonstrated that inflammatory cytokines (RANKL, OPG, IL-6) and energy regulatory signaling (Insulin, IGF-1, and OC) are integral to the

TABLE 15.1
Key Bone-Building Nutrients

Nutrient	Adult RDA or AI	Common Therapeutic Range for Bone Health*	Dietary Considerations
Calcium	1,000–1,300 mg	1,000–1,500 mg	Typical diet is inadequate, averages approximately 800 mg, with lower intake in men, ethnic minorities, and people with low social income [8, 9]
Phosphorus	700 mg	700–1,200 mg	Inadequate intake is rare except in the elderly and malnourished; excessive intake is common with the use of processed foods and soft drinks [10, 11]
Magnesium	420 mg men 320 mg women	400–800 mg	On average magnesium intake is inadequate, with lower intake in African Americans, elderly, and women compared with men [12]
Fluoride	4.0 mg men 3.0 mg women –	—	Fluoride overdose has occurred through ingestion of fluoride toothpaste and high fluoride waters [13]
Silica	No values yet set	5–20 mg	Intake is unknown. Silica is removed in food processing, current intake is suspected to be low
Zinc	11 mg men 8 mg women	20–30 mg	Marginal zinc deficiency is common, especially among the elderly [14]
Manganese	2.3 mg men 1.8 mg women	10–25 mg	Intakes are variable but on the lower end of recommended, from 0.5 to 5.3 mg/day [15]
Copper	900 mcg men and women	2–3 mg	Daily intake average for men is 1.3 mcg and women 1.0, with lower intake in the elderly [14]
Boron	No RDA established	3–4 mg	Average intake for men is 1.1 mg and for women 0.9 mg, optimal intake is considered 3 mg [16]
Potassium	4,700 mg men and women	4,700–5,000 mg	Adult intake averages 2,300 mg for women and 3,100 mg for men [17]
Vitamin D	600-until age 70; then 800 IU, men and women	1,000–2,000 IU & up as needed	Deficiency is common especially among the elderly, dark skinned, and those with little UV sunlight exposure
Vitamin C	90 mg men 75 mg women	Oral 500 mg–to bowel tolerance as needed	Average daily intake is about 84 mg for women and 105 for men [18]
Vitamin A	900 mcg men 700 mcg adult women	3000 mcg/day or less	Highest median intake for any gender and life stage is 895 mcg/day [19]
Vitamin B_6	1.7 mg men 1.5 mg women	25–50 mg	Studies indicate widespread inadequate vitamin B_6 consumption among all sectors of the population [20]
Folic Acid	400 mcg men and women	800–1,000 mcg	Inadequate intake was common among all age groups, but is improving with food fortification [21]
Vitamin K	120 mcg men 90 mcg women	1,000 mcg	The average intake for women is 122 mcg and men 138 mcg, those at risk for vitamin K deficiency are newborns not treated with vitamin K at birth and those with malabsorption [22]
Vitamin B_{12}	2.4 mg men and women	100–1,000 mcg	Most people have adequate B12 from their dietary intake, although older people and vegans are at risk of deficiency, which has improved with fortified foods [23]

(Continued)

TABLE 15.1 (CONTINUED)
Key Bone-Building Nutrients

Nutrient	Adult RDA or AI	Common Therapeutic Range for Bone Health*	Dietary Considerations
Fats	Should comprise 7% of calories minimum, General recommendation is not to exceed 30% of calories	20%–30% of total calories is perhaps more ideal	The average American consumes 33% of his/her calories in fat [24]. The consumption of essential fatty acids, however, is frequently inadequate [25]

Note: Table 15.1 highlights key nutrients in food, their recommended dietary allowance (RDA) or adequate intake (AI), the common therapeutic range that is recommended for bone health, and information on dietary considerations. The authors acknowledge Susan Brown, PhD who authored the table for this book's first edition.

balance of bone resorption and formation. And while estrogen deficiency has been recognized as a cause of osteoporosis, it may do so not only as a deficiency of a growth factor but as a consequence of increasing systemic inflammation associated with increased IL-6 levels [26–28]. RANKL and its downstream cytokines have important roles in bone, metabolic and vascular disease [29].

In a clinical setting, it may be helpful to classify osteoporosis as primary or secondary. In a postmenopausal woman, estrogen deficiency results in primary osteoporosis. Whereas suppressed estrogen levels due to an adolescent girl receiving a GnRH agonist as contraception or a premenopausal woman receiving chemotherapy for breast cancer often lead to secondary osteoporosis. Secondary osteoporosis occurs in patients who are less likely to be screened for the disease because they may not present as a prototypic osteoporosis patient. Recognizing the pathophysiology of secondary osteoporosis (Table 15.1) increases "clinical suspicion" and offers the opportunity to intervene earlier.

DETERMINANTS OF PEAK BONE MASS

Peak Bone Mass (PBM) is an essential factor in preventing osteoporosis, with an increase of PBM of 10% (one standard deviation) considered to reduce the fracture risk by 50%. PBM has been defined as "the amount of bone acquired when accrual ceases or plateaus at some point after the completion of growth and development" [30]. The greatest gains in bone mass occur during and after adolescent growth spurt in females aged 11–13 years and in males aged 14–17 years; increases in bone mass continue with PBM normally achieved late in the second decade or early in the third decade of life [31, 32]. Osteoporosis does have a strong genetic and hereditability component, contributing 60–80% to PBM [30, 33]. A recent review identified 56 loci associated with bone mineral density (BMD), 14 loci associated with osteoporotic fracture and other genetic determinants of BMD including vitamin D receptor, LDL receptor protein and collagen 1 alpha [30]. Acquisitional osteopenia is the failure to achieve the genetically determined peak bone mass and can be the result of chronic illness, use of certain medications, malnutrition, malabsorption, or the disruption of key metabolic pathways [34–36].

Failure to attain peak bone mass can be caused by:

- *Neonatal factors*, of which gestational age is the most important affecting BMD, as the majority of fetal bone is gained in the third trimester. Other factors include environmental, with winter months associated with lower vitamin D levels, and possibly maternal smoking, alcohol, caffeine intake, and diabetes mellitus [37].

- *Early life nutrition*, has been demonstrated to be associated with bone development [37]. Prospective studies show that there is likely not an association with breastfed children and bone mass [38, 39].
- *Adolescent eating disorders*, including both anorexia and bulimia, are medical conditions that have serious risks for developing osteopenia and osteoporosis. Anorexia nervosa purge/bingeing type being the most significant with over 50% of patients developing osteopenia and 20% osteoporosis [40]. In addition to decreased mineral and protein availability because of insufficient intake, contributing factors to osteoporosis include amenorrhea, and calcium and vitamin D deficiency, increased endogenous steroid production, and low levels of growth factors including IGF. In these patients, nutritional rehabilitation with weight gain, adequate calcium and vitamin D intake, moderate weight-bearing exercise, and resumption of normal menses has been shown to improve but not normalize bone mineral density [41].
- *Depo-Provera as contraception* produces estrogen deficiency. Adolescent females who use Depo-Provera are at risk for low bone mass due to failure to achieve peak bone mass [33, 42]. Although weight gain and calcium supplementation may reduce some risk, caution should be given to the use of Depo-Provera in adolescents, as the effects on skeletal health may not be fully reversible [33].
- *Lead exposure* may be a risk factor for osteoporosis, there has been an inverse association in lead exposure and BMD in white subjects using NHANES survey data, although causality cannot be established [43].

DECREASED MINERAL AVAILABILITY

- *Inflammatory bowel disease (IBD)* is associated with a high prevalence of both osteopenia and osteoporosis. Risk factors include the use of corticosteroids, malnutrition, low BMI, malabsorption of vitamin D, calcium and vitamin K, immobilization, and chronic inflammatory state with an imbalance of the RANK-RANKL-OPG system [44]. Therefore effective disease management including calcium and vitamin D supplementation, risk factor reduction, and avoidance of glucocorticoids are equally important aspects of treatment [44, 45].
- *Primary biliary cirrhosis* (PBC) is an autoimmune liver condition that mainly affects women and is associated with high rates (20%–50%) of osteoporosis. Although the exact mechanism is not clear, hormone imbalance, genetics, and cholestasis may contribute [46, 47]. Although vitamin D and K, fat-soluble vitamins have been implicated, many patients have normal vitamin D levels and replacing D and K has not shown to make an improvement on BMD [46].
- *Lactase deficiency* appears to be associated with the development of osteoporosis, through reduced calcium intake (patients avoiding milk and dairy products) and possibly through effecting calcium absorption [48].
- *Morbid obesity* has historically been viewed as having a protective effect against the development of BMD, mainly through increased mechanical load increasing BMD. However, recent research has revealed that many obese individuals have inadequate nutrition status, vitamin D deficiency, elevated parathyroid hormone levels, and are at risk for low bone mass [49].
- Postoperatively, *bariatric surgery* patients experiencing significant weight loss, severely restricted oral intake, calcium malabsorption, and concomitant vitamin D deficiency are at extremely high risk for the development of metabolic bone disease (MBD). Several factors are likely involved. Primarily, malabsorption plays a critical role with malabsorption of calcium, magnesium, fat-soluble vitamins including vitamin D, protein, B_{12}, and folic acid all being reported. Essentially all *post-gastrectomy patients* have an increased risk of

fracture and should be routinely evaluated for the presence of MBD and have had reported higher rates of osteomalacia and osteoporosis [50].

- *Gastric hypoacidity* because of atrophy, proton-pump inhibitors, and H_2 blockers is implicated in mineral malabsorption. Gastroesophageal reflux disease (GERD) does not share a causal relationship with MBD. Long-term use of proton-pump inhibitors has been shown to be associated with increased risk for fractures and osteoporosis [51].
- *High sodium intake* produces a calciuretic effect but investigations attempting to define the association of sodium with bone loss and BMD have produced conflicting results [52].
- *Caffeine* is known to increase urinary calcium losses and may reduce absorption of calcium. A prospective study demonstrated that drinking more than 330 mg caffeine day (4 cups of coffee) and having low calcium intake may be associated with osteoporotic fracture [53].
- *High protein diet* has been shown in a randomized trial not to affect urinary calcium excretion or skeletal changes [54]. However, it has been recommended to avoid very high protein diets (more than 2.0 g/Kg body weight/day) when associated with low calcium intake (less than 600 mg calcium/body weight/day) [55].
- *Phosphorus* is plentiful in the food supply predominantly due to the increased use of phosphate salts in food additives and cola beverages. Excessive phosphate intake associated with low calcium intake has been considered to be detrimental to bone health [56]. A large study examining carbonated beverages in children and adolescents found that they were associated with deceased bone mineral density but these subjects also had low protein intake [57].
- *Hypovitaminosis D* interferes with absorption of calcium. Vitamin D plays a role both in intestinal adsorption of calcium as well modifying the speed of bone turnover. Vitamin D is essential for calcium and phosphate absorption in the gut, stimulation of osteoblast activity, calcium reabsorption in the renal tubules, and normal bone mineralization throughout the life span. Absorption of vitamin D occurs mainly by passive diffusion in the proximal and mid small intestine and is highly dependent on bile salts [34].

DECREASED OSTEOBLAST ACTIVITY

- *Diabetes mellitus* (DM) is associated with increased fracture risk. Although in type 2 diabetes mellitus, BMD is normal or high, there is reduced bone strength due to microarchitectural bone changes. With type 1 diabetes mellitus, the lack of insulin, which stimulates osteoblasts, and insulin-like growth factor-1 (IGF-1) leads to lower peak bone mass. In diabetes mellitus, there is increased serum osteroprotegerin (OPG), which prevents RANKL binding resulting in suppression of osteoclastogenesis thus inhibiting remodeling and repair [58].
- *Tobacco use* has direct toxic effects on osteoblasts and also acts indirectly by modifying estrogen metabolism. Cigarette smokers on average reach menopause earlier than nonsmokers [59]. Tobacco abuse also leads to an increase in illnesses and earlier frailty by decreasing exercise capacity and increasing the likelihood of requiring corticosteroids for treatment of pulmonary diseases.
- Excessive *alcohol use* has been shown to decrease osteoblast activity. However, a non-linear relationship has been shown between alcohol consumption and hip fracture with light alcohol consumption a lower fracture risk (less than 12.5 g/day or 1.25 standard drink) [60]. Higher consumption, especially in men, however, increased the rate of fracture, perhaps related to increased falls or nutritional compromise related to alcohol abuse. Daily alcohol consumption of 50 g (approximately three standard drinks) results in a dose-dependent decrease in osteoblast activity; daily consumption of greater than 100 g eventually results in an osteopenic skeleton and an increased risk for the development of osteoporosis [61].

One drink per day for women and two drinks per day for men is the recommended safe upper limit for consumption.

- *Corticosteroid excess*, whether exogenous or endogenous, can result in deleterious effects on healthy bone. Glucocorticoid-induced osteoporosis is the most common cause of secondary osteoporosis and the first cause before 50 years [62]. Even at low doses of prednisone (5 mg daily), there is a decrease in serum P1NP and osteocalcin levels, which are markers of bone formation; with the changes reversed on discontinuation of prednisone [63]. At high doses, glucocorticoids dramatically decrease bone formation rate, decrease osteoblast numbers, and osteocyte numbers and activity [62]. There is also an increase in the expression of RANKL and decrease in OPG, which, in turn, increases the lifespan of osteoclastic cells [62]. Glucocorticoids suppress 1-hydroxylase activity and function as a 1,25(OH)D antagonist thereby blunting calcium absorption [34]. Glucocorticoids decrease sex hormones, inducing bone absorption and myopathy, therefore increasing the risk of falls. Patients on glucocorticoids have a two-fold increase risk for fractures, with the risk of vertebral fractures higher as glucocorticoids reduce BMD more in the trabecular (e.g. spine) than the cortical bone (e.g. femur) [64]. There is an alteration in bone quality as a patient on glucocorticoids with a similar BMD as a patient not on glucocorticoids will have a higher fracture risk. The cumulative dose of glucocorticoids correlates with the severity of the bone disease and the incidence of fracture. Of note, patients maintained on corticosteroid replacement due to adrenal insufficiency do not appear to be at increased risk [34]. The diagnosis of osteoporosis can be the presenting symptom of Cushing's disease. Patients with Cushing's disease have a 30% to nearly 70% increased risk of fractures [65]. Persistent physical and psychological stress can induce endogenous corticosteroids excess and increase BMD losses. Depression has been associated with elevated cortisol levels [66].

INCREASED OSTEOCLAST ACTIVITY

- In *hyperparathyroidism*, parathyroid hormone (PTH) stimulates a release of calcium from bone by an increase in osteoclast activity. It does so by increasing activation of 25-hydroxy vitamin D_3 to 1.25-dihydroxy vitamin D_3 which increases bone resorption. Primary hyperparathyroidism is frequently a consequence of a benign adenoma, yet may also be caused by a malignant tumor. In secondary hyperparathyroidism, the major causes are vitamin D deficiency and chronic kidney disease. Secondary hyperparathyroidism is the response to a lowered serum calcium level resulting in an increase in PTH levels and increased bone resorption. Consequences of hyperparathyroidism include hypercalciuria, hypercalcemia, hypophosphatemia, osteopenia/osteoporosis, osteomalacia, and kidney stones [67, 68].
- Postmenopausal *estrogen deficiency* and other *hypogondal states*, both primary and secondary are associated with osteoporosis. Estrogen deficiency increases the population of pre-B cells, a subset of bone marrow stromal cells, which in turn increases production of IL-1 and TNFα. These cytokines induce cyclo-oxygenase 2 activity increasing prostaglandin E_2 production by osteoblasts and a subsequent increase in RANKL expression and resultant osteoclastogenesis [69]. Many cancer therapies for breast, ovarian, and prostate cancer patients produce hypogonadal states. Tamoxifen has been shown to produce osteoporosis in premenopausal women. Aromatase inhibitors and GnRH agonists also produce estrogen deficiency. Estrogen deficiency may also be associated with the genetic hypogonadal states such as Turner's syndrome.
- Mature osteocytes, by sensing the mechanical forces exerted on bone by physical activity, directly influence bone remodeling. Conditions, including *inactivity, immobilization, spinal cord injury* and *sarcopenia*, that decrease these forces will have a negative effect on bone strength. Physical immobilization after trauma or due to neural damage due to cerebrovascular accident, poliomyelitis, and multiple sclerosis has been associated with

osteoporosis. A reduction in compressive mechanical forces because of immobilization reduces the canalicular fluid flow in bone with resultant osteocyte hypoxemia and death, leading to increased osteoclast activity [70]. Spinal cord injury (SCI) patients almost all develop osteopenia and osteoporosis with an increased rate of fracture. Along with the reduction of mechanical loading, the factors involved with the development of osteoporosis in SCI patients are complex. These include poor nutritional status, hypercortisolism, disordered vasoregulation, and changes in gonadal function [71].

- *Hyperthyroidism* is associated with both increased osteoblastic and osteoclastic activities. Resorption is favored overall, however, as increased formation cannot keep pace with increased resorption. The overall effect on bone homestasis of hyperkalemia, hyperphosphatemia, raised alkaline phosphate and reduced BMD [72]. Treatment of thyrotoxicosis has been shown to increase bone density but fails to restore BMD to healthy norms. The effect of exogenous subclinical hyperthyroidism on BMD in women is unclear with mixed reports of normal and decreased BMD [73]. However, a small uncontrolled case series, following women treated for thyroid hormone resistance, revealed increased BMD with thyroid hormone supplementation [74].

- *Cadmium exposure*, which is a toxic metal commonly found in industrial workplaces, in chronic low doses has been associated with the development of osteoporosis [75, 76]. Long-term cadmium exposure causes tubular renal dysfunction and increased urinary excretion of calcium [76]. Historically, there was mass cadmium poisoning due to mining in the Toyama Prefecture, Japan, which caused severe osteomalacia and osteoporosis, with the term *itai-itai* disease coined by locals for the severe pains in spine and joints [75].

IMPAIRED PROTEIN METABOLISM

- *Protein-calorie malnutrition* (PCM) occurs as a result of many chronic diseases and left uncorrected, results in MBD. Protein intake helps provide the structural matrix of bone, optimize levels of IGF-1, an important hormone in bone metabolism, and also is reported to increase urinary calcium and intestinal calcium absorption [77]. In the NHANES 1 study, hip fractures were associated with low energy intake, low serum albumin, and decreased muscle strength; all reflecting protein and caloric deficit [78]. A 10% decrease in body weight typically results in a 1%–2% bone loss, and more severe weight loss and malnutrition are considered risk factors for osteoporosis which is likely due to low protein intake [79]. Although high-protein diets have been shown to increase urinary calcium losses, there have been mixed study findings on the long-term effects on BMD [77]. Conversely, a low protein diet has been found to be related to low bone mass and increased fracture risk [77]. In two interventional trials examining graded levels of protein intake on calcium homeostasis, decreased calcium absorption and an acute rise in PTH were noted by day four of the 0.7 and 0.8 g/kg diets but not during the 0.9 or 1.0 g/kg diets [80, 81].

- *Cushing's syndrome* whether primary or secondary to exogenous long-term administration of glucocorticoids can cause decreased deposition of protein throughout the body in addition to increasing protein catabolism.

- Increasing *age* is marked by decreasing levels of growth hormones and decreased protein anabolic activity.

- *Vitamin C (Ascorbic acid)* is necessary for collagen formation and therefore bone development. Vitamin C deficiency has been associated in some subgroups, although studies are inconsistent, with reduced BMD and increased self-reported fracture risk.

- Osteocalcin in bone matrix preferentially binds *lead* resulting in decreased calcium binding and failure to bind hydroxyapatite, resulting in decreased bone formation [82]. Serum lead levels increase by 25–30% due to mobilization as bone is resorbed in postmenopausal women with osteoporosis contributing to lead toxicity and resultant illnesses late in life [83].

- *Liver Disease.* Cholestatic disease, autoimmune hepatitis, chronic viral hepatitis, and alcoholic liver disease can result in osteoporosis. Approximately 40% of patients with chronic liver disease may experience a fracture [84]. Vitamin D levels are typically low in patients with alcoholic liver disease, autoimmune hepatitis treated with glucocorticoids, and primary biliary cirrhosis, thereby increasing the risk of osteoporosis as well as osteomalacia [84, 85]. Osteoporosis can be one of the first clinical manifestations of cholestatic disease [86, 87]. Advanced chronic cholestatic disorders such as primary sclerosing cholangitis also place the patient at significant risk of developing low bone mass [84, 87].

SYSTEMIC INFLAMMATION

Given the role of inflammatory messengers and cytokines in the cell-to-cell communication vital to the balanced remodeling process, systemic inflammatory diseases with resultant increases in proinflammatory messengers have direct effects on bone leading to increased risk for the development of osteoporosis. These cytokines have been associated with increased osteoclastogenesis in multiple conditions including rheumatoid arthritis, periodontal disease, and multiple myeloma for example. RANKL-induced osteoclastogenesis has been directly implicated in osteoporosis in cell-culture work [88] and clinical work [89]. Denosumab, which is approved by the Food and Drug Administration for the treatment of osteoporosis, is a monoclonal antibody to RANKL [90]. Evidence exists that protection against inflammation and oxidative stress offered by hydroxyl methylglutaryl CoA reductase inhibitors (the statin class of cholesterol-lowering agents) may also benefit bone health [91]. A recent meta-analysis demonstrated that hydroxyl methylglutaryl CoA reductase inhibitors increased BMD, but failed to show a decrease in fracture risk [92].

- *Inflammatory bowel disease.* Patients with inflammatory bowel disease (IBD) have a high prevalence of decreased bone mineral density and an increased rate of vertebral fractures. Circulating proinflammatory cytokines increase osteoclast activity. Indeed, TNFα decreases differentiation of osteoblasts, increases differentiation of osteoclasts, and increases osteoclast survival by decreasing apoptosis. High levels of IL-6 have been found in osteoporotic patients suffering from Crohn's disease compared to non-osteoporotic patients and there is an inflammatory state with an imbalance of the RANK-RANKL-OPG system [44].
- *Gluten-sensitive enteropathy (Celiac disease).* Celiac disease is an autoimmune disorder of varying severity characterized by small bowel enteropathy resulting from exposure to wheat gluten in genetically susceptible individuals and is frequently diagnosed in patients presenting with osteoporosis [36]. Auto-antibodies to OPG have been identified in subjects with celiac disease [93].
- Several *chronic diseases of aging* have been noted to be comorbid conditions with osteoporosis. These conditions, including atherosclerosis, osteoarthritis, and periodontal disease, share inflammation as an underlying pathophysiological derangement [94].

UNCERTAIN ETIOLOGIES

- Osteoporosis has been recognized as a complication of *parenteral nutrition* (PN) for more than 25 years and appears to be multifactorial. Early studies found intravenous nutrition solutions to contain excess aluminum, but despite newer formulations that limit this element, osteoporosis continues to occur, likely through suppressing parathyroid hormones and secondary suppression of vitamin D signaling [95]. A longitudinal study conducted in Denmark noted an absence of accelerated bone lost but found the BMD of many long-term PN patients substantially reduced, making them susceptible to fragility fractures and in need of preventive strategies [96].

- *Vitamin A (retinol)* in excess with vitamin D deficiency has been found to be an additional risk for osteoporosis [97]. Although, when vitamin D is maintained at a moderate level of 50–75 nmol/L, vitamin A does not affect BMD [98].

PATIENT EVALUATION

Risk factors for osteoporosis are present in susceptible patients prior to disease manifestation. Table 15.2 organizes these risk factors as commonly encountered in a patient's chart and *medical history*.

- Many commonly used *medications* including serotonin reuptake inhibitors [99], loop diuretics, amiodarone [100], heparin [101], thiazolidinediones [102, 103], methotrexate [104], and antiepileptic drugs [105] have negative impacts on bone health.
- *Bisphosphonates* have been shown to be effective in increasing BMD [106]. However, there have been concerns regarding two uncommon long-term side effects; osteonecrosis of the jaw and atypical fractures [106, 107]. Due to these concerns, it is recommended to have a therapeutic pause of 3–5 years after treatment with bisphosphonates with patients with low risk (minor bone deficiencies and no recent fragility fracture) and moderate risk (moderate bone deficiencies and and/no recent fragility fracture) [107, 108]. New research has shown that the beneficial effects of bisphosphonates can decline after about seven years of use [109].

The *physical exam* also provides opportunities for early detection. Osteoporosis can be identified by using a stadiometer to measure height and monitor for height changes. When height is discordant with prior measured height or the patient's stated height by greater than one inch, this should prompt further evaluation. The FRAX® tool has been developed by the World Health Organization (WHO) to evaluate fracture risk of patients. Based on individual patient models that integrate the risks associated with clinical risk factors as well as bone mineral density (BMD) at the femoral neck, it can assist in making treatment choices for individual patients [110].

Laboratory diagnosis (Table 15.2) can point to modifiable risk factors for osteoporosis, particularly assays for gluten sensitivity and hypovitaminosis D. Gluten sensitivity may be a silent disease and it predisposes to calcium malabsorption. Celiac disease is estimated to be 5–10 fold more common among those with osteoporosis. Asking about bowel habits can provide clues, and utilizing common laboratory assays for gluten antibody (serum or stool anti-gliadin IgG and IgA, anti-transglutaminase IgG and IgA, and anti-endomysial IgG and IgA) can lead to diagnosis of celiac disease. Screening for hypovitaminosis D by checking a serum 25-hydroxyvitamin D (25(OH)D) is indicated in the evaluation of osteoporosis and osteomalacia. Osteomalacia, an abnormal mineralization of cartilage and bone, is most commonly caused by vitamin D deficiency. Vitamin D deficiency can occur as a result of inadequate intake of vitamin D, inadequate exposure to sunlight, or malabsorption syndromes, and is frequently found in patients following gastrectomy, small bowel resection, and bariatric procedures [86, 111]. Unlike osteoporosis, osteomalacia affects primarily cortical bone; therefore, bone densitometry testing (DXA) is unlikely to confirm the diagnosis. Clinically, these patients can present with bone pain and proximal muscle weakness; however, distinguishing osteomalacia from osteoporosis can be difficult. Diagnosis can be guided by clinical presentation and treatment can be guided by biochemical indices including 25(OH)D, calcium, phosphate, bone-specific alkaline phosphatase, parathyroid hormone, and urine calcium and phosphate [34]. However, osteoporosis is underdiagnosed and more frequently found after an osteoporotic fracture [112].

Imaging studies are an important, although not initial, screening tool but are limited by evaluating bone density rather than bone strength. Bone strength is an integration of bone density and bone quality [113]. Central DXA is the most common study used to determine bone density and can be used to evaluate current bone status and risk stratification for future fractures. The World

TABLE 15.2
Common Risk Factors for the Development of Metabolic Bone Disease

Diagnosis
- Anorexia nervosa
- Morbid obesity
- Inflammatory bowel disease
  - Crohn's disease
  - Ulcerative colitis
- Gluten-sensitive enteropathy (Celiac disease)
- Severe liver disease

Current or Previous Medical Interventions
- Glucocorticoid use >3 months or multiple courses
- Antacids containing aluminum
- Excess thyroid hormone
- Methotrexate
- Lithium
- Cholestyramine
- Gonadotropin releasing hormone (GnRH) and agonists
- Anticonvulsants
- Heparin – high dose
- Parenteral nutrition >6 months
- Aromatase inhibitors
- Cyclosporine, tacrolimus, pimecrolimus
- Bisphosphonates
- Proton-pump inhibitors

Surgical History
- Gastrectomy
- Bariatric surgery
- Organ transplant

Medical History
- Female >age 65; Male >age 70
- Fragility fracture(s)
- Post-menopausal
- Early estrogen deficiency (<45 years of age)
- Hypogonadism
- Chronic obstructive pulmonary disease
- Significant weight loss

Family History
- First degree relative with a fragility fracture

Social History
- Cigarette smoking
- Alcohol in excess of two drinks daily
- Little or no physical activity
- Low calcium intake (lifelong)
- Poor dietary habits or chronic dieting
- Cadmium exposure
- Lead exposure

Nutrition History
Insufficient intake or malabsorption:
- Protein-calorie malnutrition & weight loss
- Calcium
- Magnesium
- Vitamin B12
- Vitamin D
- Vitamin K

Excess Intake of:
- Alcohol
- Caffeine
- Phosphorus
- Protein
- Sodium
- Vitamin A (retinol)

Health Organization (WHO) has defined normal bone density, osteopenia, and osteoporosis based on the T-score. DXA results also quantify the standard deviation from that of an age and gender matched control, reported as the Z-score. If bone loss is exclusively due to the normal process of aging, the Z-score will be near zero; therefore, a secondary disease should be suspected when there is a negative deviation of greater than -1.5 [114]. Despite the strengths of DXA as the gold standard radiographic study, screening seems to be most efficacious (cost effective) for white women aged 65 and older and for those women, though younger, who are at similar risk [115, 116]. Given the slow change noted despite efficacious therapy on DEXA scans, follow-up scans at 2 year intervals are not unreasonable.

The use of *biomarkers* including osteocalcin, urinary N-telopeptide of type 1 collagen (NTX), IGF-1, and N-terminal propeptide of type 1 procollagen (P1NP), offer assistance in the diagnosis of osteoporosis, overall bone quality and about efficacy of intervention, although the exact role in clinical practice is still to be determined [117, 118].

TREATMENT

Nutrition and lifestyle changes should be considered as an integral first step in a therapeutic program for osteoporosis. A review of the patient's medical history and individual needs will identify at-risk behavioral, dietary, and nutritional choices. An individualized plan can then be created. Aerobic and resistance exercise are important constituents of a lifestyle program with beneficial changes in osteoporosis, sarcopenia, and insulin resistance [119].

Nutrients should be obtained primarily from a healthful diet. In a carefully crafted nutritional approach, supplements are reserved for nutrients whose level cannot be achieved in the diet either as a consequence of insufficiency in consumed foods or as a consequence of an individual's unique biochemical needs and underlying pathophysiology [120].

Calcium intake should be considered first when building a patient's individualized nutritional plan. Broccoli and leafy greens, such as kale, collards, parsley, and lettuce, are rich in calcium. However, calcium contained in dark leafy greens is often not biologically available due to the presence of phytates that irreversibly bind the calcium and vitamin K. Citrus fruits are a good source of *vitamin C* necessary for collagen formation and of *potassium* which helps regulate calcium absorption. Eating 5–9 servings of fruits and vegetable rich in potassium daily produces a net alkaline load and offsets the net calcium loss induced by the typical American diet's high sodium and acid load [121]. Other sources of potassium are seaweed, nuts and seeds, leafy greens, potatoes, and bananas.

Seaweed, nuts and seeds, and some grains are good sources of *magnesium* which also contributes to the formation of healthy bone. Dried plums (previously referred as prunes) are rich in many nutrients that have been shown to beneficial for bone including fiber, vitamin K, boron, copper, magnesium, and polyphenols, with studies showing a positive effect on bone density in animal models and on bone formation biomarkers in human studies [122]. Onion consumption has been found to be beneficial to BMD in perimenopausal and post-menopausal non-Hispanic white women 50 years or older [123]. *Fiber* is an important component of the alkaline diet. Some forms of fiber can impair mineral absorption, but this is not uniformly the case and a diet high in fiber is recommended. One specific group of fibers found in fruits and vegetables are the inulin-type fructans, a subclass of fructooligosaccharides, which have been shown to improve calcium absorption in adolescents and adults [124]. Fruits and vegetables are also the primary dietary source of boron, a trace element which is beneficial for trabecular bone microarchitecture and cortical bone strength [125].

Caffeine, commonly found in coffee, tea, carbonated soft drinks, and chocolate, can increase urinary excretion of calcium. However, tea drinkers have higher bone density compared to non-drinkers. Research demonstrates that the flavonoids found in tea may offset caffeine's effect and actually increase bone density. Caffeine intake of greater than 300 mg/day has been shown to cause higher spine bone loss in elderly postmenopausal women [126]. The deleterious effects of caffeine on bone can be negated by consuming adequate calcium [127].

The evidence regarding the role of phosphoric acid in *high-phosphate-containing carbonated beverages* is mixed in regards to direct bone effects. Despite the lack of conclusive evidence for the role of phosphoric acid, soft drinks contain minimal calcium and displace calcium-containing beverages from the diet [8, 128]. Cola intake has been associated with low BMD in women [8]. This problem is expected to have a significant impact on the prevalence of osteoporosis in the future as children raised with this habit reach adulthood with acquisitional osteopenia. *Calorie-restriction induced weight loss* has been associated with reductions in BMD while exercise-induced weight loss appears to minimize bone loss [129].

NUTRITIONAL SUPPLEMENTS

The bone-building nutrients presented in Table 15.1 provide a template for dietary nutrient needs. When patients are unable to achieve these goals through diet, especially when nutrient demands change with medications and underlying supplemental medical conditions, nutrients are an effective adjunct. There are numerous over-the-counter and over-the-internet supplements targeting bone health and while many are indeed beneficial, some may be ineffective or indeed detrimental. When choosing nutritional supplements, purchasing products with Good Manufacturing Practice Certification reduces the risk of adulterated or contaminated products.

The Institute of Medicine recommends as the recommended dietary allowances for *calcium*; 1300 mg daily for children ages 9–18 years old; 1,000 mg for men ages 19–70 years old and women ages 19–50 years old; and 1,200 mg for men ages >70 years old and women ages >50 years old [10]. Dietary sources are still considered the best, though the standard diet of western commerce generally falls far short of supplying adequate calcium. In comparing the amount of elementary calcium in the most common calcium preparations, calcium carbonate (40%) and calcium phosphate (21%) have the highest amounts. Calcium citrate has been reported to have slightly higher absorption than calcium carbonate, especially when taken on an empty stomach [130], although other studies have shown that they are of equal bioavailability [131]. The literature supports up to 1800 mg daily for patients who are actively losing weight and for patients who have undergone bariatric surgery [132, 133]. However, there have been recent concerns about possible over supplementation of calcium with an increased risk of cardiovascular disease, therefore, emphasizing the importance of dietary calcium intake and evidence-based use of calcium supplements in the appropriate patients [134].

Epidemiological studies have shown a positive association of *magnesium* with bone density. Magnesium appears to affect bone remodeling and strength, has a positive association with hip BMD in both men and women, and plays an important role in calcium and bone metabolism [135]. Hypomagnesemia blunts parathyroid hormone activity resulting in altered calcium metabolism, hypocalcemia, vitamin D abnormalities, and further decreased jejunal magnesium absorption [136]. Patients with low magnesium levels have found to have lower BMD, but no higher rates of fractures [137]. Magnesium oxide supplementation in a small cohort of adolescent healthy girls has been found to improve BMD [138].

In 222 consecutive hip fracture patients evaluated for *vitamin D* deficiency, 60% were noted to be severely deficient with 25-hydroxy vitamin D levels below 12 ng/ml [139]. A meta-analysis of calcium supplementation or calcium and vitamin D supplementation revealed treatment was associated with a 12% reduction in overall fracture rates and 24% in studies with a high compliance rate [140]. In addition to diminished outdoor time for vitamin D synthesis and low population-wide intake, common medications decrease the absorption of dietary vitamin D: cholestyramine, colestipol HCL, orlistat, mineral oil, and the fat substitute olestra [141]. Other drugs can induce activation of the pregnane X receptor (PXR), which likely enhances CYP24 expression and catabolism of 25(OH)D, leading to vitamin D deficiency. These drugs include antiepileptics, rifampcin, and taxol and HIV protease inhibitors such as ritonavir and saquinavir [142].

Seniors and those diagnosed with osteopenia or osteoporosis should be evaluated with a 25-hydroxy vitamin D level and treated to optimize levels. Most experts agree that optimal levels of 25-hydroxy-vitamin D levels are 50–70 ng/ml. Patients with vitamin D deficiency require immediate and aggressive therapy. Repletion with over-the-counter multivitamins is ineffective and not recommended due to the risk of concomitant vitamin A excess. Adequate tissues stores can be repleted by initially providing oral doses of 2,000–5,000 international units (IU) of vitamin D_3 daily. Efficacy of the treatment should be determined by repeat serum levels. Maintenance dosing is recommended and should be based upon The Institute of Medicine recommendations: the recommended dietary allowances are 600 IU daily for children and adults ages 9–70 years old and 800 IU daily for adults ages >70 years old [8]. The tolerable upper intake level for vitamin d is 4,000 IU daily. For patients, unable to tolerate or adequately absorb oral supplements, exposure to sunlight (UVB radiation) is an excellent source of vitamin D and is an effective alternative. Sun exposure twice a week of the arms and legs for 5–30 minutes (depending on time of day, season, latitude, skin pigmentation) has been shown to give adequate vitamin D3 [143].

Increasingly, the medical literature demonstrates that *botanicals* modulate signaling pathways important to bone health. Berberine, a natural alkaloid with antioxidant, anti-inflammatory, and glucose and lipid-lowering actions, actively modulates protein kinases active in osteoclastogenesis [144–146]. Hop extracts, specifically rho-iso-alpha acids (RIAA), also by modifying kinases have been shown in vitro to inhibit osteoclastogenesis and in vivo animal models to reduce bone and cartilage degradation [147]. In a 12 week study of women with and without metabolic syndrome, biomarkers of bone turnover were favorably impacted by a combination of RIAA, berberine, and vitamins D and K [148, 149].

Isoflavones, found in soy and red clover, have attracted the most research interest to date for the prevention and treatment of osteoporosis. Epidemiologic studies have demonstrated beneficial effects in premenopausal, perimenopausal, and postmenopausal women [150]. The research demonstrated a dose-dependent benefit curve. Despite these findings, soy isoflavones have been marketed in relatively high doses with resultant concerns regarding their safety noted. Specifically, at higher than dietary levels, there are concerns that because of their estrogenic effects they may be procarcinogenic as well as goitrogenic. However, research has shown that across a broad range of hormonal parameters including thyroid function tests, follicle stimulating hormone and luteinizing hormone levels, and total estrogen levels, one serving of soy food per day had no demonstrable negative effects [151, 152]. Given the current data, soy supplementation as a food is considered an advantageous strategy [153, 154], but supplementation with isolated isoflavones should be evaluated on a case-by-case basis.

CLINICAL SUMMARY

When, despite a healthful lifestyle, there remains an imbalance between bone formation and resorption, further dietary changes and targeted nutraceuticals are clinically-assessed tools to address the unique needs of patients with osteopenia and osteoporosis. Throughout this chapter, we have outlined analyzing potential risk factors including medical conditions, nutritional deficiencies, and lifestyle factors. Better orthopedic outcomes have been shown in early identification of these risk factors with appropriate screening tools such as detailed medical history, physical examination, laboratory testing, and imaging. For example, a young female patient who is 40 years old and suffers a hip fracture from a fall may have a medical history on review inclusive of an eating disorder as a teenager, prior bariatric surgery in her 30s, vitamin D deficiency, and use of glucocorticoids for frequent asthma exacerbations. In making a treatment plan for improved orthopedic outcomes for this patient and others, we must address the underlying risk factors to improve bone health and prevent further long-term complications associated with osteopenia and osteoporosis.

REFERENCES

1. Matthews GDK, Huang CL, Sun L, and Zaidi M. Translational Musculoskeltal science: Is Sarcopenia the next clinical target after osteoporsis? *Ann NY Acad Sci.* 2011;1237:95–105.
2. U.S. Preventive Services Task Force. Screening for osteoporosis: U.S. preventive services task force recommendation statement. *Ann Intern Med.* 2011;154(5):356–64.
3. Seeman E. Bone quality: The material and structural basis of bone strength. *J Bone Mineral Metab.* 2008;26:1–8.

4. Liedert A, Kaspar D, Blakytny R, Claes L, and Ignatus A. Signal transduction pathways involved in mechanotransduction in bone cells. *Biochem Biphysiol Res Commun.* 2006;349:1–5.

5. Hadjidakis DJ and Androulakis II. Bone remodeling. *Ann N Y Acad Sci.* 2006;1092:385–396.

6. Lau RY and Guo X. A review on current osteoporosis research: With special focus on disuse bone loss. *J Osteoporos.* 2011;2011:293808. doi:10.4061/2011/293808.

7. Meier C, Nguyen TV, Handelsman DJ, Schindler C, Kushnir MM, Rockwood AL, Meikle AW, Center JR, Eisman JA, and Seibel MJ. Endogenous sex hormones and incident fracture risk in older men: The Dubbo osteoporosis epidemiology study. *Arch Intern Med.* 2008;168(1):47–54.

8. Institute of Medicine (US) Committee to Review Dietary Reference Intakes for Vitamin D and Calcium; Ross AC, Taylor CL, Yaktine AL, Del Valle HB, editors. *Dietary Reference Intakes for Calcium and Vitamin D.* Washington (DC): National Academies Press (US); 2011.

9. Ma J, Johns RA, and Stafford RS. Americans are not meeting current calcium recommendations. *Am J Clin Nutr.* 2007;85(5):1361–1366.

10. Tucker KL, Morita K, Qiao N, Hannan MT, Cupples LA, and Kiel DP. Colas, but not other carbonated beverages, are associated with low bone mineral density in older women: The Framingham Osteoporosis Study. *Am J Clin Nutr.* 2006;84(4):936–942.

11. Institute of Medicine (US) Standing Committee on the Scientific Evaluation of Dietary Reference Intakes. *Dietary Reference Intakes for Calcium, Phosphorus, Magnesium, Vitamin D, and Fluoride.* Washington (DC): National Academies Press (US); 1997. 5, Phosphorus.

12. Ford ES and Mokdad AH. Dietary magnesium intake in a national sample of US adults. *J Nutr.* 2003;133(9):2879–2882.

13. World Health Organization. Inadequate or excess fluoride: A public health concern. Public Health and the Environment 2010. Available online at www.who.int/ipcs/features/fluoride.pdf?ua=1 (accessed July 14, 2017).

14. Ma J and Betts NM. Zinc and copper intakes and their major food sources for older adults in the 1994–96 continuing survey of food intakes by individuals (CSFII). *J Nutr.* 2000;130(11):2838–2843.

15. Institute of Medicine (US) Panel on Micronutrients. *Dietary Reference Intakes for Vitamin A, Vitamin K, Arsenic, Boron, Chromium, Copper, Iodine, Iron, Manganese, Molybdenum, Nickel, Silicon, Vanadium, and Zinc.* Washington (DC): National Academies Press (US); 2001. 10, Manganese.

16. Rainey CJ, Nyquist LA, Christensen RE, Strong PL, Culver BD, and Coughlin JR. Daily boron intake from the American diet. *J Am Diet Assoc.* 1999;99(3):335–340.

17. Hoy MK and Goldman JD. Potassium Intake of the U.S. Population. *What We Eat In America*, NHANES 2009–2010. Food Surveys Research Group Dietary Data Brief No. 10. September 2012.

18. Moshfegh A, Goldman J, and Cleveland L. Usual Nutrient Intakes from Food Compared to Dietary Reference Intakes. *What We Eat in America*, NHANES 2001–2002. Washington DC: U.S. Department of Agriculture Research Service, 2005.

19. Institute of Medicine (US) Panel on Micronutrients. *Dietary Reference Intakes for Vitamin A, Vitamin K, Arsenic, Boron, Chromium, Copper, Iodine, Iron, Manganese, Molybdenum, Nickel, Silicon, Vanadium, and Zinc.* Washington (DC): National Academies Press (US); 2001. 4, Vitamin A.

20. Institute of Medicine (US) Standing Committee on the Scientific Evaluation. *Dietary Reference Intakes and its Panel on Folate, other B Vitamins, and Choline. Dietary Reference Intakes for Thiamin, Riboflavin, Niacin, Vitamin B6, Folate, Vitamin B12, Pantothenic Acid, Biotin, and Choline.* Washington (DC): National Academies Press (US); 1998. 7, Vitamin B6.

21. Bailey RL, Dodd KW, Gahche JJ, Dwyer JT, McDowell MA, Yetley EA, Sempos CA, Burt VL, Radimer KL, and Picciano MF. Total folate and folic acid intake from foods and dietary supplements in the United States: 2003–2006. *Am J Clin Nutr.* 2010;91(1):231–237.

22. U.S. Department of Agriculture, Agricultural Research Service. What we eat in America. 2009–2010. 2012.

23. Ervin RB, Wright JD, Wang CY, and Kennedy-Stephenson J. *Dietary Intake of Selected Vitamins for the United States Population: 1999–2000 External Link Disclaimer. Advance Data from Vital and Health Statistics*; no 339. Hyattsville, Maryland: National Center for Health Statistics. 2004.

24. Centers for Disease Control and Prevention. National Center for Health Statistics. Diet/Nutrition. 2017. Available online at www.cdc.gov/nchs/fastats/diet.htm (Accessed July 17, 2017).

25. Papanikolaou Y, Brooks J, Reider C, and Fulgoni VL. U.S. adults are not meeting recommended levels for fish and omega-3 fatty acid intake: Results of an analysis using observational data from NHANES 2003–2008. *Nutrition J.* 2014;13:31.

26. Yasui T, Maegawa M, et al. Changes in serum cytokine concentrations during the menopausal transition. *Maturitas.* 2007;56(4):396–403.

27. Kim OY, Chae JS, Paik, JK, Seo HS, Jang Y, Cavaillon JM, and Lee JH. Effects of aging and menopause on serum interleukin-6 levels and peripheral blood mononuclear cell cytokine production in healthy nonobese women. *Age (Dordr)* 2012;34(2):415–25.

28. Mundy GR. Osteoporosis and inflammation. *Nutrition Rev* 2007(II);65(12):S147–S151.

29. Hofbauer LC and Schoppet M. Clinical implications of the osteoprotegerin/RANKL/RANK system for bone and vascular disease. *JAMA* 2004;292:490–495.

30. Gordon CM, Zemel BS, Wren TA, Leonard MB, Bachrach LK, Rauch F, Gilsanz V, Rosen CJ, and Winer KK. The determinants of peak bone mass. *J Pediatr.* 2017;180:261–269.

31. Theintz G, Buchs B, Rizzoli R, Slosman D, Clavien H, Sizonenko PC, and Bonjour JP. Longitudinal monitoring of bone mass accumulation in healthy adolescents: Evidence for a marked reduction after 16 years of age at the levels of lumbar spine and femoral neck in female subjects. *J Clin Endocrinol Metab.* 1992;75(4):1060–1065.

32. Baxter-Jones AD, Faulkner RA, Forwood MR, Mirwald RL, and Bailey DA. Bone mineral accrual from 8 to 30 years of age: An estimation of peak bone mass. *J Bone Miner Res.* 2011;26(8):1729–1739.

33. Weaver CM, Gordon CM, Janz KF, Kalkwarf HJ, Lappe JM, Lewis R, O'Karma M, Wallace TC, and Zemel BS. The National Osteoporosis Foundation's position statement on peak bone mass development and lifestyle factors: A systematic review and implementation recommendations. *Osteoporos Int.* 2016;27(4):1281–1386.

34. Shoback D, Marcus R, and Bilke, D. Metabolic bone disease. In: Greenspan FS and Gardner DG, eds. *Basic and Clinical Endocrinology* (7th edn). New York, NY: McGraw-Hill; 2004. p. 295–361.

35. Dennisson E. Osteoporosis. In: Pinchera A, Bertagna X, and Fischer J, eds. *Endocrinology and Metabolism.* London: McGraw-Hill International (UK) Ltd.; 2001. p. 271–282.

36. Fiore CE, Pennisi P, Ferro G, Ximenes B, Privitelli L, Mangiafico RA, Santoro F, Parisi N, and Lombardo T. Altered osteoprotegerin/RANKL ratio and low bone mineral density in celiac patients on long-term treatment with gluten-free diet. *Horm Metab Res* 2006;38:417–422.

37. Javaid MK and Cooper C. Prenatal and childhood influences on osteoporosis. *Best Pract Res Clin Endocrinol Metab.* 2002;16(2):349–367.

38. Muniz LC, Menezes AM, Assunção MC, Wehrmeister FC, Martínez-Mesa J, Gonçalves H, Domingues MR, Gigante DP, Horta BL, and Barros FC. Breastfeeding and bone mass at the ages of 18 and 30: Prospective analysis of live births from the Pelotas (Brazil) 1982 and 1993 cohorts. *PLoS One.* 2015;10(4):e0122759.

39. Muniz LC, Menezes AM, Buffarini R, Wehrmeister FC, and Assunção MC. Effect of breastfeeding on bone mass from childhood to adulthood: A systematic review of the literature. *Int Breastfeed J.* 2015;10:31.

40. Zipfel S, Seibel MJ, Löwe B, Beumont PJ, Kasperk C, and Herzog W. Osteoporosis in eating disorders: A follow-up study of patients with anorexia and bulimia nervosa. *J Clin Endocrinol Metab.* 2001;86(11):5227–5233.

41. Mehler PS, Krantz MJ, and Sachs KV. Treatments of medical complications of anorexia nervosa and bulimia nervosa. *J Eat Disord.* 2015;3:15.

42. Lange HL, Manos BE, Gothard MD, Rogers LK, and Bonny AE. Bone mineral density and weight changes in adolescents randomized to 3 doses of depot medroxyprogesterone acetate. *J Pediatr Adolesc Gynecol.* 2017;30(2):169–175.

43. Campbell JR and Auinger P. The association between blood lead levels and osteoporosis among adults–results from the third national health and nutrition examination survey (NHANES III). *Environ Health Perspect.* 2007;115(7):1018–1022.

44. Ali T, Lam D, Bronze MS, and Humphrey MB. Osteoporosis in inflammatory bowel disease. *Am J Med.* 2009;122 (7):599–604.

45. Lima CA, Lyra AC, Rocha R, and Santana GO. Risk factors for osteoporosis in inflammatory bowel disease patients. *World J Gastrointest Pathophysiol.* 2015;6(4):210–218.

46. Glass LM and Su GL. Metabolic bone disease in primary biliary cirrhosis. *Gastroenterol Clin North Am.* 2016;45(2):333–343.

47. Raszeja-Wyszomirska J and Miazgowski T. Osteoporosis in primary biliary cirrhosis of the liver. *Przegląd Gastroenterologiczny.* 2014;9(2):82–87.

48. Newcomer AD, Hodgson SF, McGill DB, and Thomas PJ. Lactase deficiency: Prevalence in osteoporosis. *Ann Intern Med.* 1978;89(2):218–220.

49. Gonnelli S, Caffarelli C, and Nuti R. Obesity and fracture risk. *Clin Cases Mineral Bone Metab.* 2014;11(1):9–14.

50. Tovey FI, Hall ML, Ell PJ, and Hobsley M. A review of postgastrectomy bone disease. *J Gastroenterol Hepatol.* 1992;7(6):639–645.

51. Andersen BN, Johansen PB, and Abrahamsen B. Proton pump inhibitors and osteoporosis. *Curr Opin Rheumatol.* 2016;28(4):420–425.

52. Teucher B and Fairweather-Tait S. Dietary sodium as a risk factor for osteoporosis: Where is the evidence? *Proc Nutr Soc.* 2003;62(4):859–866.

53. Hallström H, Wolk A, Glynn A, and Michaëlsson K. Coffee, tea and caffeine consumption in relation to osteoporotic fracture risk in a cohort of Swedish women. *Osteoporos Int.* 2006;17(7):1055–1064.

54. Cao JJ, Pasiakos SM, Margolis LM, Sauter ER, Whigham LD, McClung JP, Young AJ, and Combs GF Jr. Calcium homeostasis and bone metabolic responses to high-protein diets during energy deficit in healthy young adults: A randomized controlled trial. *Am J Clin Nutr.* 2014;99(2):400–407.

55. Bonjour JP. Protein intake and bone health. *Int J Vitam Nutr Res.* 2011;81(2–3): 134–142.

56. Nieves JW. Osteoporosis: The role of micronutrients. *Am J Clin Nutr.* 2005;81(5):1232S–1239S.

57. Libuda L, Alexy U, Remer T, Stehle P, Schoenau E, and Kersting M. Association between long-term consumption of soft drinks and variables of bone modeling and remodeling in a sample of healthy German children and adolescents. *Am J Clin Nutr.* 2008;88(6):1670–1677.

58. Jackuliak P and Payer J. Osteoporosis, fractures, and diabetes. *Int J Endocrinol.* 2014;2014:820615.

59. Bijelic R, Milicevic S, and Balaban J. Risk factors for osteoporosis in postmenopausal women. *Med Arch.* 2017;71(1):25–28.

60. Zhang X, Yu Z, Yu M, and Qu X. Alcohol consumption and hip fracture risk. *Osteoporos Int.* 2015;26(2):531–542.

61. Chakkalakal DA. Alcohol-induced bone loss and deficient bone repair. *Alcohol Clin Exp Res* 2005;29(12):2077–2090.

62. Briot K and Roux C. Glucocorticoid-induced osteoporosis. *RMD Open.* 2015;1(1):e000014.

63. Ton FN, Gunawardene SC, Lee H, and Neer RM. Effects of low-dose prednisone on bone metabolism. *J Bone Miner Res* 2005;20:464–470.

64. van Staa TP, Leufkens HG, and Cooper C. The epidemiology of corticosteroid-induced osteoporosis: A meta-analysis. *Osteoporos Int* 2002;13:777–787.

65. Kaltsas G and Makras P. Skeletal diseases in Cushing's syndrome: Osteoporosis versus arthropathy. *Neuroendocrinology* 2010;92(suppl 1):60–64.

66. Cizza G, Ravn P, Chrousos GP, and Gold PW. Depression: A major, unrecognized risk factor for osteoporosis? *Trends Endocrinol Metab.* 2001;12(5):198–203.

67. Cormier C, Souberbielle JC, and Kahan A. Primary hyperparathyroidism and osteoporosis in 2004. *Joint Bone Spine.* 2004;71(3):183–189.

68. Mosekilde L. Primary hyperparathyroidism and the skeleton. *Clin Endocrinol (Oxf).* 2008;69(1):1–19.

69. Theriault RL. Pathophysiology and implications of cancer treatment-induced bone loss. *Oncology (Williston Park).* 2004;18(5 Suppl 3):11–15.

70. Epstein S, Inzerillo AM, Caminis J, and Zaidi M. Disorders associated with acute rapid and severe bone loss. *J Bone Miner Res.* 2003;18(12):2083–2094.

71. Maïmoun L, Fattal C, and Sultan C. Bone remodeling and calcium homeostasis in patients with spinal cord injury: A review. *Metabolism.* 2011;60(12):1655–1663.

72. Dhanwal DK. Thyroid disorders and bone mineral metabolism. *Indian J Endocrinol Metab.* 2011;15(Suppl 2):S107–S112.

73. Stein E and Shane E. Secondary osteoporosis. *Endocrinol Metab Clin North Am.* 2003;32(1):115–134, vii.

74. Hurlock, DG. Personal communication.

75. Alfvén T, Elinder CG, Carlsson MD, Grubb A, Hellström L, Persson B, Pettersson C, Spång G, Schütz A, and Järup L. Low-level cadmium exposure and osteoporosis. *J Bone Miner Res.* 2000;15(8):1579–1586.

76. Nawrot T, Geusens P, Nulens TS, and Nemery B. Occupational cadmium exposure and calcium excretion, bone density, and osteoporosis in men. *J Bone Miner Res.* 2010;25(6):1441–5.

77. Heaney RP and Layman DK. Amount and type of protein influences bone health. *Am J Clin Nutr.* 2008;87(5):1567S–1570S.

78. Huang Z, Himes JH, and McGovern PG. Nutrition and subsequent hip fracture risk among a national cohort of white women. *Am J Epidemiol.* 1996;144:124–234.

79. Ilich JZ and Kerstetter JE. Nutrition in bone health revisited: A story beyond calcium. *J Am Coll Nutr* 2000;19(6):715–737.

80. Kerstetter J, Svastisalee C, Caseria DM, Mitnick ME, and Insogna KL. A threshold for low-protein-diet-induced elevations in parathyroid hormone. *Am J Clin Nutr.* 2000;72:168–173.
81. Giannini S, Nobile M, et al. Acute effects of moderate dietary protein restriction in patients with idiopathic hypercalciuria and calcium nephrolithiasis. *Am J Clin Nutr.* 1999;69:267–271.
82. Dowd, TL, Rosen, JF, Mirts, L, and Gundberg, CM, The effect of Pb(2+) on the structure and hydroxyapatite binding properties of osteocalcin. *Biochimica Biophysica Acta.* 2001;1535:153–163.
83. Nash, D., Magder, LS, Sherwin, R, Rubin, RT, and Silbergeld, EK. Bone density related predictors of blood lead levels among peri- and post-menopausal women in the United States, 3rd National Health Nutritional Examination Survey 1988–1994. *Am J Epidemiol.* 2004; 160: 901–911.
84. Nakchbandi IA. Osteoporosis and fractures in liver disease: Relevance, pathogenesis and therapeutic implications. *World J Gastroenterol.* 2014;20(28):9427–9438.
85. Cijevschi C, Mihai C, Zbranca E, and Gogălniceanu P. Osteoporosis in liver cirrhosis. *Rom J Gastroenterol.* 2005;14(4):337–341.
86. Bernstein CN, Leslie WD, and Leboff MS. AGA Technical review: Osteoporosis in gastrointestinal diseases. *Gastroenterology* 2003;124(3):795–841.
87. Sanchez AJ and Aranda-Michel J. Liver disease and osteoporosis. *Nutr Clin Prac* 2006;21:273–278.
88. To TT, Witten PE, Renn J, Bhattacharya D, Huysseune A, and Winkler C. Rankl-induced osteoclastogenesis leads to loss of mineralization in a medaka osteoporosis model. *Development.* 2012;139(1):141–150.
89. Jabbar S, Drury J, Fordham JN, Datta HK, Francis RM and Tuck SP. Osteoprotegerin, RANKL, and bone turnover in postmenopausal osteoporosis. *J Clin Pathol* 2011;64(4):354–357.
90. Cummings SR, San Martin J, et al. Denosumab for prevention of fractures in postmenopausal women with osteoporosis. *NEJM* 2009;361(8):756–765.
91. Yin H, Shi ZG, Hu J, Wang R, Luan ZP, and Guo DH. Protection against osteoporosis by statins is linked to a reduction of oxidative stress and restoration of nitric oxide formation in aged and ovariectomized rats. *Eur J Pharmacol* 2012;674(2–3):200–206.
92. Wang Z, Li Y, Zhou F, Piao Z, and Hao J. Effects of statins on bone mineral density and fracture risk: A PRISMA-compliant systematic review and meta-analysis. *Medicine.* 2016;95(22):e3042.
93. Riches PL, McRorie E, Fraser WD, Determann C, van't Hof R, and Ralston SH. Osteoporosis associated with neutralizing autoantibodies against osteoprotegerin. *NEJM* 2009;361:1459–1465.
94. Serhan, CN. Clues for new therapeutics in osteoporosis and periodontal disease: A new role for lipoxygenase. *Expert Opin Ther Targets.* 2004;8:643–654.
95. Hernández-Sánchez A, Tejada-González P, and Arteta-Jiménez M. Aluminium in parenteral nutrition: A systematic review. *Eur J Clin Nutr.* 2013;67(3):230–238.
96. Haderslev KV, Tjellesen L, Haderslav PH, and Staun M. Assessment of the longitudinal changes in bone mineral density in patients receiving home parenteral nutrition. *JPEN.* 2004;28(5):289–294.
97. Mata-Granados JM, Cuenca-Acevedo JR, Luque de Castro MD, Holick MF, and Quesada-Gómez JM. Vitamin D insufficiency together with high serum levels of vitamin A increases the risk for osteoporosis in postmenopausal women. *Arch Osteoporos.* 2013;8:124.
98. Joo NS, Yang SW, Song BC, and Yeum KJ. Vitamin A intake, serum vitamin D and bone mineral density: Analysis of the Korea National Health and Nutrition Examination Survey (KNHANES, 2008–2011). *Nutrients.* 2015;7(3):1716–1727.
99. Richards JB, Papaioannou A, et al. Effect of selective serotonin reuptake inhibitors on the risk of fracture. *Arch Intern Med.* 2007;167(2):188–194.
100. Rejnmark L. Cardiovascular drugs and bone. *Curr Drug Saf.* 2008;3(3):178–184.
101. Stein, E. and Shane, E. Secondary osteoporosis. *Endocrinol Metab Clin North Am.* 2003;32:115–134.
102. Sardone LD, Renlund R, Willett TL, Fantus IG, and Grynpas MD. Effect of rosiglitazone on bone quality in a rat model of insulin resistance and osteoporosis. *Diabetes.* 2011;60:3271.
103. Wan Y, Chong LW, and Evans RM. PPAR-γ regulates osteoclastogenesis in mice. *Nat Med.* 2007;13(12):1496–1503.
104. Pfeilschifter J and Diel IJ. Osteoporosis due to cancer treatment: Pathogenesis and management. *J Clin Oncol.* 2000;28:1570–1593.
105. Pack, A.M., Gidal, B., and Vasquez, B., Bone disease associated with antiepileptic drugs, *Cleveland Clinic Journal of Medicine,* 71, s42–s48, 2004.
106. Davis S, Martyn-St James M, et al. A systematic review and economic evaluation of bisphosphonates for the prevention of fragility fractures. *Health Technol Assess.* 2016;20(78):1–406.
107. Whitaker M, Guo J, Kehoe T, and Benson G. Bisphosphonates for osteoporosis—where do we go from here? *N Engl J Med.* 2012;366(22):2048–2051.

108. Villa JC, Gianakos A, and Lane JM. Bisphosphonate treatment in osteoporosis: Optimal duration of therapy and the incorporation of a drug holiday. *HSS J.* 2016;12(1):66–73.

109. Ward J, Wood C, Rouch K, Pienkowski D, Malluche HH. Stiffness and strength of bone in osteoporotic patients treated with varying durations of oral bisphosphonates. *Osteoporos Int.* 2016;27(9):2681–2688.

110. Kanis JA, Oden A, Johansson H, Borgström F, Ström O, and McCloskey E. FRAX® and its applications to clinical practice. *Bone.* 2009;44:734–743.

111. Mason EM, Jalagani H, and Vinik AI. Metabolic complications of bariatric surgery: Diagnosis and management issues. *Gastroenterol Clin N Am.* 2006;34:25–33.

112. Weaver J, Sajjan S, Lewiecki EM, and Harris ST. Diagnosis and treatment of osteoporosis before and after fracture: A side-by-side analysis of commercially insured and medicare advantage osteoporosis patients. *J Manag Care Spec Pharm.* 2017;23(7):735–744.

113. National Institutes of Health Consensus Development Panel on Osteoporosis Prevention, Diagnosis, and Therapy. Osteoporosis prevention, diagnosis, and therapy. *JAMA.* 2001 Feb 14; 285(6): 785–95.

114. Bernabei R, Martone AM, Ortolani E, Landi F, and Marzetti E. Screening, diagnosis and treatment of osteoporosis: A brief review. *Clin Cases Miner Bone Metab.* 2014;11(3):201–207.

115. Nayak S, Roberts MS, and Greenspan SL. Cost-effectiveness of different screening strategies for osteoporosis in postmenopausal women. *Ann Intern Med.* 2011;155(11):751–761.

116. Schousboe JT and Gourlay ML. Comparative effectiveness and cost-effectiveness of strategies to screen for osteoporosis in postmenopausal women. *Ann Intern Med.* 2011;155(11):788–789.

117. Eastell R and Hannon RA. Biomarkers of bone health and osteoporosis risk. *Proc Nutr Soc.* 2008;67(2):157–162.

118. Botella S, Restituto P, Monreal I, Colina I, Calleja A, and Varo N. Traditional and novel bone remodeling markers in premenopausal and postmenopausal women. *J Clin Endocrinol Metab.* 2013;98(11):E1740–E1748.

119. Sundell J. Resistance training is an effective tool against metabolic and frailty syndrome. *Adv Prev Med.* 2011;2011:984683.

120. Schulman RC, Weiss AJ, and Mechanick JI. Nutrition, bone, and aging: An integrative physiology approach. *Curr Osteoporos Rep.* 2011;9:184–195.

121. New SA. Intake of fruits and vegetables: Implications for bone health. *Proc Nutr Soc.* 2003;62(4):889–899.

122. Arjmandi BH, Johnson SA, Pourafshar S, Navaei N, George KS, Hooshmand S, Chai SC, and Akhavan NS. Bone-protective effects of dried plum in postmenopausal women: Efficacy and possible mechanisms. *Nutrients.* 2017;9(5):E495.

123. Matheson EM, Mainous AG 3rd, and Carnemolla MA. The association between onion consumption and bone density in perimenopausal and postmenopausal non-Hispanic white women 50 years and older. *Menopause.* 2009;16(4):756–759.

124. Coxam V. Current data with inulin-type fructans and calcium, targeting bone health in adults. *J Nutr.* 2007;137:2527S–2533S.

125. Zofkova I, Davis M, and Blahos J. Trace elements have beneficial, as well as detrimental effects on bone homeostasis. *Physiol Res.* 2017;66(3):391–402.

126. Rapuri PB, Gallagher JC, Kinyamu HK, and Ryschon KL. Caffeine intake increases the rate of bone loss in elderly women and interacts with vitamin D receptor genotypes. *Am J Clin Nutr.* 2001;74(5):694–700.

127. Massey LK. Is caffeine a risk factor for bone loss in the elderly? *Am J Clin Nutr.* 2001;74:569–570.

128. Fernando GR, Martha RM, and Evangelina R. Consumption of soft drinks with phosphoric acid as a risk factor for the development of hypocalcemia in postmenopausal women. *J Clin Epidemiol.* 1999;52(10):1007–1010.

129. Villareal DT, Fontana L, Weiss EP, Racette SB, Steger-May K, Schechtman KB, Klein S, and Holloszy JO. Bone mineral density response to caloric restriction-induced weight loss or exercise-induced weight loss. *Arch Intern Med.* 2006;166:2502–2510.

130. Apgar B. Comparison of common calcium supplements. Am Apgar B. Comparison of common calcium supplements. *Am Fam Physician.* 2000;62(8):1895–1896.

131. Heaney RP, Dowell MS, Bierman J, Hale CA, and Bendich A. Absorbability and cost effectiveness in calcium supplementation. *J Am Coll Nutr.* 2001;20(3):239–246.

132. Jensen LB, Kollerup G, Quaade F, and Sørensen OH. Bone mineral changes in obese women during moderate weight loss with and without calcium supplementation. *J Bone Miner Res.* 2001;16:141–147.

133. Ricci TA, Chowdhury HA, Heymsfiled SB, Stahl T, Pierson RN Jr, and Shapses SA. Calcium supplementation suppresses bone turnover during weight reduction in postmenopausal women. *J Bone Miner Res.* 1998;13:1045–1050.

134. Tankeu AT, Ndip Agbor V, and Noubiap JJ. Calcium supplementation and cardiovascular risk: A rising concern. *J Clin Hypertens (Greenwich)*. 2017;19(6):640–646.

135. Farsinejad-Marj M, Saneei P, and Esmaillzadeh A. Dietary magnesium intake, bone mineral density and risk of fracture: A systematic review and meta-analysis. *Osteoporos Int*. 2016;27(4):1389–1399.

136. Castiglioni S, Cazzaniga A, Albisetti W, and Maier JA. Magnesium and osteoporosis: Current state of knowledge and future research directions. *Nutrients*. 2013;5(8):3022–3033.

137. Orchard TS, Larson JC, Alghothani N, Bout-Tabaku S, Cauley JA, Chen Z, LaCroix AZ, Wactawski-Wende J, and Jackson RD. Magnesium intake, bone mineral density, and fractures: Results from the Women's Health Initiative Observational Study. *Am J Clin Nutr*. 2014;99(4):926–933.

138. Carpenter TO, DeLucia MC, Zhang JH, Bejnerowicz G, Tartamella L, Dziura J, Petersen KF, Befroy D, and Cohen D. A randomized controlled study of effects of dietary magnesium oxide supplementation on bone mineral content in healthy girls. *J Clin Endocrinol Metab*. 2006;91(12):4866–4872.

139. Bischoff-Ferrari HA, Can U, Staehelin HB, Platz A, Henschkowski J, Michel BA, Dawson-Hughes B, and Theiler R. Severe vitamin D deficiency in Swiss hip fracture patients. *Bone*. 2008;42(3):597–602.

140. Tang BMP, Eslick GD, Nowson C, Smith C, and Bensoussan A. Use of calcium or calcium in combination with vitamin D supplementation to prevent fractures and bone loss in people aged 50 years and older: a meta-analysis. *Lancet* 2007;370:657–666.

141. Hendler SS and Rorvik DR, eds. *PDR for Nutritional Supplements*. Montvale: Medical Economics Company, Inc; 2001.

142. Gröber U and Kisters K. Influence of drugs on vitamin D and calcium metabolism. *Dermato-endocrinology*. 2012;4(2):158–166. doi:10.4161/derm.20731.

143. Holick MF. Vitamin D deficiency. *N Engl J Med*. 2007;357(3):266–281.

144. Cicero AF and Baggioni A. Berberine and its role in chronic disease. *Adv Exp Med Biol*. 2016;928:27–45.

145. Hu JP, Nishishita K, Sakai E, Yoshida H, Kato Y, Tsukuba T, and Okamoto K. Berberine inhibits RANKL-induced osteoclast formation and survival through suppressing the NF-kappaB and akt pathways. *Eur J Pharmacol*. 2008;580(1–2):70–79.

146. Lee YS, Kim YS, et al. AMP kinase acts as a negative regulator of RANKL in the differentiation of osteoclasts. *Bone*. 2010;47(5):926–937.

147. Konda VR, Desai A, Darland G, Bland JS, and Tripp ML. META060 inhibits osteoclastogenesis and matrix metalloproteinase in vitro and reduces bone and cartilage degradation in a mouse model of rheumatoid arthritis. *Arthritis Rheumatism*. 2010;62(6):1683–1692.

148. Lamb JJ, Holick MF, et al. Nutritional supplementation of hop rho iso-alpha acids, berberine, vitamin D, and vitamin K produces a favorable bone biomarker profile supporting healthy bone metabolism in postmenopausal women with metabolic syndrome. *Nutr Res*. 2011;31(5):347–355.

149. Holick MF, Lamb JJ, et al. Hop rho iso-alpha acids, berberine, vitamin D3 and vitamin K1 favorably impact biomarkers of bone turnover in postmenopausal women in a 14-week trial. *J Bone Miner Metab*. 2010;28(3):342–350.

150. Taku K, Melby MK, Nishi N, Omori T, and Kurzer MS. Soy isoflavones for osteoporosis: An evidence based approach. *Maturitas*. 2011;70(4):333–338.

151. Kurzer MS. Hormonal effects of soy in premenopausal women and men. *J Nutr*. 2003;132(3):570S–573S.

152. Persky VW, Turyk ME, Wang L, Freek S, Chatterton R Jr, Barmes S, Erdman J Jr, Sepkovic DW, Bradlow HL, and Potter S. Effect of soy protein on endogenous hormone in postmenopausal women. *Am J Clin Nutr*. 2002;75(1):145–153.

153. Matthews VL, Knutsen SF, Beeson WL, and Fraser GE. Soy milk and dairy consumption is independently associated with ultrasound attenuation of the heel bone among postmenopausal women: The adventist health study-2. *Nutr Res*. 2011;31(10):766–775.

154. Reinwald S and Weaver CM. Soy components vs. whole soy: Are we betting our bones on a long shot? *J Nutr*. 2010;140(12):2312S–2317S.

16 Nutritional Status and Interventions for Reducing Stress Fracture Risk among Military Personnel

James McClung, PhD

INTRODUCTION

Military service results in unique occupational demands that often require significant physical training and performance. Exposure to the physical demands of military service results in an increased risk of injury, including overuse injuries to bone, such as stress fractures, which may occur in association with unaccustomed repetitive physical activities. Initial military training (IMT) is the initial indoctrination of civilians to military service. During this 8–10-week course, military recruits are exposed to a series of physical training activities, including road marching with weighted packs, distance running, sprinting, and muscle strength training exercises. These activities, often repetitive and unaccustomed, result in an increased risk of stress fracture, as recruits engaging in IMT are up to 18 times more likely to experience a stress fracture than other active-duty personnel. The relative risk of fractures during IMT is significantly higher for women than for men.

Although many of the risk factors for stress fracture, such as gender, genetics, and race, are not modifiable, others, including nutrition, provide the opportunity for intervention. Recent studies have detailed relationships between nutritional status and risk of stress fracture. Iron and vitamin D status have been linked to stress fracture risk, and calcium and vitamin D supplementation has been linked to the optimization of bone health and reduction in stress fracture incidence during IMT. This chapter will review the evidence linking a series of nutrients, such as iron, calcium, and vitamin D, to stress fracture risk and will highlight how these nutrients affect bone health in active populations.

PATHOPHYSIOLOGY AND EPIDEMIOLOGY OF STRESS FRACTURES IN MILITARY RECRUITS

Stress fractures, incomplete fractures of bone, typically occur in association with unaccustomed repetitive physical activities, particularly activities that result in the mechanical loading of bone. Ideally, mechanical loading results in adaptations to bone geometry that result in improved bone strength. However, a stress fracture may occur when the bone is repeatedly loaded beyond its ability to adapt and withstand the associated strains. IMT is a period during which new military recruits participate in a series of physical activities to which they are generally unaccustomed, such as load carriage (i.e., marching with body armor and boots). These activities, associated with repetitive mechanical loading, result in increased bone turnover due to modeling and remodeling, and may result in temporarily weakened bone, as mineralization occurs only after the formation of new bone matrix (Hughes and Petit, 2010). Stress fractures may occur when the process of bone repair does not occur quickly enough to overcome the fatigue damage resulting from repetitive loading.

Stress fractures come with significant fiscal and personnel cost to the US military. Although estimates of the incidence of stress fracture in recruits enduring IMT vary significantly, stress fractures are among the most common overuse injuries, affecting up to 5% of male recruits and 21% of female recruits (Jones et al., 2002; Rauh et al., 2006; Gaffney-Stomberg et al., 2014). Notably, more than half of female recruits that experience a stress fracture may attrite from military service (Jones et al., 2002). This comes at a great cost to the military and to the service member: The military loses the prior investment in the recruitment and training of the service member and endures the medical and rehabilitation costs associated with the injury; the service member loses the opportunity to serve and to gain the vocational experience and other benefits associated with a career in the military. Notably, stress fracture is a significant concern for civilian populations, including athletes participating in sports such as track and field (Changstrom et al., 2015). In fact, incidence rates may exceed 20% in such populations, highlighting the importance of developing interventions for stress fracture prevention (Bennell et al., 1996).

NUTRITION AND BONE HEALTH

IRON

Iron is a nutritionally essential trace element that confers function through incorporation into a series of proteins and enzymes. Iron incorporates into hemoglobin and myoglobin, essential for the transport and storage of oxygen. Iron also incorporates into enzymes that participate in metabolic pathways, such as cytochrome c, NADH dehydrogenase, and succinate dehydrogenase. Given the necessity of iron for oxygen transport and storage as well as energy metabolism, the effects of poor iron status on physical and neurocognitive performance in humans have been well-described (McClung and Murray-Kolb, 2013).

New research points to the role of iron in bone health. Iron is a mineral component of bone, although in far lesser abundance than other minerals such as calcium, magnesium, and phosphorous. Iron contributes to the protein content of bone, including the synthesis of collagen, which comprises up to 90% of total bone protein (Toxqui and Vaquero, 2015). Animal studies indicate a relationship between iron status and the mechanical strength, density, and mineralization of bone (Katsumata et al., 2006; Medeiros et al., 2002, 2004).

Human clinical trials linking iron status and bone health are limited. One study indicates a link between dietary iron and bone mineral density in healthy postmenopausal women (Harris et al., 2003). Another study demonstrates a link between iron deficiency anemia (IDA) and bone resorption, and a beneficial effect of recovery from IDA on bone remodeling in premenopausal women (Wright et al., 2013).

Poor iron status affects a significant portion of the population, including military service members. Iron deficiency (ID, depleted iron stores) and IDA (ID and hemoglobin levels below a clinical cut-off value) affects billions of people worldwide (DeMaeyer and Adiels-Tegman, 1985). In the developed world, poor iron status affects premenopausal women more than men due to factors including poor dietary intake, menstrual blood loss, and gestational requirements. Population studies conducted in the United States indicate that ID may affect over 15% of girls between the ages of 16 and 19, and that IDA may affect up to 4% of women between the ages of 20 and 49 (Looker et al., 1997). Data from the US military indicate that over 13% of women that begin military service arrive for training with ID (McClung et al., 2006).

The recommended dietary allowance (RDA) for iron is 15 mg/day for girls between the ages of 14 and 18 and 18 mg/day for women between the ages of 19 and 50 (IOM, 2001). The RDA for boys and men is less, 11 mg/day and 8 mg/day, respectively.

Iron occurs in two forms in the diet, *heme* and *non-heme*. Heme iron, which is more bioavailable for absorption than non-heme iron, is found in meat sources such as beef and other red meats.

Non-heme iron is found in fortified foods, such as breakfast cereals; and vegetable sources, including spinach and other leafy green vegetables.

Iron is a nutrient of concern for women military personnel for a number of reasons. First, a significant proportion of women beginning military training enter with poor iron status, and iron status declines significantly during IMT. In a cross-sectional study, the incidence of ID climbed from 13.4% at the start of IMT to 32.8% at the end of training (McClung et al., 2006). Similarly, the incidence of IDA climbed from 5.8% at the start of training to 20.9% at the end of training. Longitudinal studies have confirmed the decline in iron status associated with IMT and have demonstrated an association between the decline in iron status and aerobic performance (McClung et al., 2009b). It is important to note that IMT-related declines in iron status occur in both men and women recruits, although the decline is steeper among women. This is compounded by the data indicating that men begin training with more robust iron stores (Yanovich et al., 2015).

Poor iron status, particularly IDA, affects both neuropsychological and physical performance (McClung et al., 2009a; McClung and Murray-Kolb, 2013). Further, poor iron status may be associated with injury, to include stress fracture (Yanovich et al., 2011).

Few studies have carefully investigated the link between iron status, bone health, and stress fracture incidence in military personnel. One study conducted with women military recruits in the Israeli Defense Force (IDF) found that 12% of women trainees experienced stress fracture, and that trainees with stress fractures had reduced levels of serum iron and transferrin saturation as compared to women who did not experience fractures (Merkel et al., 2008). Another assessment conducted with women recruits in the IDF found that the women who suffered stress fractures had elevated incidence of IDA (Yanovich et al., 2011).

CALCIUM AND VITAMIN D

Calcium and vitamin D are the two micronutrients most commonly associated with the formation and metabolism of bone. Calcium is the largest mineral component of bone; more than 99% of total body calcium occurs as calcium hydroxyapatite in bones and teeth. Beyond the role of calcium in providing bone with hard tissue and strength, calcium is essential for mediating vascular contraction and vasodilation, nerve transmission, muscle function, intracellular signaling, and hormonal secretion.

Importantly, bone serves as the reservoir for calcium to support the functions of calcium in the circulatory system, muscles, and other tissues. This process is regulated by parathyroid hormone (PTH, a calcium sensor) and vitamin D. Increased secretion of PTH from the parathyroid gland occurs in response to reductions in circulating ionic calcium, which are detected by calcium-sensing receptors expressed on parathyroid cells. PTH secretion induces 1α-hydroxylase in the kidney, which converts vitamin D to calcitriol, its active hormonal form, which then stimulates calcium absorption in the gut. PTH secretion also increases renal tubular resorption of calcium and activates osteoclastic bone resorption, thereby increasing circulating ionic calcium levels.

Vitamin D is a unique nutrient in that it may be consumed through the diet and also synthesized endogenously from cholesterol precursors in response to UVB radiation of the skin. 25-hydroxylation of dietary and endogenous vitamin D in the liver results in 25-hydroxyvitamin D 25(OH)D, the major circulating form of vitamin D. This form of vitamin D is further hydroxylated in the kidney to form 1,25-dihydroyvitamin D (calcitriol, $1,25(OH)_2D_3$), the active hormonal form of vitamin D. The best described function of vitamin D in human health occurs through calcitriol regulation of calcium homeostasis and bone health. Although beyond the scope of this chapter, vitamin D contributes to other biological functions, including the regulation of cell proliferation, cell differentiation, apoptosis, and potentially the prevention of cancer and other conditions, such as cardiovascular disease and infection.

Foods rich in calcium include dairy products, nuts, legumes, and dark green and leafy vegetables. Food products are sometimes fortified with calcium, including non-dairy milk (i.e., soy milk), breads, juices, and breakfast cereals. Foods rich in vitamin D are limited. These include fatty fishes, such as salmon; and fortified foods, such as milk and some cheeses and yogurts. When setting the RDA for calcium and vitamin D, the Institute of Medicine (IOM) focused on the maintenance of bone health, considering factors such as bone mineral density and fracture risk (IOM, 2011).

The RDA for calcium for men and women aged 19–50 is 1000 mg/day. The RDA for vitamin D for men and women aged 19–50 is 600 IU/day. Notably, some experts, including the Endocrine Society, recommend intakes of vitamin D beyond the RDA (Holick et al., 2011).

The prevalence of poor vitamin D status is dependent on cut-off values used to define deficiency. If serum 25(OH)D levels of 20 ng/mL are used to define deficiency, over 40% of the US population may be considered deficient (Forrest and Stuhldreher, 2011). Calcium deficiency is difficult to define due to the regulation of circulating ionic calcium levels through the actions of PTH; analysis of population data indicates that dietary calcium intake may be inadequate in adult men and women (Mangano et al., 2011). It is important to note that deficiency of either calcium or vitamin D results in impaired bone mineralization, known as *rickets* in children and *osteomalacia* in adults.

Calcium and vitamin D are of particular importance for military personnel due to the effects of training on bone turnover and the risk of stress fracture. Further, military personnel often wear protective clothing that prevents sunlight exposure, or operate at night or in conditions of low sunlight. Longitudinal studies have characterized vitamin D status in female US Army recruits during IMT and elucidated declines during training in the late summer months in the Southeastern United States (Andersen et al., 2010). In this study, decrements in vitamin D status were coupled with increases in PTH, indicating calcium mobilization from bone. A second longitudinal study, also conducted in female US Army recruits during IMT, confirmed elevations in PTH over the period of the training course and also described elevations in biomarkers of both bone formation (bone alkaline phosphatase and procollagen I N-terminal peptide) and bone resorption (tartrate-resistant acid phosphatase and C-terminal telopeptide) (Lutz et al., 2012). Interestingly, dietary intakes of both calcium and vitamin D were below the RDA; mean calcium intake was 882 mg/day during IMT (RDA = 1000 mg/day), and mean vitamin D intake was 164 IU/day (RDA = 600 IU/day).

Recent studies have linked vitamin D status to the risk of stress fracture during military training (Ruohola et al., 2006; Burgi et al., 2011; Dao et al., 2015). In fact, Burgi and colleagues (2011) found that there was double the risk of stress fractures of tibia and fibula during IMT among women Navy recruits with serum 25(OH)D levels less than 20 ng/mL as compared to those with concentrations of 40 ng/mL or greater. Interestingly, these authors recommend a target serum 25(OH)D concentration of 40 ng/mL for the prevention of stress fractures during IMT, which is significantly greater than the level recommended by the IOM for the avoidance of deficiency in civilian populations.

Although beyond the scope of the present chapter, recent studies have explored the relationship between genetic factors, including single-nucleotide polymorphisms (SNPs), and bone health, to include risk of stress fracture. Studies have linked SNPs in the vitamin D receptor (VDR) to bone health (Mencej-Bedrac et al., 2009) and stress fracture in military populations (Chatzipapas et al., 2009). One recent study linked SNPs in the VDR and vitamin D binding protein (DBP) to vitamin D status and bone turnover (Gaffney-Stomberg et al., 2017). Further, calculation of a genetic risk score comprised of both VDR and DBP SNPs uncovered an association between genetic risk and the biomarker response to dietary calcium and vitamin D intake.

NUTRITIONAL INTERVENTIONS TO PREVENT STRESS FRACTURES

IRON

Randomized, controlled trials have not directly tested the hypothesis that iron interventions may reduce stress fracture incidence. However, one recent study demonstrated the efficacy of an iron supplement (15 mg elemental iron/day) in preventing declines in iron status among women US Army recruits during IMT (McClung et al., 2009a). When provided daily, treatment with iron attenuated the declines in iron status observed in the placebo group, regardless of starting iron status, and resulted in significant improvements in aerobic performance in study participants beginning IMT with IDA. A second randomized, controlled trial assessed the impact of an iron-fortified food product on iron status in female recruits during US Army IMT. Although less effective than the trial providing iron as a dietary supplement, the fortified food product (56 mg elemental iron/day) attenuated the decline in iron status in volunteers beginning the trial with IDA (Karl et al., 2010).

In 2012, the US Air Force initiated a program providing a multivitamin containing iron (27 mg elemental iron/day) to women recruits at the start of IMT. Although not a research trial, metrics associated with program efficacy, such as all-cause attrition from military training, medical attrition, and stress fracture incidence data, were collected and compared to historical populations not provided with a multivitamin (Barnes et al., 2015). Although not statistically significant, all-cause attrition was reduced by 8% in female trainees who were provided with the prenatal vitamin as compared to historical controls. Similarly, medical attrition was reduced by over 25%, and stress fracture incidence was reduced by 3%. These data indicate that multivitamin use may protect against injury and attrition during IMT, although compliance data were not collected, and comparison to historical data may be difficult to accurately interpret. In 2016, the US Army began a similar multivitamin program for female recruits during IMT; this effort includes education regarding iron nutrition, including dietary guidance and perspectives regarding declines in iron status occurring during training. The multivitamin, which contains 27 mg elemental iron/day, is available to women recruits under the guidance and oversight of medical personnel and is optional during training. Similar to the Air Force program, this effort is not intended as a controlled research trial, although it may provide an opportunity to track the effects of a multivitamin containing iron on attrition and the incidence of stress fracture into the future.

CALCIUM AND VITAMIN D

Given the well-described roles of calcium and vitamin D in supporting bone health, randomized, controlled trials have investigated the efficacy of these nutrients for preventing stress fracture and optimizing bone structure and function. In a pioneering study, Lappe and colleagues (2008) provided a calcium and vitamin D–containing dietary supplement or placebo to over 5200 female US Navy recruits during IMT. The treatment contained 2000 mg/day of calcium (as calcium carbonate) and 800 IU/day of vitamin D (as vitamin D3) for the 8 weeks of training. Nearly 6% of the study population experienced a stress fracture. Intention-to-treat analyses indicated that provision of the calcium and vitamin D supplement resulted in a 20% lower incidence of stress fracture than the placebo group; there were 226 stress fractures in the treatment group and 270 fractures in the placebo group. The most common site of fracture was the tibia/fibula; at that site, there were 138 fractures in the treatment group and 179 in the placebo group. In the same study, relative risk was calculated for a number of factors independent of treatment; amenorrhea, age >25, smoking, and use of depomedroxyprogesterone contributed to the risk of stress fracture, while physical fitness/exercise prior to IMT was protective.

In a second randomized, controlled trial, Gaffney-Stomberg and colleagues (2014) assessed the effects of a calcium and vitamin D–fortified food product on nutritional status and bone structure. In this study, men ($n = 156$) and women ($n = 87$) US Army recruits consumed food products (snack bars, two/day) containing 130–140 calories with (treatment) and without (placebo) 1000 mg/day of calcium (as calcium carbonate) and 500 IU/day of vitamin D (as vitamin D3) throughout a 9-week IMT course. Although stress fracture incidence was not assessed, consumption of the calcium and vitamin D–fortified food product resulted in significant increases in circulating ionized calcium and attenuated increases in PTH observed in the placebo group. Consumption of the calcium and vitamin D–fortified food product also conferred benefits to bone health, as bone density, bone mineral content, and bone thickness were improved in the treatment group as compared to the placebo group at various sites within the tibia, as assessed using peripheral quantitative computed tomography.

Collectively, the data gleaned from these two controlled trials highlight the potential benefits of calcium and vitamin D in optimizing bone health during periods of elevated bone turnover such as IMT.

In 2017, the US Army began providing a snack item containing approximately 200 calories, 1000 mg calcium (as calcium carbonate), and 2000 IU vitamin D (as vitamin D3) to all recruits during IMT. The item is provided once per day and is intended to be served as a snack, as foods are not typically permitted to be consumed outside of the dining facility. Similar to the Army and Air Force multivitamin programs, this effort is not a randomized, controlled trial, but the incidence of injury and attrition may be considered in the context of historical data in an effort to determine the potential efficacy of calcium and vitamin D in mitigating stress fracture risk.

PATIENT EVALUATION

Stress fracture risk may be a consideration when assessing patients indicating participation in unaccustomed or repetitive physical activities, such as the start of a new exercise training program (i.e., running) or intention to begin military service. Physicians should be aware of risk factors for stress fracture, such as gender (increased risk in females), BMI (low BMI indicates increased risk), smoking status (increased risk in current and prior smokers), and fitness level (increased risk in sedentary individuals). Physicians may consider screening such patients for nutrient status, to include iron and vitamin D. Iron status should be assessed utilizing a series of biomarkers, such as indicators of iron storage (i.e., serum ferritin) in combination with hemoglobin to determine the presence of ID, IDA, or anemia not associated with poor iron status. The use of multiple biomarkers of iron status is critical due to factors (such as inflammation) that may confound any single indicator. Example biomarkers of iron status include serum ferritin, transferrin saturation, total iron binding capacity, erythrocyte protoporphyrin, and soluble transferrin receptor. Note that not all biomarkers may be available at local laboratories, and each should be interpreted using cut-off values recommended by clinical laboratories, as appropriate. Population studies typically define anemia in premenopausal women as hemoglobin <12 g/dL (Looker et al., 1997). Vitamin D status may be assessed through the measurement of serum 25(OH)D; cut-off values recommended by clinical laboratories vary significantly. Recent IOM reports indicate that individuals may be at risk of deficiency relative to bone health at serum levels <12 ng/mL (IOM 2011), although levels above 40 ng/mL may be beneficial for the avoidance of stress fracture in at-risk populations (Burgi et al., 2011).

If ID is identified through clinical assessment, improvements in dietary intake may be the most appropriate initial recommendation for improvements in iron status. Patients should be urged to consume foods rich in iron, such as meats, leafy green vegetables, and fortified cereals. Referral to a registered dietitian (RD) may be of value. Consumption of a low-dose iron supplement may be a consideration on an individual basis. If IDA or anemia without ID is identified, the patient should be treated or referred following established clinical guidelines. In cases of poor vitamin D status, again, improvements in dietary intake may be the most appropriate initial recommendation. Increased consumption of fortified food products, such as dairy, should be recommended, and consumption of a vitamin D supplement may be a consideration on an individual basis. Improvements in calcium intake may also be recommended through calcium-rich foods such as leafy green vegetables. In the case of both iron and vitamin D, IOM recommendations for tolerable upper intake levels should be considered prior to recommending supplementation.

SUMMARY AND CONCLUSION

Stress fractures are incomplete fractures of bone that occur during periods of unaccustomed physical activity. Although stress fractures affect both men and women, risk is markedly greater in women. Stress fractures are costly injuries to athletes participating in repetitive activities, such as running; and to military personnel engaged in the rigorous unaccustomed activities associated with

IMT, such as load carriage. Many unmodifiable factors affect the risk of stress fracture, such as age, sex, and genetics. Nutrition is a modifiable factor affecting the risk of stress fracture that may provide a tool for prevention. Poor iron (more common in women) and vitamin D status have been linked to stress fracture risk, and randomized, controlled trials of calcium and vitamin D supplementation have demonstrated efficacy in the prevention of stress fracture. Although further research may be required, optimizing iron, calcium, and vitamin D intake prior to and during engagement in repetitive unaccustomed activities, including military training, should be considered in efforts to reduce stress fracture risk.

DISCLAIMER

The opinions or assertions contained herein are the private views of the author and are not to be construed as official or as reflecting the views of the Army or the Department of Defense.

REFERENCES

Andersen, NE, Karl, JP, Cable, SJ, et al. 2010. Vitamin D status in female military personnel during combat training. *J. Int. Soc. Sports Nutr.* 7:38.

Barnes, KR, Tchandja, JN, Webber, BJ, Federinko, SP, and Cropper, TL. 2015. The effects of prenatal vitamin supplementation on operationally significant health outcomes in female Air Force trainees. *Mil. Med.* 180:554–558.

Bennell, KL, Malcolm, SA, Thomas, SA, Reid, SJ, Brukner, PD, Ebeling, PR, and Ward, JD. 1996. Risk factors for stress fractures in track and field athletes. A twelve-month prospective study. *Am. J. Sports Med.* 24:810–818.

Burgi, AA, Gorham, ED, Garland, CF, et al. 2011. High serum 25-hydroxyvitamin D is associated with a low incidence of stress fractures. *J. Bone Miner. Res.* 26:2371–2377.

Changstrom, BG, Brou, L, Khodaee, M, Braund, C, and Comstock, RD. 2015. Epidemiology of stress fracture injuries among US high school athletes, 2005–2006 through 2012–2013. *Am. J. Sports Med.* 43:26–33.

Chatzipapas, C, Boikos, S, Drosos, GI, et al. 2009. Polymorphisms of the vitamin D receptor gene and stress fractures. *Horm. Metab. Res.* 41:635–640.

Dao, D, Sodhi, S, Tabasinejad, R, et al. 2015. Serum 25-hydroxyvitamin D levels and stress fractures in military personnel: A systematic review and meta-analysis. *Am. J. Sports Med.* 43:2064–2072.

DeMaeyer, E, and Adiels-Tegman, M. 1985. The prevalence of anemia in the world. *World Health Stat. Q.* 38:306–316.

Forrest, KY, and Stuhldreher, WL. 2011. Prevalence and correlates of vitamin D deficiency in US adults. *Nutr. Res.* 31:48–54.

Gaffney-Stomberg, E, Lutz, LJ, Rood, JC, et al. 2014. Calcium and vitamin D supplementation maintains parathyroid hormone and improves bone density during initial military training: A randomized, double-blind, placebo-controlled trial. *Bone* 68:46–56.

Gaffney-Stomberg, E, Lutz, LJ, Scherbina, A, et al. 2017. Association between single gene polymorphisms and bone biomarkers and response to calcium and vitamin D supplementation in young adults undergoing military training. *J. Bone Miner. Res.* 32:498–507.

Harris, MM, Houtkooper, LB, Stanford, VA, et al. 2003. Dietary iron is associated with bone mineral density in healthy postmenopausal women. *J. Nutr.* 133:3598–3602.

Holick, MF, Binkley, NC, Bischoff-Ferrari, HA, et al. 2011. Evaluation, treatment, and prevention of vitamin D deficiency: An Endocrine Society clinical practice guideline. *J. Clin. Endocrinol. Metab.* 96:1911–1930.

Hughes, JM, and Petit, MA. 2010. Biological underpinnings of Frost's mechanostat thresholds: The importance of osteocytes. *J. Musculoskelet. Neuronal Interact.* 10:128–135.

Institute of Medicine. 2001. *Dietary Reference Intakes for Vitamin A, Vitamin K, Arsenic, Boron, Chromium, Copper, Iodine, Iron, Manganese, Molybdenum, Nickel, Silicon, Vanadium, and Zinc.* Washington, DC: The National Academies Press.

Institute of Medicine. 2011. *Dietary Reference Intakes for Calcium and Vitamin D.* Washington, DC: The National Academies Press.

Jones, BH, Thacker, SB, Gilchrist, J, Kimsey, CD Jr, and Sosin, DM. 2002. Prevention of lower extremity stress fractures in athletes and soldiers: A systematic review. *Epidemiol. Rev.* 24:228–247.

Karl, JP, Lieberman, HR, Cable, SJ, Williams, KW, Young, AJ, and McClung, JP. 2010. Randomized, double-blind, placebo-controlled trial of an iron-fortified food product in female soldiers during military training: Relations between iron status, serum hepcidin, and inflammation. *Am. J. Clin. Nutr.* 92:93–100.

Katsumata, S, Tsuboi, R, Uehara, M, and Suzuki, K. 2006. Dietary iron deficiency decreases serum osteocalcin concentration and bone mineral density in rats. *Biosci. Biotechnol. Biochem.* 70:2547–2550.

Lappe, J, Cullen, D, Haynatzki, G, Recker, R, Ahlf, R, and Thompson, K. 2008. Calcium and vitamin D supplementation decreases incidence of stress fractures in female Navy recruits. *J. Bone Miner. Res.* 23:741–749.

Looker, AC, Dallman, PR, Carroll, MD, Gunter, EW, and Johnson, CL. 1997. Prevalence of iron deficiency in the United States. *JAMA.* 277:973–976.

Lutz, LJ, Karl, JP, Rood, JC, et al. 2012. Vitamin D status, dietary intake, and bone turnover in female soldiers during military training: A longitudinal study. *J. Int. Soc. Sports Nutr.* 9:38.

Mangano, KM, Walsh, SJ, Insogna, KL, Kenny, AM, and Kerstetter, JE. 2011. Calcium intake in the United States from dietary and supplemental sources across adult age groups: New estimates from the National Health and Nutrition Examination Survey 2003–2006. *J. Am. Diet. Assoc.* 111:687–695.

McClung, JP, Marchitelli, LJ, Friedl, KE, and Young, AJ. 2006. Prevalence of iron deficiency and iron deficiency anemia among three populations of female personnel in the US Army. *J. Am. Coll. Nutr.* 25:64–69.

McClung, JP, Karl, JP, Cable, SJ, et al. 2009a. Randomized, double-blind, placebo-controlled trial of iron supplementation in female soldiers during military training: Effects on iron status, physical performance, and mood. *Am. J. Clin. Nutr.* 90:124–131.

McClung, JP, Karl, JP, Cable, SJ, Williams, KW, Young, AJ, and Lieberman, HR. 2009b. Longitudinal decrements in iron status during military training in female soldiers. *Br. J. Nutr.* 102:605–609.

McClung, JP, and Murray-Kolb, LE. 2013. Iron nutrition and premenopausal women: Effects of poor iron status on physical and neuropsychological performance. *Annu. Rev. Nutr.* 33:271–288.

Medeiros, DM, Plattner, A, Jennings, D, and Stoecker, B. 2002. Bone morphology, strength and density are compromised in iron-deficient rats and exacerbated by calcium restriction. *J. Nutr.* 132:3135–3141.

Medeiros, DM, Stoecker, B, Plattner, A, Jennings, D, and Haub, M. 2004. Iron deficiency negatively affects vertebrae and femurs of rats independently of energy intake and body weight. *J. Nutr.* 134:3061–3067.

Mencej-Bedrac, S, Prezelj, J, Kocjan, T, et al. 2009. The combinations of polymorphisms in vitamin D receptor, osteoprotegerin and tumour necrosis factor superfamily member 11 genes are associated with bone mineral density. *J. Mol. Endocrinol.* 42:239–247.

Merkel, D, Moran, DS, Yanovich, R, et al. 2008. The association between hematological and inflammatory factors and stress fractures among female military recruits. *Med. Sci. Sports Exerc.* 40:S691–S697.

Rauh, MJ, Macera, CA, Trone, DW, Shaffer, RA, and Brodine, SK. 2006. Epidemiology of stress fracture and lower-extremity overuse injury in female recruits. *Med. Sci. Sports Exerc.* 38:1571–1577.

Ruohola, JP, Laaksi, I, Ylikomi, T, et al. 2006. Association between serum 25(OH)D concentrations and bone stress fractures in Finnish young men. *J. Bone Miner. Res.* 21:1483–1488.

Toxqui, L, and Vaquero, MP. 2015. Chronic iron deficiency as an emerging risk factor for osteoporosis: A hypothesis. *Nutrients* 7:2324–2344.

Wright, I, Blanco-Rojo, R, Fernandez, MC, et al. 2013. Bone remodeling is reduced by recovery from iron-deficiency anaemia in premenopausal women. *J. Physiol. Biochem.* 69:889–896.

Yanovich, R, Merkel, D, Israeli, E, Evans, RK, Erlich, T, and Moran, DS. 2011. Anemia, iron deficiency, and stress fractures in female combatants during 16 months. *J. Strength Cond. Res.* 12:3412–3421.

Yanovich, R, Karl, JP, Yanovich, E, et al. 2015. Effects of basic combat training on iron status in male and female soldiers: A comparative study. *US Army Med. Dep. J.* Apr-Jun: 67–73.

Section III

Metabolic Therapies for Specific Orthopedic Conditions

17 Perioperative Metabolic Therapies in Orthopedics

Frederick T. Sutter MD, MBA

INTRODUCTION

The physiological stress of major surgical procedures has been thoroughly reviewed[1] and there have been robust studies of the influence of metabolic therapy in general surgical procedures, and outcome measures beyond the length of stay (LOS) and readmission rates are being evaluated in the current literature. Scientific literature at a meta-analysis level of recommendation[2,3] demonstrates the interrelationship between nutritional status, as a major determinant, and achieving successful general surgical outcomes when compared in enhanced recovery after surgery (ERAS) protocols, even in normally nourished patients. This chapter hones the general surgery research to orthopedic application. It details clinical and immediate metabolic therapy strategies to support patients undergoing orthopedic surgery.

Physicians are personally consuming and recommending nutrients to their patients, with a majority in the orthopedic and cardiology specialties. It appears timely, then, that they consider the abundant literature on this topic and begin prescribing specific diet, nutrient and exercise regimens to benefit patient outcomes.[4] Many of today's orthopedic surgeries are elective, providing a generous preoperative (preop) window to prepare a willing patient to achieve the best result possible. The orthopedic surgical substrate of bone, muscle, and connective tissue represents the body's stockpile of protein, pH buffering, and minerals. Metabolic intervention to support these tissues offers a strategic leverage point to improve outcomes.

Orthopedic procedures occur disproportionately among patients with preexisting deconditioning, sarcopenia, and/or obesity. Self-directed patient metabolic efforts can be focused by physician guidance in the perioperative period and could also reduce the use of dietary supplements that can create unwanted complications in the perioperative period as the use of supplemental nutrients frequently occurs unbeknownst to the treating physician despite detailed intake history.[5]

Clinical behavior changes slowly and implementation of perioperative nutrition support is compounded by the fact that most physicians have had little opportunity for training in the use of nutrient therapies. Orthopedic fast-track clinical pathways rarely include a detailed discussion on nutrition beyond identifying those who are malnourished. In today's healthcare environment shortening hospital length of stay, limiting the use of opioids, and reducing readmission through an organizational, multimodal approach creates many challenges. The combination of patient interest in optimizing their personal outcome with an impending surgical event creates a superb opportunity to spark meaningful patient compliance in a perioperative metabolic therapy program.

EPIDEMIOLOGY

With the trends of increased outpatient surgeries, shortened inpatient surgical stays, rising prevalence of obesity and bariatric surgery, published surgical results for hospitals, and a greater reliance on the primary physician for follow-up care, there is great opportunity to expand the outcomes horizon beyond the challenges of surgical technique. Engaging the support of willing non-surgical clinicians to reduce perioperative risks can facilitate recovery and meaningfully improve outcomes.

The prevalence of obesity has more than doubled in the last 30 years. There has been a concurrent increase in total calories consumed primarily in the form of carbohydrates and a slight decrease in the amount of protein calories.[6] Obesity has increased the incidence of arthritic conditions requiring orthopedic procedures in younger adults, with greater complication rates of wound infection, deep venous thrombosis, cardiac events, and anesthesia risks.[7–10] Obesogenic sarcopenia increases these risks.[11] See Chapter 10 for detailed review.

PERIOPERATIVE METABOLIC RISKS

The combination of years of nutrient depletion due to poor diet, polypharmacy[12], obesogenic sarcopenia, disease-related malnutrition, advanced age, and deconditioning creates a challenging perioperative landscape for the orthopedic patient. Even anticipation of the procedure increases stress and can interfere with sleep. Activity restriction and pain, particularly in the lower limbs commonly promotes deconditioning with secondary loss of lean body mass creating an additional risk in the form of sarcopenia, which is associated with unfavorable outcomes.[13] With inactivity, the patient frequently has a significant decline in vitamin D levels negatively influencing bone healing. Joint disease and subsequent surgery increases demand on the contralateral limb, increasing the risk of additional surgery.[14] The restriction of nutrients during the NPO period prior to surgery initiates catabolism of lean tissue and dehydration and sets the stage for postoperative insulin resistance and hyperglycemia in diabetics. Eliminating medications and nutrients targeted for pain management prior to this can increase pain, immobility, and the need for additional narcotic analgesia. Surgery induces major catabolic stress as an inflammatory response creating a hyperimmune state and the associated depletion of many conditionally essential nutrients. This is understandably followed by immunosuppression due to exhausted substrates, increasing the risk of infection[15] and postoperative complications. This severe challenge to the exquisitely balanced TH1 and TH2 immune autoregulation system deserves further consideration as the contextual foundation for further research in perioperative metabolic therapy which has been elegantly reviewed by Smit, et al.[16] The chronic pain of advanced osteoarthritis is associated with sleep complaints in 67%–88% of patients, both of which share additional co-morbidities such as obesity, type 2 diabetes, and depression.[17] Frequently, the patient has myofascial pain, which several studies found to significantly impair sleep quality as well.[18] The majority of potentially addictive prescription sleep medications actually decrease time spent in the restorative sleep stages 3 and 4. Use of these medications should be sparing and balanced with other sleep strategies to avoid long term dependence and challenging withdrawal symptoms. Non-pharmacological sleep treatments are preferable, which presents a major opportunity for perioperative pain management in this age of polypharmacy and opioid addiction.[19]

After surgery, post-anesthesia nausea and vomiting (PONV) and immobilization can advance catabolic wasting and limit nutrient intake. Wound healing and blood loss increase demand for many nutrients well in excess of normal dietary intake, so consuming a "regular diet" is highly unlikely to fully meet the metabolic demands for optimal healing.[20]

ENHANCED RECOVERY AFTER SURGERY GUIDELINES

ERAS protocols have been developed to provide multimodal clinical support pathways to address the challenges of the perioperative period and have been demonstrated worldwide to be cost-effective and improve outcomes for a variety of surgical procedures.[21] This idea was pioneered 20 years ago[22] as a method for treating patients following colonic surgery. The focus in orthopedics currently is on the high-volume procedures of total joint arthroplasty (nearly 1,000,000 knee and hip procedures in the US annually)[23] and more recently of spine surgery. ERAS protocols are grouped in three multidisciplinary guideline bundles: preoperative, intraoperative, and postoperative.

The preop phase includes education and management of patient expectations for outcomes and pain control before and after surgery as well as the ERAS process; physiotherapy functional and cardiopulmonary (6 min walk test) evaluations; dietary assessment [there are several that have been validated: Mini Nutrition Assessment (*MNA®*), Subjective Global Assessment (SGA), and Nutritional Risk Screening (NRS)] to identify nutritional deficiencies combined with preop enteral nutrition – even in normally nourished patients – and minimizing preop fasting period to 2 hours, unless there is documentation of gastroparesis. Preventive analgesia may include pharmacologic intervention with limited opioids, non-steroidal anti-inflammatory drugs (NSAIDs), acetaminophen, and non-pharmacologic interventions to include acupuncture, neuromuscular electrical stimulation for knee and hip arthroplasty (NMES),[24] pulsed electromagnetic fields therapy (PEMF)[25], and early use of metabolic therapies effective in pain management as outlined below.

Intraoperative (intraop) intervention would include minimally invasive surgery, a preference for neuraxial anesthesia, goal directed fluid management,[26] and active warming for the avoidance of hypothermia and nausea and vomiting prophylaxis. Postoperative (postop) guidelines include early physiotherapy and mobilization, aggressive managements of PONV, balanced pain control with careful attention to minimizing narcotic analgesics, gum chewing to facilitate peristalsis and early return to oral diet and nutrition support formulas for at least 7 days, early discharge to home, and dynamic postop rehab progression for early return to functional activities. Online patient education (PlanAgainstPain.com) regarding pain management with opioids has been developed by the *Choices Matter* campaign, recently launched in New York City. For greater detail regarding ERAS approaches, see Reader Resources.

PHARMACOLOGY

The use of non-steroidal anti-inflammatory drugs (NSAIDs), cyclo-oxygenase-2 inhibitors, disease-modifying anti-rheumatic drugs (DMARDs), and biologic agents (BAs) in the perioperative period should be evaluated given their impact on the wound healing process. Potential complications include wound dehiscence, infection, impaired collagen synthesis, and an enhanced side effect profile in the postop period. There is consensus on the anti-platelet effects of NSAIDs[27] and prudent limitation of NSAIDs in patients with proven stress fractures has also been recommended,[28] implying the consideration of impaired bone healing. Evidence is sparse on the use of DMARDs and BAs, however, a 2016 retrospective study of rheumatoid arthritis (RA) patients undergoing surgery concluded that continuation of DMARD monotherapy such as methotrexate (MTX), hydroxychloroquine, leflunomide, or the combination of MTX and TNFα-inhibitor therapy for RA in the perioperative setting was not associated with increased rates of overall postoperative infectious complication and wound infections in a total of 9362 surgeries among 5,544 RA patients.[29] The practitioner will need to consider disease severity, individual risk of exacerbation, and potential surgical risk factors in the context of drug pharmacokinetics prior to making recommendations for cessation of therapy.[30]

PREOPERATIVE PATIENT EVALUATION

PHYSICAL EXAM

The definition and significance of sarcopenia have been reviewed by Kohlstadt[11] and others. In general, sarcopenia can be defined as the age- or disuse-related loss of muscle and fat-free body mass, reducing muscle metabolism, strength, and mobility in older adults. Skeletal muscle mass is quantified as being less than or equal to two standard deviations (SD) below the mean. Associated risk factors for sarcopenia are cigarette smoking, chronic illnesses, underweight, physical inactivity, and a poorer sense of psychosocial well-being.[31,32]

Waist and hip circumference used alone or in combination with BMI is an anthropometric indicator of health risk and is easily performed. The combination of both is a very sensitive metric to predict health risk. The National Institute of Health[33] suggests abdominal obesity as a very high health risk indicator and can be identified with waist circumference (measured at the umbilicus) in men ≥ 102 cm (40 inches) and in women ≥ 88 cm (35 inches). The waist-to-hip ratio (WHR) is the preferred clinical measure of central obesity for predicting mortality, even in those regarded as very lean (BMI < 20), normal, and overweight (BMI > 25). Risk rises significantly for cardiovascular mortality when the WHR goes beyond 0.8 for women and 0.9 for men.[34,35]

Clinical identification of obesogenic sarcopenia demonstrates poor fat-free mass (FFM) in obese individuals and can be appreciated as pendulous adiposity in the arms, abdomen, and even the thighs and legs. Gentle palpation over the triceps area (as if performing a skin-fold fat measurement) and estimating the remaining muscle can also be clinically revealing. This is opposed to the more stout or solid individual with considerable muscle mass, despite being identified as obese by BMI. Bench research on age-related sarcopenia and fatigability demonstrated the presence of enhanced reactive oxygen species, systemic inflammation, apoptotic susceptibility, and reduced mitochondrial biogenesis.[36,37] Obesogenic sarcopenia in the frail elderly presenting for total joint arthroplasty presents a great challenge; however, simple interventions with nutrition, exercise, and weight loss have been demonstrated to ameliorate these risk factors over longer periods of time (up to 6 months) so it is imperative to identify these individuals early to anticipate a longer preoperative interval.[38]

Nutrition-Specific Preoperative Laboratory Evaluation

With the usual preoperative lab studies, several additional laboratory studies can be very useful in assessing potential nutritional deficiencies or surgical risks (see Table 17.1). Supplementing a low normal nutrient value prepares the patient for the catabolic stress of healing. Scientific literature has described "metabolic therapy" as that which involves the administration of a substance normally found in the body to enhance a metabolic reaction. This can be achieved in two ways: one, by giving a substance to achieve greater than normal levels in the body to drive a biochemical reaction in the desired direction; two, by using a substance to correct the relative or absolute deficiency of a cellular component. This concept is useful in the context of prescribing nutrients to improve surgical outcomes.

Elevated high-sensitivity C-reactive protein has been associated with higher complications and greater length of stay for orthopedic patients. To address this, removing sugar, consuming low arachidonic acid food groups, targeting protein intake, and taking antioxidants are best (see Tables 17.2 and 17.3). Patients with low albumin were twice as likely to require prolonged hospitalization (>15 days) for elective total hip replacement compared with those in whom the albumin level was 3.9 g/dl or greater. A recent meta-analysis[40] of over 112,000 orthopedic surgical patients demonstrated that those with an albumin level < 3.5 g/dL had an almost 2.5-fold increased risk of surgical site infection.[39,40] Following transferrin and albumin levels perioperatively has also been used to predict delayed wound healing after total hip arthroplasty.[50]

Prealbumin is a sensitive, cost-effective serum marker for protein malnutrition that responds quickly to increasing protein intake, particularly in the form of branched chain amino acids (BCAAs) and can be monitored bi-weekly in acute situations. In critically ill patients, lower levels are associated with increased hospital length of stay, morbidity, and mortality.[1]

The incidence of healing complications was three times more frequent in individuals with preoperative total lymphocyte count (TLC) <1500 cells/mm compared with normals[45] and in surgical treatment of hip fractures in the elderly, TLC and the Mini Nutrition Assessment (MNA®) were more predictive compared with several other parameters in predicting delayed wound healing.[46] The MNA takes 10–15 min to implement and the MNA short form (MNA®-SF) is a 5 minute, inexpensive clinical preop evaluation to determine nutritional risk in the surgical patient and can be predictive of functional decline during the year after surgery.[47]

TABLE 17.1

Preoperative Laboratory Assessment for Enhanced Recovery After Surgery

Lab	Optimal Range	Indicator	Note	References
Albumin	3.9 g/dL or greater	↑ LOS and 2.5× infection rates when <3.5	↑ dietary intake 0.8–1.4 g protein/kg body wt/day	39,40
hsCRP	<3 mg/L	If >3 mg/L, associated with ↑ complication and LOS for ortho pts	Treat with anti-inlfammatory diet, curcumin See Tables 17.2, 17.5	41
Folate	>5.4 ng/mL	Lowers Hcy with B6,B12	Use activated form See Table 17.3	42
Iron, Ferritin	Per lab	Supports blood element formation	Support if <NL range; See Table 17.3	43
Homocysteine (Hcy)	4–8 µM/L	↑levels associated with ↑ risk of CVA, CAD, DVT	↑ risk 9–17 µM/L ↑↑ risk >17 µM/L; See Table 17.2	40, 44–46
Total lymphocyte count	>1500 cells/mm³	3X ↑ in healing complications	Predicts fxn ↓ 1 yr postop	47–49
Magnesium	↑NL range	Bone healing, ↓ in obesity, chronic pain	Rx depletion in combination with low intake in typical diet	50
Prealbumin	>15 mg/dL	↓cost, early marker for ↓ protein	Rapid response to correction	1
Transferrin	>200 mg/dL	Predictor of slow wound healing in THA	Acute marker; may be ↑ in chronic Fe deficiency anemia	51
Vitamin B6	>50 nmol/L	↑ DVT <23 nmol/L	See Table 17.3	52
Vitamin B12	>500 pg/mL	10%–15% over age 60 are deficient	IM injection typically not covered by insurances; pts usually willing to pay minor cost	50
Vitamin D (25-OH D3)	50–70 ng/dL	Bone healing, ↓ in obesity, chronic and nonspecific	See Table 17.3	53

Abbreviations: CAD, Coronary Artery Disease; CVA, Stroke; DVT, Deep Vein Thrombosis; fxn, Function; hsCRP, high sensitivity C-reactive Protein; LOS, Length of Stay; Pts, Patients; THA, Total Hip Arthroplasty.
Lifestyle Medicine Consultants, Inc. Copyright 2017.

TREATMENT RECOMMENDATIONS

DIET

Adequate caloric intake is essential, especially in the form of protein. It is a key macronutrient in wound healing and managing complications related to sarcopenia along with exercise,[54] and is critical to help promote muscle protein synthesis and decrease inflammation-associated loss of lean body mass and function. Instruct the patient to target at least the recommended daily allowance of 0.8 g/kg body weight of protein intake, provided there is no concomitant liver, renal disease, or history of gout. Protein sources in the form of seafood and organ meats can be high in purines (some examples include: adenine, guanine, hypoxanthine, xanthine, theobromine, caffeine, uric acid, and isoguanine), usually restricted in treating gout. However, consumption of these in the presence of caffeinated or alcoholic beverages (especially beer) is more likely to precipitate a gout attack at the RDA level for protein.[55] Higher dietary protein (up to 1.6 g protein/kg/day or up to 30% of total caloric intake) can enhance response to resistance exercise in the elderly.[53,56] Protein intake will be metabolized best if consumed evenly throughout the day, particularly with the midday meal or for

TABLE 17.2

Dietary Guidelines to Modulate Perioperative Inflammation

Food Category	Serving Size	Servings per Day	Calories per Serving	Choices[a]
Concentrated protein	3.5 oz (after cooking)	3–4	150	Poultry (remove all skin), turkey and chicken; lean, grass fed meats; sliced, boiled ham, pork tenderloin, beef steak, ground beef (5% fat); fish (avoid farmed fish); veggie burger; dairy (if tolerated): cottage cheese 1% fat, ¾ cup ricotta reduced fat, ½ cup; Tofu products: tofu, 1 cup, tempeh ½ cup, soy burger 4 oz
Vegetables	½ cup	5–7	10–25	All vegetables are allowed except white potato, turnip, parsnip, rutabaga, and corn. Fresh vegetable juice or green beverages are allowed: note sugar content
Fruits	½ cup	3–4	80	All whole fruits except: banana, oranges, grapes, pineapple, and papaya. Fruit juices not recommended
Dairy substitutes	6 oz	1–2	80–100	Non-GMO almond, rice, coconut, hemp "milks" with no added sugar
Legumes	½ to 1 cup	1–2	100–200	All peas and beans, hummus, bean soups
Grains, Spelt	½ cup	1–3	75–100	Gluten free, whole grains such as; quinoa, farro, millet, chia, flax, amaranth, buckwheat, brown rice, gluten free whole oats with at least 3 grams or more of fiber per serving
Nuts, Seeds	1 small handful	1 per day	150–200	All nuts except cashews, macadamias, pistachios; 1–2 tbsp of nut butter
Oils	1 tsp	4–6	40	Olive, coconut, avocado, macadamia oils for cooking; flax seed, and walnut oils for salads, mayonnaise from olive oil (no sugar added), avocado, green or black olives (8–10)
Beverages	*Ad libitum*	Water intake per day to equal ½ body wt, in oz	0	Water, organic herbal tea, decaffeinated coffee or tea, mineral water, club soda or selzer, plain or flavored (no added artificial sweeteners)
Condiments	*Ad libitum*, except salt	*Ad libitum*	0	Cinnamon, carob, mustard, horseradish, vinegar, lemon, lime, flavored extracts, herbs/spices; apple cider vinegar (organic unfiltered); no refined sugars or artificial sweeteners are advised

[a] Patients should be advised to avoid foods to which they have a history of intolerance.
Lifestyle Medicine Consultants, Inc. Copyright 2017.

convenience in the form of protein beverages. A meta-analysis of 36 randomized controlled trials (RCT) (3790 patients) showed that the use of high-protein supplements (>20% of calories from protein) was associated with reduced complications and readmission to hospital, improved grip strength, increased intake of protein and energy, and improvements in weight.[57] Specific dietary recommendations are listed in Table 17.2.

Closer to surgery, ERAS protocols advise minimizing preoperative fasting and clear liquids containing nutrient formulas can safely be offered up to 2 hours before surgery.[58] Carbohydrate loading using complex carbohydrates can improve the incidence of postoperative insulin resistance and hyperglycemia which is associated with higher rates of postsurgical infection, as well as reducing PONV and initial pain scores.[59]

TABLE 17.3
Better Quality Supplements

The product demonstrates:

- Independent lab testing
- Chelated minerals
- Fish Oils: label states free of heavy metals, PCBs
- No artificial colors, sweeteners, preservatives
- Use of health conscious fillers like vegetable based cellulose
- Avoid fillers and binders: glycols, sucrose, etc.
- No common allergens such as wheat, gluten, corn protein, soy, or dairy products
- "Nutrition Facts" labeling and complete label disclosure of contents

Manufacturing guidelines:

- cGMP (Current Good Manufacturing Practices)
- NSF™ (NSF International, The Public Health and Safety Company™)
- ISO 9000 or ISO 9001:2000 (International Organization for Standardization)
- TGA (Therapeutic Goods Administration Australian Government)

The anabolic response to increased protein intake is less robust in the elderly compared with younger individuals, but can be improved with exercise and increased protein intake. "Anabolic resistance" to muscle protein synthesis (MPS) in age-related sarcopenia[60] can be addressed by using branched chain amino acids (leucine, isoleucine, valine) or leucine alone, along with specific exercise prescription (see Table 17.3). The notion of a "leucine threshold" has been postulated for the blunted response to MPS in elderly muscle. In addition, exercise is most effective with a focus on structural appropriateness (e.g., arthritis or tendonitis in the area to be exercised) and intensity. For the elderly, low-load (30% of a one repetition maximum (1RM)), higher repetition (to fatigue or "shakiness") exercise has been demonstrated to produce MPS. Readers are referred to a more detailed review of exercise prescriptions.[61]

In order to quell the surgically induced inflammatory cascade, some general dietary guidelines limiting animal fat content, arachidonic acid, refined carbohydrates, and simple sugars should be offered to the patient. Arachidonic acid is the physiologic precursor of proinflammatory eicosanoids such as prostaglandins and leukotrienes which are best limited in the preop period (Table 17.2). These molecules can then go on to produce superoxide, which promotes a feed-forward, or propagated lipid peroxidation chain reaction, increasing antioxidant demand for the body. Appreciable results occur within 10 days, although the first 5–7 days may be challenging if considerable sugar consumption has been habitual prior to initiating dietary changes. Supplemental oral nutrition supplements (ONS) or immunonutrition (IN) beverages will help balance blood sugar during this transition.

European Society for Clinical Nutrition and Metabolism has recently defined consensus diagnostic criteria for malnutrition according to two options: BMI less than 18.5 kg/m² or combined weight loss > 10% or > 5% weight loss over 3 months plus reduced BMI; or a low fat free mass index indicating sarcopenia.[3] Treating malnourished patients is beyond the scope of this chapter, requires longer periods of preop preparation, and in acute circumstances necessitates stabilization with total parenteral nutrition.

PAIN CONTROL

Implementing metabolic therapy for pain management takes time, some patience, and patient education. Symptomatic slow acting drugs for osteo-arthritis (SYSADOA), a term coined about 20 years ago, include products such as glucosamine sulfate and chondroitin sulfate which have been available as prescription medications in Europe. Therapeutic benefit requires 1–3 months which needs to be considered in advance of any weaning from pharmaceuticals. These two nutrients have been demonstrated in randomized, double-blind, placebo-controlled trials to be effective not only with symptom management, but also preventive for arthritis progression; hence, the newer term structure/disease-modifying anti–oa drug (S/DMOAD).[62–64]

Distinction is made with regard to the use of pharmaceutical-grade crystalline glucosamine sulfate (GS) and chondroitin sulfate (CS) that are prescribed medications in Europe as opposed to some commercial products available in North America as over-the-counter (OTC) products, which demands careful attention to product quality (see Table 17.3). Also, results obtained with glucosamine sulfate may not be extrapolated to other salts, such as the hydrochloride (HCl) formulation. Grade A level of evidence [at least one randomized controlled trial (RCT)] and Grade 1a level of recommendation (meta- analysis of RCT's) exists that glucosamine sulfate and chondroitin sulfate therapies offer symptomatic and disease-modifying influence in osteoarthritis.[65] Controversy has waxed and waned over the years about GS and CS effectiveness with varying levels of consensus recommendations; however, the consensus appears to be influenced by the availability of quality supplements in North America and economic drivers in Europe where they are prescription items.

CS has been shown in a two-year RCT to be superior to celecoxib at reducing cartilage volume loss as measured by quantitative MRI, with similar efficacy in pain management[64] and to be effective in the treatment of osteoarthritis and concomitant psoriasis.[66] The value of SYSADOA medications is not only are they comparable to anti-inflammatories such as celecoxib and diclofenac sodium with symptom relief, but, as a study over 20 years ago revealed, the slow acting component of the therapeutic response, although appearing later in time than the NSAIDs, lasted up to 3 months after the end of treatment.[67] This weighs heavily in the favor of using glucosamine sulfate and chondroitin sulfate preop, as a therapeutic benefit is highly likely to persist through the perioperative nutrient withdrawal phase. This is particularly important in joint surgery with regard to the increased demands on the contralateral limb.[14]

Curcumin is the active compound present in turmeric rhizomes (*curcuma longa*) that has both antioxidant and anti-inflammatory properties. Turmeric has been safely consumed for thousands of years and has been studied extensively in a wide variety of clinical conditions. It has been shown to significantly lower CRP ($p < 0.001$) and other inflammatory markers versus placebo in a RCT/meta-analysis in patients with metabolic syndrome, over 8 weeks at a dose of 500 mg twice daily, with a 95% confidence interval.[68] In smaller studies it has been compared with diclofenac in active rheumatoid arthritis, showing superior pain management and no adverse effects[69] and in knee OA with similar results.[70] Most formulations are well tolerated; however, the author has noted greater patient intolerance to preparations that include a black pepper fruit extract or other excipients. It has demonstrated efficacy and safety in combination with SYSADOA medications to help pain and mobility in knee OA.[71]

In the last four years, in the author's experience, high molecular weight sodium hyaluronic acid (HA) in combination with hydrolyzed collagen and polysaccharides has been an effective clinical tool for metabolic management of osteoarthritis in hundreds of patients. It significantly reduced pain in as early as 2 months and, more impressively, at 3 months ($p < 0.001$) it increased the endogenous hyaluronic acid secreted by synoviocytes, reduced synovial effusion, and improved muscle function about the knee joint in several small but elegant studies. It has been demonstrated to be more effective than extracted and fermented HA.[72–74] For patients with rheumatoid arthritis, encouraging responses have been demonstrated with the use of undenatured collagen type II (UC-II) (see Case Study 2).[75,76]

Fish oil-derived omega-3 fatty acids displacing the arachidonic acid of the cell membrane of immune cells attenuate the production of inflammatory prostaglandins and prostacyclins and reduce the cytotoxicity of inflammatory cells.[2] The essential fatty acids eicosapentaenoic (EPA) and docosahexaenoic acids (DHAs) are the precursors of resolvins, protectins, and maresins: mediators that aid in the resolution of the inflammatory arachidonic acid cascade and are shown to reduce cellular inflammation by inhibiting the transportation of inflammatory cells and mediators to the site of inflammation.[77]

One fish oil study raises the possibility that the anti-inflammatory actions of omega-3 fatty acids may play a role in the prevention of sarcopenia.[78] A review by Bays[79] of clinical trials demonstrated high-dose omega-3 fatty acid consumption to be safe, even when concurrently administered with other agents that may increase bleeding, such as aspirin and warfarin. For the management of preop pain, particularly before the withdrawal of NSAIDs or other prescription drugs, the author suggests that patients use 2000–2500 mg of EPA and DHA (combined dose) for about 3–4 weeks prior to withdrawal of the prescription drugs. Following the precaution of one week of abstinence from all added nutrients remains a safe margin until further studies are done in humans on wound healing and bleeding diathesis.

Additional treatment options for managing preoperative pain, particularly during pharmaceutical withdrawal, include specific diets for weight loss and dysinflammation,[80] acupuncture, and physical therapy. Rakel's *Integrative Medicine* is an excellent reference source for other integrative medicine approaches for effective pain management.[81]

METABOLIC AGENTS TO OPTIMIZE OUTCOMES

The following is a limited discussion in the context of metabolic therapy to highlight a few of the agents listed in Table 17.4. Research is looking beyond the notion of treating or preventing deficiency disease states and limiting hospital length of stay. It is moving to evaluate safe and economical nutrient applications in specific clinical environments that will promote a desired, measurable result, particularly with regard to nutrients that support healthy immune autoregulation in the perioperative period. Food sources for most agents are included; however, nutrient levels in foods typically do not contain an adequate quantity to support a clinical impact in the acute setting.

Recent surgical literature studying immunonutrition (IN) in the perioperative period has demonstrated improvements in outcomes and postop nutritional values over oral nutrition supplements (ONS) when measuring serum proteins, albumin, and zinc despite being consumed for only 7 days preop, and in normally nourished patients. IN formulas add higher levels of nutrients, particularly selenium, zinc, and omega-3 fatty acids in addition to arginine, glutamine, N-acetyl cysteine, beta-glucans, and glycine and probiotics, among others and demonstrated greater increases in serum prealbumin and decreases in hsCRP than the control group.[88,92,126–130] There is a discussion that perioperative immunonutrition for elective surgery should be the current standard of care.[131] A few IN commercial products are available (see Reader Resources). Recommending high-quality, professional grade nutrients in the perioperative period insures dose and absorption. (see Table 17.3).

AMINO ACIDS

Glutamine is the most abundant free amino acid in the cytosol and during stress it constitutes 70% of amino acids released by skeletal muscle, and provides metabolic fuel to T-lymphocytes, enterocytes, and other rapidly proliferating cells. Arginine and glutamine are "semi-essential" or "conditionally essential" amino acids during critical illness and severe trauma. Combination products of amino acids have been studied in an effort to avoid loss of quadriceps muscle strength after total knee arthroplasty (TKA).[88]

Studies have shown that arginine deficiency occurs as a result of surgical injury. Supplementation in the periop period has great utility; arginine is considered to be a direct nitric oxide precursor, inducing nitric oxide release to inhibit smooth muscle contraction; stimulating collagen deposition in wound healing[81]; increasing blood flow, nutrient uptake, and glucose utilization in muscle, particularly during exercise. It dramatically increases strength in trained men compared with controls.[13] It has also shown promise along with proper diet and exercise in patients with insulin

TABLE 17.4

Metabolic Agents to Optimize Orthopedic Outcomes

Agent	Dose	Support	Notes	Food Sources	Adult DRI	References
N-Acetyl Cysteine	500–600 mg bid	Antiox, ↓LOS/pain mgt	Precursor to glutathione	NMA	ND	82
L-Arginine	3–6 g bid	Collagen formation, supports synthesis of protein and mitochondria	Start at lower doses in DM and HTN, HSV infections	Dairy, beef, pork, nuts	ND	83–85
Calcium	1200–1500 mg Ca carbonate; 800–1000 Chelated or MCHC products	Typical diet 500–600 mg/day, supports bone healing	Monitor for constipation; citrate, maleate are best forms; Balance 2 Ca:1 Mg	Dairy, kale, broccoli	800–2500 mg[a]	51
L-Carnitine	0.5–2 g bid	Sarcopenia, muscle/cardiac support, ↑ mitochondrial efficacy	Can be low in vegans, helpful in DM wounds	Red meats	ND	86
Chondroitin Sulfate	400–600 mg bid	Improves pain in OA, may be disease-modifying	Reduces proinflammatory cytokines in chondrocytes	Limited	ND	61–65
Coenzyme Q 10	0.5–1200 mg/day	Antiox, higher doses with CHF, monitor INR with warfarin pts	Reduced by statins, helps fatigue and muscle recovery	NMA	ND	87
Native Collagen Type II	10 mg/day	Oral "tolerization" with gut immune structures; pain mgt RA and OA	Take away from food dose is critical	Bovine/porcine sources	ND	73
Copper	1–4 mg/day	Collagen cross-linking	Use with zinc, dietary intake is low; avoid in active cancer pts	Organ meats, seafood, nuts and seeds	0.9–10 mg	88
Creatine	3–5 g/day	Supports muscle protein synthesis with ATP recharge	Best used after exercise, can help fatigue and tx sarcopenia in frail elderly	NMA	ND	89
Curcumin	1–4 g/day	Antiox/anti-inflamm for pain mgt	Lowers CRP	Tumeric spice	ND	14,67–69
EFA's: EPA/DHA	2–3 g/day EPA+DHA	Reduces inflammation, prevents sarcopenia	Take with food; tolerance can vary with different oil forms	Coldwater fish	ND	76,77
Folate	0.8–5 mg/day	lowers ↑ Hcy	Use with B6, B12; Bioactive forms best: Quatrefolic®, Metafolin®	Dark greens, grains, beans	0.4–1.0 mg	40,42–44
Glucosamine Sulfate	750 mg bid	Pain mgt in OA, may be disease-modifying	Use caution in shellfish allergy	NMA	ND	60–63
Glutamine	5 g bid	Supports GI integrity, prevents loss of muscle mass	Monitor for constipation	"Conditionally essential" amino acid	ND	90
Hyaluronic acid	80 mg/day	Pain mgt OA with effusion	Hyal-Joint® (author's experience)	NMA	ND	71, 72
Iron	Practitioner directed to tolerance at UL	Use gluconate, bis-glycinate chelate, vitamin C↑↑ absorption	GI upset, constipation, judicious use for cancer pts	Meats, fish, poultry, and dark greens	8–45 mg/day	48

(Continued)

TABLE 17.4 (CONTINUED)

Metabolic Agents to Optimize Orthopedic Outcomes

Agent	Dose	Support	Notes	Food Sources	Adult DRI	References
L-Leucine	4–5 g bid	Stimulates muscle protein synthesis in elderly > protein alone	Use if renal compromise prevents ↑ protein intake, substitute BCAA's 6–7 g bid	Soy, lentils, beef, salmon	1–3 g/day (WHO)	19, 91
Alpha-Lipoic Acid	300–600 mg bid	Diabetic neuropathy, ↓damage ischemic reperfusion	May lower blood glucose levels, monitor in DM, regenerates Vits C and E	Kidney, heart, liver, broccoli, spinach, potatoes	ND	92–95
Magnesium	400–800 mg/day	Bone healing, use 2:1 Ca:Mg, Intake is generally inadequate	Can loosen stools, supports muscle pain	Leafy greens, grains, nuts	320–770 mg[b]	96
Manganese	5–10 mg/day	Bone healing, enzyme and protein metabolism	Limit with liver disease/cholestasis	Grains, tea, greens	1.8–11 mg	97
Melatonin	0.5–3 mg, 30 min before hs	Sleep and pain support postop	Studies done with lower doses, avoid in leukemia, Hodgkin's disease	Tart cherries	ND	98–100
MSM	1–6 g/day	Pain mgt in OA	Limited studies GI intolerance	NMA	ND	101
Probiotics	10–100 B CFU's/ day L.acidophilus, B. bifidum, S.boulardii	Supports GI integrity post- antibiotic diarrhea, associated with inflammation	Flatulence Use 10–14 days pre and postop shown to reduce postop complications	Yogurt (Note: Food sources offer limited therapeutic outcomes)	ND	102, 103
Protein	0.8–1.6 g/kg/day in equally divided doses	Essential for wound healing, common deficiency worldwide	Poorly digested in hypochlorhydric elderly, use hydrolyzed protein shakes, limit in severe renal disease	Meat, poultry, fish, eggs, milk, yogurt, nuts, legumes, seeds	0.66–1.52 g/kg/day	40, 53, 54
S-Adenosyl Methionine	400–600 mg bid	Pain mgt joint disease, fatigue	GI intolerance, use earlier in day, may activate bipolar pts	Metabolite in the body of B vitamin metabolism	ND	104–108
Selenium	50–400 µg/day	Antioxidant, supports healing, ↓intake associated with sarcopenia, in most IN formulas	Hair loss, brittle nails in doses > 1 mg/day	Brazil nuts, meat, seafood, grains, vegetables	55–400 µg/day	86,109
Silicon	5 mg bid	Deficiency leads to bone defects	Use caution in renal lithiasis; Best as orthosilicic acid	Cereal and unrefined grain products	ND	110
L-Theanine	50–200 mg/day	Aids anxiety, sleep	Well tolerated	Green tea (*Camellia Sinensis*)	ND	111
5-Hydroxy Tryptophan (5-HTP)	50–300 mg/day	Precursor of serotonin, supports sleep, aids anxiety	Theoretical risk of serotonin syndrome if given with SSRI Rx, use hs	Chocolate, oats, dried dates, turkey, pumpkin seeds	ND	112

(Continued)

TABLE 17.4 (CONTINUED)
Metabolic Agents to Optimize Orthopedic Outcomes

Agent	Dose	Support	Notes	Food Sources	Adult DRI	References
Vitamin A	15,000–25,000 IU/day	Antioxidant, wound healing, osteoporosis, sarcopenia	Use combination of mixed carotenoids	Retinol in animal based foods, carotenoids in vegetables, fruits	2310–9900 IU	113
Vitamin B2 (Riboflavin)	10–100 mg/day	↑intake - ↓hip fx	Supplement sensitive to light exposure	Fortified cereals, organ meats	1.1–1.3 mg/day	114
Vitamin B5 (Pantothenate)	500–750 mg bid	Wound healing	No toxicity and safe	Chicken, beef, potatoes	5 mg/day	95
Vitamin B6 (Pyridoxine)	10–100 mg/day	Lowers ↑Hcy, Low serum B6 associated with DVT	Few reports of neurotoxicity in sustained, high doses; caution in idiopathic neuropathy	Cereals, beef liver, organ meats	1.3–100 mg/day	110, 115, 116
Vitamin B12 (Cobalamin)	500–5000 µg/day	Lowers ↑Hcy, preferably as methylcobalamin, can improve disrupted sleep	Well tolerated	Shellfish, organ meats, sardines	2.4 µg	48
Vitamin C (Ascorbate)	1–2 g bid	Wound/bone healing, prevents sarcopenia, ↑need in smokers, ↓ risk RSD in Colles fx	If GI intolerance, use buffered or ester C	Citrus fruits, vegetables, tomato, theoretical risk of renal lithiasis with higher doses	75–2000 mg	117, 118
Vitamin D3	800–10,000/day	Bone metabolism, low in chronic pain, may influence seasonal affective disorder	Well tolerated, hypercalcemia at 160–500 ng/dL, monitor levels Q8–12 wks with loading dose	Enriched food sources likely inadequate for surgical patients	600–4000 IU/day[a]	119–122
Vitamin E (alpha-Tocopherol)	100–200 IU/day mixed tocopherols	Prevents sarcopenia, supports high EFA intakes	Use caution in warfarin therapy or vitamin K deficiency	Vegetable oils, grains, vegetables, meats, nuts, avocados	12–15 mg (8–10 IU)	123
Zinc	30–50 mg/day	Essential in wound healing	Take with copper, can cause GI upset	Seafood (oysters and sardines), organ meats, sunflower seeds	8–40 mg	124,125

Note: DRIs obtained from Dietary Reference Intakes, Institute of Medicine (IOM 2006). DRI is a range from RDA (Recommended Daily Allowance = average daily dietary nutrient intake level sufficient to meet requirements of 97%–98% healthy individuals), or AI (Adequate Intake = recommended daily intake estimates when RDA cannot be determined) to UL (Tolerable Upper Limit = Highest daily intake that is likely to pose no risk of adverse health effects to almost all individuals in the general population).

DRI, Dietary Reference Intakes; AI, Adequate Intakes; UL, Upper Limit; ND, Not Determined; NMA, No Meaningful Amount; CFU, Colony-Forming Units; Adult, 19 years and older

[a] Dietary Reference Intakes for Calcium and Vitamin D, Institute of Medicine (2011); Vitamin D as cholecalciferol and assumes minimal exposure to sunlight, Antiox, Antioxidant; Anti-inflamm, Anti-Inflammatory; B, Billions; BCAA, branched chain amino acids; Ca, calcium;DM, Diabetes Mellitus; DVT, deep vein thrombosis; EFA, Essential Fatty Acids; Fx, fracture; HCY, homocysteine; hs, bedtime; 5-HTP, 5-Hydroxytryptophan; LOS, length of stay; OA, Osteoarthritis; HTN, Hypertension; HSV, Herpes Simplex Virus; MCHC, Micro Crystalline Hydroxyapatite Concentrate; CHF, Congestive Heart Failure; MSM, Methylsulfonylmethane.

[b] 770 mg magnesium assumes maximum dietary intake of 420 mg plus maximum supplemental intake of 350 mg

Lifestyle Medicine Consultants, Inc. Copyright 2017.

resistance and obesity, while sparing lean body mass.[82] Use with caution and lower starting doses if the individual is diabetic, on blood pressure medicine, or has a history of herpes simplex virus (HSV) infections. History of HSV infection is a concern because arginine shares transport proteins with lysine and relative deficiencies of lysine can be a trigger for an outbreak. Arginine should be avoided in the perioperative period in individuals with acute respiratory distress syndrome or septicemia.[132]

Immunonutrition supplements have varying concentrations of these key ingredients and the ideal dosages are not well defined. In fact, the relative dosages of the immune-modulating ingredients even vary from country to country in products made by the same manufacturer. There is no broad-based consensus about standard dosages for immunonutrients and they are frequently included (typically in lower quantities) in ONS formulas. In addition to being more effective at stimulating muscle protein synthesis (MPS) in the elderly compared with younger subjects, L-leucine alone or BCAAs may also be an acceptable strategy for patients with renal impairment who cannot tolerate higher total protein intakes.[19,89]

N-acetylcysteine (NAC) has been studied with attention to ischemia/reperfusion of orthopedically operated limbs. It appears to lessen the need for postoperative analgesics, and can decrease hospital stay.[80] Along with other dietary amino acids such as glutamine and glycine, and antioxidants such as vitamins C and E, selenium, and lipoic acid, NAC provides cysteine as a substrate for the recycling of glutathione, which is frequently depleted in the presence of oxidative stress. Glutathione is recognized as the final pathway for the reduction of reactive oxygen species (ROS). L-Carnitine is important for vegetarians or those with metabolic syndrome and has been shown to enhance cardiac performance and increase exercise tolerance in humans with ischemic heart and peripheral vascular disease.[133,134]

Creatine can also be useful in the frail elderly as an adjunctive support to increase muscle strength and mass with an exercise program.[87] It can be mixed with the patient's favorite juice or nonalcoholic beverage and consumed 1–2 times per day. When taken along with caffeinated beverages, a stimulating effect may be experienced, so it is best taken earlier in the day.

S-adensosylmethionine (SAMe) is a naturally occurring combination of the amino acid methionine and adenosine triphosphate (ATP). It is a methyl donor and inhibits synthesis of proinflammatory interleukens and TNF-alpha. It upregulates proteoglycan synthesis and the proliferation rate of chondrocytes, promoting cartilage formation and repair in doses ranging from 400 to 1600 mg/day in divided doses. In a double-blind crossover study at 1200 mg/day compared with celecoxib (200 mg), it had the same efficacy and a lower incidence of side effects over a 2-month period.[103] Other research has shown similar or better efficacy with fewer side effects at 8–12 weeks compared with naproxen,[102] indomethacin,[105] ibuprofen,[104] and nabumetone.[106] It can also elevate mood and help with anxiety. Supportive nutrients such as B6, B12, folate, and trimethylglycine may be given simultaneously in the presence of elevated homocysteine(Hcy) and monitor Hcy levels if recommending higher doses of SAMe for more than 3 months as it can theoretically drive serum levels above recommended normals.

ANTIOXIDANTS

Coenzyme Q10 (CoQ10) has been safely prescribed for individuals with congestive heart failure and severe neurological conditions in daily doses of 400–1200 mg. In times of severe oxidative stress, CoQ10 along with lipoic acid can be viewed as conditionally essential nutrients, because the body cannot make enough of them. There has been a case report of the reduced effectiveness of warfarin drugs with CoQ10 use. Therefore, more frequent international normalized ratio(INR) testing is indicated when initiating therapy in this patient group. This coenzyme produces a favorable response in treating fatigue on a very consistent basis. For individuals taking statin prescription medications (as well as red yeast rice, the natural form of lovastatin), myopathy and the more common myalgias may be supported by the use of CoQ10.[135]

Alpha-lipoic acid is a potent, multifunctional antioxidant that improves tissue glutathione levels, reduces lipid peroxides, increases insulin sensitivity, and helps regenerate vitamins C and E. It has been used effectively in Germany for decades orally and intravenously for the treatment of diabetic polyneuropathy.[90] It can be a useful adjunct for improving insulin sensitivity in as little as two weeks[91] and treatment over 90 days with 300 mg daily decreased mean hemoglobin A1c from 11.49 to 9.96.[92] In the author's experience, it also improves neuopathic symptoms during surgical recovery involving compromised neural structures and has been shown to help rehabilitation efforts for back pain.[136] Alpha-lipoic acid was used in combination with CoQ10, magnesium, and omega-3 fatty acids preoperatively, up until the day of surgery and for 1 month thereafter, and was demonstrated to enhance several heart surgery recovery parameters.[93]

MINERALS

Minerals in the form of inorganic mineral salts such as carbonates, oxides, phosphates, and sulfates compete with one another for absorption in the gut. When minerals are consumed in this form they can also be blocked by the intake of natural fiber found in cereals and fruits.[137] While there are other considerations influencing absorption when patients are taking a specific mineral such as iron preoperatively, an important clinical application is to supplement calcium and magnesium together. Generally, a ratio of two parts calcium to one part magnesium is recommended. Apart from any pain medications that alter bowel motility, patients may find calcium to be constipating and magnesium to have a laxative effect. Calcium citrate and magnesium citrate may be better absorbed in patients with hypochlorhydria (higher in the elderly) and can also confer an alkalinizing effect. Microcrystalline hydroxyapatite is a blend of minerals found in bone. Studies have shown magnesium intake and levels are strongly and independently associated with the anabolic hormones testosterone and IGF-1.[94]

Zinc is an essential component of over 100 key enzymes and plays a central role in cellular growth and differentiation, particularly in rapid turnover tissues like those of the immune system and gastrointestinal tract. Zinc carnosine is a preparation that has been helpful with relieving mild gastric upset, while supporting zinc levels.[121]

Selenium has antioxidant properties and is a key constituent of multiple selenoproteins, particularly the glutathione peroxidases, which are part of the antioxidant defense system of cells, and iodothyronine deiodinase, an enzyme which converts the inactive precursor of thyroxine, tetraiodothyronine (T4) into the active form, tri-iodothyronine (T3). It protects the body against oxidative stress and infection. Zinc and selenium are key trace minerals found in most immunonutrition formulas.[86,107]

HORMONES

Melatonin is a safe and effective sleep aid when studied as a preoperative anxiolytic in 9 of 10 studies reviewed. Five studies showed opioid sparing or reduced pain scores and reduced pediatric emergence delirium. Its antioxidant properties are also being studied for use in sepsis and reperfusion injuries.[96–98] For more detailed discussion on hormones, see Chapter 9.

VITAMINS

Vitamin B12 absorption is inadequate in approximately 15% of individuals over 65 due to the lack of gastric acidity, decreased intrinsic factor, and in *Helicobacter pylori* infections.[51] For individuals with low serum B12 levels and where intramuscular dosing is not an option, doses of 5000 µg/day are acceptable in a sublingual form of methylcobalamin for shorter term use. Low serum B6 is associated with an increased risk of DVT[1,113,114] and is best supplemented in its activated form of pyridoxal-5'-phosphate. B5 (pantothenic acid) enhanced wound healing in a human study with a dosage of 200–900 mg/day.[95] There is a much higher incidence of heart disease and elevated Hcy levels compared with healthy controls for individuals with rheumatoid arthritis treated with methotrexate, which inhibits B6 metabolism. B6 therapy is frequently prescribed, however, when associated with elevated Hcy, the addition of B12 and folate is indicated.

Vitamin C therapy after distal radius fracture has been shown to reduce the incidence of complex regional pain syndrome (CRPS) from 10.1% to 2.4% studied in 427 fractures at doses of 500 mg/day, which is well above what can be consumed in a healthy diet of 5 vegetables and fruits per day.[112]

Of all the nutrients involved in orthopedic metabolic therapy, vitamin D3 is pivotal for bone health and immune regulation. It is a metabolically active hormone and preoperative guidelines for treatment of 25-hydroxyvitamin D3 (25(OH)D3) deficiency/insufficiency to quickly optimize physiologic levels in the preoperative setting are included in Table 17.5. The recommended form for treatment is cholecalciferol (D3) as opposed to ergocalciferol (D2), which has been shown in one calculation to have a relative potency of D3:D2 of 9.5:1; in another, D2 was one-third that of D3.[138] The guide is intentionally accelerated for achieving near term results and minimizing retesting expense[117,118,139,140] and represents the author's clinical approach based on experience. Optimal serum level for individuals with osteoporosis, osteopenia, and sarcopenia is 50–70 ng/mL. If these target levels appear alarming, current data suggest that 25(OH) D3 concentrations must rise above 300 ng/ml to produce hypercalcemia and toxicity, and maintaining levels below 100 ng/ml will ensure a wide safety margin. Attention to timely lab studies and physician follow-up is recommended for supplementation over 4000 IU/day, particularly in patients with renal insufficiency where much lower starting doses should be used and levels carefully monitored.

The Institute of Medicine increased the RDA and UL for vitamin D in 2010 and current peer review medical literature continues to demonstrate links between deficiency states and an expanding list of medical conditions and recommends laboratory assessment and advises correction to optimal levels as a part of current medical therapy. Patients with persistent, nonspecific musculoskeletal pain, particularly those with darker pigmented skin in more northern latitudes have shown extraordinarily high incidences of severe hypovitaminosis D, even in younger individuals.[120] The long list of disease states associated with low vitamin D in very large cohorts ($n > 300,000$ men and women) should command the clinician's attention and, with a wide safety margin, be the first line approach to orthopedic metabolic therapy.[119] General guidelines for treatment of vitamin D3 deficiency/insufficiency to quickly optimize physiologic levels in the perioperative setting are included in Table 17.5.

TABLE 17.5
Perioperative Metabolic Guidelines to Optimize 25-Hydroxy Vitamin D3

Starting 25-OH D3 Level (ng/mL)	Starting Daily Dose	Testing Interval[a]	Next Daily Dose	Retest	Maintenance
<0	5000–10,000IU	6–8 weeks	3000–5000IU	Q 8–12 weeks until level stable	Per lab values to maintain 50—70 ng/ml level
20–32	5000IU	6–8 weeks	2000–5000IU	Q16 weeks	As above
32–50	2000–5000IU	Q 3–4 months until stable	2000IU	Q 6 months	As above
50–75	800–2000IU	Annually in winter			As above

[a] Retest 25-OH D3 and Ionized Calcium.
Lifestyle Medicine Consultants, Inc. © 2017.

PROBIOTICS

Simple use of preop and postop probiotics in doses of 10 million to 10 billion colony-forming units (CFU) *Lactobacillus* and *Bifidobacter* species/day for 1–2 weeks before and after surgery, in 8 of 12 randomized controlled trials, showed a significant reduction in bacterial infection rates in non-critically ill surgical patients.[101] In clinical experience, 30–100 billion CFU are well tolerated and potentially more influential. The obese surgical patient is particularly at risk for local and systemic inflammation based on microbiota composition in the gut. They demonstate reduced bacterial diversity, a decreased Bacteroidetes/Firmicutes ratio, an increased abundance of potential proinflammatory Proteobacteria, and elevated fecal calprotecin (a measure of neurtrophil migration to the intestinal muscosa) and hsCRP, even in the absence of intestinal permeability.[127] A recent RCT also demonstrated the influence of preop Saccharomyces boulardii in lowering intestinal inflammatory cytokines.[128] In the future, greater research focus in this domain is inevitable as the influence of inflammation and oxidative stress on outcomes in the surgical arena becomes more evident.

APPLICATION TO REGENERATIVE MEDICINE PROCEDURES

In the domain of regenerative medicine procedures involving stem cell therapies, the preop (prehabilitation) and postop (rehabilitation) concept is still applicable as with major surgical procedures, however, there is a relative paucity of published research. The understanding of how stem cells are influenced by systemic inflammation, microenvironment, and their paracrine function is growing and will be fertile ground to evaluate metabolic therapy influence. Aberrations in autoregulation of biological communication systems, particularly at an advanced age can detrimentally influence stem cell harvest and engraftment. The term "inflamma-aging" [141] suggests that influence and one can view disease states as reflecting chronic autoregulatory imbalance resulting in stem cell failure. Very few metabolic therapy studies have been published in this clinical area; however, those nutrients studied demonstrating some benefit include glucosamine sulfate, chondroitin sulfate, curcumin, carnosine, resveratrol, vitamins C and D, fish oil omega-3 fatty acids, curcumin, ellagic acid, beta-glucans, Green tea catechins, quercetin, hesperidin, lysine, proline, arginine, and N-acetyl cysteine.[142–145]

Holding the view that aging, senescence, and degenerative disease is a failure of stem cell health may prove useful for studying predictability of regenerative medicine procedures. A more robust preop assessment of inflammatory and oxidative stress biomarkers such as 8-hydroxy-2'-deoxyguanosine (8-OHdG), F2-Isoprostane, and lipid peroxides along with lifestyle choices and assessing the microbiome could provide some estimate of healing capacity.

SUMMARY AND CLINICAL RECOMMENDATIONS

The scientific assessment of metabolic therapy in the perioperative period is difficult due to the wide variety of nutrients that can influence healing. This generates a greater number of variables to evaluate, which meta-analysis attempts to reduce, making specific consensus nutrient recommendations much more difficult. However, meaningful future research is likely to assume a systems biology framework to allow for this challenge and the rising demand for personalized therapeutic intervention in medicine. There is consistent evidence that, at the very least, ONS formula should contain a broad spectrum of conditionally essential macro and micronutrients to support the physiologic challenges of the perioperative period: adequate protein intake to facilitate healing in the pre and postoperative periods; complex carbohydrate loading in the immediate preoperative period; well-studied key nutrients such as selenium, fish oil-derived omega-3 fatty acids; conditionally essential amino acids arginine and glutamine; fat and water-soluble vitamins and trace and macro minerals.

Clinicians are well positioned to initiate ERAS protocols including immunonutrition to optimize surgical outcomes given the timing of elective orthopedic surgery. The key points are

- Metabolic therapy is safe and can measurably improve outcomes
- The distinctive circumstance of impending surgical threat, combined with patient interest in metabolic therapy creates a superb opportunity for the physician to spark motivated patient compliance in a preoperative program, particularly with lifestyle choices of diet and exercise
- The nutrient status of many surgical patients is surprisingly poor, particularly the obese elderly
- Sarcopenia is underdiagnosed and treatable with guided exercise and nutrient support
- Perioperative enteral immunonutrition beverages have been shown to improve primary outcomes, even in a normally nourished patient
- Limit or eliminate negative pharmaceutical and poor dietary influences on healing
- Jump start bone metabolism with focused treatment of vitamin D insufficiency/deficiency, and supplement with balanced, chelated minerals for orthopedic patients
- Dietary advice can be simple: eliminate or avoid refined flour, sugar, soft drinks/juices-diabetics need to follow blood sugar closely; consume lean, healthy protein portions with every meal; 5 half-cup servings of vegetables and one fruit serving/day; take a high-quality multivitamin

CASE STUDIES

CASE 1

History of Present Illness

72-year-old man who is a retired engineer presented on July 21 stating that he "wants to lose weight" in anticipation of total knee replacement in 3 months. He was having difficulty controlling his blood pressure and the pain in his right knee was becoming unbearable, limiting his mobility and social life. He has gained 50 pounds in the last 10 years, has been using CPAP for 15 years with a long-standing history of hypertension, elevated cholesterol, and prediabetes with a fasting blood sugar 114 and hemoglobin A1c of 6.0, and mildly elevated microalbuminuria.

Past Medical History

Significant for torn meniscus in the right knee 1997; left knee 1999. States he has "bone-on-bone" in both his knees and recent venous ablation bilaterally in the lower extremities that did not help the swelling in his left leg down by his ankle.

Medications

losartan 100 mg, lisinopril 40 mg, Crestor 40 mg, aspirin 81 mg

Habituants

10 glasses of wine a week, 4 cups of green tea a day, and varying amounts of soda on a daily basis.

Physical exam

Central obesity with BMI 36, blood pressure 180/100, waist circumference 45.5 inches. Range of motion (ROM) of left knee was -12 degrees of extension and 102 degrees of flexion; and right knee -10 degrees of extension and 98 degrees of flexion, no effusion, some ligamentous laxity from joint space narrowing and tenderness over the pes and semitendinosus tendons bilaterally; 1+ edema about the ankles bilaterally. There were no other noteworthy abnormalities on examination.

Assessment and Plan

Comprehensive preoperative guidelines were recommended to include a lifestyle medicine program of walking as tolerated, a structured nutrition program with weekly accountability to focus on healthy weight loss and education about the impact of his daily lifestyle choices on his blood pressure and prediabetes and associated risks with surgery due to his obesity. The patient was advised to start SYSADOA supplementation to include a combination of hyaluronic acid, glucosamine sulfate, and chondroitin sulfate in therapeutic doses, CoQ10 100 mg a day, omega-3 fatty acids (monoglyceride form) 1300 mg twice daily, curcumin 500 mg twice daily and increasing to 1000 mg three times a day as needed for exacerbation of pain. The patient elected to discuss these recommendations with his PCP and surgeon who were in agreement. Blood pressure medication was subsequently augmented with amlodipine 10 mg daily.

Lifestyle counseling started on Sept 8, 6 weeks before his scheduled right TKA. He was seen for five visits losing a total of 18.5 pounds prior to surgery; blood pressure was 132/68; he lost 3 inches from his waist and 1.5 inches from his hips. He was able to eliminate the added amlodipine for blood pressure control prior to surgery.

For 2 weeks prior to his surgical date, he was advised to discontinue any further weight loss from calorie restriction but to continue with healthy food choices consisting of a wide variety of vegetables and lean protein sources with each meal, and to continue with the elimination of cow dairy, refined sugar, and refined flour and grains.

He underwent uneventful right TKA surgery on October 23, participated in a postoperative rehabilitation program, and returned to the lifestyle medicine program 3 months after surgery. He had maintained his weight during the course of rehabilitation and with another 10 weeks of supervision lost another 10 pounds with a total waist circumference loss of 5.5 inches, 3 inches from his hips and a total weight loss of 28 lbs. Discharge blood pressure 120/64, hemoglobin A1c 5.7, fasting blood sugar 92. The range of motion of his right knee was 100 degrees but nontender and nonpainful at that point. Blood pressure medication remained unchanged and Crestor was reduced to 20 mg. The patient remained stable and underwent successful left TKA the following year, requiring manipulation under anesthesia due to longstanding contracture, but otherwise surgery was uncomplicated and biometrics and medications remained unchanged.

Case 2

History or Present Illness

29-year-old Caucasian female presented on September 27 with a 3–4-month exacerbation of RA which was initially diagnosed in 2006 and treated until 2013 with a wide variety of DMARDs and BAs to include methotrexate and Plaquenil over 7 years. The patient chose to discontinue medications due to a wide variety of unacceptable side effects, although the medications were significantly helpful. She had not seen her rheumatologist in over 3 years. In the interim, she had done very well using a wide variety of integrated and lifestyle approaches and had done reasonably well until that summer when some increased stress around her daily activities at work exacerbated her pain. She presented with severely swollen joints, right greater than left knee, right great toe, volar left index finger, and diffuse morning stiffness lasting about 3 hours. She has a family history of cancer and her mother has elevated cholesterol but no autoimmune disease. Initial subjective WOMAC score: Pain 7/20; stiffness 6/8; difficulty with ADLs 38/68. Other PMH is non-contributory.

Physical exam

BMI 19.4, BP 100/64, synovitis and effusion about the carpal row bilaterally, worse on the left with 70% decrease in range of motion globally and a 3 cm cystic structure on the volar aspect of the left index finger MCP joint. Bilateral knees had 2+ effusions, extension lags bilaterally with flexion at

140 degrees. Left ankle had a 2+ effusion and a 60% global loss of range of motion, similarly in the right great toe.

Laboratory studies

Total cholesterol 296, triglycerides 71, HDL 78, LDL 204, normal thyroid functions, rheumatoid factor 257 IU/dl (nl < 14), CCP (IgG) >250 units (nl < 20), hsCRP 0.3 mg/dL. 25-hydroxy D3 24 ng/mL.

Imaging studies

X-rays of the bilateral knees demonstrate effusion, slight narrowing of the medial femorotibial joint bilaterally but no erosions. MRI of the left hand demonstrated chronic erosive disease of the carpometacarpal joints and a large effusion of the flexor tendon sheath of the second ray with a partial tear of the superficial flexor tendon and erosive arthropathy of the wrist. The patient was advised to recommit to her previous dietary plan excluding dairy, soy, and wheat; she was started on a probiotic 100 billion CFU of Lactobacillus/Bifidobacter, undenatured collagen type II (40 mg, chicken source) on an empty stomach daily, vitamin D3 5000 IU (no soy), curcumin 500–1000 mg twice a day, omega-3 fatty acids (monoglyceride form) 1300 mg twice a day and naproxen 220 mg for breakthrough pain.

Treatment

The patient was referred for surgical consultation, given the tendon tear and her active lifestyle, and back to her rheumatologist whom she had not seen for several years for reconsideration of pharmaceutical treatment because of the worsening of wrist erosions on comparison to previous films.

A follow-up in 6 weeks demonstrated noteworthy pain relief and stiffness that the patient reports to be about 50%–60% with significant lessening of the effusion in her knees, wrists, ankle, and great toe. Surgical consultation was performed and surgery was scheduled for the following week. Rheumatologic consultation recommended to continue on with current treatment in anticipation of tendon reconstruction surgery and improvement, but to reconsider pharmacotherapy after rehabilitation.

The three-month follow-up showed considerable improvement on WOMAC score: pain 2/20; stiffness 0/8; difficulty with ADLs 5/68. The patient was participating in postop rehabilitation for the hand surgery. Wrist ROM is largely unchanged from initial visit, ROM in both knees without extension lags, some bogginess on the right but no effusion, no effusions in the left ankle. Labs: ESR, CRP normal, unchanged rheumatoid factor 254.5 IU/mL, 25-hydroxy D3 59.1 ng/ml.

Follow-up at 7 months demonstrated fully healed flexor tendon repair of the left index finger, persistent mild bogginess of the synovium of the left knee, ROM 136 degrees, right knee 144 degrees. ROM of bilateral wrists is unchanged but there are no joint effusions or synovitis obvious. The patient reports overall improvement at about 80% and morning stiffness is an hour or less. Patient had been consistent with her diet and her metabolic therapy program. At that point she elected to continue watchful waiting and routine follow-up with her rheumatologist.

READER RESOURCES

ERAS Information

- http://erasusa.org
- http://aserhq.org
- http://espen.org
- PlanAgainstPain.com
- Subjectiveglobalassessment.com

Perioperative Nutrient Beverages

- https://drinkclearfast.com/nutrition-preparing-for-surgery/
- https://abbottnutrition.com/juven/
- https://www.nestlehealthscience.us/brands/impact/impact-advanced-recovery-hcp

REFERENCES

1. Kavalukas, S.L., Barbul, A. 2011. Nutrition and wound healing: And update. *Plast Reconstr Surg* Jan;127(Suppl 1):38S–43S.
2. Hegazi, R.A., Hustead, D.S., Evans, D.C. 2014. Preoperative standard oral nutrition supplements vs. immunonutrition: Results of a systematic review and meta-analysis. *J Am Coll Surg* Nov;219(5):1078–1087.
3. Weimann, A., Braga, M., Carli, F., et.al. 2017. ESPEN guideline: Clinical nutrition in surgery. *Clin Nutr* Jun;36(3):623–50.
4. Dickinson, A., Shao, A., Boyon, N., Franco, J.C. 2011. Use of dietary supplements by cardiologists, dermatologists and orthopedists: Report of a survey. *Nutr J* Mar;3;10:20.
5. Eisenberg, D.M., Kessler, R.C., Foster, C., Norlock, F.E., Calkins, D.R., Delbanco, T.L. 1993. Unconventional medicine in the United States. Prevalence, costs, and patterns of use. *N Engl J Med* Jan 28;328(4):246–52.
6. Wright, J., Kennedy-Stephenson, M., Wang, C. 2004. Trends in intake of energy and macronutrient-United States, 1971–2000. *MMWR* Feb 6;53(4):80–2.
7. Patel, N., Bagan, B., Vadera, S., et.al. 2007. Obesity and spine surgery: Relation to perioperative complications. *J Neurosurg Spine* Apr;6(4):291–7.
8. Harms, S., Larson, R., Sahmoun, A.E., Beal, J.R. 2007. Obesity increases the likelihood of total joint replacement surgery among younger adults. *Int Orthop* Feb;31(1):23–6.
9. Liu, B., Balkwill, A., Banks, E., Cooper, C., Green, J., Beral, V. 2007. Relationship of height, weight and body mass index to the risk of hip and knee replacements in middle-aged women. *Rheumatology* May;46(5):861–7.
10. Stürmer, T., Günther, K.P., Brenner, H. 2000. Obesity, overweight and patterns of osteoarthritis: The Ulm Osteoarthritis Study. *J Clin Epidemiol* Mar 1;53(3):307–13.
11. Kohlstadt, I. 2006. *Scientific Evidence for Musculoskeletal, Bariatric, and Sports Nutrition.* Boca Raton: CRC Press/Taylor & Francis, p.427.
12. Pelton, R., LaValle, J. 2004. *The Nutritional Cost of Drugs: A Guide to Maintaining Good Nutrition While Using Prescription and Over-the-counter Drugs.* Engelwood, CO: Morton Publishing Company.
13. Cosquéric, G., Sebag, A., Ducolombier, C., Thomas, C., Piette, F., Weill-Engerer, S. 2006. Sarcopenia is predictive of nosocomial infection in care of the elderly. *Br J Nutr* Nov;96(5):895–901.
14. McMahon, M., Block, J.A. 2003. The risk of contralateral total knee arthroplasty after knee replacement for osteoarthritis. *J Rheumatol* Aug;30(8):1822–4.
15. Calder, P.C. 2007. Immunonutrition in surgical and critically ill patients. *Br J Nutr* Oct;98(Suppl 1):S 133–9.
16. Smit, A., O'Byrne, A., Van Brandt, B., Bianchi, I., Kuestermann, K. 2009. *Introduction to Bioregulatory Medicine.* Stuttgart: Thieme.
17. Finan, P., Goodin, B., Smith, M. 2013. The association of sleep and pain: An update and a path forward. *J Pain* Dec;14(12):1539–52.
18. Lentz, M.J., Landis, C.A., Rothermel, J., Shaver, J.L. 1999. Effects of selective slow wave sleep disruption on musculoskeletal pain and fatigue in middle aged women. *J Rheumatol* Jul;26(7):1586–92.
19. Tang, N., Sanborn, A. 2014. Better quality sleep promotes daytime physical activity in patients with chronic pain? A multilevel analysis of the within-person relationship. *PLoS ONE* 9(3): e92158. Available online at https://doi.org/10.1371/journal.pone.0092158
20. Stohs, S.J., Dudrick, S.J. 2011. Nutritional supplements in the surgical patient. *Surg Clin North Am* Aug;91(4):933–44.
21. Roulin, D., Donadini, A., Gander, S., et.al. 2013. Cost-effectiveness of the implementation of an enhanced recovery protocol for colorectal surgery. *Br J Surg* Jul;100(8):1108–14.
22. Kehlet, H. 1997. Multimodal approach to control postoperative pathophysiology and rehabilitation. *Br J Anaesth.* May;78(5):606–17.
23. Kremers, H., Larson, M., Crowson, M., Kremers, W., Washington, R., Steiner, C., et al. 2015. Prevalence of total hip and knee replacement in the United States. *J Bone Joint Surg Am* 97:1386–97.

24. Moretti, B., Notarnicola, A., Moretti, L., et.al. 2012. I-ONE therapy in patients undergoing total knee arthroplasty: A prospective, randomized and controlled study. *BMC Musculoskelet Disord* Jun 6;13:88.

25. Dallari, D., Fini, M., Giavaresi, G., et.al. 2009. Effects of pulsed electromagnetic stimulation on patients undergoing hip revision prostheses: A randomized prospective double-blind study. *Bioelectromagnetics* Sep;30(6):423–30.

26. Thacker, J.K., Mountford, W.K., Ernst, F.R., Krukas, M.R., Mythen, M.M. 2016. Perioperative fluid utilization variability and association with outcomes: Considerations for enhanced recovery efforts in sample U.S. surgical populations. *Ann Surg* Mar;263(3):502–10.

27. Busti, A.J., Hooper J.S., Amaya C.J., Kazi S. 2005. Effects of perioperative antiinflammatory and immunomodulating therapy on surgical wound healing. *Pharmacotherapy* Nov;25(11):1566–91.

28. Wheeler, P., Batt, M.E. 2005. Do non-steroidal anti-inflammatory drugs adversely affect stress fracture healing? A short review. *Br J Sports Med* Feb;39(2):65–9.

29. Juo, H.H., Peck, A., Gove, N., Ng, B. 2016. Perioperative use of synthetic disease-modifying anti-rheumatic drugs or tumor necrosis factor α inhibitors does not associate with increased rates of post-operative infections. *Arthritis Rheumatol* 68(Suppl 10).

30. Goodman, S.M. 2015. Optimizing perioperative outcomes for older patients with rheumatoid arthritis undergoing arthroplasty: Emphasis on medication management. *Drugs Aging* May;32(5):361–9.

31. Petersen, A.M., Magkos, F., Atherton, P., et.al. 2007. Smoking impairs muscle protein synthesis and increases the expression of myostatin and MAFbx in muscle. *Am J Physiol Endocrinol Metab* Sep;293(3):E843–8.

32. Lee, J.S., Auyeung, T.W., Kwok, T., Lau, E.M., Leung, P.C., Woo, J. 2007. Associated factors and health impact of sarcopenia in older Chinese men and women: A cross-sectional study. *Gerontology* 53(6):404–10.

33. National Heart, Lung, and Blood Institute. 1998. Clinical guidelines on the identification, evaluation, and treatment of overweight and obesity in adults: The evidence report. *Obes Res* 6:S51–S210.

34. Welborn, T.A., Dhaliwal, S.S. 2007. Preferred clinical measures of central obesity for predicting mortality. *Eur J Clin Nutr* Dec;61(12):1373–9.

35. Yusuf, S., Hawken, S., Ounpuu, S., et.al. 2005. Obesity and the risk of myocardial infarction in 27,000 participants from 52 countries: A case-control study. *Lancet* Nov 5;366(9497):1640–9.

36. Chabi, B., Ljubicic, V., Menzies, K.J., Huang, J.H., Saleem, A., Hood, D.A. 2008. Mitochondrial function and apoptotic susceptibility in aging skeletal muscle. *Aging Cells* Jan;7(1):2–12.

37. Degens, H. 2010. The role of systemic inflammation in age-related muscle weakness and wasting. *Scand J Med Sci Sports* Feb;20(1):28–38.

38. Villareal, D.T., Banks, M., Sinacore, D.R., Siener, C., Klein, S. 2006. Effect of weight loss and exercise on frailty in obese older adults. *Arch Intern Med* Apr 24;166(8):860–6.

39. Del Savio, G.C., Zelicof, S.B., Wexler, L.M., et.al. 1996. Preoperative nutritional status and outcome of elective total hip replacement. *Clin Orthop relat Res* May;(326):153–61.

40. Yuwen, P., Chen, W., Lv, H., et.al. 2017. Albumin and surgical site infection risk in orthopaedics: A meta-analysis. *BMC Surg* Jan 16;17(1):7.

41. Ackland, G.L., Scollay, J.M., Parks, R.W., de Beaux, I., Mythen, M.G. 2007. Pre-operative high sensitivity C-reactive protein and post operative outcome in patients undergoing elective orthopaedic surgery. *Anaesthesia* Sep;62(9):888–94.

42. McCully, K.S. 2007. Homocysteine, vitamins, and vascular disease prevention. *Am J Clin Nutr* Nov;86(5):1563S–8S.

43. Theusinger, O.M., Leyvraz, P.F., Schanz, U., Seifert, B., Spahn, D.R. 2007. Treatment of iron deficiency anemia in orthopedic surgery with intravenous iron: Efficacy and limits: A prospective study. *Anesthesiology* Dec;107(6):923–7.

44. Gerdhem, P., Ivaska, K.K., Isaksson, A., et.al. 2007. Associations between homocysteine, bone turnover, BMD, mortality, and fracture risk in elderly women. *J Bone Miner Res* Jan;22(1):127–34.

45. Selhub, J., Jacques, P.F., Wilson, P.W., Rush, D., Rosenberg, I.H. 1993. Vitamin status and intake as primary determinants of homocysteinemia in an elderly population. *JAMA* Dec 8;270(22):2693–8.

46. Spence, J.D. 2007. Homocysteine-lowering therapy: A role in stroke prevention? *Lancet Neurol* Sep;6(9):830–8.

47. Marin, L.A., Salido, J.A., López, A., Silva, A. 2002. Preoperative nutritional evaluation as a prognostic tool for wound healing. *Acta Orthop Scand* Jan;73(1):2–5.

48. Guo, J.J., Yang, H., Qian, H., Huang, L., Guo, Z., Tang, T. 2010. The effects of different nutritional measurements on delayed wound healing after hip fracture in the elderly. *J Surg Res* Mar;159(1):503–8.

49. Chu, C.S., Liang, C.K., Chou, M.Y., Lu, T., Lin, Y.T., Chu, C.L. 2017. Mini-nutritional assessment short-form as a useful method of predicting poor 1-year outcome in elderly patients undergoing orthopedic surgery. *Geriatr Gerontol Int* Dec; 17(12):2361–8.

50. Institute of Medicine. 2006. *Dietary Reference Intakes*. Washington, D.C.:The National Academy Press, p. 343.

51. Gherini, S., Vaughn, B.K., Lombardi, A.V. Jr., Mallory, T.H. 1993. Delayed wound healing and nutritional deficiencies after total hip arthroplasty. *Clin Orthop Relat Res* Aug;(293):188–95.

52. Hron, G., Lombardi, R., Eichinger, S., Lecchi, A., Kyrle, P.A., Cattaneo, M. 2007. Low vitamin B6 levels and the risk of recurrent venous thromboembolism. *Haematologica* Sep;92(9):1250–3.

53. Bischoff-Ferrari, H.A., Dietrich, T., Orav, E.J., et.al. 2004. Higher 25-hydroxyvitamin D concentrations are associated with better lower-extremity function in both active and inactive persons aged > or = 60 y. *Am J Clin Nutr* Sep;80(3):752–8.

54. Campbell, W.W. 2007. Synergistic use of higher-protein diets or nutritional supplements with resistance training to counter sarcopenia. *Nutr Rev* Sep;65(9):416–22.

55. Helman, T.G. In: Kohlstadt, I. (ed.), *Scientific Evidence for Musculoskeletal, Bariatric, and Sports Nutrition*. 2006, Boca Raton, FL: CRC, Taylor & Francis, p. 427.

56. Evans, W.J. 2004. Protein nutrition, exercise and aging. *J Am Coll Nutr* Dec;23(6 Suppl):601S–609S.

57. Cawood, A.L., Elia, M., Stratton, R.J. 2012. Systematic review and meta-analysis of the effects of high protein oral nutritional supplements. *Ageing Res Rev* Apr;11(2):278–96.

58. Pogatschnik, C., Steiger, E. 2015. Review of preoperative carbohydrate loading. *Nutr Clin Pract* Oct;30(5):660–4.

59. Ata, A., Lee, J., Bestle, S.L., Desemone, J., Stain, S.C. 2010. Postoperative hyperglycemia and surgical site infection in general surgery patients. *Arch Surg* Sep;145(9):858–64.

60. Breen, L., Phillips, S.M. 2011. Skeletal muscle protein metabolism in the elderly: Interventions to counteract the 'anabolic resistance' of ageing. *Nutr Metab (Lond)* Oct 5;8:68.

61. Jonas, S., Phillips, E.M. 2009. *ACSM's Exercise is Medicine™ A Clinician's Guide to Exercise Prescription*. Philadelphia: Lippincott Williams & Wilkins.

62. Reginster, J.Y., Bruyere, O., Neuprez, A. 2007. Current role of glucosamine in the treatment of osteoarthritis. *Rheumatology (Oxford)* May;46(5):731–5.

63. Kahan, A., Uebelhart D., De Vathaire F., et al., 2009. Long term effects of chondroitins 4 and 6 sulfate on knee osteoarthritis. The study on Osteoarthritis progression, prevention, a two-year randomized, double-blind, placebo-controlled trial. *Arthritis Rheum* Feb;60(2):524–33.

64. Pelletier, J.P., Raynauld, J.P., Beaulieu, A.D., et.al. 2016. Chondroitin sulfate efficacy versus celecoxib on knee osteoarthritis structural changes using magnetic resonance imaging: A 2-year multicentre exploratory study. *Arthritis Res Ther* Nov 3;18(1):256.

65. Zeng, C., Wei, J., Li, H., et.al. 2015. Effectiveness and safety of glucosamine, chondroitin, the two in combination, or celecoxib in the treatment of osteoarthritis of the knee. *Sci Rep* Nov 18;5:16827.

66. Möller, I., Pérez, M., Monfort, J., et.al. 2010. Effectiveness of chondroitin sulphate in patients with concomitant knee osteoarthritis and psoriasis: A randomized, double-blind, placebo-controlled study. *Osteoarthritis Cartilage* Jun;18(Suppl 1):S32–40.

67. Morreale, P., Manopulo, R., Galati, M., et al. 1996. Comparison of the anti-inflammatory efficacy of glucosamine, chondroitin sulfate, and collagen hydrolysate. *J Rheum* Aug;23(8): 1385–91.

68. Panahi, Y., Hosseini, M.S., Khalili, N., Naimi, E., Majeed, M., Sahebkar, A. 2015. Antioxidant and anti-inflammatory effects of curcuminoid-piperine combination in subjects with metabolic syndrome: A randomized controlled trial and an updated meta-analysis. *Clin Nutr* Dec;34(6):1101–8.

69. Chandran, B., Goel, A. 2012. A randomized, pilot study to assess the efficacy and safety of curcumin in patients with active rheumatoid arthritis. *Phytother Res* Nov;26(11):1719–25.

70. Kizhakkedath, R., Antony, B., Benny, M., Kuruvilla, B.T. 2011. Clinical evaluation of an herbal formulation, Rhulief®, in the management of knee osteoarthritis. *Osteoarthritis Cartilage* 19(1):S145–S146.

71. Sterzi, S., Giordani, L., Morrone, M., et.al. 2016. The efficacy and safety of a combination of glucosamine hydrochloride, chondroitin sulfate and bio-curcumin with exercise in the treatment of knee osteoarthritis: A randomized, double-blind, placebo-controlled study. *Eur J Phys Rehabil Med* Jun;52(3):321–30.

72. Sanchez, J., Bonet, M., Keijer, J., et al. 2013. Blood cell transcriptomics as a source of potential biomarkers of articular helath improvement: Effects of oral intake of a rooster combs extract rich in hyaluronic acid. *Genes Nutr* Sep;9(5):417.

73. Martinez-Puig, D., Moller I., Fernandez C., et al. 2013. Efficacy of oral administration off yoghurt supplemented with a preparation containing hyaluronic acid in adults with mild joint discomfort: A randomized, double-blind, placebo controlled intervention study. *Med J Nutrition Metab* 6:63–8.

74. Moriña, D., Sola, R., Valls R., et al. 2013. Efficacy of a low-fat yogurt supplemented with a rooster comb extract on joint function in mild knee pain patients: A subject-level meta-analysis. *Ann Nutr Metab* 63(S1):1386.

75. Woo, T., Lau, L., Cheng, N., Chan, P., Tan, K., Gardner, A. 2017. Efficacy of oral collagen in joint pain - osteoarthritis and rheumatoid arthritis. *J Arthritis* Feb;6:233.

76. Bakilan, F., Armagan, O., Ozgen, M., Tascioglu, F., Bolluk, O., Alatas, O. 2016. Effects of native type II collagen treatment on knee osteoarthritis: A randomized controlled trial. *Eurasian J Med* Jun;48(2):95–101.

77. Serhan, C.N., Petasis, N.A. 2011. Resolvins and protectins in inflammation resolution. *Chem Rev* Oct 12;111(10):5922–43.

78. Robinson, S.M., Jameson, K.A., Batelaan, S.F., et.al. 2008. Diet and its relationship with grip strength in community-dwelling older men and women: The Hertfordshire cohort study. *J Am Geriatr Soc* Jan;56(1):84–90.

79. Bays, H. 2007. Safety considerations with omega-3 fatty acid therapy. *Am J Card* Mar;99(6A):35C–43C.

80. Christensen, R., Bartels, E.M., Astrup, A., Bliddal, H. 2007. Effect of weight reduction in obese patients diagnosed with knee osteoarthritis: A systematic review and meta-analysis. *Ann Rheum Dis* Apr;66(4):433–9.

81. Rakel, D. 2018. *Integrative Medicine*, 4th Edition. Philadelphia: Elsevier.

82. Orban, J.C., Levraut, J., Gindre, S., et.al. 2006. Effects of acetylcysteine and ischaemic preconditioning on muscular function and postoperative pain after orthopaedic surgery using a pneumatic tourniquet. *Eur J Anaesthesiol* Dec;23(12):1025–30.

83. Witte, M.B., Barbul, A. 2003. Arginine physiology and its implication for wound healing. *Wound Repair Regen* Nov-Dec;11(6):419–23.

84. Lucotti, P., Setola, E., Monti, L.D., et.al. 2006. Beneficial effects of a long-term oral L-arginine treatment added to a hypocaloric diet and exercise training program in obese, insulin-resistant type 2 diabetic patients. *Am J Physiol Endocrinol Metab* Nov;291(5):E906–12.

85. Preli, R.B., Klein, K.P., Herrington, D.M. 2002. Vascular effects of dietary L-arginine supplementation. *Atherosclerosis* May;162(1):1–15.

86. Thorne Research, Inc. 2005. Monograph. L-Carnitine. *Altern Med Rev* Mar;10(1):42–50.

87. Spigset, O. 1994. Reduced effect of warfarin caused by ubidecarenone. *Lancet* Nov 12;344(8933):1372–3.

88. Berger, M.M., Shenkin, A. 2008. Trace element requirements in critically ill burned patients. *J Trace Elem Med Biol* 21(Suppl 1):44–8.

89. Candow, D.G., Chilibeck, P.D. 2007. Effect of creatine supplementation during resistance training on muscle accretion in the elderly. *J Nutr Health Aging* Mar-Apr;11(2):185–8.

90. Nishizaki, K., Ikegami, H., Tanaka, Y., Imai, R., Matsumura, H. 2015. Effects of supplementation with a combination of β-hydroxy-β-methyl butyrate, L-arginine, and L-glutamine on postoperative recovery of quadriceps muscle strenth after total knee arthroplasty. *Asia Pac J Clin Nutr* 24(3):412–20.

91. Nicastro, H., Artioli, G.G., Costa Ados, S., et.al. 2011. An overview of the therapeutic effects of leucine supplementation on skeletal muscle under atrophic conditions. *Amino Acids* Feb;40(2):287–300.

92. Ziegler, D. 2004. Thioctic acid for patients with symptomatic diabetic polyneuropathy: A critical review. *Treat Endocrinol* 3(3):173–89.

93. Zhang, Y., Han, P., Wu, N., et.al. 2011. Amelioration of lipid abnormalities by α-lipoic acid through antioxidative and anti-inflammatory effects. *Obesity (Silver Spring)* Aug;19(8):1647–53.

94. Udupa, A., Nahar, P., Shah, S., Kshirsagar, M., Ghongane, B. 2013. A comparative study of effects of omega-3 fatty acids, alpha lipoic acid and Vitamin E in type 2 diabetes mellitus. *Ann Med Health Sci Res* Jul;3(3):442–6.

95. Hadj, A., Esmore, D., Rowland, M., et al. 2006. Pre-operative preparation for cardiac surgery utilizing a combination of metabolic, physical and mental therapy. *Heart Lung Circ* Jun;15(3):172–81.

96. Maggio, M., Ceda, G.P., Lauretani, F., et al. 2011. Magnesium and anabolic hormones in older men. *Int J Androl* Dec; 34(6 Pt 2):e594–600.

97. Vaxman, F., Olender, S., Lambert, A., Nisand, G., Grenier, J.F. 1996. Can the wound healing process be improved by vitamin supplementation? Experimental study on humans. *Eur Surg Res* Jul-Aug;28(4):306–14.

98. Brzezinski, A., Vangel, M.G., Wurtman, R.J., et.al. 2005. Effects of exogenous melatonin on sleep: A meta-analysis. *Sleep Med Rev* Feb;9(1):41–50.

99. Yousaf, F., Seet, E., Venkatraghavan, L., Abrishami, A., Chung, F. 2010. Efficacy and safety of melatonin as an anxiolytic and analgesic in the perioperative period: A qualitative systematic review of randomized trials. *Anesthesiology* Oct;113(4):968–76.

100. Jarratt, J. 2011. Perioperative melatonin use. *Anaesth Intensive Care* Mar;39(2):171–81.
101. Butawan, M., Benjamin, R.L., Bloomer, R.J. 2017. Methylsulfonylmethane: Applications and safety of a novel dietary supplement. *Nutrients* Mar 16;9(3):e290.
102. Gionchetti, P., Rizzello, F., Venturi, A., Campieri, M. 2000. Probiotics in infective diarrhoea and inflammatory bowel diseases. *J Gastroenterol Hepatol* May;15(5):489–93.
103. Rayes, N., Soeters, P.B. 2010. Probiotics in surgical and critically ill patients. *Ann Nutr Metab* 57(Suppl):29–31.
104. Caruso, I., Pietrogrande, V. 1987. Italian double-blind multicenter study comparing S-adenosylmethionine, naproxen and placebo in the the treatment of degenerative joint disease. *Am J Med* Nov 20; 83(5A):66–71.
105. Najm, W.I., Reinsch, S., Hoehler, F., Tobis, J.S., Harvey, P.W. 2004. S-adenosyl methionine (SAMe) versus celecoxib for the treatment of osteoarthritis symptoms: A double-blind cross-over trial. *BMC Musculoskelet Disord* Feb 26;5:6.
106. Müller-Fassbender, H. 1987. Double-blind clinical trial of S-adenosylmethionine versus ibuprofen in the treatment of osteoarthritis. *Am J Med* Nov 20;83(5A):81–3.
107. Vetter, G. 1987. Double-blind comparative clinical trial with S-adenosylmethionine and indomethacin in the treatment of osteoarthritis. *Am J Med* Nov 20;83(5A):78–80.
108. Kim, J., Lee, E., Koh, E., et al. 2009. Comparative clinical trial of S-adenosylmethionine versus nabumetone for the treatment of knee osteoarthritis: An 8-week, multicenter, randomized, double-blind, double-dummy, Phase IV study in Korean patients. *Clin Ther* Dec;31(12):2860–72.
109. Chaput, J.P., Lord, C., Cloutier, M., et.al. 2007. Relationship between antioxidant intakes and class I sarcopenia in elderly men and women. *J Nutr Health Aging* Jul-Aug;11(4):363–9.
110. Jugdaohsingh, R., Tucker, K.L., Qiao, N., Cupples, L.A., Kiel, D.P., Powell, J.J. 2004. Dietary silicon intake is positively associated with bone mineral density in men and premenopausal women of the Framingham Offspring cohort. *J Bone Miner Res* Feb;19(2):297–307.
111. Juneja, L.R., Chu, D.C., Okubo, T., Nagato, Y., Yokogoshi, H. 1999. L-theanine - a unique amino acid of green tea and its relaxation effect in humans. *Trends Food Sci Technol* Jun;10(6–7):199–204.
112. Thorne Research, Inc. 2006. L-Tryptophan. Monograph. *Altern Med Rev* Mar;11(1):52–6.
113. Wicke, C., Halliday, B., Allen, D., et.al. 2000. Effects of steroids and retinoids on wound healing. *Arch Surg* Nov;135(11):1265–70.
114. Yazdanpanah, N., Zillikens, M.C., Rivadeneira, F., et.al. 2007. Effect of dietary B vitamins on BMD and risk of fracture in elderly men and women: The Rotterdam study. *Bone* Dec;41(6):987–94.
115. Cattaneo, M., Lombardi, R., Lecchi, A., Bucciarelli, P., Mannucci, P.M. 2001. Low plasma levels of vitamin B(6) independently associated with a heightened risk of deep-vein thrombosis. *Circulation* Nov 13;104(20):2442–6.
116. Cattaneo, M. 2006. Hyperhomocysteinemia and venous thromboembolism. *Semin Thromb Hemost* Oct;32(7):716–23.
117. Alcantara-Martos, T., Delgado-Martinez, A.D., Vega, M.V., Carrascal, M.T., Munuera-Martinez, L. 2007. Effect of vitamin C on fracture healing in elderly Osteogenic Disorder Shionogi rats. *J Bone Joint Surg Br* Mar;89(3):402–7.
118. Shah, A.S., Verma, M.K., Jebson, P.J. 2009. Use of oral vitamin C after fractures of the distal radius. *J Hand Surg Am* Nov;34(9):1736–8.
119. Holick, M.F. 2005. The vitamin D epidemic and its health consequences. *J Nutr* Nov;135(11):2739S–48S.
120. Cannell, J.J., Hollis, B.W., Zasloff, M., Heaney, R.P. 2008. Diagnosis and treatment of vitamin D deficiency. *Expert Opin Pharmacother* Jan;9(1):107–18.
121. Wei, M.Y., Giovannucci, E.L. 2010. Vitamin D and multiple health outcomes in the Harvard cohorts. *Mol Nutr Food Res* Aug;54(8):1114–26.
122. Plotnikoff, G.A., Quigley, J.M. 2003. Prevalence of severe hypovitaminosis D in patients with persistent, nonspecific musculoskeletal pain. *Mayo Clin Proc* Dec;78(12):1463–70.
123. Khor, S.C., Abdul Karim, N., Ngah, W.Z., Yusof, Y.A., Makpol, S. 2014. Vitamin E in sarcopenia: Current evidences on its role in prevention and treatment. *Oxid Med Cell Longev* 2014:914853.
124. Williams, J.Z., Barbul, A. 2003. Nutrition and wound healing. *Surg Clin North Am* Jun;83(3)571–96.
125. Mahmood, A., FitzGerald, A.J., Marchbank, T., et.al. 2007. Zinc carnosine, a health food supplement that stabilises small bowel integrity and stimulates gut repair processes. *Gut* Feb;56(2):168–75.
126. Moya, P., Soriano-Irigaray, L., Ramirez, J.M., et.al. 2016. Perioperative standard nutrition supplements versus immunonutrition in patients undergoing colorectal resection in a n enhanced recovery (ERAS) protocol: A multicenter randomized clinical trial (SONVI Study). *Medicine (Baltimore)* May;95(21):e3704.
127. Xu, J., Yunshi, Z. 2009, Immunonutrition in surgical patients. *Curr Drug Targets* Aug;10(8): 771–7.

128. Lee, J.G., Kim, Y.S., Lee, Y.J., et.al. 2016. Effect of immune-enhancing nutrition enriched with or without beta-glucan on immunomodulation in critically ill patients. *Nutrients* Jun 2;8(6):e336.

129. Verdam, F.J., Fuentes, S., de Jonge, C., et.al. 2013. Human intestinal microbiota composition is associated with local and systemic inflammation in obesity. *Obesity (Silver Spring)* Dec;21(12):E607–15.

130. Consoli, M.L., da Silva, R.S., Nicoli, J.R., et.al. 2016. Randomized clinical trial: Impact of oral administration of saccharomyces boulardii on gene expression of intestinal cytokines in patients undergoing colon resection. *JPEN J Parenter Enteral Nutr* Nov;40(8):1114–21.

131. Bharadwaj, S., Trivax, B., Tandon, P., Alkam, B., Hanouneh, I., Steiger, E. 2016. Should perioperative immunonutrition for elective surgery be the current standard of care? *Gastroenterol Rep (Oxf)* May;4(2):87–95.

132. Zhu, X., Herrera, G., Ochoa, J.B. 2010. Immunosuppression and infection after major surgery: A nutritional deficiency. *Crit Care Clin* Jul;26(3):491–500.

133. Cherchi, A., Lai, C., Angelino, F., et.al. 1985. Effects of L-carnitine on exercise tolerance in chronic stable angina: A multicenter, double-blind, randomized, placebo controlled crossover study. *Int J Clin Pharmacol Ther Toxicol* Oct;23(10):569–72.

134. Brevetti, G., Chiariello, M., Ferulano, G., et.al. 1988. Increases in walking distance in patients with peripheral vascular disease treated with L-carnitine: A double-blind, cross-over study. *Circulation* Apr;77(4):767–73.

135. Rundek, T., Naini, A., Sacco, R., et al. 2004. Atorvastatin decreases the coenzyme Q10 level in the blood of patients at risk for cardiovascular disease and stroke. *Arch Neurol* Jun;61(6):889–92.

136. Ranieri, M., Sciuscio, M., Cortese, A.M. 2009. The use of alpha-lipoic acid (ALA), gamma linolenic acid (GLS) and rehabilitation in the treatment of back pain: Effect on health-related quality of life. *Int J Immunopathol Pharmacol* Jul-Sep;22(3 Suppl):45–50.

137. Knudsen, E., Sandström, B., Solgaard, P. 1996. Zinc, copper and magnesium absorption from a fibre-rich diet. *J Trace Elem Med Biol* Jun;10(2):68–76.

138. Armas, L.A., Hollis, B.W., Heaney, R.P. 2004. Vitamin D2 is much less effective than Vitamin D3 in humans. *J Clin Endocrinol Metab* Nov;89(11):5387–91.

139. Adams, J., Kantorovich, V., Wu, C., et al., 1999. Resolution of vitamin D insufficiency in osteopenic patients results in rapid recovery of bone mineral density. *J Clin Endocrinol Metab* Aug;84(8):2729–30.

140. Hollis, B.W. 2005. Circulating 25-hydroxyvitamin D levels indicative of vitamin D sufficiency: Implications for establishing a new effective dietary intake recommendation for vitamin D. *J Nutr* Feb;135(2):317–22.

141. Lepperdinger, G. 2011. Inflammation and mesenchymal stem cell aging. *Curr Opin Immunol* Aug;23(4):518–24.

142. Derfoul, A., Miyoshi, A.D., Freeman, D.E., Tuan, R.S. 2007. Glucosamine promotes chondrogenic phenotype in both chondrocytes and mesenchymal stem cells and inhibits MMP-13 expression and matrix degradation. *Osteoarthritis Cartilage* Jun;15(6):646–55.

143. Ivanov, V., Cha, J., Ivanova, S., et.al. 2008. Essential nutrients suppress inflammation by modulating key inflammatory gene expression. *Int J Mol Med* Dec;22(6):731–41.

144. Mikirova, N.A., Jackson, J.A., Hunninghake, R., et.al. 2009. Circulating endothelial progenitor cells: A new approach to anti-aging medicine? *J Transl Med* Dec 15;7:106.

145. Peltz, L., Gomez, J., Marquez, M., et.al. 2012. Resveratrol exerts dosage and duration dependent effect on human mesenchymal stem cell development. *PLoS One* 7(5):e37162.

18 Metabolic Therapies for Muscle Injury

Ana V. Cintrón, MD and Kenneth Cintron, MD, MBA

INTRODUCTION

Skeletal muscle injuries are among the most common forms of trauma that occur during competitive and recreational sports, comprising 10%–55% of all injuries [1]. Direct and indirect trauma are the responsible mechanisms, strain being the most common indirect injury encountered by health care providers. Eccentric-induced muscle strains are among the most common, the musculotendinous junction being the segment most commonly involved, with an incidence that varies among different sports. Most strains occur when the muscle is stretched during an active contraction, resulting from mechanical stresses which exceed the parameters that induce adaptations, producing instead acute injury [2].

A comprehensive evaluation including a complete history and physical exam considering the mechanism of injury and the biomechanics of the sport is essential to reach an accurate diagnosis. The classic therapeutic approach involves PRICE – protection, rest, ice, compression and elevation – followed by the use of non-steroidal anti-inflammatory drugs (NSAIDs)/corticosteroids, therapeutic modalities and progressive exercise programs rendering functional movements, which in the case of athletes are directed at their specific sport.

Although this classic approach may be helpful for short-term pain reduction and early recovery of function, it does not typically reverse the structural changes associated with degenerative conditions and may contribute to worse long-term outcomes [3]. Optimal therapeutic strategies for muscle injury are still to be reached.

This chapter provides evidence-based information on emerging therapeutic modalities available for muscle injury and the specific effects of them on muscle recovery and regeneration. The authors apply the scientific evidence to individual patients in order to optimize outcomes.

CLINICAL EVALUATION

INJURY CLASSIFICATION

Muscle injury classifications and grading systems have undergone a continuous advancement and change towards more objective evidence-based approaches. By tradition and simplicity of use, the symptoms and signs present after injury constituted the basis for grading it as "mild" or "grade one" (strain), "moderate" or "grade two" (partial tear) and "severe" or "grade three" (complete tear). New and more complete grading classifications have been developed in the recent years including the Munich Classification, the British Athletic Classification and most recently in 2015 the MLG-R Classification [4]. The latter, proposed by Aspetar and Barcelona Football Club's medical staff is to our understanding the most comprehensive. It describes the injury mechanism whether it is direct or indirect, its location whether proximal, middle or distal in direct injuries, or within tendon, muscle-tendon junction or muscle periphery if indirect. It also classifies severity on a 0–4 grading scale based on cross-sectional involvement seen on MRI as well as its evolution, whether this is the first injury or re-injury [4]. Most importantly, however, given the changing nature of medical knowledge and understanding of muscle injury, further studies are needed to validate the new grading systems.

PREDISPOSING FACTORS

Extrinsic Factors

Management of musculoskeletal injuries must include the identification of factors which may have contributed to the injury, especially those which may be modified to affect the outcomes of recovery and risk for re-injury.

Extrinsic risk factors vary for upper and lower extremity muscular injuries and the specific type of exercise/sport involved. Among the most common are training variables including intensity, frequency, techniques and equipment, duration and intensity of play, and environmental factors. Functional deficits in the kinetic chain may lead to compensating subclinical biomechanical deficits. Once identified, these deficits can often be corrected to minimize the risk for re-injury. Obesity can also change the biomechanical forces that lead to injury.

Intrinsic Factors

Intrinsic factors include older age, sex, muscle imbalances or functional deficits in the kinetic chain, low back pathology and previous muscle injury. The literature is conflicting regarding some factors associated with a predisposition to muscle injuries. Some of these are modifiable and closely related to metabolism.

Aging is associated with a decrease in antioxidant efficiency and an increase in oxidative stress damage after incremental exhaustive exercises [5]. Compared with skeletal muscle of young people, the number of macrophages is lower, the gene expression of several cytokines is higher, and stress signaling proteins are activated in skeletal muscle of elderly people at rest. Sarcopenia may also result from inadequate repair and chronic maladaptation following muscle injury in the elderly. Macrophage infiltration and the gene expression of certain cytokines are reduced in skeletal muscle of elderly people compared with young people, following exercise-induced muscle injury [6, 7]. Obesity can also change the biomechanical forces that lead to injury.

Flexibility is important. A study performed in male professional soccer players showed that an increased tightness of the hamstring or quadriceps muscles have a statistically higher risk for a subsequent musculoskeletal lesion. A simple preseason hamstring and quadriceps muscle flexibility testing can identify patients at risk of developing hamstring and quadriceps muscle injuries [8].

Genetic predisposition is among the intrinsic factors. Single nucleotide polymorphisms (SNPs) are an exciting and new field of investigation in orthopedics, sports medicine and regenerative medicine. Another study on an elite professional soccer club found a statistically significant association between the degree of injury and recovery time for non-contact musculoskeletal muscle injuries in SNPs in the IGF2, CCL2, and ELN genes. Players that present these types of SNPs are now involved in specific prevention programs [9].

Other studies have demonstrated an association of the COL5A1 rs12722 and the Apal genotype of the Vitamin D receptor SNP with the severity of musculoskeletal injuries and the MCT1 rs1049434 polymorphism with an increased incidence of musculoskeletal injuries in the group studied, respectively [10, 11].

Genetics exerts influence on regulators of inflammation in skeletal muscle, including the key regulators nuclear factor kappa-light-chain-enhancer of activated B cells (NF-kB), suppressor of cytokine signaling 3 (SOCS3) and peroxisome proliferator-activated receptor gamma coactivator 1 (PGC-1). Heat shock proteins and reactive oxygen and nitrogen species regulate inflammation indirectly by altering the activity of these transcription factors and genes.

The genetic profile based on the SNPs can be used to enhance and describe, as objectively as possible, the risks of injury for everyone, leading to an improved selection process and a personalized preventative care and treatment options.

The Hormone Balance

One way in which male and female sex hormones influence muscle mass and strength is by attenuating muscle damage after eccentric exercise. Skeletal muscle does not regenerate without satellite cells, confirming their pivotal and non-redundant role [12]. Studies have shown that estrogens and androgens impact positively on satellite cell activation and proliferation *in vivo*. Sex hormones establish adult quiescent satellite cell populations by regulating the myofiber niche at puberty and re-establishing them during regeneration [13].

They are able to upregulate their own receptor in muscle cells and satellite muscle cells, the latter being muscle multipotent stem cells whose activation is imperative for muscle regeneration and adaptation to exercise [14].

Thyroid hormone (TH) plays a critical role in regulating the function of satellite cells, the bona fide skeletal muscle stem cells. Deiodinases (D2 and D3) have been found to modulate the expression of various TH target genes in satellite cells [15]. Thyroid hormone signaling is required for skeletal muscle development, contractile function and muscle regeneration. Current studies suggest that the dynamic control of thyroid hormone activity through the regulation of deiodinase expression can be harnessed to optimize myogenesis in patients with muscle diseases or injury [16].

Impaired glucose tolerance is associated with increased serum concentrations of interleukin 6 (IL-6) [17]. Increased levels of IL-6, however, have been suggested to have a detrimental effect on muscle growth and in general, higher levels of IL-6 were found in frail older men and were negatively associated with reported levels of physical activity, fitness, and IGF-I. In addition, higher levels of IL-6 were found in several inflammatory conditions associated with insulin resistance. In this regard, it was reported that IL-6 levels rather than TNF or leptin were strongly associated with obesity and insulin resistance.

In summary, exercise, maintenance of the metabolic properties of the muscle tissue, and the balance of anabolic hormones are powerful, and to some extent modifiable, factors for muscle adaptation and regeneration.

PHASES OF MUSCLE RECOVERY

Research has shown that the natural progression of muscle injury proceeds through a highly interdependent sequence of steps, leading to the restoration of tissue architecture and function. Three main phases have been identified in the process of muscle regeneration: a destruction phase with the initial inflammatory response, a regeneration phase with activation and proliferation of satellite cells and a remodeling phase with the maturation of the regenerated myofibers and functional recovery [18].

The importance of the initial inflammatory phase has been emphasized, during which the influx of neutrophils and pro-inflammatory macrophages play an important role in the phagocytosis of damaged muscle, and the secretion of many growth factors which play an important role in muscle regeneration [19]. Anti-inflammatory macrophages follow in the process, promoting the activation of satellite cells, which proliferate and produce new myofibers, while angiogenesis, innervation and fibrotic tissue production complete the regeneration phase.

An essential role in the process of regeneration is played by growth factors, among which are insulin-like growth factor-1 (IGF-1), which promotes myoblast proliferation and muscle growth, vascular endothelial growth factor (VEGF), which promotes angiogenesis, and transforming growth factor-β1 (TGF-β1), which is responsible for collagen deposition and fibrosis formation, while inhibiting satellite cell proliferation [19]. While the role of TGF-β1 is important in the process of restoring tissue architecture, the deposition of fibrous tissue in muscle has been implicated in the lack of full restoration of muscle function and as a possible cause of re-injury. The use of an anti-fibrotic therapy which blocks TGF-β1 (such as antihypertensive Losartan), has been shown to improve muscle regeneration by decreasing the amount of fibrous tissue within the muscle, decreasing muscle loss and improving muscle remodeling [20].

As the role of the initial inflammatory response to muscle injury has gained importance, the greater the concern over the use of NSAIDs, especially in the initial phases of recovery. NSAIDs have been found to decrease prostaglandin E2, slowing the proliferation and maturation of differentiated myogenic precursor cells, and increase the expression of TGF-β1, therefore increasing the production of fibrotic/scar tissue.

TREATMENT MODALITIES

PHYSICAL

Cryotherapy and Heat

Heat and cold therapy are considered part of the standard of care for acute musculoskeletal pain. However, most recommendations for use of heat and cold therapy in acute musculoskeletal injury are based on empirical experience or unconfirmed information because the evidence base supporting the efficacy of these modalities is quite limited. Cold treatment or "cryotherapy" produces vasoconstriction with vasodilatation following reflexively, decreased local metabolism and blood flow, and minimized enzymatic activity and the subsequent demand for oxygen, thereby limiting the extent of injury to the uninjured tissue. Additionally, cryotherapy is able to decrease pain by desensitizing nociceptive sensory nerves, which according to studies by Nadler et al. [21], allows for the recovery of pain-free movements and accelerates the healing process. Cryotherapy is most commonly used during the first 48 hours of acute musculoskeletal injuries such as sprains, strains and contusions, while use beyond the initial acute phase is directed towards continued pain control, muscle re-education and control of swelling when utilized with compression. On the other hand, physiological effects of heat therapy include pain relief, increases in blood flow and metabolism, and increased elasticity of connective tissue. Increasing tissue temperature stimulates vasodilation and increases tissue blood flow, which is thought to promote healing by increasing the supply of nutrients and oxygen to the site of injury [21].

In a systematic review, Collins [22] showed limited evidence in humans suggesting treatment with cold may improve pain and function in muscle strains. In animal models, nonetheless, cryotherapy has been shown to decrease inflammation, tissue necrosis, and hematoma size after muscle injury. Furthermore, icing of the injured skeletal muscle for an extended period of six hours was shown to obtain a substantial effect on hemorrhage limitation and tissue necrosis at the site of the muscle injury in rats [23]. Despite the limited evidence of cryotherapy's long-term benefits after muscle strain in humans, its different effects – acute pain control, low cost, ease of application in its different forms (e.g. cold packs with or without compression, ice immersion, ice massage, etc.) – in addition to its low risk of adverse effects if used correctly mean that this modality is still recommended overall by clinicians and authors in the first 48 hours after acute muscle strains. Important to note, the contraindications for cryotherapy include ischemia, cold intolerance, Raynaud's phenomenon, cold allergy, inability to communicate and insensate skin.

Superficial Heat

There are numerous types of superficial heat delivery, such as those imparted by convection, conduction, radiation and conversion, exerting its effects no deeper than the skin and subcutaneous fat [24]. Clinical studies using superficial heat in muscle injury are limited. Interestingly, however, Hassan et al. [25] showed evidence of bio-metabolic principles to support its use after comparing warm vs. cold water immersion vs. a no-treatment control, 15 minutes after eccentric hamstring exercises in sixty young athletic males. Warm water significantly decreased markers of muscle stress reaction, including skeletal troponin I, creatine kinase, and myoglobin levels, compared with cold water or control ($P < 0.05$), suggesting a decrease in muscle stress reaction markers when compared to cold. Nonetheless, the clinical significance of these findings applied to prevention of muscle strains or accelerating muscle repair after a strain is questioned.

Moreover, a clinical study [26] using a specialized MRI technique provided the first objective evidence that therapeutic application of superficial heat does not enhance the recovery of damaged muscle fibers after eccentric exercise, as evidenced by specific muscle imaging. In summary, there is no clear evidence to support that superficial heat after muscle strains positively affects outcomes.

Deep Heat: Ultrasound

Ultrasound has both thermal and non-thermal effects, by which the proposed treatment for wounds and inflammation is based on the belief that either its heat production (by increasing blood flow and metabolic or enzymatic activity) or non-thermal effects (by changing cell wall permeability) accelerate healing [27]. Even so, there are few studies specifically evaluating its use in muscle strains. A systematic review by Van der Windt et al. [28] from well-designed trials evaluating ultrasound therapy concluded that there is little evidence to show efficacy in the treatment of musculoskeletal disorders. Similarly, a literature review by Shanks et al. [29] from studies dating from 1975 to 2009 found that there is currently no high-quality evidence available to suggest that therapeutic ultrasound is effective for musculoskeletal conditions of the lower limb.

High Galvanic Electrical Stimulation (HVPGS)

High-voltage pulsed galvanic stimulation of tissue is gaining widespread use for wound healing, especially diabetic ulcers, edema reduction and pain relief, by combining very short pulse duration (of constant intensity) and high peak voltage, yet low total current per second, to give relative comfort and avoid tissue damage while stimulating muscle contraction [30]. Although the main use of HVPGS in sports rehabilitation is for the relief of pain, it can also be used to aid in tissue healing when used post-operatively. The muscle contraction elicited by HVPGS is sought to stimulate circulation by pumping blood through venous and lymphatic channels after acute injuries, when fluid accumulation is significant, while keeping an injured joint protected. Despite the limitation of studies specifically investigating this modality after muscle strains, a review by Lake [31] concluded that electrical muscle stimulation may be helpful in controlling edema after injury, preventing loss of muscle bulk and strength associated with immobilization, selective strengthening and enhancing motor control. Therefore, its use after muscle strains may be considered in view of the aforementioned proposed mechanisms, although high-quality strain-specific studies are lacking.

Transcutaneous Electrical Nerve Stimulation (TENS)

TENS is usually defined as the application of an electric current therapy through the skin to a peripheral nerve or nerves for the control of pain. Three theories have been put forward to explain the analgesic effects of electrical stimulation, the gate-control theory being the most widely recognized in the literature [32]. Nonetheless, there are very few studies evaluating TENS-associated muscle repair or outcomes after muscle strain. There is, however, a large, randomized, placebo-control study that showed that TENS may be as effective as acetaminophen/codeine for pain control in acute traumatic disorders such as contusions, sprains and strains [33]. A review by Robinson et al. [34] concluded that TENS appears to give the best benefit in the treatment of early postoperative pain or pain from acute injuries such as sprains/strains and contusions. However, the response can be variable, unpredictable and short lived. All in all, studies have shown that TENS is generally unharmful, may sometimes provide pain relief above the placebo response, is more effective in acute pain relief with short-term benefit, and is more effective at higher stimulation intensities. In summary, despite lack of evidence studying direct outcome measures of TENS use after muscle injury, the authors believe this is a safe and effective modality for acute pain relief after acute soft tissue injuries and, in our experience, helps the patient tolerate more evidence-based treatments such as therapeutic exercise during the rehabilitation process.

Micro-Electric Nerve Stimulation (MENS)

Micro-electric nerve stimulation is a relatively new modality currently being studied in both laboratory and clinical scenarios, which, as the name implies, transmits through small surface electrodes small electric currents to stimulate nerves. The MENS bio-physiologic mechanism is still not well understood; however, it has been reported to increase the synthesis of adenosine triphosphate (ATP) by stimulating the electron transport system of mitochondria in rat skin under electrical stimulation with a 500 μA current, but to depress it with a current of 1000 μA or higher. In addition, animal studies have shown that the use of MENS using 0.3 Hz, 10 μA stimuli facilitated the regeneration of injured skeletal muscles of rats via stimulating the proliferative potential of muscle satellite cells, a key player in muscle regeneration, and accelerated muscle regeneration by stimulating muscle protein synthesis [35]. Moreover, recent human studies have shown that MENS confers reductions in delayed-onset muscle soreness (DOMS) and signs and symptoms of muscle damage following eccentric exercise in human subjects, strongly suggesting that the therapy facilitates the regeneration of injured skeletal muscle [36]. Despite the few studies available, there is evidence of safety and efficacy enough to consider the application of MENS after acute muscle strain injuries to promote muscle repair.

Extracorporeal Shock Wave Therapy (ESWT)

Extracorporeal shock wave therapy has been widely employed in the treatment of enthesopathy with good clinical response; however, studies on its benefits after acute muscle injury are limited, although promising. For example, Zissler et al. [37] recently showed that the use of ESWT after acute cardiotoxin-induced injury to the quadriceps femoris muscle of rats, was associated with significantly higher contents of pax7-positive satellite cells, mitotically active H3P+ cells, and of cells expressing the myogenic regulatory factors myoD and myogenin, indicating enhanced proliferation and differentiation rates of satellite cells. Moreover, a clinical study by Costa et al. [38] showed that ESWT associated with physical therapy proved to be effective at treating long-term muscle injury, with good performance and the ability to return to sport practice for all patients in the trial, suggesting there may be a space for ESWT after both acute and chronic muscle injury.

Photobiomodulation (PBMT)

A systematic review by Bjordal, et al. [39] evaluates the available literature regarding the use of PBMT for treatment of acute pain from soft tissue injury and sums up the most evidenced mechanisms by which PBMT exerts its effects: angiogenetic and local microcirculation increase, local anti-inflammatory effects as well as direct effects on cells, soft tissue and biochemical markers in a dose-dependent manner. Additionally, the review presents multiple laboratory trials showing PBMT has anti-inflammatory effects by decreasing prostaglandin E_2, reducing interleukin 1 levels, reducing TNF levels (associated with tissue fibrosis in injured skeletal muscle) and reducing cyclooxygenase 2 levels. These anti-inflammatory effects are also seen at a cellular level, as demonstrated by a local decrease in edema, hemorrhage, neutrophil influx and reduced cell apoptosis. There is strong evidence in animal trials that PBMT improves functional outcomes compared to both systemic and intralesional diclofenac in controlled muscle strains in rats. Clinical testing, however, is controversial as there is a lack of appropriately controlled trials. Many health professionals use PBMT for both chronic and acute inflammatory conditions, and there is consistent evidence for improvement of functional outcome measures vs. placebo in trials studying musculoskeletal injuries such as acute ankle sprains, acute Achilles tendonitis and medial tibial shin splints. Nonetheless, in a comprehensive summary of PBMT mechanisms and its use, expert in the field Dr. Michael Hamblin [40] presents unresolved questions that remain to date: using laser vs. non-coherent light? What is the correct dosage of light? Use either continuous or pulsed treatment? The optimal wavelength is also controversial; however, it is the most agreed among clinicians, using 600–700 nm range for treating superficial tissue, and wavelengths between 780 and 950 nm for deeper tissues due to longer optical penetration. In summary, PBMT shows promise for use in acute muscle strain injury by the mechanisms outlined in this section; however, more research to determine optimal treatment for muscle recovery after strains is needed.

Massage

In athletes, massage as a preparation prior to sports has been suggested to accelerate recovery after exercise and is commonly used as therapy intervention after sports-related musculoskeletal injuries. The specific mechanisms of action are still under study; however, they include: increased lymph flow, a shift from sympathetic to parasympathetic response, prevention of fibrosis, increased clearance of blood lactate, and effects on the immune system, cognition and pain [41]. More specifically, studies have shown that muscle can perceive mechanical stimuli and respond by the generation of corresponding intracellular signals in a magnitude-dependent manner, leading to qualitative and quantitative changes in gene expression that initiate muscle damage or muscle repair. For example, Agarwal and colleagues [42] showed that 20%–50% mechanical stretch applied to muscle *ex vivo* results in activation of nuclear factor kappa B (NF-KB)-mediated transcription factors and pro-inflammatory gene induction, suggesting that critical levels of mechanical forces are necessary for tissue homeostasis. Furthermore, there is evidence of a dose-dependent effect of massage-like loading (MLL) on the recovery of mechanical properties as well as histological evidence for MLL to decrease muscle fiber damage [43]. In addition, the clinical effects of immediate vs. delayed massage 48 hours following eccentric exercise showed that both strategies led to an accelerated recovery of muscle function (isometric torque) compared with a control, exercised and non-massaged muscle [44]. The same author showed that four days of massage-like loading at a predetermined magnitude, duration and frequency of tissue loading, led to an accelerated recovery of muscle function. The exact mechanisms by which massage may aid in the recovery of muscle function following intense exercise are currently being studied but remain unresolved. Nonetheless, clinical studies have generally shown positive outcomes and potential benefits from massage therapy as means of muscle injury rehabilitation. Further research on massage-directed muscle recovery and the conditions necessary (i.e. type of massage, applied forces, duration of therapy, etc.) are needed to fully understand the clinical utility of the available research.

Acupuncture

Acupuncture is widely used to relieve persistent pain and to treat many disorders, including both acute and chronic pain. It entails the stimulation of specific acupoints on the body with acupuncture needles, typically chosen by the practitioner based on the patients' individual characteristics and their treating condition. Acupuncture is traditionally used after injuries including sprains, strains, contusions, bone and joint injury as well as chronic pain. However, well-designed, controlled, high-quality evidence-based studies for improving recovery or functional outcomes after muscle injury are unavailable. There is, however, evidence that may support the promotion of muscle recovery by increasing local blood flow to skin and muscle after acupuncture treatment [45]. There is more evidence, however, regarding acupuncture and its use for pain control. In 2007, Taguchi reviews acupuncture's analgesic and anesthetic use on acute clinical pain in Japan [46], reviewing different studies supporting its effect by increasing pain threshold and by increasing endogenous opioids and receptors. The author later presents positive clinical outcomes of acupuncture for post-operative pain, dental procedure analgesia, post-herpetic neuralgia and reflex sympathetic dystrophy. A recent individual patient data meta-analysis [47] restricted to high-quality trials showed acupuncture is associated with reductions in chronic pain as compared to sham acupuncture and as compared to no acupuncture control for non-specific musculoskeletal pain, osteoarthritis, chronic headache and shoulder pain. All in all, medicine is moving towards individualized or personalized treatments by identifying intrinsic factors that may constitute if and how a patient will respond to certain treatments. A recent review supports this notion by showing that the levels of signaling molecules associated with acupuncture analgesia, including those of descending inhibitory system, endogenous opioids, and CCK-8, may be differentially expressed in responders and non-responders [48]. This may suggest an explanation for the variation of results in many of the available clinical studies. At this time, there is limited evidence regarding acupuncture's specific effect on functional outcomes and muscle recovery after muscle strain; however, there is some evidence to support its use in acute pain and chronic musculoskeletal conditions. Despite its common use in sports injuries, controlled studies are still needed to better elucidate and recommend its use after muscle injury.

Exercise

Rehabilitation protocols for muscle strains incorporate exercise programs in accordance to the three different phases of recovery. Phase one, or the inflammatory phase exercise program, incorporates range of motion (ROM) exercise as well as pain-free isometric exercise to avoid loss of range of motion and to prevent muscle atrophy, while at the same time protecting the injured tissue. Phase two and three progress to isotonic and/or isokinetic exercise programs aiming to increase strength and improve neuromuscular control, while progressing to functional exercise programs which are sport-specific [49].

At the cellular level, many of the growth factors and cytokines which activate the pathway to muscle growth and hypertrophy can be found in an inactive form bound to regulatory proteins in the muscle extracellular matrix. These proteins have been found to be activated not only in response to muscle injury but also to stretching and exercise [50]. Valero et al. demonstrated that mesenchymal-like stem cells, mainly pericytes, rapidly appear in skeletal muscle post-exercise, revealing an event which may be necessary for effective repair and/or growth following exercise and/or injury.

Multiple systematic reviews have shown that the current standard of care, which is largely driven by concentric exercise, does not adequately restore muscle strength after joint or muscle injury, as measured by high rates of re-injury and the low percentage of individuals who return to their pre-injury level of sport.

The use of eccentric exercise as part of a rehabilitation program has been avoided due to the association of this lengthening muscle contraction to muscle injury. Eccentric exercise has been used as an experimental model for muscle injury in multiple research studies, commonly using lengthening stretches of a very high magnitude, up to 20%–60% beyond optimal fiber length, which exceeds physiological fiber strains during *in vivo* muscle contractions. In addition, limiting the number of sarcomeres in many of these experiments eliminates the largest myofilament titin (connectin), responsible for most of passive tension within the sarcomere and involved in signaling pathways that regulate tissue growth and adaptation in skeletal muscle during lengthening contractions [51].

Research has shown several effects related to eccentric exercise that favor its use in the rehabilitation of muscle injuries. As compared to concentric exercise, eccentric exercise is capable of directly promoting the growth of sarcomeres in series at a reduced metabolic rate as measured by lower levels of electromyographical activity during exercise. This finding has been associated with the rightward shift of the torque-joint angle relationship in animal models that are exposed to repeated bouts of eccentric exercise, indicating an improvement in muscle force at longer muscle lengths [52]. Studies in the clinical/athletic settings which have incorporated eccentric exercises as part of the rehabilitation protocols for hamstring muscle strains have shown a significant mechanical benefit, with a rightward shift in the optimum angle of hamstring torque-angle relationship [51]. Tyler et al. found that athletes who engaged in a rehabilitation protocol focused on performing eccentric contractions could return to sport stronger, with no recurrent hamstring strains, while those who did not comply with the program returned to sport with a 50% re-injury rate [51].

Additional morphological changes in response to eccentric exercise are gains in muscle cross-sectional area, increase in pennation angle [53] and increase in type II fibers [54]. Lengthening of the sarcomere has also been found to trigger a signaling complex which regulates and triggers tissue growth and adaptation [51], and to improve peripheral and central neural adaptations associated with poor neuromuscular control, with a resultant improvement in the recruitment and/or firing rate of alpha-motor neurons [55].

Muscle inhibition commonly occurs after a traumatic muscle or joint injury, where reduced alpha-motor neuron recruitment and/or firing rates are responsible for the lack of volitional control of the muscle. Some investigators hypothesize that the inhibition originates from several triggers, such as pain, effusion or altered afferent input from the damaged tissues, as well as central mechanisms [56]. Several studies using eccentric exercise protocols have shown improvement in muscle fiber recruitment in patients with slow/incomplete recovery attributed to this inhibition [57].

In addition to the direct effects in muscle, exercise in general has also been shown to increase the secretion of follistatin by hepatocytes, an autocrine glycoprotein which is a potent inhibitor of both activin and myostatin, factors that suppress muscle hypertrophy and impair muscle regeneration [49].

The importance of exercise in muscle injury rehabilitation cannot be over-emphasized. Interventions regarding exercise programs for muscle rehabilitation should be targeted to the individual's specific physiological needs/deficits and to sport-specific functional needs.

The traditional therapy of rest must be prescribed with caution, taking into consideration that in some instances of muscle injury rest may jeopardize the opportunity to locally recruit stem cells to the zone of injury and enhance regeneration through controlled and monitored exercise regimens, starting prior to the completion of the regeneration phase [58].

Concentric exercise has an important role in specific clinical scenarios in which overloading of the muscle or tendon are contraindicated, where range of motion is limited and in the presence of joint effusions [57]. However, the addition of eccentric exercise as rehabilitation progresses should be highly considered as a tool which research has shown improves muscle recovery and decreases re-injury.

Direct mechanical stimulation has been studied to stimulate and regenerate injured muscle tissue. Despite insufficient evidence to endorse or discontinue routine stretching before or after exercise to prevent injury among competitive or recreational athletes [59], there are multiple studies which have shown that stretching triggers an intracellular cellular cascade of events, including nitric oxide synthesis, which results in hepatocyte growth factor (HGF) release and satellite activation [60], which favors early stretching in the rehabilitation of muscle injuries. The use of low-intensity resistance exercise [20%–30%, one repetition maximum (1 RM)] with blood flow restriction has gained increasing interest because of increasing satellite cell activation, promoting marked proliferation of myogenic stem cells with resultant muscle hypertrophy and marked increase in rapid force capacity, revealing a potential technique which can be important for muscle atrophy recovery [61].

Nutritional Interventions

Proper nutritional intervention, very often ignored, is a strategy that can reduce or minimize the impact of a musculoskeletal injury and can enhance the rate of full recovery [62]. There are several reasons nutrition is specifically important for muscle injury recovery [63, 64].

Loss of muscle mass, strength and function are common consequences of immobilization resulting from musculoskeletal injuries. There is an increased need for enzymatic cofactors and precursor molecules to facilitate and speed up the metabolic machinery that leads to recovery.

Decreased energy requirement is a consequence of immobilization due to muscle injury. Voluntary diminished energy intake can be a common consequence of physical inactivity, especially in those exercisers that are very concerned about body weight and composition [65, 66]. During recovery, especially phase one, daily energy requirements can increase up to 20% above basal needs. Adequate energy supply is essential to prevent energy malnutrition, to overcome and prevent longer periods of inflammation and to promote anabolism.

Poor carbohydrate intake is associated with wasting, loss of unwanted body fat and poor wound healing [67]. The primary reason for this is because when carbohydrates are not metabolically available, protein is catabolized to meet energy demands rather than being available for muscle anabolism and structural repair. Meanwhile, excessive carbohydrate intake can provoke hyperinsulinemia, which can also prevent adequate healing process and can provoke alterations in immune system function and increments in the infectious process [67].

Some strategies to enhance muscle protein synthesis (MPS) after exercise have been proposed. Distribution of the total amount of protein throughout the day seems to promote MPS in a more efficient manner than eating big amounts of protein in fewer meals. Two protocols have been proposed to help and maintain MPS for longer periods of time, 20 g/protein/meal [63] and 0.25–0.30 g of protein/kg [64]. Although these protocols are recommended for recuperation after exercise, it's a reasonable strategy to implement it in both stages to promote wound and bone healing, muscle hypertrophy and strength gain.

Adequate water consumption is often overlooked. Water is very important to maintain skin turgor, oxygenation and tissue perfusion [67]. It also serves as the main transport of nutrients, waste removal, maintenance of body temperature and blood pressure [65]. The estimated fluid for recovering patients is approximately 1ml/kcal/day. Requisites must be adjusted due to insensible losses and the presence of vomiting and diarrhea [68]. Water, soups, milk, juices, fresh fruits and vegetable consumption are recommended to accomplish hydration needs.

The inflammatory response starts immediately after an exercise injury [65]. This response has a variable duration, from a few hours up to many days. An adequate inflammatory process is essential for muscle recovery [67]. In this matter, nutritional intervention must be done cautiously. The consumption of anti-inflammatory nutrients must be made with precaution, to safeguard the natural healing process and help maintain the inflammation period under the expected duration (Table 18.1).

Omega-3 fatty acids act as a potent reductor of the inflammatory stage through a myriad cascade of reactions that interferes with or reduces the formation and influence of arachidonic acid [69]. The best sources are coldwater fish, fish oils and commercial supplements, while other sources such as seed (flax, chia) can be incorporated into daily consumption. Omega-3 fatty acids are highly recommended to reduce inflammation status in chronic situations such as rheumatoid arthritis [70]. At this moment, there is no specific recommendation of Omega-3 fatty acids consumption for exercise-related muscle injury. Taking into account all reported benefits of this fatty acid [71], low-moderate intake is advisable. In this regard, pro-inflammatory substances like alcohol, saturated and trans-fat must be avoided.

Curcumin, a low molecular weight polyphenol, is derived from the rhizomes of the plant turmeric (*Curcuma longa*). It is a potent antioxidant that protects body cells and tissues by blocking free radical attacks by toxins in food, the environment and those produced internally, such as superoxide, hydrogen peroxide and nitric oxide. Curcumin protects deoxyribonucleic acid (DNA) from oxidation, reducing the risk of mutations and supports immunity by inhibiting the proliferation of damaging cells and toxins and by boosting macrophage and antibody activity [68].

TABLE 18.1

Anti-Inflammatory/Anti-Oxidant Supplementation for Muscle Injury

Supplement	Proposed Mode of Action	Suggested Dose
Omega-3 fatty acids	Anti-inflammatory Reduced joint pain	1.5–3 g/day
Curcumin	Anti-oxidative, anti-apoptotic and anti-inflammatory	2–4 g/day
Bioflavonoids(Quercetin, Polyphenols, Epicatechin)	Anti-oxidant activity	200–1000 mg/day
Bromelain	Anti-inflammatory Anti-edematous, analgesic Anti-thrombotic	200–400 mg/tid

Source: Table by Nevarez C, Sports Nutritionist; The Center for Sport Health and Exercise Science, San Juan, Puerto Rico.

Quercetin is a flavonoid that, like turmeric, possesses great anti-inflammatory activity but does so with a different mechanism of action. It works by reducing TNF-induced recruitment of pro-inflammatory genes. However, in a double-blind laboratory study, quercetin supplementation had no effect on markers of muscle damage or inflammation after eccentric exercise [72].

Bromelain, the enzyme in pineapple, has a mechanism of anti-inflammatory action which is mediated by increasing serum fibrinolytic activity, reducing plasma fibrinogen levels and decreasing bradykinin levels, which results in reduced vascular permeability and, hence, reduced edema and pain. Bromelain has been demonstrated to reduce exercise-induced muscle damage and inflammation, enhancing recovery. In a recent randomized, double-blind, placebo-controlled trial, bromelain supplementation reduced subjective feelings of fatigue and was associated with a trend to maintain testosterone concentration in competitive cyclists [73].

Antioxidant nutrients help to reduce the inflammation process and have also been connected to reduced joint pain [74]. Moderate consumption of these components on a daily basis can contribute to accelerating the healing process. Fresh fruits, especially pineapple and papaya, dark chocolate and blueberries are a few examples of foods that can reduce inflammation without inhibiting the natural course of inflammation process after bone-muscle trauma.

Orthobiologics

Clinical research is moving rapidly to cell-based therapies and biomaterials that promote healing, such as platelet-rich plasma, stem cells and biologic scaffolds. Research on their role in muscle injury and repair will be discussed.

Stem Cells

Pluripotent mesenchymal stem cells (MSC) have the capacity to differentiate into diverse mesodermal lineages, including muscle, bone, tendon and ligament, acting to modulate the body's response to injury, facilitating replacement with healthy tissue by way of environmental modification or direct differentiation into local components [75]. Stem cell therapy involves re-implanting autologously and allogenically, with the advantage of avoiding the triggering of an immune response, and therefore having a key role in tissue healing and immunomodulation [76]. However, research and treatment of musculoskeletal conditions with MSC has been focused mainly on tendon, ligament and cartilage injuries, and is still limited in its evidence-based support [69].

Research has been focused on muscle satellite cells (SC) and their role in muscle repair and regeneration. They are skeletal muscle mononuclear stem cells, which remain in a quiescent state until activation occurs in response to different physiological and pathological stimuli, including exercise, stretching, electrical stimulation and injury such as post-training micro-injuries [77]. Activation results in the formation of precursor myogenic cells known as myoblasts, which are responsible for muscle fiber hypertrophy through the addition of nuclei to existing myofibers [18]. They also have an important implication in cell therapy due to their self-renewal as well as their capability to differentiate into myofibers, processes which depend on a number of factors, including the microenvironment and the presence of myogenic regulatory factors.

Research has shown that the response of SC to exercise and treatment modalities is multifactorial, and has been described in the previous sections. Muscle-derived stem cells (MDSC) are believed to be precursors of satellite cells and could self-proliferate as well as differentiate down non-muscle lineages to contribute to tissue repair. Research in animal muscle injury models has shown that intramuscular injection of MDSC greatly enhanced muscle healing by increasing angiogenesis through the increase of vascular endothelial growth factor (VEGF) and decreasing scar tissue formation [70]. This MDSC autocrine and paracrine function has been shown to be one of the determining factors in their ability to promote tissue repair [76].

Transplantation of satellite cell-derived myoblasts has also been explored as a promising approach for the treatment of skeletal muscle disorders. However, as for other myogenic cell therapies, experiments have raised concerns about the limited migratory and proliferative capacities of the cells, as well as their limited lifespan *in vivo* [78]. Controlling the microenvironment of injected myogenic cells using biological scaffolds has been found to enhance muscle regeneration by providing structural support, facilitating cell adhesion and migration during the repair process [79]. Combining myogenic cells, biomaterial-based scaffolds and growth factors may provide a therapeutic option to improve regeneration of injured skeletal muscles [18]. The potential risk of colonization of nontarget tissues, stimulation of cancer, and transmission of infections must be kept in mind [80].

Platelet-Rich Plasma

The use of platelet-rich plasma (PRP) has been considered by many authors as a possible alternative approach based on the ability of autologous growth factors and cytokines to facilitate tissue repair, regeneration and remodeling [81]. Once activated, the alpha granules of platelets release cytokines, signaling a cascade that promotes inflammation and neovascularization and the release of multiple growth factors essential for recovery, among them platelet-derived growth factor (PDGF), TGF-β1, IG-1, and VEGF. However, there has been concern due to PRP's addition of TGF-β1 to that already present in the healing process, negatively promoting the formation of fibrotic tissue and decreasing satellite cell activation [82].

The use of an anti-fibrotic agent in combination with PRP has significantly improved healing when compared to PRP alone. Losartan, an angiotensin II receptor antagonist, blocks the effect of TGF-β1 and reduces fibrosis, improving the effectiveness of the PRP on muscle healing, an effect which is suspected to be mediated through the increase of angiogenesis [83]. Decorin, a growth factor antagonist for tumor growth which has an antifibrotic, anti-inflammatory and anticancer effect, has also been found to neutralize the negative effect of TGF-β1 when combined with PRP [82].

Conflicting results have emerged from human clinical studies done on hamstring strains and the use of PRP. In a randomized controlled trial in athletes with grade two hamstring strains, Hamid et al., found that a single autologous PRP injection combined with a rehabilitation program had a significant decrease in the time for full recovery (almost 50%) as compared to patients in the control group receiving only the rehabilitation program [84]. On the other hand, Hamilton et al. conducted a randomized, three-arm (double-blind for the injection arms), parallel group trial, in which 90 professional athletes with MRI positive hamstring injuries were randomized to injection with PRP-intervention, platelet-poor plasma or no injection, followed by an intensive standardized rehabilitation program, and found no benefit of PRP injection over intensive rehabilitation [85]. Reurink et al. found no significant difference in time for return to sports or rate of re-injury in a double-blind, placebo-controlled trial conducted in three study centers, in which 80 competitive and recreational athletes with acute hamstring muscle injuries were randomly assigned to receive intramuscular injections of PRP or isotonic saline as a placebo, followed by the same rehabilitation program [86].

A recent Cochrane review concluded that there is currently insufficient evidence to support the use of PRP for treating musculoskeletal soft tissue injuries, highlighting the importance of randomized controlled studies on specific conditions and standardization of PRP preparation methods to make significant conclusions [87].

Multiple explanations have been given for the variable study results, among those the variability of preparations and techniques, conflicting optimal number of platelets, the need for activation, time frame before additional interventions and questions regarding the optimal post-treatment rehabilitation [88]. There have been animal studies that have shown increased satellite cell activation and contractile force in repetitive (overuse) injury models, as compared to single event injury, raising the question whether the efficacy of PRP may be related to the type of injury [81].

Case Study

This is a 53 y/o male, a retired pitcher from Major League Baseball after 16 seasons, who has been recently involved in cross-fit training and injured his right hamstring during a sprinting session. Physical exam revealed tenderness in the proximal musculotendinous junction (MTJ) and a

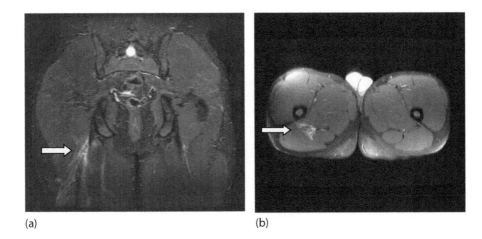

(a)   (b)

FIGURE 18.1 T2 weighted images in the coronal (a) and axial (b) planes demonstrate edema and a partial disruption at the proximal myotendinous junction of the biceps femoris consistent with a grade two injury.

resolving hematoma, classified as a grade two MTJ strain. MRI confirmed an area of hyperintensity at the biceps femoris muscle consistent with a grade two partial tear from its origin into the MTJ (Figure 18.1a,b). Ultrasonography revealed a corresponding transverse image with a hypoechoic area of edema surrounding the MTJ, slight flexion of the knee demonstrating continuity of muscle and ruling out a complete tear.

TABLE 18.2
Classification and Evaluation of Muscle Injury and Predisposing Factors

Initial Clinical Evaluation

Classify Injury:

- *Traditional*: Mild "grade one", moderate "grade two" or severe "grade three".
- *Comprehensive*: MLG-R classification – explore the mechanism of injury, location, grade, and determine if re-injury.

Classify Phase of Injury:

- *Phase one*: Destruction/Acute Inflammation (0–3 days) – inflammatory response.
- *Phase two*: Regeneration (3–21 days) – activation and proliferation of satellite cells.
- *Phase three*: Remodeling (3–60 days) – maturation of the regenerated myofibers and functional recovery.

Identify Predisposing Factors:

Intrinsic

Modifiable:

- *Biomechanical*: Look for history of previous injury, agonist/antagonist muscle weakness or inflexibility.
- *Bio-metabolic*: Consider evaluating growth hormone, testosterone, estrogen, thyroid, insulin levels and inflammation biomarkers.
- *Nutritional*: Consider nutritionist evaluation and diet modifications.

Non-modifiable:

- *Genetic*: Consider *individual-based* profile based on SNPs to determine if personalized prevention program needed.

Extrinsic

- Explore other causes such as training errors, change in intensity, frequency, technique, equipment and duration of training and play.

Source: Table by Romeu, R. Physical Medicine and Rehabilitation, VACHS, San Juan, Puerto Rico.

The extrinsic risk factor identified was a progressive intensity of the sports activity in a short period of time, without proper rest and evident generalized fatigue. The intrinsic factors identified were the previous history of injury, age and hamstring tightness.

During the initial inflammatory phase, the rehabilitation program consisted of relative rest with the use of crutches and touch-weight bearing, compression, elevation, cold therapy and gentle ROM. After ten days, he was able to place full weight with minimal pain. On the initial visit, the patient was started with an anti-inflammatory/antioxidant diet consisting of a Mediterranean diet supplemented with a multivitamin, 2000 mg per day of fish oil, 1000 mg of vitamin C per day and 200 mg of a bromelain three times a day. During the regenerative phase, a gentle stretching program was

TABLE 18.3
Summary of Proposed Treatment Modalities for Muscle Injury

Treatment Modalities

Physical

- *Cryotherapy*: May consider in the acute phase for edema and pain control.
- *High Voltage Galvanic (HVGES)*: May consider in acute phase for edema and pain control.
- *Transcutaneous Electrical Nerve Stimulation (TENS)*: May consider during all phases for pain control.
- *Micro-electrical Nerve Stimulation (MENS)*: May consider during regeneration and remodeling phases for satellite cell stimulation.
- *Extracorporeal shockwave therapy (ESWT)*: May consider in regeneration and remodeling phases.
- *Photobiomodulation Therapy (PBMT)*: May consider in regeneration and remodeling phases.
- *Massage*: May consider in all phases of muscle injury if tolerated.
- *Acupuncture*: May consider in all phases of injury if tolerated.

Exercise

Targeted to the individual's specific physiological needs/deficits and to sport-specific functional needs & according to injury phase:

- *During phase one*: Pain-free isometric exercises.
- *During phase two and three*: Isotonic and/or isokinetic exercise & progression to functional exercise programs. Consider eccentric over concentric exercise.
- *Concentric*: Used if limited range of motion and joint effusion.
- *Eccentric*: Shown to increase sarcomere growth, type II fibers, muscle force, improve neuromuscular control and decrease re-injury.

Nutritional Interventions

- *Energy requirements*: Consider increasing total daily caloric intake up to 20% above basal needs, accounting for stress and activity factors.
- *Carbohydrates*: Adequate quantity of non-processed carbs preferred.
- *Proteins*: Recommend 0.25–0.30 g/kg or 20 g/protein/meal of good quality amino acid source taken after exercise to promote muscle protein synthesis.
- *Fat*: Mono-unsaturated recommended over saturated fats.
- *Water*: Recommend 1 ml/kcal/day and adjusted to insensible losses.
- Moderate intake of essential O-3 fatty acid foods and anti-oxidant nutrients are recommended.
- Avoid pro-inflammatory food (e.g. alcohol, saturated fats).

Orthobiologics

Insufficient evidence to support standard use:

- *Stem cells*: Muscle-derived stem cells with biomaterial-based scaffolds and growth factors show greatest promise.
- *Platelet rich plasma*: Conflicting evidence, however an anti-fibrotic agent in combination with PRP has shown good results.

Source: Table by Romeu, R. Physical Medicine and Rehabilitation, VACHS, San Juan, Puerto Rico.

added, followed by isometric strengthening contractions to reach 50%–70% maximal. The modalities used included MENS and massage, followed by PBMT and TENS. After two weeks, minimal weight eccentric hamstring exercises were incorporated, progressing throughout the next four weeks. By week six, hamstring strength was 85% of contralateral side, and the patient was started in functional/agility and jogging drills. By the end of the final remodeling phase, the flexibility of both hamstrings had improved and were symmetric. The patient gradually progressed from jogging to running, and eventually to sprinting to progressive participation in sport within 14 weeks.

SUMMARY

Musculoskeletal injuries are an undesirable but common part of physical activity, regardless of the level of participation and intensity for the elite or recreational athlete. Lessening the impact of these consequences and boosting the recovery from these injuries are major goals for physical activity participants. The approach outlined in Tables 18.2 and 18.3 is a practical way the authors have developed to implement emerging research into the clinical treatment of athletes with muscle injury.

ACKNOWLEDGMENT

The authors would like to express their gratitude to Dr. Rafael Romeu, PMR senior resident at the Veterans Administration Caribbean Healthcare System and Ms. Carmen Nevarez, MHSN, LND and professor of the Center for Sport Health and Exercise Science, PMR Department, University of Puerto Rico School of Medicine, for their important collaboration in the completion of this chapter.

REFERENCES

1. U.S. Bone & Joint Decade. The Burden of Musculoskeletal Diseases in the United States. 2008–2012. Available at http://www.boneandjointburden.org/.
2. Tidball, J. G. (2011). Mechanisms of muscle injury, repair, and regeneration. *Compr Physiol*. doi:10.1002/cphy.c100092.
3. Sepúlveda, F., Baerga, L., & Micheo, W. (2015). The role of physiatry in regenerative medicine: The past, the present, and future challenges. *PM&R*, 7(4): 76–80. doi:10.1016/j.pmrj.2015.01.004.
4. Grassi, A. (2016). An update on the grading of muscle injuries: A narrative review from clinical to comprehensive systems. *Joints*, 4(1): 39–46. doi:10.11138/jts/2016.4.1.039.
5. Bouzid, M. A., Hammouda, O., Matran, R., Robin, S., & Fabre, C. (2014). Changes in oxidative stress markers and biological markers of muscle injury with aging at rest and in response to an exhaustive exercise. *PLoS ONE*, 9(3). doi:10.1371/journal.pone.0090420 (accessed Jul 16, 2017).
6. Thorborg, K. (2014). What are the most important risk factors for hamstring muscle injury? *Clin J Sport Med*, 24(2): 160–161. doi:10.1097/jsm.0000000000000091.
7. Hägglund, M., Waldén, M., & Ekstrand, J. (2012). Risk factors for lower extremity muscle injury in professional soccer. *Am J Sports Med*, 41(2): 327–335. doi:10.1177/0363546512470634.
8. Witvrouw, E., Danneels, L., Asselman, P., Dhave, T., & Cambier, D. (2003). Muscle flexibility as a risk factor for developing muscle injuries in male professional soccer players. *Am J Sports Med*, 31(1): 41–46. doi:10.1177/03635465030310011801.
9. Pruna, R., Ribas, J., Montoro, J. B., & Artells, R. (2015). The impact of single nucleotide polymorphisms on patterns of non-contact musculoskeletal soft tissue injuries in a football player population according to ethnicity. *Med Clínica (English Edition)*, 144(3): 105–110. doi:10.1016/j.medcle.2013.09.003.
10. Massidda, M., Bachis, V., Corrias, L., Piras, F., Scorcu, M, Calò, C. M. (2015) Influence of the MCT1 rs12722 on musculoskeletal injuries in professional soccer players. *J Sports Med Phys Fitness*, 55(11):1348–1353.
11. Massidda, M., Eynon, N., Bachis, V., Corrias, L., Culigioni, C., Piras, F., Cugia, P., Scorcu, & Calò, C. M. (2015). Vitamin D receptor gene polymorphisms and musculoskeletal injuries in professional football players. *Exp Ther Med*, 1(1): 33. doi.org/1 0.3892/etm.2015.2364.
12. Relaix, F. & Zammit, P. S. (2012). Satellite cells are essential for skeletal muscle regeneration: The cell on the edge returns centre stage. *Development*, 139(16): 2845–2856. doi:10.1242/dev.069088.

13. Kim, J., Han, G., Seo, J., Park, I., Park, W., Jeong, H., . . . Kong, Y.(2016). Erratum: Sex hormones establish a reserve pool of adult muscle stem cells. *Nature Cell Biol*, 18(10): 1109–1109. doi:10.1038/ncb3416.

14. Adams, G. R. (2002). Invited review: Autocrine/paracrine IGF-I and skeletal muscle adaptation. *J Appl Physiol*, 93(3): 1159–1167. doi:10.1152/japplphysiol.01264.2001.

15. Ambrosio, R., Stefano, M. A., Girolamo, D. D., & Salvatore, D. (2017). Thyroid hormone signaling and deiodinase actions in muscle stem/progenitor cells. *Mol Cell Endocrinol*, 459: 79–83. doi:10.1016/j.mce.2017.06.014.

16. Salvatore, D., Simonides, W. S., Dentice, M., Zavacki, A. M., & Larsen, P. R. (2013). Thyroid hormones and skeletal muscle—new insights and potential implications. *Nature Rev Endocrinol*, 10(4): 206–214. doi:10.1038/nrendo.2013.238.

17. Müller, S., Martin, S., Koenig, W., Hanifi-Moghaddam, P., Rathmann, W., Haastert, B., . . . Kolb, H.(2002). Impaired glucose tolerance is associated with increased serum concentrations of interleukin 6 and co-regulated acute-phase proteins but not TNF-α or its receptors. *Diabetologia*, 45(6): 805–812. doi:10.1007/s00125-002-0829-2.

18. Laumonier, T., & Menetrey, J. (2016). Muscle injuries and strategies for improving their repair. *J Exp Orthopaedics*, 3(1). https://doi.org/10.1186/s40634-016-0051-7.

19. Dueweke, J. J., Awan, T. M., & Mendias, C. L. (2017). Regeneration of skeletal muscle after eccentric injury. *J Sport Rehabilitation*, 26(2): 171–179. doi:10.1123/jsr.2016-0107.

20. Burks, T. N., Andres-Mateos, E., Marx, R., Mejias, R., Erp, C. V., Simmers, J. L., . . . Cohn, R. D. (2011). Losartan restores skeletal muscle remodeling and protects against disuse atrophy in sarcopenia. *Sci Translational Med*, 3(82). https://doi.org/10.1016/j.exger.2014.07.017.

21. Nadler S. F., Weingand K., & Kruse R. J. (2004). The physiologic basis and clinical applications of cryotherapy and thermotherapy for the pain practitioner. *Pain Physician*, 7(3): 395–399.

22. Collins, N. C. (2008). Is ice right? Does cryotherapy improve outcome for acute soft tissue injury? *Emergency Med J*, 25(2): 65–68. doi:10.1136/emj.2007.051664.

23. Schaser, K., Disch, A. C., Stover, J. F., Lauffer, A., Bail, H. J., & Mittlmeier, T. (2007). Prolonged superficial local cryotherapy attenuates microcirculatory impairment, regional inflammation, and muscle necrosis after closed soft tissue injury in rats. *Am J Sports Med*, 35 (1): 93–102. doi:10.1177/0363546506294569.

24. Frontera, W. R. et al., (2010). Physical inactivity: Physiological and functional impairments and their treatment. In *DeLisa's Physical Medicine & Rehabilitation: Principles and Practice*, 5th edn., vol. 1.

25. Hassan E. S. (2011). Thermal therapy and delayed onset muscle soreness. *J Sports Med Phys Fitness*, 51(2): 249–254.

26. Jayaraman, R. C., Reid, R. W., Foley, J. M., Prior, B. M., Dudley, G. A., Weingand, K. W., & Meyer, R. A. (2004). MRI evaluation of topical heat and static stretching as therapeutic modalities for the treatment of eccentric exercise-induced muscle damage. *Eur J Appl Physiol*, 93(1–2): 30–38. doi:10.1007/s00421-004-1153-y.

27. Young, S., & Dyson, M. (1990). Effect of therapeutic ultrasound on the healing of full-thickness excised skin lesions. *Ultrasonics*, 28(3), 175–180. doi:10.1016/0041-624x(90)90082-y.

28. van der Windt, D., van der Heijden, G., van den Berg, S., ter Riet, G., de Winter, A. & Bouter, L. (1999). Ultrasound therapy for musculoskeletal disorders: A systematic review. *Pain* 81 (3): 257–272.

29. Shanks, P., Curran, M., Fletcher, P., & Thompson, R. (2010). The effectiveness of therapeutic ultrasound for musculoskeletal conditions of the lower limb: A literature review. *Foot*, 20(4): 133–139. doi:10.1016/j.foot.2010.09.006.

30. High Voltage Pulsed Current (HVPC). N.p., n.d. Web. 20 June 2017. http://www.electrotherapy.org/modality/high-voltage-pulsed-current-hvpc.

31. Lake, D. (1992). Neuromuscular electrical stimulation: An overview and its application in the treatment of sports injuries. *Sports Med*, 13 (5): 320–336.

32. Press, J. M., Plastaras, C. T., & Wiesner, S. L. (n.d.). Physical modalities and pain management. *Rehabilitation Sports Injuries Sci Basis*, 204–231. doi:10.1002/9780470757178.ch10.

33. Ordog, G. J. (1987). Transcutaneous electrical nerve stimulation versus oral analgesic: A randomized double-blind controlled study in acute traumatic pain. *Am J Emergency Med*, 5(1): 6–10. doi:10.1016/0735-6757(87)90281-6.

34. Robinson, A. J. (1996). Transcutaneous electrical nerve stimulation for the control of pain in musculoskeletal disorders. *J Orthopaedic Sports Phys Therapy*, 24(4): 208–226. doi:10.2519/jospt.1996.24.4.208.

35. Fujiya, H., Ogura, Y., Ohno, Y., Goto, A., Nakamura, A., Ohashi, K., Uematsu, D., Aoki, H., Musha, H. and Goto, K. (2015). Microcurrent electrical neuromuscular stimulation facilitates regeneration of injured skeletal muscle in mice. *J Sports Sci Med* 14(2): 297–303.

36. Curtis, D., Fallows, S., Morris, M. and McMakin, C. (2010). The efficacy of frequency specific micro-current therapy on delayed onset muscle soreness. *J Bodyw Mov Ther,* 14(3): 272–279. doi:10.1016/j.jbmt.2010.01.009.

37. Zissler, A., Steinbacher, P., Zimmermann, R., Pittner, S., Stoiber, W., Bathke, A. C., & Sänger, A. M. (2016). Extracorporeal shock wave therapy accelerates regeneration after acute skeletal muscle injury. *Am J Sports Med,* 45(3): 676–684.

38. Astur, D. C., Santos, B., Moraes, E. R., Arliani, G. G., Santos, P. R., & Pochini, A. D. (2015). Extracorporeal shockwave therapy to treat chronic muscle injury. *Acta Ortopédica Brasileira,* 23(5): 247–250. doi:10.1590/1413-785220152305142211.

39. Bjordal, J. M., Johnson, M. I., Iversen, V., Aimbire, F., & Lopes-Martins, R. A. (2006). Low-level laser therapy in acute pain: A systematic review of possible mechanisms of action and clinical effects in random-ized placebo-controlled trials. *Photomed Laser Surgery,* 24(2): 158–168. doi:10.1089/pho.2006.24.158.

40. Hamblin, M. R. (2008). The role of nitric oxide in low level light therapy. Proc. of SPIE Vol. 6846. Mechanisms for Low-Light Therapy III, 684602; doi:10.1117/12.764918.

41. Bar, P. R., Reijneveld JC, Wokke JHJ, et al. (1997). Muscle damage induced by exercise: Nature, preven-tion, and repair. In: Salmons S., ed. *Muscle Damage.* Oxford, Oxford University Press, 1–27.

42. Agarwal, S., Long P, Seyedain A (2003). A central role for the nuclear factor-kappaB pathway in anti-inflammatory and proinflammatory actions of mechanical strain. *FASEB J,* 17(8): 899–901.

43. Crane JD, Ogborn DI, Cupido C, et al. (2012) Massage therapy attenuates inflammatory signaling after exercise-induced muscle damage. Sci. Transl. Med. 4:119ra113. doi:10.1126/scitranslmed.3002882.

44. Best, T. M., Gharaibeh, B., and Huard, J. (2012). Stem cells, angiogenesis and muscle healing: A poten-tial role in massage therapies? *Br J Sports Med,* 47(9): 556–560.

45. Sandberg, M., Lundeberg, T., Lindberg, L., & Gerdle, B. (2003). Effects of acupuncture on skin and mus-cle blood flow in healthy subjects. *Eur J Appl Physiol,* 90(1–2): 114–119. doi:10.1007/s00421-003-0825-3.

46. Taguchi, R. (2008). Acupuncture anesthesia and analgesia for clinical acute pain in Japan. *Evidence-Based Complementary Alternative Med,* 5(2): 153–158.

47. Vickers, A. J. and Klaus L. (2014). Acupuncture for chronic pain. *JAMA,* 311(9): 955–956.

48. Kim, Y., Park, J., Kim, S., Yeom, M., Lee, S., Oh, J., Park, H. (2017). What intrinsic factors influence responsiveness to acupuncture in pain?: a review of pre-clinical studies that used responder analysis. BMC Complement. Alter. Med, 17: 281. doi:10.1186/s12906-017-1792-2.

49. Hansen, J., Brandt, C., Nielsen, A. R., Hojman, P., Whitham, M., Febbraio, M. A., . . . Plomgaard, P. (2011). Exercise induces a marked increase in plasma follistatin: Evidence that follistatin is a contrac-tion-induced hepatokine. *Endocrinology,* 152(1): 164–171. doi:10.1210/en.2010-0868.

50. Valero, M. C., Huntsman, H. D., Liu, J., Zou, K., & Boppart, M. D. (2012). Eccentric exercise facili-tates mesenchymal stem cell appearance in skeletal muscle. *PLoS ONE,* 7(1). doi:10.1371/journal.pone.0029760.

51. Puchner, E. M., Alexandrovich A., Kho A.L., Hensen U., Schäfer L.V., Brandmeier B.,…Gautel, M. (2008). Mecha- noenzymatics of titin kinase. *Proc Natl Acad Sci USA,* 105(36): 13385–13390.

52. Butterfield, T. A. & Herzog W. (2006). The magnitude of muscle strain does not influence serial sarco-mere number adaptations following eccentric exercise. *Pflugers Arch.* 451(5): 688–700.

53. Aagaard, P., Andersen, J. L., & Dyhre-Poulsen, P. (2001). A mechanism for increased contractile strength of human pennate muscle in response to strength training: Changes in muscle architecture. *J Physiol,* 534: 613–623.

54. Hather, B. M., Tesch, P. A., Buchanan, P., & Dudley, G. A. (1991). Influence of eccentric actions on skeletal muscle adaptations to resistance training. *Acta Physiol Scand,* 143: 177–185.

55. Lepley, L. K., Wojtys, E. M., & Palmieri-Smith, R. M. (2015). Combination of eccentric exercise and neuromuscular electrical stimulation to improve quadriceps function post–ACL reconstruction. *Knee,* 22(3): 270–277.

56. Rice, D. A. & McNair P. J. (2010). Quadriceps arthrogenic muscle inhibition: Neural mechanisms and treatment perspectives. *Semin Arthritis Rheum,* 40(3): 250–266.

57. Lepley, K. & Butterfield, T. (2017). Shifting the current clinical perspective: Isolated eccentric exercise as an effective intervention to promote the recovery of muscle after injury. *J Sport Rehabilitation,* 26(2): 122–130.

58. Nielsen, J. L., Aagaard P, Bech RD, Nygaard T, Hvid LG, Wernbom M, Suetta C, Frandsen U. (2012). Proliferation of myogenic stem cells in human skeletal muscle in response to low load resistance train-ing with blood flow restriction. *J Physiol,* 590(17): 4351–4361.

59. Quintero, A., Wright, V., Fu, F., & Huard, J. (2009). Stem cells for the treatment of skeletal muscle injury. *Clin Sports Med.,* 28 (1): 1–11.

60. Tatsumi, R., Hattori, A., Ikeuchi, Y., Anderson, J. E., & Allen R. E. (2002). Release of hepatocyte growth factor from mechanically stretched skeletal muscle satellite cells and role of PH and nitric oxide. *Mol Biol Cell*, 13(8): 2909–2918.

61. Nielsen, J. L., Frandsen, U., Prokhorova, T., Bech R. D., Nygaard, T., Suetta, C., & Aagaard P. (2017). Delayed effect of blood flow-restricted resistance training on rapid force capacity. *Med Sci Sports Exerc*, 49(6): 1157–1167.

62. Demling, R. H. (2009). Nutrition, anabolism, and the wound healing process: An overview. *ePlasty*, 9: 69.

63. Witard, O. C., Jackman, S. R., Breen, L., Smith, K., Selby, A., and Tipton, K. D. (2014). Myofibrillar muscle protein synthesis rates subsequent to a meal in response to increasing doses of whey protein at rest and after resistance exercise. *Am J Clin Nutr*, 99(1): 86–95.

64. Moore, D. R., Churchward-Venne, T. A., Witard, O., Breen, L., Burd, N. A., Tipton, K. D., and Phillips, S. M. (2014). Protein ingestion to stimulate myofibrillar protein synthesis requires greater relative protein intakes in healthy older versus younger men. *J Gerontol A Biol Sci Med Sci* 70(1): 57–62.

65. Dunford, M. & Doyle, J.A. (2015). *Nutrition for Sport and Exercise*. 3rd edn.

66. Tipton, K. D. (2017). Nutritional support for injuries requiring reduced activity. *Sports Sci Exchange*, 28(169): 1–6.

67. Tipton, K. D. (2009). Nutrition for acute exercise-induced injuries. *Ann Nutr Metab*, 57 (2): 43–53. doi: 10.1159/000322703.

68. Calder, P. C. (2013). n-3 fatty acids, inflammation and immunity: New mechanisms to explain old actions. *Proc Nutr Soc*, 72(3): 326–336.

69. Marcel, C. (2017). Curcumin. *CINAHL Nursing Guide*, Persistent link to this record (Permalink): http://search.ebscohost.com/login.aspx?direct=true&db=nrc&AN=T707485&site=nrc-live.

70. O'Fallon, K. S., Kaushik, D., Michniak-Kohn, B., Dunne, C. P., Zambraski, E. J., & Clarkson, P. M. (2012). Effects of quercetin supplementation on markers of muscle damage and inflammation after eccentric exercise. *Int J Sport Nutrition Exercise Metab*, 22(6), 430–437. doi:10.1123/ijsnem.22.6.430.

71. Shing, C. M., Chong, S., Driller, M. W., & Fell, J. W. (2016). Acute protease supplementation effects on muscle damage and recovery across consecutive days of cycle racing. *Eur J Sport Sci*, 16(2), 206–212. doi:10.1080/17461391.2014.1001878.

72. He, Y., Yue, Y., Zheng, X., Zhang, K., Chen, S., & Du, Z. (2015). Curcumin, inflammation, and chronic diseases: How are they linked? *Molecules*, 20(5): 9183–9213. doi:10.3390/molecules20059183.

73. Ahmad, Z., Wardale, J., Brooks, R., Henson, F., Noorani, A., & Rushton, N. (2012). Exploring the application of stem cells in tendon repair and regeneration. *Arthroscopy*, 28(7): 1018–1029.

74. Jamil Bashir, M. D., Andrew Sherman, M. D., Henry Lee, D. O., Lee Kaplan, M. D., Hare, J. M., & Mesenchymal Stem, M. D. (2014). Cell therapies in the treatment of musculoskeletal diseases. *PM R*, 6(1): 61–69.

75. Bazgir, B., Fathi, R., Rezazadeh Valojerdi, M., Mozdziak, P., & Asgari, A. R. (2017). Satellite cells contribution to exercise mediated muscle hypertrophy and repair. *Cell J*, 18(4): 473–484.

76. Ota, S., Uehara, K., Nozaki, M., Kobayashi, T., Terada, S., Tobita, K., Fu, F. H., & Huard, J. (2011). Intramuscular transplantation of muscle-derived stem cells accelerates skeletal muscle healing after contusion injury via enhancement of angiogenesis. *Am J Sports Med*, 39(9): 1912–1922.

77. Gharaibeh, B., Lavasani, M., Cummins, J. H., & Huard J. (2011) Terminal differentiation is not a major determinant for the success of stem cell therapy–cross-talk between muscle-derived stem cells and host cells. *Stem Cell Res Ther*, 2: 31–43.

78. Borrelli, C., Cezar, C. A., Shvartsman, D., Vandenberg, H. H., & Mooney, D. J. (2011). The role of multifunctional delivery scaffold in the ability of cultured myoblasts to promote muscle regeneration. *Biomaterials*, 32(34): 8905–8914.

79. Jeon, O. H. & Elisseeff, J. (2016). Orthopedic tissue regeneration: Cells, scaffolds, and small molecules. *Drug Deliv Transl Res*, 6(2): 105–120.

80. Mandelbaum, B. (2017). Stem cells in sports medicine: Ready for prime time? *Medscape*.

81. Hammond, J. W., Hinton, R. Y., Curl, L. A., Muriel, J. M., & Lovering, R. M. (2009). Use of autologous platelet-rich plasma to treat muscle strain injuries. *Am J Sports Med*, 37(6): 1135–1142.

82. Kelc, R., Trapecar, M., Gradisnik, L., Slak Rupnik, M., & Vogrin M. (2015). Platelet-rich plasma, especially when combined with a TGF-β inhibitor promotes proliferation, viability and myogenic differentiation of myoblasts in vitro. *PLoS ONE*. 10(2). doi:10.1371/journal.pone.0117302.

83. Terada, S, Ota S, Kobayashi M, Kobayashi T, Mifune Y, Takayama K, Witt M, Vadala G, Oyster N, Otsuka T, Fu FH, Huard J (2013). Use of an antifibrotic agent improves the effect of platelet-rich plasma on muscle healing after injury. *J Bone Joint Surg Am*, 95(11): 980–988.

84. A Hamid, M. S., Mohamed Ali, M. R., Yusof, A., George, J., & Lee L. P. (2015). Platelet-rich plasma injections for the treatment of hamstring injuries: A randomized controlled trial. *Am J Sports Med*, 42(10): 2410–2418.

85. Hamilton, B., Tol, J. L., Almusa, E., Boukarroum, S., Eirale, C., Farooq, A., Whiteley, R. & Chalabi, H. (2015). Platelet-rich plasma does not enhance return to play in hamstring injuries: A randomized controlled trial. *Br J Sports Med*, 49(14): 943–950.

86. Reurink, G., Goudswaard, G, Moen, M., Weir, A, Verhaar, J, Bierma-Zeinstra, S., Maas, M., & Tol, J. (2014). Platelet-rich plasma injections in acute muscle injury. *N Engl J Med*, 370(26): 2546–2547.

87. Moraes, V., Lenza, M., Tamaoki, M., Faloppa, F., & Belloti, J. (2014). Platelet-rich therapies for musculoskeletal soft tissue injuries. Cochrane Bone, Joint and Muscle Trauma Group. 29 April.

88. Mautner, K., Malanga, G., & Colberg, R. (2011). Optimization of ingredients, procedures and rehabilitation for platelet-rich plasma injections for chronic tendinopathy. *Pain Manag*, 1(6): 523–532.

19 Tendinopathy
Addressing the Chronic Pain and Pathophysiology

David Musnick, MD

INTRODUCTION

Tendinopathy has distinguishing features in regard to clinical presentation, pathophysiology, imaging options and treatment options. Since tendinopathies often co-exist with other musculoskeletal conditions, they are overlooked and the underlying pathophysiology is not completely treated. Integrative approaches to clinical diagnosis and treatment are presented in this chapter.

CLINICAL PRESENTATION AND DIAGNOSIS

The most common tendons that present with tendinopathy are: supraspinatus, infraspinatus, subscapularis, long head of the biceps, quadriceps, patella, hamstring and Achilles tendons. Lateral and medial epicondylitis are also forms of tendinopathy.

Patients with tendinopathy and tendinitis will both present with the following symptoms: pain in the area of a tendon that is worse with use, palpation pressure and muscle testing. There may be visible tendon thickening in Achilles tendinopathy. In advanced cases, there may be muscle atrophy, but this is unusual. Both conditions are usually worse with eccentric loads. Patients with tendinopathy usually have had pain in a tendon that has gone on for more than 6–8 weeks. The tenderness in the tendon can become quite easily provoked with little pressure or use. The tendon area becomes sensitized and demonstrates low threshold characteristics in regard to pressure and pain with use. There is also a possibility of the development of secondary hyperalgesia, in which the receptive field for pain processing in the cord expands and the patient perceives a wider area of pain that is larger than the tendon itself. Patients with tendinopathy may have had strain injuries of the muscle or tendon that did not heal. Tendinopathy pain is usually not constant but is usually intermittent but easily set off or aggravated. Patients may also have pain, spasm or trigger points in the muscle belly of the tendon. Muscle testing of the muscle with the tendinopathy can show poor recruitment or breakaway weakness.

If a patient has had an undiagnosed tendinopathy they are at risk of straining or tearing the tendon because the tendon is degenerative and cannot handle the mechanical stress of athletic endeavors. In that case, the clinician may be seeing a presentation of second- or third-degree strains.

Regional findings that increase risk for tendinopathy should be evaluated, including: poor motor recruitment of the joint and surrounding joints, shortening of muscles, joint laxity, spinal facet and nerve syndromes, abnormal movement patterns, etc.

Tendinopathy should be suspected in any patient having intermittent pain in a tendon in which it has been occurring more than 2 months. Physical exam should involve palpation of the tendon and muscle, joint range of motion testing, resisted motor testing and testing of any possible involved or contributing joint regions (facet joints in the spine extremity joints etc.) Tests for ligament laxity should be done on exam. Of note is that muscle testing of a suspected tendinopathy should not be too aggressive as it may lead to significant pain or even tear of the tendinopathy tendon.

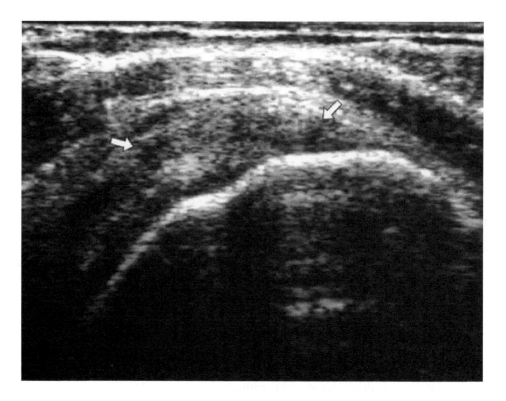

FIGURE 19.1   The following ultrasound study demonstrates mild thickening and decreased echo of a supraspinatus tendinopathy.

The definitive diagnosis should be made with imaging studies, either ultrasound or MRI. Ultrasound is preferable in most cases because it is much less expensive and a second study can be ordered once treatment is concluded to determine if there is radiological evidence of healing. Ultrasound may show evidence of decreased echo or thickening in tendinopathy areas. Anechoic areas or extra fluid may be strains and tears. Confirmation ultrasound is important to identify residual tendinopathy, which leaves the patient susceptible to injury from sports and maximum loads. It is recommended that an ultrasound be obtained prior to starting injection treatments as treatment. Also, at least 8 weeks should pass before a second ultrasound is obtained (Figure 19.1).

Tendinopathy on MRI shows an increased signal in the tendon. The increased signal is related to increased water content associated with increased blood flow and excessive proteoglycans, and is more effective at distinguishing partial tears. MRI is recommended if one is also looking for labral pathology in the shoulder and hip. It is a more expensive study and would not be used as a follow-up study to document healing.

PATHOLOGY AND ETIOLOGIES

Tendinopathy is mostly a degenerative tissue condition of part or all of a tendon. (Abate et al., 2009). There is an increase in tenocytes, increase in proteoglycans, vascular hyperplasia and collagen disorganization (Scott, Khan, Cook and Duronio, 2007). Tendinopathy is more likely in the mid aspect of a tendon. Most tendons with tendinopathy exhibit thickening. Tendon thickening can be fusiform, diffuse or nodular. Degenerative changes may be hypoxic, mucoid, hyaline, myxoid, fatty and fibrinoid degeneration (Hashimoto, Nobuhara and Hamada, 2003; Khan, Maffulli, Coleman, Cook & Taunton, 1998).

Although the tendon may be thickened it is weaker than normal tendon. There are numerous biochemical changes in tendinopathy. There is an upregulation of vascular endothelial growth factor (VEGF) and an increase in metalloproteinases (MMPs). MMPs lead to the degradation of the extracellular matrix. There may be some upregulation of prostaglandin E_2 (PGE2), which can inhibit Type 1 collagen synthesis. There appears to be repetitive microtrauma with failure of repair. This repetitive overload may overcome the ability of the tendon to repair. Cumulative microtrauma may weaken collagen cross-linking and also affect the non-collagenous matrix and the vascular elements of the tendon. Neovascularity and associated nerve proliferation occurs in tendinopathy and is the primary reason for the condition's sensitization and pain (Yang, Coleman, Pugh and Nokes, 2012).

There may be more than one contributing cause in the development of tendinopathy. Contributing factors include: overuse, compressive forces such as from ligament or bone such as from the acromion and the coracoacromial ligaments in the shoulder that can cause friction forces on the tendon. Other causes can be a contusion and a strain that does not adequately heal.

Other causes may contribute to degeneration of the tendon, including diabetes, certain systemic infections, SLE, rheumatoid arthritis and reactive arthritis. Aging contributes to tendinopathy because there is a deleterious effect on mechanical properties of tendons. Aging can lead to reduced arterial blood flow, impaired metabolism and damage from advanced glycosylated end products (Langberg, Olesen, Skovgaard and Kjaer, 2001).

COMORBIDITIES

Patients with tendinopathy often have *spasm or trigger points* in the muscle proximal to the tendon. Trigger points can cause a constant tension on a tendon and aggravate or be a cause of tendinopathy and need to be treated. Trigger points may also exist in other muscles that move a joint related to the tendon and these should be treated.

Tendon and muscle strains are a common coexisting condition. It is important to identify a partial or *total tendon tear* by ultrasound or MRI because they need to be managed with the goals of pain relief and function recovery and, if possible, healing the tears. Most commonly, total or 3rd degree tears will need to be operated on. *Partial tears* may often be treated without surgery by using physical therapy, low-level laser therapy (LLLT), also called photobiomodulation (PBMT), and frequency specific microcurrent (FSM). If they do not show evidence of healing by ultrasound within 3–4 months, then they should be treated with platelet-rich plasma (PRP) or other emerging regenerative injection therapies aimed at regenerating and filling in the tear. If the clinician is dealing with a high-level athlete they may decide to accelerate the timetable and use PRP or another regenerative injection sooner. To emphasize the clinical significance of therapy, it is of note that tendinopathy may start off as a grade one or two strain that does not heal and only subsequently turns into a tendinopathy.

Joint laxity or hypermobility may be an underlying cause of tendinosis. The reason for this is that muscles that are involved in stabilizing a joint that is hypermobile can be overworked, leading to trigger points or overuse of a tendon. For example, if there is glenohumeral laxity in a shoulder joint, rotator cuff and biceps tendinopathy are more likely to develop over time.

Patients that have generalized joint laxity syndromes are at higher risk of tendinopathy. These include Marfan, Ehlers–Danlos and Benign Hypermobile Joint syndromes. Stabilizing a hypermobile joint may be part of a treatment program for the tendinopathy. If tendinopathy was to be treated with PRP, prolotherapy or another injection method to regenerate the tendon, then thought should be given to treat a hypermobile joint concurrent with the tendon injection.

Facet joint dysfunction with inflammation, subluxation, sensitization or all of the above may be associated with tendinopathy. This is usually with a facet joint in the neck for shoulder, elbow, wrist tendinopathy and a facet region of the lumbar spine for lower extremity tendinopathy. Sometimes the only symptoms may be spine stiffness, restriction of range of motion or tenderness over the facet capsule. There may be more significant facet dysfunction if there is actual facet hypermobility, which can be a cause of sensitization of the joint and aberrant signaling from the facet joint.

Enthesopathy conditions like reactive arthritis and ankylosing spondylopathy can predispose to tendinopathy because of the enthesis inflammation in these conditions. This would be suspected with tendon pain at multiple locations with or without sacroiliac or other joint area pain. If this is suspected, a clinician should order blood work to evaluate an autoimmune inflammatory condition.

Hormone levels, especially testosterone, may affect the development or healing from tendinopathy. Receptors for testosterone have been found in tendons (Khalkhali-Ellis et al., 2002). Concentrations of dihydrotestosterone may increase concentration of tenocytes (Denaro et al., 2010). Testosterone may regulate differentiation in mesenchymal pluripotent cells and lineage determination in a tendon (Denaro et al., 2010). Men with low testosterone levels show a significant reduction in endothelial and circulating progenitor cells. Testosterone replacement therapy may induce an increase in these progenitor cells (Abate et al., 2016). This effect can be important during tendon-healing and repair in men with low testosterone, when active proliferation is required.

The author has had favorable results using small amounts of aqueous testosterone (5–10 mg) when combined with dextrose when using prolotherapy to treat tendinopathy. There are, however, no clinical trials comparing tendinopathy treatment with or without testosterone when using prolotherapy. The author has also found it efficacious to assess and treat low testosterone levels in male patients with suspected low testosterone as well as with any individual that has had more than one tendon involved with tendinopathy or strains. Anabolic hormones should not be used in the competitive athlete unless a medically prescribed therapy exception is obtained. It is also important to assess and treat thyroid hormone status.

Thyroid hormone may affect the proliferation of tenocytes (Oliva et al., 2016). It is important in any patient with tendinopathy to make sure that their thyroid function is normal.

Local levels of growth hormone(GH)/insulin-like growth factor 1(IGF-1) facilitate increased collagen production, increased stem cells and increased tenocyte proliferation in tendons (Nielsen et al., 2014; Abate et al., 2016). This has been demonstrated in patients with classic Ehlers–Danlos syndrome (Nielsen et al., 2014). In patients with Ehlers–Danlos syndrome, the addition of growth hormone might be considered to improve tendinopathy. Injection of GH in the patellar tendons of elderly men showed increased tendon collagen synthesis (Doessing et al., 2010).

Consideration should be given to *antibiotic* selection. Fluoroquinolone antibiotics' use can predispose to tendinopathy and tendon rupture. Since some causes of reactive arthritis have developed resistance to fluoroquinolones, these antibiotics are used less frequently in association with tendinopathy comorbidities. Further, this class of antibiotics should be avoided in athletic individuals (van der Linden et al., 2001), as well as in the elderly, diabetic or the renal-function compromised patient. Cyclosporin and erythromycin are associated with rhabdomyolysis and may through this mechanism be anticipated to contribute to tendinopathy.

The adverse effects can be confirmed on the product information known as drug labels. Drug labels can be accessed on two U.S. federal websites – the Food and Drug Administration's (FDA's) website and the National Institutes of Health's (NIH's) resource entitled DailyMed.

Other potential *adverse drug effects* should be noted. All statin lipid-lowering therapies are associated with tendinopathy and tendon rupture. Corticosteroids are not advised to be injected into the tendon for treatment of tendinopathy but if used systemically can also interfere with the tendon's regenerative processes. Colchicine is a medication used to treat gout. Especially in the initial phase of treatment, it has been implicated in muscle weakness including tendinopathy. Cocaine, LSD, amphetamines and ecstasy have been demonstrated to contribute to tendon pathology.

Comorbid *metabolic conditions* include diabetes, obesity, heat stress, ketoacidosis from diabetes and other causes, various electrolyte imbalances, hypothyroidism, carnitine deficiency and lactate dehydrogenase deficiency. Some clinicians take the view that obstructive sleep apnea, prevalent yet underdiagnosed and undertreated, merits consideration as a comorbidity given its association with inadequate muscle oxygenation even in the mild form.

TREATMENT

PHYSICAL THERAPY

Tendinopathy has been treated for many years with physical therapy. An important use of physical therapy is to use Scientific Therapeutic Exercise Progression (STEP) to improve the strength and organization of the collagen in the tendon. This is usually done with high repetition (35–45 reps) lower resistance exercises 2–3 times a day for the first 4 weeks of treatment. In this type of exercise, there is a slight tugging on the tendon. This type of exercise can be demonstrated to a patient and can be used concurrently with injection therapies. A common approach in physical therapy has been to use eccentric exercises for the tendon and to strengthen muscles in regions that are related to the tendinopathy (Norregaard, Larsen, Bieler and Langberg, 2007; Ohberg, Lorentzon and Alfredson, 2004; Holmgren, Bjornsson-Hallgren, Oberg, Adolfsson and Johannson, 2012).

These approaches work reasonably well but may not fully resolve a tendinopathy. It is important to demonstrate healing on an ultrasound study as being pain-free is not always associated with full tendon healing. A type of treatment, mobilization with movement has shown efficacy, especially with epicondylitis (Bisset et al., 2006; Backstrom, 2002). Physical therapy with eccentric exercise may flare up a patient with rotator cuff tendinopathy or with any tendinopathy.

Physical therapy approaches may work on strengthening, working on muscle imbalances and movement patterns. Clinicians should also evaluate and treat the facet regions of the spine related to the tendon to see if there is an improvement in pain or recruitment.

Other physical therapy methods involve STEP to stimulate tissue repair with high repetition exercises. STEP and eccentric loading can be integrated together in a therapy program. The author's clinical experience here is that tendinopathy patient outcomes from physical therapy benefit from combined STEP and eccentric exercise.

Physical therapy can be used concurrently with modalities such as low-level laser therapy and/or frequency specific microcurrent. It can also be used concurrently with injection techniques such as PRP and prolotherapy.

LOW-LEVEL LASER THERAPY (PHOTOBIOMODULATION) AND FREQUENCY SPECIFIC MICROCURRENT

Low-level laser therapy may have very beneficial effects to treat tendinopathy when used 2–3 times per week for 4–6 weeks along with exercise therapy (Tumilty et al., 2010).

It appears that low-level laser therapy alone is not as effective as low-level laser therapy with exercise therapy. Also, exercise therapies may not be as effective alone as when combined with low-level laser therapy (Xiao-Guang, Cheng and Song, 2014).

Low-level laser therapy should be used to deliver 5–9 joules at the tendon in the area of documented tendinopathy. Also, the periosteal attachment should be treated. The clinician should be careful to not rub the laser at the periosteum or the tendon as it may flare up sensitization. It is the author's opinion that the 904 nm laser may offer benefits for both pain relief and tendon healing compared to the 808 nm which may be fine for pain relief but may not be as efficacious for tissue healing. It appears that frequent treatments with the laser are indicated, such as 2–3 times a week for 4–6 weeks (Haslerud, Magnussen, Joensen, Lopes-Martins & Bjordal, 2015).

Frequency specific microcurrent is a modality that can be used by itself or combined with a program with exercise therapy to decrease pain sensitization and heal tendinopathy. Microcurrent has been reported to increase adenosine triphosphate (ATP) production, protein synthesis and membrane transport, all contributing to the energy status of tissue. There are yet no published studies researching the effects on tendinopathy. Given the pathophysiology of the disease, the mechanism of action of the modality and the clinical response from our patient series with tendinopathy, we anticipate that when studies are conducted specifically in tendinopathies that they will demonstrate healing. Chapter 18 introduces the use of a microcurrent modality for muscle strain, a common comorbidity of tendinopathy. The repair frequency (124) on the A channel is a time-dependent frequency and must be used for a minimum of 45 minutes at least once over the course of the treatment and usually more than one time. Frequency specific microcurrent (Figure 19.2) can be combined with LLLT to decrease pain and encourage healing of tendinopathy (McMakin, 2011).

Topical Treatments

Topical nonsteroidal anti-inflammatory drug (NSAID) creams or gels have limited efficacy since tendinopathy is not an inflammatory condition. There may be a role for topical lidocaine as an agent to provide some pain relief. Clinically, it appears that pain processing and sensitization can improve if the patient has a localized prolonged numbing effect.

Nitric oxide may play a role in collagen and protein synthesis repair in tendinopathy. Glyceryl trinitrate has been studied in supraspinatus tendinopathy and has shown efficacy in reducing pain and improving function (Assem 2015) where its benefit is theorized to be increasing regional blood flow. Doses ranged from 1.25 mg to 5 mg/24 hours. Topical glyceryl trinitrate treatment decreased pain scores, improved range of motion and improved muscular force. The study followed patients for up to 6 months (Paoloni, Appleyard, Nelson & Murrell, 2005). It should be used with caution in any patient that has low blood pressure and also noted that headache is a frequent side effect. Transderm nitro patches should not be used as an isolated treatment but could be added to a patient's treatment regimen to decrease pain and improve function in tendinopathy. The studies are varied in terms of duration and length of dosage. It would be reasonable to try a patch at 8–12 hours per day and use it for at least six weeks.

Injection Therapies

It is the author's clinical judgment and experience that any injection therapy should be done along with the use of highly skilled physical therapy.

Injection of cortisone near a tendon is not only not helpful but it may weaken the tendon and should be avoided. In some cases, the subacromial space may be injected under ultrasound guidance if the clinician determines that there is a significant subacromial bursitis.

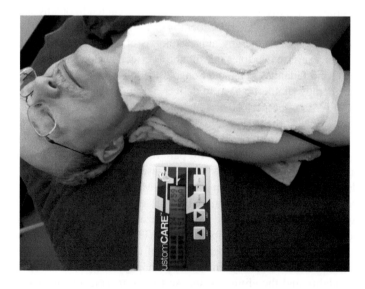

FIGURE 19.2   Setup and device for Frequency Specific Microcurrent of the tendinopathy of the shoulder.

Regenerative injections are the injections of substances into a tendon, ligament or joint for the purpose of regenerating the degenerative tissue. In the case of tendinosis, it would be injection into the tendon. The current injection therapies that fall into this category are: prolotherapy (also called regenerative injection therapy), platelet-rich plasma, amniotic membrane solution injection and stem cell injections.

Prolotherapy is the injection of local anesthetic and dextrose with or without other agents to stimulate tendon repair or to treat ligament laxity. A number of studies have shown efficacy in treating lateral epicondylitis, rotator cuff tendinopathy and Achilles tendinopathy (Scarpone, Rabago, Zgierska, Arbogest & Snell 2008; Yelland et al., 2011; Bertrand, Reeves, Bennett, Bicknell & Cheng 2016). There was a review in 2015 that indicated possible benefit but that the treatment method was not well supported by studies (Sanderson & Bryant, 2015).

In our clinical experience, prolotherapy can decrease pain and can stimulate tissue regeneration. These conclusions are based on a reduction in symptoms, improvement in function and ultrasound verification of healing. It is generally recommended that prolotherapy be done once monthly and repeated 3–5 times to treat tendinopathy. It is significantly less expensive and less uncomfortable than PRP but also less effective than PRP. Prolotherapy should not be used if there are areas of defect or partial tears. PRP would be better to treat tendinopathy to fill in a tear. Prolotherapy may be thought of as a treatment of simpler, less extensive cases of tendinopathy without tears. It should only be used if combined with physical therapy and STEP exercise approaches.

Platelet-rich plasma is an injection treatment that has been used extensively to treat all tendon areas of tendinopathy for the past 10 years. PRP contains growth factors, including platelet-derived growth factor (PDGF), transforming growth factor beta (TGF-β), VEGF, epidermal growth factor (EGF), IGF-I, fibroblast growth factor (FGF) and hepatocyte growth factor (HGF), which can aid in the healing of tendinopathy (Anitua, 2005). Because of this concentration of growth factors, PRP is thought to be more effective than dextrose prolotherapy for tendinopathy.

PRP has proven reasonably efficacious but may not relieve all of the pain or may leave some residual pain in the tendon or periosteum. For tendinopathy documented by ultrasound or MRI, injections with PRP are a very reasonable treatment approach. In general, PRP should be guided by ultrasound to improve the accuracy of the treatment. Numerous studies have shown the efficacy of this injection technique (Filardo et al., 2014; Oloff, Elmi, Nelson & Crain, 2015; Zhou & Wang, 2016). Most of the studies have been done regarding Achilles tendinopathy.

PRP forms a fibrin gel which can act as a structural platform for migrating cells and tissue healing in tendinopathy. PRP appears to induce proliferation of tendon cell types: tendon stem/progenitor cells and tenocytes (Wang et al., 2012; Zhang & Wang, 2010). PRP may only need to be done one time or may be repeated after an interval of 6–8 weeks. If pain remains despite ultrasound evidence of healing then the author would suggest using a modality such as low-level laser therapy or frequency specific microcurrent to relieve the pain which is due to sensitized tissue in the tendon or the periosteum.

Stem cell injections are also studied in tendinopathy. Tendons have some stem cells in their structure (Xu & Murrell, 2008). There have been a number of studies evaluating stem cell injection for certain regional tendinopathies. The theory is that injecting stem cells may increase the population of healthy tenocytes. There can be methodological challenges in that stem cells would need to differentiate into tenocytes. There may be some efficacy for lateral epicondylitis and for patellar tendinopathy. Because stem cell injections are somewhat invasive and very costly, other injection approaches should be initiated early in the course of the treatment. Stem cell therapy would be reasonable for refractory cases of tendinopathy (Chong et al., 2007; Pas, Moen, Haisma & Winters, 2017).

CLINICAL SUMMARY

A comprehensive history and physical exam should be done as outlined previously looking for factors that need to be addressed to help to heal the tendinopathy. The patient should be advised to modify use of the region but to maintain motion. They should be advised to minimize eccentric loads except during physical therapy. They should maintain aerobic exercise to decrease stress and continue the benefits of aerobic exercise. They may need to modify the exercise so as to not overuse the tendon. An example would be to not use the arms of the elliptical equipment in a patient with shoulder tendinopathy.

It is best to use imaging such as musculoskeletal ultrasound soon after suspecting tendinopathy. Patients are much more likely to be adherent to treatment plans if there is an imaging study that confirms a diagnosis.

The patient should be referred to a very skilled physical therapist who has had training in manual physical therapy, STEP, eccentric exercise and, if possible, mobilization with motion techniques. If the patient is already sensitized in the tissue, friction massage or other similar techniques that scrape the tissue should be avoided. One should present different options to the patient, an option that does not involve injections and one that does. The patient should be involved in decisions regarding care.

Low-level laser therapy (photobiomodulation) possibly combined with frequency specific micro-current if available can be administered at least twice a week for 4–6 weeks. If there is a tear with the tendinopathy, then one should elect to go right to PRP unless the tear is too large for PRP. Other types of injection that can provide scaffolding for a partial tear can also be considered, including the use of stem cell therapy.

With prolotherapy, at least 3 treatment sessions are needed and one may consider adding small amounts of testosterone and/or growth hormone depending on the patient's medical history. If one uses PRP or another regenerative injection, only one to two injections might be necessary.

Ultrasound should be used to determine if the tendon is actually healed at least 6 weeks after an injection or at the end of a course of physical therapy with or without modalities. If there is residual pain after treatment one should consider that there is pain at the periosteum and this should be treated with either frequency specific microcurrent or low-level laser therapy or both.

REFERENCES

Abate M, Gravare-Silbernagel K, Siljeholm C, Di Iorio A, De Amicis D, Salini V, Werner S, and Paganelli R. Pathogenesis of tendinopathies: Inflammation or degeneration? *Arthritis Res Ther.* 2009; 11(3): 235.

Abate M, Guelfi M, Pantalone A, Vanni D, Schiavone C, Andia I, and Salini V. Therapeutic use of hormones on tendinopathies: A narrative review. *Muscles Ligaments Tendons J.* 2016; 6(4): 445–452.

Anitua E, Andía I, Sanchez M, Azofra J, del Mar Zalduendo M, de la Fuente M, and Nurden AT. Autologous preparations rich in growth factors promote proliferation and induce VEGF and HGF production by human tendon cells in culture. *J Orthopaedic Res.* 2005; 23(2): 281–286.

Assem, Y Glyceryl trinitrate patches—An alternative treatment for shoulder impingement syndrome. *J Orthopaedic Translation.* 2015; 3(1): 12–20.

Backstrom KM. Mobilization with movement as an adjunct intervention in a patient with complicated de Quervain's tenosynovitis: A case report. *J Orthop Sports Phys Ther.* 2002; 32(3): 86–94.

Bisset L, Beller E, Jull G, Brooks P, Darnell R, and Vicenzino B. Mobilisation with movement and exercise, corticosteroid injection, or wait and see for tennis elbow: Randomised trial. *BMJ.* 2006; 333: 939.

Bertrand H, Reeves KD, Bennett CJ, Bicknell S, and Cheng AL. Dextrose prolotherapy versus control injections in painful rotator cuff tendinopathy. *Arch Phys Med Rehabil.* 2016; 97(1):17–25.

Chong AK, Ang AD, Goh JC, Hui JH, Lim AY, Lee EH, and Lim BH. Bone marrow-derived mesenchymal stem cells influence early tendon-healing in a rabbit Achilles tendon model. *J Bone Joint Surg Am.* 2007; 89: 74–81.

Denaro V, Ruzzini L, Longo UG, Franceschi F, De Paola B, Cittadini A, Maffulli N, and Sgambato A. Effect of dihydrotestosterone on cultured human tenocytes from intact supraspinatus tendon. *Knee Surg Sports Traumatol Arthrosc.* 2010; 18: 971–976.

Doessing S, Heinemeier KM, Holm L, et al. Growth hormone stimulates the collagen synthesis in human tendon and skeletal muscle without affecting myofibrillar protein synthesis *J Physiol.* 2010; 588: 341–351.

Filardo G, Kon E, Di Matteo B, Di Martino A, Tesei G, Pelotti P, Cenacchi A, and Marcacci M. Platelet-rich plasma injections for the treatment of refractory Achilles tendinopathy: results at 4 years. *Blood Transfus*. 2014; 12(4): 533–540.

Hashimoto T, Nobuhara K, and Hamada T. Pathologic evidence of degeneration as a primary cause of rotator cuff tear. *Clin Orthop Relat Res*. 2003; 415: 111–120.

Haslerud S, Magnussen LH, Joensen J, Lopes-Martins RA, and Bjordal JM. The efficacy of low-level laser therapy for shoulder tendinopathy: A systematic review and meta-analysis of randomized controlled trials. *Physiother Res Int*. 2015; 20(2):108–125. doi:10.1002/pri.1606.

Holmgren T, Björnsson-Hallgren H, Öberg B, Adolfsson L, and Johansson K. Effect of specific exercise strategy on need for surgery in patients with subacromial impingement syndrome: Randomised controlled study. *BMJ*. 2012; 344: e787.

Khalkhali-Ellis Z, Handa RJ, Price RH, Jr, Adams BD, Callaghan JJ, and Hendrix MJ. Androgen receptors in human synoviocytes and androgen regulation of interleukin 1beta (IL-1beta) induced IL-6 production: A link between hypoandrogenicity and rheumatoid arthritis? *J Rheumatol*. 2002; 29(9): 1843–1846.

Khan KM, Maffulli N, Coleman BD, Cook JL, and Taunton JE. Patellar tendinopathy: Some aspects of basic science and clinical management. *Br J Sports Med*. 1998; 32(4): 346–355.

Langberg H, Olesen J, Skovgaard D, and Kjaer M. Age related blood flow around the Achilles tendon during exercise in humans. *Eur J Appl Physiol*. 2001; 84: 246–248.

McMakin, C. *Frequency Specific Microcurrent in Pain Management*.

Nielsen RH, Holm L, Jensen JK, Heinemeier KM, Remvig L, and Kjaer M. Tendon protein synthesis rate in classic Ehlers-Danlos patients can be stimulated with insulin-like growth factor-I. *J Appl Physiol*. 2014; 117(7): 694–698.

Nørregaard J, Larsen CC, Bieler T, and Langberg H. Eccentric exercise in treatment of Achilles tendinopathy. *Scand J Med Sci Sports*. 2007; 17(2): 133–138.

Ohberg L, Lorentzon R, and Alfredson H. Eccentric training in patients with chronic Achilles tendinosis: Normalised tendon structure and decreased thickness at follow up. *Br J Sports Med*. 2004; 38(1): 8–11.

Oliva F, Piccirilli E, Berardi AC, Frizziero A, Tarantino U, and Maffulli N. Hormones and tendinopathies: The current evidence. *Br Med Bull*. 2016; 117(1): 39–58.

Oloff LM, Elmi E, Nelson J, and Crain J. Retrospective analysis of the effectiveness of platelet-rich plasma in the treatment of Achilles tendinopathy: Pretreatment and posttreatment correlation of magnetic resonance imaging and clinical assessment. *Foot Ankle Spec*. 2015; 8(6): 490–497.

Paoloni JA, Appleyard RC, Nelson J, and Murrell GA. Topical glyceryl trinitrate application in the treatment of chronic supraspinatus tendinopathy: A randomized, double-blinded, placebo-controlled clinical trial. *Am J Sports Med*. 2005; 33(6): 806–813.

Pas HIMFL, Moen MH, Haisma HJ, and Winters M. No evidence for the use of stem cell therapy for tendon disorders: A systematic review. *Br J Sports Med*. 2017; 51(13): 996–1002.

Sanderson LM, and Bryant A. Effectiveness and safety of prolotherapy injections for management of lower limb tendinopathy and fasciopathy: A systematic review. *J Foot Ankle Res*. 2015; 8: 57.

Scarpone M, Rabago DP, Zgierska A, Arbogest J, and Snell E. The efficacy of prolotherapy for lateral epicondylosis: A pilot study. *Clin J Sport Med*. 2008; 18(3): 248–254.

Scott A, Khan KM, Cook J, and Duronio V. Human tendon overuse pathology: Histopathologic and biochemical findings. In: *Tendinopathy in Athletes*, Woo SL, Arnoczky SP, and Renstrom P (Eds). Malden, MA: Wiley-Blackwell, 2007.

Tumilty S, Munn J, McDonough S, Hurley DA, Basford JR, and Baxter GD. Low level laser treatment of tendinopathy: A systematic review with meta-analysis. *Photomed Laser Surg*. 2010; 28(1): 3–16. doi:10.1089/pho.2008.2470.

van der Linden PD, van Puijenbroek EP, Feenstra J, Veld BA, Sturkenboom MC, Herings RM, and Stricker BH. Tendon disorders attributed to fluoroquinolones: A study on 42 spontaneous reports in the period 1988 to 1998. *Arthritis Rheum*. 2001; 45(3): 235–239.

Wang X, Qiu Y, Triffitt J, Carr A, Xia Z, and Sabokbar A. Proliferation and differentiation of human tenocytes in response to platelet rich plasma: An *in vitro* and *in vivo* study. *J Orthopaedic Res*. 2012; 30(6): 982–990.

Xiao-Guang L, Cheng L, and Song JM. Effects of low-level laser therapy and eccentric exercises in the treatment of Patellar tendinopathy. *Int. J Photoenergy*. 2014; 2014: 6. http://dx.doi.org/10.1155/2014/785386.

Xu Y, and Murrell GA. The basic science of tendinopathy. *Clin Orthop Relat Res*. 2008; 466(7): 1528–1538.

Yang X, Coleman DP, Pugh ND, and Nokes LD. The volume of the neovascularity and its clinical implications in Achilles tendinopathy. *Ultrasound in Med. and Biol*. 2012; 38(11): 1887–1895.

Yelland MJ, Sweeting KR, Lyftogt JA, Ng SK, Scuffham PA, and Evans KA. Prolotherapy injections and eccentric loading exercises for painful Achilles tendinosis: A randomised trial. *Br J Sports Med.* 2011; 45(5): 421–428.

Zhang J, and Wang JHC. Platelet-rich plasma releasate promotes differentiation of tendon stem cells into active tenocytes. *Am J of Sports Med.* 2010; 38(12): 2477–2486.

Zhou Y, and Wang JHC. PRP treatment efficacy for tendinopathy: A review of basic science studies. *BioMed Res Int.* 2016; 2016: 8. http://dx.doi.org/10.1155/2016/9103792.

20 Metabolic Therapies in the Management of Heel Pain

Emily M. Splichal, DPM, MS

INTRODUCTION

The body is deeply interconnected, which means that compensation patterns or dysfunction in one area of the body can have a profound effect on another area. This interconnectedness is mediated throughout the anatomy including the highly innervated fascial system, which is covered in depth in Chapters 5 and 21. This interconnectedness of the human body lies not only within the musculo-skeletal system but also exists metabolically, with every disease, medication and lifestyle decision affecting the entire body.

The human foot is a complex network of crossing nerves, blood vessels and myofascial tissue all of which undergo unique stress due to their distal proximity and repetitive stress during dynamic movement. According to the American Podiatric Medical Association (APMA), more than 77% of adults will experience foot pain with only one-third of them seeking medical attention. This means that over 50% of adults have the belief that foot pain is normal. Despite the prevalence of foot pain, pain should not be the only trigger to evaluate the health of your patient's feet. A foot exam provides system-wide information and can often be the first indication of medication side effects or systemic metabolic compromise. For example, arthritis, diabetes, nerve and circulatory disorders can present their initial symptoms in the feet. Similarly, adverse effects of prescription medications can some-times manifest first in the feet.

This chapter elaborates on the diagnosis and management of heel pain in light of the integrated nature of the human foot. It is an introduction to the science of metabolic therapies in podiatry and a call for collaboration between medical doctors and podiatrists for the future management of foot health from a metabolic perspective.

Heel pain is one of the most common pathologies presented to the podiatrist office and it has been estimated that plantar fasciitis occurs in approximately 2 million Americans each year and affects as much as 10% of the population over the course of a lifetime.[1] Of the causes of heel pain, mechanical plantar fasciitis is the most frequently encountered diagnosis; however, this is not the only cause of plantar heel pain. The differential diagnosis of medication-induced heel pain and the systemic effects on connective tissue must always be considered in the patient presenting with foot pain and must be considered before the effects even present.

PATHOANATOMICAL FEATURES OF THE PLANTAR FASCIA

The plantar aponeurosis or fascia consists of 3 bands: lateral, medial and central all of which are further divided into superficial and deep fibers (see Figure 20.1).[1,2] The central band originates from the medial tubercle of the plantar surface of the calcaneus and travels toward the toes as a solid band of tissue dividing into 5 slips, each of which inserts into the proximal phalanx of each toe. When the toes are extended, the plantar fascia is functionally stiffened, creating stability in the foot and engaging the "windlass mechanism" of the plantar fascia. The windlass mechanism assists in supi-nating the rear foot and releasing elastic energy during the push-off phase of gait.

In many cases, plantar fasciitis is the result of repetitive tensile overload or stress. This repetitive stress causes changes in the plantar aponeurosis that can be either acute or chronic.

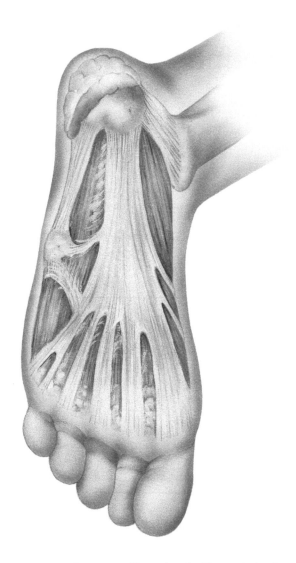

FIGURE 20.1 Plantar aponeurosis anatomy. (Reproduced with permission from Shutterstock.)

In a 2003 study, Lemont introduced the term plantar fasciosis to de-emphasize the idea that inflammation is the cause of pain.[3] Histopathologic studies have shown that patients with diagnosed plantar fasciitis have more disorganization of fibrous tissue similar to degenerative tendinosis rather than inflammation.

The most common site of pain in patients complaining of heel pain diagnosed as plantar fasciitis is near the origin or enthesis of the central band of the plantar aponeurosis at the medial plantar tubercle of the calcaneus with occasional pain in the mid-portion of the central band just prior to it splitting into the 5 slips. Patients typically report pain with their first step in the morning or after a period of rest, also known as post-static dyskinesia. The pain will often subside with activity only to return toward the end of the day; it is described as sharp or burning and is localized to the plantar surface of the heel, with paresthesias uncommon.

Although conservative treatments for plantar fasciitis (see Table 20.1) have been in use for decades, the understanding and fine-tuning of these treatments continue to evolve. The most

---

TABLE 20.1

Conservative Treatment Protocol for Plantar Fasciitis

Anti-inflammatory agents (NSAIDs, corticosteroid injections, icing)

Stretching (calf, plantar fascia specific)

Orthotics (custom-molded, over the counter)

Night splints

---

common conservative treatment protocol includes NSAIDs or corticosteroid injections, calf and plantar fascia stretching, custom-molded orthotics and night splints.[1,3] With 90% of plantar fasciitis responding to the conservative treatment, it is in the best interest of the patient to seek a comprehensive treatment program as opposed to a one-size-fits-all approach to treatment.

HEEL PAIN CASE STUDY

A 54-year-old post-menopausal woman with a history of relapsing-remitting multiple sclerosis (RRMS) was referred to podiatry for evaluation of left plantar heel pain non-responsive to conservative treatment. The patient stated that the left heel pain began 6 months prior during her last RRMS flare up, which happened to coincide with a trip to Europe. This was not her first bout of plantar heel pain and she reported a diagnosis 1 year prior of plantar fasciitis. Currently, her pain is described as sharp and burning localized to the plantar heel and is 8 out of 10 on the pain scale.

The patient first presented to her medical doctor 3 months prior, when an x-ray was taken and calcaneal spur and fracture were ruled out. She was advised to start the standard conservative treatment of NSAIDs, stretching, icing, supportive footwear and decreased activity. The patient was not able to take the NSAIDs due to gastric irritation and her use of Omeprazole, but she did follow the rest of the recommended treatment. After not responding to conservative treatment, she returned and was referred to physical therapy for 6 weeks of manual therapy and foot strengthening. The patient noted a slight improvement; however, when she increased her activity the pain returned to 8/10. The patient sought additional treatment options.

QUESTIONS TO BE CONSIDERED

1. Why is this patient not responding to conservative treatment options? Is there something systemically (diagnosis or medication) that is preventing her plantar fascia from healing?
2. Has all appropriate imaging been done to rule out all possible different diagnosis?
3. What advanced treatment options are available to this patient based on the chronicity of the condition?

METABOLIC CONSIDERATIONS IN PLANTAR FASCIITIS

If a patient is non-responsive to conservative treatment, the systemic-wide effects of medications and inflammatory levels must be taken into consideration. In diabetes, for example, the prevalence of systemic-wide inflammation is high due to the effects of advanced glycation end products, which has a deleterious effect on the collagen of tendons and ligaments.[4] The five most common systemic conditions that have an effect on the elasticity and inflammation of the plantar aponeurosis include diabetes mellitus, menopause, hypercholesterolemia, autoimmune conditions such as rheumatoid arthritis and lupus, and cancer[4] (see Table 20.2).

In patients presenting with heel pain and a subsequent medical condition or taking a medication that places increased risk on the plantar aponeurosis, balancing both mechanical and metabolic

TABLE 20.2

Medical Conditions Associated with Heel Pain

Diabetes mellitus Type I, Type II

Hypercholesterolemia

Pre-post menopause

Autoimmune conditions (rheumatoid arthritis, lupus)

Cancer (cancer therapy)

stress is paramount to the recovery of the patient. For example, in the case of familial hypercholesterolemia, tendon xanthomas or lipomatosis are commonly observed in the Achilles tendon, which is due to the fascial continuity between the Achilles tendon and the plantar aponeurosis. This can place undue stress on the plantar foot, increasing the risk for Achilles tendinitis or plantar fasciitis.[5]

Similarly, physiological changes occur in the musculoskeletal system during aging, including a decrease in muscle mass and strength, and an alteration of the tendon and bone structure. It has been observed that these changes are due to a decrease in collagen synthesis, an increase in free radical expression and a shift in metabolism in favor of catabolic activity. It is suggested that in females the level of estrogen, which decreases drastically in the post-menopause period, plays a crucial role in tendon metabolism and altering the production of different growth factors.[6] The presence of estrogen receptors in tenocytes may indicate that tendon health is influenced by estrogen levels with a reduction in blood estrogen levels associated with a reduction in tensile strength, collagen synthesis and fiber diameter and an increase in the degradation of tendon tissue.

Due to the systemic nature of medications, possible side effects and metabolic disruption to connective tissue must always be considered in the patient presenting with foot pain (see Table 20.3). Widely used medications associated with foot pain are the lipid-lowering statins. Worldwide, statins have quickly become one of the most widely prescribed families of drugs. The increasing use of statins does not come without risk. One of the most common side effects that is of concern to foot health includes myopathies.[7] The correlation of myopathies and plantar fasciitis is due to the repetitive stress placed on the foot during ambulation.

Another common medication that causes complications in foot health are chemotherapeutic agents, including platinum drugs, taxanes, epothilones and vinca alkaloids.[8] Chemotherapy-induced peripheral neuropathy is the most common podiatric side effect that is not only painful and uncomfortable for the patient but can lead to overuse of the plantar fascia and weakness in the intrinsic foot muscles. This can be quite distressing for patients; however, recent evidence from several small pilot studies has shown that the use of vitamin E might help prevent or lessen the side effects of chemotherapy-induced peripheral neuropathy and thus the risk of plantar fasciitis. Other agents that look promising in preliminary studies include glutamine, glutathione, N-acetylcysteine, oxcarbazepine and xaliproden.[8]

TABLE 20.3

Medications that Complicate the Management of Heel Pain

Statins

Chemotherapy

Oral contraceptives

Proton pump inhibitors

Quinolones

For younger female patients, the use of oral contraceptives and exogenous estrogen must also be considered in the health of the plantar fascia and connective tissue. Research has shown that women taking oral contraceptives, thereby having higher exogenous estrogen levels, would be more susceptible to muscle and tendon damage and have an attenuated recovery from exercise-induced muscle damage.[9] It has also been shown that oral contraceptives have an inhibiting effect on collagen synthesis in tendon, bone, muscle and connective tissue, which may be related to a lower bioavailability of insulin-like growth factor 1 (IGF-I).[9]

The final two medications to consider are proton pump inhibitors (PPIs) and quinolones. Many consider PPIs to be devoid of adverse effects; however, PPIs can cause serious adverse effects. PPIs are initially overlooked as a cause of hyponatremia, myopathy and rhabdomyolysis.[10]

The pathophysiology of quinolone-induced tendinopathy is not fully clear; however, some concepts have been suggested. It is a well-accepted multifactorial pathophysiology and very documented. Recommendations for use avoidance in certain patients can also be added. *In vitro* studies in cultured tendon cells have confirmed the clinical observation that quinolones can increase the risk of tendon rupture.

The pathogenesis of tendon rupture is secondary to fluoroquinolone therapy.[11] Under normal circumstances, the rate of matrix turnover and tendon fibroblast is low. It has been theorized that quinolones disproportionately affect human tendons that have a limited capacity for repair, namely the Achilles tendon, and in tissue affected by structural compromise (pre-existing tendinopathy or trauma).

ADVANCED IMAGINING OF THE PLANTAR APONEUROSIS

Advanced imaging is required in the case of non-responsive heel pain or in a patient with metabolic conditions such as diabetes, arthritis or autoimmune disease. An assessment of the plantar fascia with ultrasound is a well-established method in podiatry and provides a more thorough assessment of the plantar aponeurosis health. Plantar fascia thickness is one finding observed on ultrasound with trends noted in increasing pulmonary function test (PFT) and age. A normal PFT is 3 mm as opposed to 5 mm in those patients with symptomatic plantar heel pain.[13] Diabetes has also been associated with greater plantar fascia thickening and collagen glycation.[13] Due to the long half-life of collagen in tendons and ligaments, PFT assessed by ultrasound is a relevant measure of tissue glycation and metabolic burden. Glycation and oxidation of collagen in soft tissues may be independent risk factors for microvascular complications.

When considering advanced imaging, the benefit of differentiating between acute and chronic plantar fasciitis may have a sound contribution in patient treatment. The management of plantar fasciitis is primarily conservative; however, in the case of non-responding heel pain, differential diagnosis or more advanced tissue degeneration must be considered. Magnetic resonance imaging (MRI) provides a means to determine the possible cause of a nerve entrapment, a plantar fascial tear or even a missed calcaneal stress fracture. A detailed history and physical examination should guide your differential diagnosis (see Table 20.4).

TABLE 20.4
Differential Diagnosis in Plantar Heel Pain

Plantar fibroma
Plantar fascial tear
Baxter's nerve entrapment
Inflammatory arthropathy
Radiculopathy
Bone bruise or calcaneal fracture

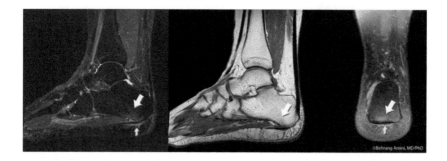

FIGURE 20.2   MRI demonstrating plantar fasciitis. (Reproduced with permission from Dr. Behrang Amini.)

Common MRI findings include increased signal intensity consistent with edema in the perifascial soft tissue depicted on T2-weighted images (see Figure 20.2). This finding is consistent with the finding that perifascial edema was considered to be the most common manifestation of plantar fasciitis.[14] In chronic plantar fasciitis (symptoms >6 months), soft tissue edema both superficial and deep to the plantar aponeurosis was the dominant abnormal imaging finding in 70% of cases.[14] The second most common MRI finding of plantar fasciitis, seen in 58% of patients, was mild to moderate thickening of the plantar aponeurosis, which presumably corresponded to the presence of granulation tissue.[14] The third most common MRI finding of plantar fasciitis, observed in 33% of our cases, was increased signal intensity within the involved plantar fascia on T2-weighted and short-TI inversion recovery (STIR) images; this finding presumably was consistent with edema and intrasubstance microtears.[14]

ADVANCED CONCEPTS IN CHRONIC PLANTAR FASCIOSIS

Advanced concepts in regenerative medicine should be considered in the case of degeneration and plantar fascia thickening. Interventions such as platelet-rich plasma (PRP), amniotic stem cells or umbilical cord stem cells may provide benefit in select patients as technologies progress. Shockwave therapy and acupuncture may also be of benefit for selected patients.

All regenerative treatment options use the science of tissue healing to bring chronic tissue into an acute inflammatory state. PRP was one of the first regenerative medicine options in the orthopedic and sports medicine industries, and research continues to broaden its effective use. PRP provokes an elevated release of growth factors in an attempt to jumpstart the healing of a chronic injury. Increased concentrations of autologous platelets yield high concentrations of growth factors, leading to healing of the soft tissue on a cellular level. A 2014 study by Monto *et al.* demonstrated increased efficacy in the application of PRP injections versus corticosteroids in chronic, non-responding plantar fasciitis. Monto *et al.* demonstrated faster and prolonged pain reduction in the PRP group with a 2 year follow-up demonstrating a continued decrease of symptoms.[15]

FUNCTIONAL PODIATRY APPROACH TO HEEL PAIN CASE STUDY

We now return to the initial case presentation and the questions to be considered. In our 54-year-old woman, the recurrent and persistent nature of her plantar heel pain carries the suspicion of possible plantar fascial thickening, degeneration and tear compounded by systemic inflammation secondary to MS and gastritis.

Ultrasound and MRI should be ordered to further evaluate the condition of the plantar fascia. In this specific patient, a plantar fascial thickening of 4.5 mm and a superficial tear of the central band of the plantar fascia were observed on MRI (Figure 20.2). All treatment options were discussed with the patient and her medical doctor and the decision was made to undergo a series of two PRP injections 2 weeks apart, followed by 4 weeks of immobilization in a walking boot. During her immobilization period, the patient was carefully monitored for acute symptoms of her MS. Eight weeks after the initial injection, the patient reported an 80% improvement in her symptoms with full return to activities.

CONCLUSION

Treating feet has whole-body implications requiring podiatry to work closely with medical doctors and vice versa. Although this was a brief introduction to the importance of systemic inflammation and glycation levels on peripheral nerve health and fascial elasticity, it should begin to challenge conventional approaches to foot health. In my podiatric experience, patients are most effectively approached from a metabolic perspective and in collaboration with a team of medical doctors. Optimal foot health lays the foundation for ensuring movement longevity and the integration of movement as medicine for cardiovascular, neurological and musculoskeletal health.

REFERENCES

1. Roxas, M. Plantar fasciitis: Diagnosis and therapeutic considerations. *Altern Med Rev.* 2005; 10(2): 83–93.
2. Chandler, TJ et al. A biomechanical approach to the prevention, treatment and rehabilitation of plantar fasciitis. *Sports Med.* 1993; 15(5): 344–352.
3. Lemont H, Ammirati KM, Usen NJ. Plantar fasciitis: A degenerative process (fasciosis) without inflammation. *J Am Podiatr Med Assoc.* 2003; 93(1): 234–237.
4. Abate, M et al. Occurrence of tendon pathologies in metabolic disorders. *Rheumatology.* 2013; 52(4): 599–608.
5. Dagistan, E et al. Multiple tendon xanthomas in patient with heterozygous familial hypercholesterolaemia: Sonographic and MRI findings. *BMJ Case Rep.* 2013: bcr2013200755.
6. Frizziero, A et al. Impact of oestrogen deficiency and aging on tendon: A concise review. *Muscle Ligaments Tendons J.* 2014; 4(3): 324–328.
7. Phillips, P et al. Statin-associated myopathy with normal creatine kinase levels. *Ann Intern Med.* 2012; 137(7): 581–585.
8. Wolf, S et al. Chemotherapy-induced peripheral neuropathy: Prevention and treatment strategies. *Eur J Cancer.* 2008; 44(11): 1507–1511.
9. Hansen, M et al. Effect of administration of oral contraceptives *in vivo* on collagen synthesis in tendon and muscle connective tissue in young women. *J Appl Phys.* 2009; 106(4): 1435–1443.
10. Colmenares, EW et al. Proton pump inhibitors: Risk for myopathy? *Ann Pharmacother.* 2017; 51(1): 66–71.
11 Childs SG. Pathogenesis of tendon rupture secondary to fluoroquinolone therapy. *Orthop Nurs.* 2007; 26(3): 175–182.
12. Kim, G. The risk of fluoroquinolone-induced tendinopathy and tendon rupture. *J Clin Aesthet Dermatol.* 2010; 3(4): 49–54.
13. Craig, ME et al. Plantar fascia thickness, a measure of tissue glycation, predicts the development of complications in adolescents with type 1 diabetes. *Diabetes Care.* 2008; 31(6): 1201–1206.
14. Theodorou, D et al. Plantar fasciitis and fascial rupture: MR imaging findings in 26 patients supplemented with anatomic data in cadavers. *Radiographics.* 2000; 20(1): 42–46.
15. Monto, R et al. Platelet-rich plasma efficacy versus corticosteroid treatment for chronic, severe plantar fasciitis. *Foot Ankle Int.* 2014; 35(4): 313–318.
16. Zelen, C et al. Prospective, randomized, blinded, comparative study of injectable micronized dehydrated amniotic/chorionic membrane allograft for plantar fasciitis: A feasibility study. 2013; 34(10): 1332–1339.
17. Garras, D et al. Particulate umbilical cord/amniotic membrane for the treatment of plantar fasciitis. *AOFAS 2017 Meeting.* 2017.

21 Fascial Syndromes
Emerging, Treatable Contributors to Musculoskeletal Pain

David Lesondak, BCSI, ATSI, FST, FFT

INTRODUCTION

Fascia is essential to the overall health and function of the human body and is a key component to understanding the human structure. Fascia is both a tissue and a system. The collagen content of fascia is capable of slowly remodeling itself over time, based on the mechanical forces to which it is subjected. This has both positive and negative ramifications. Understanding how the complexities of repetitive force transmission through the body's fascial web can affect posture and function will guide the physician or clinician to a new understanding of the complexities of chronic pain and physical dysfunction where traditional musculoskeletal models prove insufficient.

This chapter details the emerging integral role of fascia in chronic musculoskeletal pain, as well as improving fluid flow to enhance metabolic function.

DEFINING OUR TERMS

For most of medical history, fascia was thought to be an inert, biologic packing material and, as such, it held very little medical interest; however, that view is rapidly changing. In the year 2000, PubMed showed 364 new papers under the topic. By contrast, in 2017, 475 articles were listed for the first 6 months alone. This growing trend can be traced back to the First International Fascia Research Congress, which took place at the Harvard School of Medicine in 2007 and drew over 500 researchers and clinicians. The fifth such conference is to be held in Berlin, Germany, in 2018. Significant was their definition of fascia not just as a tissue, but also as a system: *The fascial system consists of the three-dimensional continuum of soft, collagen containing, loose and dense fibrous connective tissues that permeate the body. It incorporates elements such as adipose tissue, adventitae and neurovascular sheaths, aponeuroses, deep and superficial fasciae, epineurium, joint capsules, ligaments, membranes, meninges, myofascial expansions, periostea, retinacula, septa, tendons, visceral fasciae, and all the intramuscular and intermuscular connective tissues including endo-/peri-/mysium.*

The fascial system interpenetrates and surrounds all organs, muscles, bones and nerve fibers, endowing the body with a functional structure, and providing an environment that enables all body systems to operate in an integrated manner [1].

COMPONENTS AND RECENT RESEARCH

Fascia is composed of fiber and fluid, collagen and ground substance, also collectively referred to as the extracellular matrix (ECM). The fiber is predominantly collagen, of which there are at least 15 distinctive types [2]. The most abundant in connective tissue is collagen Type I, which accounts for 90% [3]. These fibers wind together in a triple helix, giving the fascia tremendous tensile strength that, gram for gram, is stronger than steel [4]. Like steel, collagen is highly ductile, meaning that when subjected to extreme forces it will slowly deform, rather than break like porcelain or glass.

Ground substance is host to a variety of proteoglycans, which are composed of smaller molecules called glycosaminoglycans (GAGs). One specific GAG worth clinical consideration is hyaluronan. Hyaluronan is the hydraulic fluid that keeps the muscles and joints gliding properly and is produced in the sliding layers between the epimysium of the muscles by a class of cells called fasciacytes. Changes in the viscosity of hyaluronan could compromise the sliding behaviors of the underlying muscles and fascia, creating symptomatic pain [5].

It is further theorized that the ECM, with its abundance of hydrophilic GAGs, acts very much like a sponge. While drinking water is necessary for proper metabolic function, it is not enough. It is the mechanical stimulation of the fascial tissues via compression stretching, and upping the core body temperature, serving to wring out the sponge, allowing old waste water to be carried away and new fresh water to be taken up by the tissue, helping to clean up any metabolic traffic jams. Whether that happens via movement or manual therapy is considered moot at this point.

The fascia also contains an abundance of cell types including mast cells, T cells, macrophages, lymphocytes, adipocytes and the recently discovered telocytes [6]. Telocytes are mechanosensitive cells that are vital to many physiological processes like stem cell upkeep, tissue repair and immune function. Telocytes share genetic material with other cells via extracellular vesicles. This discovery lends additional credence to the theory that the fascial system is a body-wide, cellular signaling network [7,8].

The most abundant cell in the fascia is the fibroblast, the custodian of the ECM. Along with producing cytokines, interleukins and other immune function cells, the fibroblast also synthesizes and remodels collagen based on the tension between the cell and the ECM. So, when the tension is low, there is little collagen production. When under high tension, the fibroblast will increase collagen production and cell proliferation [9]. Direction sensitive, the fibroblast will organize itself based on the pull of the underlying matrix [10]. Subjects with low back pain (LBP) showed a 25% greater thickness in their lumbar fascia when compared to pain-free controls [11]. The lack of regular movement or total immobility will give the fibroblasts little to no stimulation, which has a negative impact on the formation of healthy collagen and also causes a loss of crimp (Figure 21.1).

Crimp is the two-directional, lattice-like collagen weave that accounts for the springy, elastic movements that are a property of the fascia [12]. Animals studies show that immobilization promotes the development of crosslinks among the fibers, inhibiting natural movement [13].

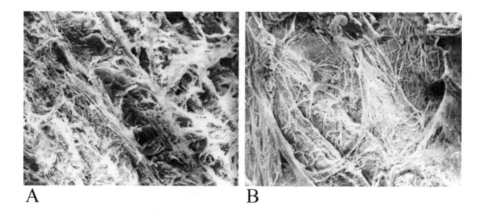

A   B

FIGURE 21.1 (a) Electron microscope image showing collagen fibers in a normal soleus perimysium running in three different distinct orientations. (b) How immobilization destroys the collagen network and renders the orientations indistinguishable. (Reproduced from Jarvinen et al. with permission.)

Appropriate fibroblast stimulation through movement and manual therapy can restore healthy crimp formation [14].

An in vitro study subjected an active culture of fibroblasts to sufficient repetitive strain to incur hardening of the collagenous elements of the cytoskeleton. These stressed cells had a 30% higher rate of apoptosis non-stressed controls. Moreover, stressed cells treated to compression with stretch, the core components of myofascial release, reduced apoptosis to slightly below the level of the control group and restored other negative factors to near their pre-stressed levels [15].

ANATOMY AND THE FASCIAL SYSTEM

While anatomy books like to divide fascia into discrete units and aggregates, it is vital to remember that all these parts, pieces and layers are part of one system. Starting just under the skin with the more superficial or areolar layer to the deep fascia or fascia profunda. The deep fascia comprises all the layers that interact with the musculoskeletal body (Figure 21.2). The deep fascia is highly organized and very much like an elastic, full-length body stocking – the innermost layer peeling away to form an epimysium, a pocket around each muscle. These epimysial pockets are free to glide due to hyaluronan [5]. This layer continues to the bundled perimysium, down to each individual muscle fiber wrapped in its own endomysium. This honeycomb arrangement allows for load sharing among the individual myofibers. Electron microscope studies have also revealed collagen fibers running in a more perpendicular fashion, creating a longitudinal network through the epimysium to the adjacent antagonistic muscle [16]. Other imaging studies clearly show the collagen fibers getting smaller and smaller, going all the way down to and through individual cell walls [17].

The deep fascia also includes the dynaments, which are highly specialized connective tissue structures organized in series with muscle fascicles, rather than in parallel, as has traditionally been thought. This calls into question the idea that ligaments are only active during the end ranges of joint movement [18].

Another significant development was a series of body-wide maps organized around the mostly vertical lines of fascial force transmission [19]. These maps, known as the anatomy trains [20,21], adhere to specific rules regarding direction, depth and direct and mechanical connections in certain planes of movement (via shared skeletal connections) and the fact that muscles also "attach" to other muscles via the fascia, and not just bone (Figure 21.3). The anatomy trains have survived the scrutiny of the cadaver laboratory [22]. A recent systematic review of anatomical dissection studies [23] looked for independent evidence for 6 of the 12 maps, finding sufficient corroboration for 3. The most verified map is the superficial back line (SBL) (Figure 21.4).

Covering the dorsal aspect of the body, the SBL comprises the plantar fascia to the periostea of the calcaneus, which has a fascial connection to the gastrocnemius via the Achilles tendon. From the gastrocnemius, we have a functional coupling with the hamstring, making an important distinction. Functionally, when the knee is flexed, the fascia of the upper and lower leg functions separately. When extended, they link, rather like two pairs of hands linked at the wrist (think of trapeze artists) to form one functional unit. Fascial crosslinks have also been observed at this junction [23]. The hamstrings continue to the ischial tuberosity, which continues across to the lateral border of the sacrum via the sacrotuberous ligament. Numerous dissections have revealed that the superficial aspects of the ligament are continuous with the tissue on either side of the ischial tuberosity; and have shown the ability to lift the superficial fibers of the sacrotuberous ligament away from the body while still maintaining a strong continuity with the hamstrings and the fascia of the erector spinae [21,22]. From the erector spinae, we travel up to the galea apoeneurotica to the epicranial fascia. Though we have started from the ground and worked our way up, this is arbitrary. Fascial force transmission works in both directions.

While not meant to supplant the traditional origin/insertion model, the anatomy trains present a model for holistic anatomy, the understanding of which can lead the clinician or physician to different insights, and a model for understanding biotensegrity.

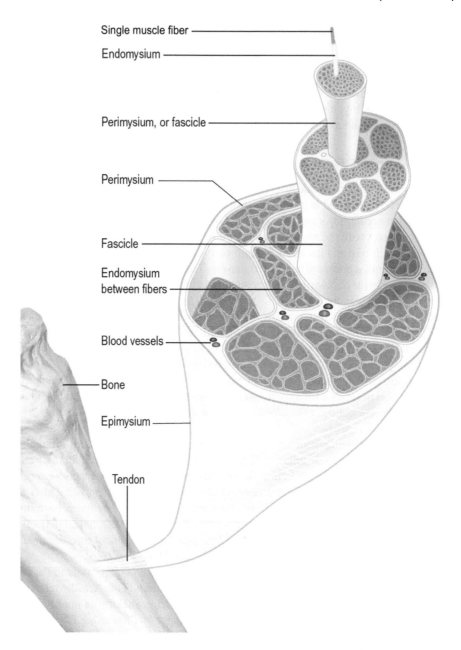

FIGURE 21.2 The layers of the deep fascia from the epimysium of the muscle to the endomysium; the individual wrapping for each muscle fiber. (Reproduced with permission from Handspring Publishing Ltd, taken from *Fascia: What It Is and Why It Matters* by David Lesondak, 2017.)

BIOTENSEGRITY

Biotensegrity is a biomechanical first proposed by orthopedic surgeon Stephen Levin [24,25]; it leverages the truss or the three-dimensional triangle model. Trusses can withstand tensile forces much better than a square frame design. The Saint Louis Arch is constructed on the truss model. So is the arch of the foot.

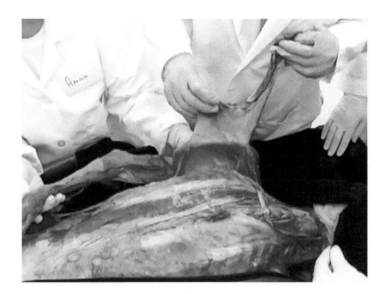

FIGURE 21.3 Does muscle really "attach" to bone? In this fresh tissue dissection, viewed from the profound side, there is no clear distinction or border between the splenius, rhomboid and serratus muscles. Screen capture from video by author. (Photo courtesy of Thomas Myers and the Laboratories for Anatomical Enlightenment.)

Arising from the worlds of art and architecture, tensegrity is defined as any structure that employs contiguous tensional members and discontinuous compression members in such a way that each member operates with maximum efficiency and economy. In the biotensegrity model, the bones are the discontinuous compression members and the surrounding connective tissue, the fascial system, provides the tensional framework. Clinically, subjects who have undergone massage for shoulder pain utilizing tensegrity principles showed a statistically significant increase in both passive and active range of motion (ROM) during flexion and abduction [26].

Tensegrity is also the basic property of the cellular structure. Experiments have shown that mechanical restructuring of the cell via the cytoskeleton tells the cell what to do [27–29]. In short, when cells were stretched, they thrived. And, similar to Meltzer's study [15], cells prevented from stretching went into apoptosis. This process happens via integrins, a cell receptor that binds the cell to the ECM with collagen fibers. When stimulated by pressure and vibration, the integrin transmits this tension directly to the nucleus, altering gene expression and activating mechanotransduction.

Clinically, a massage after strenuous exercise was shown to both increase the production of anti-inflammatory agents and create new mitochondria by inducing mechanotransduction [30]. There is now little doubt that manual therapies can alter genetic expression [31]. While joint degeneration can still occur even in the absence of inflammatory agents [32], it is worth noting that such studies do not take into account strain hardening and repetitive motion syndromes.

RELEVANT METABOLIC PATHWAYS

While not much is known about the fascia and nutrition, adequate amounts of Vitamin C are vital for collagen Type I synthesis [33]. Otherwise, the basics of an anti-inflammatory diet are recommended, including essential omega-3 fatty acids with an overall low ratio of omega-6 to omega (3:1 or 5:1), though the typical intake ratio in the diet of most Americans is much higher [34]. Omega-3 supplements offer a safe alternative in helping balance this ratio [35], but certain doses can lower platelet aggregation [36].

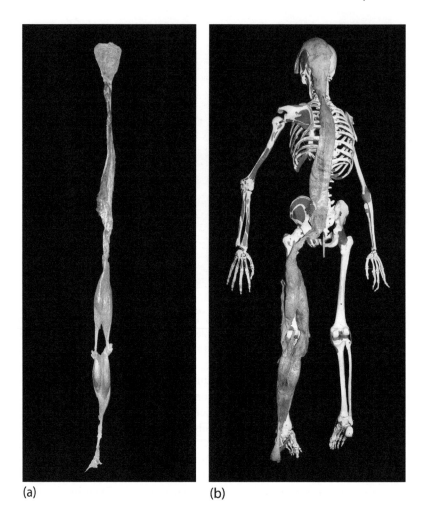

(a)   (b)

FIGURE 21.4 The superficial back line (SBL) in both unembalmed (a) and embalmed (b) dissections. (b) Overlaid on the skeleton model for clarity. Photos by author. (Photo courtesy of Thomas Myers and the Laboratories for Anatomical Enlightenment.)

Certain spices and herbs also contain bioactive substances shown to reduce inflammation. They have the added benefit of regulating inflammation through multiple pathways, as opposed to modifying just a single enzyme of an inflammatory cascade. These spices and herbs include capsaicin, curcumin, ginger, licorice, saffron and turmeric [37,38], although high doses of these can create toxicity and also interfere with certain medications.

Olive oil is a good source of oleocanthol, which inhibits the production of pro-inflammatory COX-1 and COX-2 enzymes, with 3.5 tbsp the equivalent of 200 mg of ibuprofen [39]. Individuals whose diets are rich in olive oil generally exhibit reduced inflammatory markers [40]. The catechins found in green tea and red wine also protect against free radicals and oxidative cell damage [41], further inhibiting inflammatory markers and responses.

DIAGNOSING FASCIAL CONDITIONS

The question remains as to how to diagnose fascial conditions. Ultrasound has proven a reliable diagnostic tool. Studies have correlated areas of pain with differences in fascial thickness when compared to control groups [11,42]. But not all of us have access to ultrasound equipment, or the appropriate time to use it on every patient if we do.

The most common symptoms of fascial dysfunction include:

- Decrease in local and/or general ROM
- Soft tissue pain when performing simple movements
- Compromised motor control, coordination in activities of daily living (ADLs)
- Reduced flexibility, lack of resilience
- Bad posture/body-wide patterns of compensation
- Dull aches or pains that never truly go away and/or do not respond to conventional ortho-pedic treatments
- Diminished proprioception and/or interoception that often manifests as a perceived clumsiness/bumping into things and uncertainty about physiological feelings

While each of these conditions could indicate a non-fascial condition, one of the simplest ways to assess if it is a fascial problem is patho-anatomical assessment. Bony landmarks related to the area of pain are palpated to look for asymmetries that would correlate with the symptoms. For example, in the case of LBP, is one iliac crest higher than the other? Does the anterior superior iliac spine (ASIS) deviate more than 7° with the posterior superior iliac spine (PSIS) in the sagittal plane? And so on.

Upon discovering such asymmetries and pointing them out to the patient, are they capable of easily correcting them? Or does the correction create further distortion and/or pain? A good rule of thumb is as follows: If asymmetries are present, manual therapy is indicated. If asymmetries are not present or are easily corrected when pointed out, a more movement-based solution is indicated.

These distinctions are important to accurately refer the patient to the proper fascia-based therapist.

FASCIAL THERAPIES

Fascia-related therapies are multiplying rapidly. They can be most easily categorized as manual or movement therapy. Many therapists combine elements of both, but that does not necessarily indicate a more efficacious treatment. The following is a list of some of the therapies with a reputation for achieving results.

Manual therapy: Structural integration including Rolfing, anatomy trains structural integration drop (kinesis myofascial integration) and Hellerwork; Myofascial Release, Trigger Point Therapy, Fascial Manipulation; and Visceral Manipulation.

Movement therapy: Fascial movement; MELT method; fascial fitness; and yoga. Recommended yoga modalities include therapeutic, yin, Iyengar and restorative.

Other: Fascial stretch therapy, which combines assisted stretching with traction and proprioceptive neuromuscular facilitation (PNF); and acupuncture. While not generally recognized as a fascial modality, acupuncture has been shown to interact with the fascia in ways that induce mechanotransduction [43] and influence the behavior of fibroblasts [44]. A preliminary investigation has also revealed the likelihood that the meridian system of traditional Chinese medicine organizes itself along fascial planes [45]. Regional treatment for musculoskeletal disorders are also referred to as dry needling.

While certain aspects of treatment differ, they all share the quality of increasing proprioception and tactile discrimination, the diminishment of which has been shown to be involved with many pain syndromes [46,47]. To minimize adhesions, treatment is recommended by 3 weeks after surgery, sooner if superficial soreness has diminished.

The following table serves only as a general guideline. On an individual basis, therapists may be more highly skilled with treating certain conditions than others, and as such may have higher individual effectiveness ratings. It is recommended that you seek out and assess qualified practitioners in your area.

Therapies/ Conditions	Manual Therapies				
	Structural Integration	Myofascial Release	Trigger Point Therapy	Fascial Manipulation	Visceral Manipulation
Low back pain	●	●	●	●	
Fibromyalgia	●[a]	✔[a]	●[a]		
Thoracic outlet/carpal tunnel	●	✔	●	●	
"Smartphone neck"	●	●	●	●	
Concussion	●[a]		✔		
Scoliosis	●[a]	✔		✔	✔[a]
GERD, IBS, reflux, etc.					●
Running/sports injuries	●	●	●	●	
Post organ replacement	●[a]		✔	✔	●[a]
Post joint replacement	●	✔	✔		
Stroke contractures	✔	✔	●	●	

Note: ●, very effective; ✔, effective.
[a] Indicates modalities work well in conjunction for this condition.

Therapies/ Conditions	Movement Therapies				Other	
	Fascial Movement	MELT Method	Fascial Fitness	Yoga	Fascial Stretch Therapy	Acupuncture
Low back pain	✔	●		●	●	✔
Fibromyalgia	●[a]	●[a]		✔[a]	●[a]	●[a]
Thoracic outlet/carpal tunnel		✔			●	✔
"Smartphone neck"	●	●		●	●	✔
Concussion	✔	✔		✔		●[a]
Scoliosis	●[a]	●[a]		●		
GERD, IBS, reflux, etc.						●
Running/sports injuries	●	●	●		●	
Post organ replacement	✔		✔			✔
Post joint replacement	●	●	●	●	●	
Stroke contractures					✔	✔

Note: ●, very effective; ✔, effective.
[a] Indicates modalities work well in conjunction for this condition.

CASE STUDY

PATIENT PROFILE

This is the case of a 46-year-old businesswoman who likes to practice yoga, initially complaining of numbness in her left lateral forefoot in March 2016. The symptoms were mild and intermittent until 6 months later when she felt a "pull" in her low back while performing a backbend in class. After several weeks of constant LBP, she began treatment with a chiropractor who diagnosed her with a "low left pelvis". Her relief was "occasional", but after 6 weeks of care her foot numbness spread to the whole forefoot. She also reported an apparent redness and mild swelling of the left foot. There was a recurring feeling like her legs and the soles of both feet were "on fire".

She began to receive acupuncture treatments that helped initially, but overall the symptoms began to worsen. Chiropractic treatment was placed on hold, an anti-inflammatory diet was recommended and x-rays of the lumbar spine ordered.

The x-rays revealed narrowing of the disc space from L3 to S1 and a sacral anteversion. A magnetic resonance image (MRI) was ordered, but was not done due to insurance issues. A week later, tingling and numbness radiculopathies in the lower extremities worsened and the patient now had irradiation to her arms as well. A neurologist was consulted, who ordered an MRI that was again denied. After three physical therapy treatments, her left leg radiculopathy persisted. Finally, a year after her symptoms started and on the advice of her physician, she was referred to our office for evaluation and further treatment.

CLINICAL OBSERVATIONS

Overall, the patient is a healthy individual of great physicality, given her longevity in the fitness industry. Patho-anatomical assessment revealed relevant postural anomalies: the left hemipelvis had a pronounced anterior tilt in the sagittal plane. Likewise, the left leg showed a hyperextended knee. The right hip, by comparison, was within 7° of neutral. There was a lateral rotation in the left hip in the transverse plane and the left hip had a left tilt (meaning the right iliac crest appeared higher) in the frontal plane. A very slight right bend of the lumbar spine could also be seen and palpated. All of these anomalies fit with her presenting symptoms. Pain was self-rated as 6–7 on the pain scale. Neuropathy/radiculopathy 7–8 on the left leg and 4–5 on the right leg.

TREATMENT PLAN

The basic plan was for a series of weekly visits with the objective of horizontalizing the pelvis to reduce uneven tension and wear in the lower back. This would occur in a logical progression from superficial to deep. Each session would be designed to deal with the most presenting symptoms while at the same time preparing her for subsequent treatments. The duration of treatment in specific areas does not have a specific dose response, but rather is dictated by "endfeel" – the pliability of the tissue and the degree of change in the patient's comfort and mobility.

First treatment: The SBL (see section titled 'Anatomy and the Fascial System') was chosen to provide immediate relief and gauge the patient's response. As the right side of the lower SBL was locked long and the left side was locked short, lengthening and differential techniques to promote glide between muscles were used on the left. Sacral multifidi treated with appropriate compression and slow nutation and counter-nutation. Given the probability of herniation, the erector spinae group was treated by putting the patient in supported spinal flexion with deep breathing providing the requisite stretch. Sub-occipitals release.

Results: While no visible changes were present, the patient reported an ease in tension.

Recommendations: The patient revealed that she still teaches hot yoga, which seems to exacerbate her symptoms. I suggested reducing the heat by 5° in the classes.

Second treatment – Subjective: The patient reported "feeling great" for 1 hour past treatment, followed by a gradual onset of symptoms. Pain remained at 6–7. She reduced the heat in the hot yoga classes by 5° and reported a 50% reduction in burning sensation post class. The patient also shared information regarding a "difficult childbirth" in 2012 when a tailgut cyst was removed post-partum. *Treatment:* Left quadriceps in a cephalad direction. Lower deep front line. Deep posterior compartment released with slow active flexion/extension of foot bilaterally. Left thigh anterior intermuscular septum treated in cephalad direction, posterior septum caudally. Right thigh septa treated cephalad and differentially to free adhesions caused by compression due to favoring. Left quadratus. Supported erector spinae. Quadratus lumborum. *Results*: While no visible changes were present, the patient reported feeling "different" with ease in overall tension.

Third treatment – Subjective report: The patient reported feeling the "best I've felt in a long time" on the first day following the previous treatment. The second day, she still felt "good" with a gradual return of symptoms, but not as intense, by Day 3. The pain was self-rated as 5–6 on the pain scale. Neuropathy/radiculopathy 5–6 on the left leg and 2–3 on the right leg. *Treatment*: Left side: pectineus, adductor longus, gluteus medius, quadratus femoris. Bi-lateral psoas with the patient going into bridge. Erector spinae and sub-occipitals.

Fourth treatment – Subjective: Overall, the patient felt "better" for most of the week. The perception of "nerve stuff" was more prevalent for the first 2 days, but had now diminished to neuropathy/radiculopathy 4–5 on the left leg and 1–2 on the right leg. *Objective*: The left pelvis was visibly less rotated and closer to horizontal. The overall pain level, especially LBP was reported at 4–5, with brief spikes to 6–7. *Treatment*: The focus was on refining left-side restrictions. Pectineus psoas tendon, obturator externus. Multifidi on both sides. AMPs were based on the pelvic clock. Erector spinae.

Fifth treatment – Subjective: Neuropathy/radiculopathy 3–4 on the left leg and 0–1 on the right leg. The left pelvis was within 7° of horizontal. LBP was reported at 2–3. *Treatment*: The focus was on the back functional line, which links the latissimus dorsi on the right with the gluteus maximus on the left via the lumbodorsal fascia. Bi-lateral psoas releases coupled with slow spinal extension. Coccygeal ligaments. Erector spinae were treated with the patient seated with AMP of slow extension while treatment proceeded caudally.

Sixth treatment – Subjective report: The patient reported a good week. Her check up with the neurologist was positive. An MRI was now considered unnecessary. *Treatment:* Peroneals, edges of the illiotibial band as necessary where adhesions to the vastus lateralis and biceps femoris were palpated. Iliac crest and quadratus lumborum, lattissimus. Bi-lateral with left side focus.

At this point, the next three treatments were scheduled 2–3 weeks apart. These last few treatments involved some fine-tuning of the previous sessions. By the end of the ninth and last treatment, the patient reported an 85%–90% improvement. She returned to the gym and resumed some light running. She is scheduled for a routine 6-month check-up.

CONCLUSION

Healthy fascia is vital to the regulation, maintenance and overall function of the human body. Improving tissue quality, hydration and function improves musculoskeletal performance, enhances metabolic uptake and restores resiliency and intracellular communication. Fascia-oriented interventions are suggested in cases of chronic pain as an alternative to surgery and/or medication. Even as this chapter goes to press a new space has just been discovered [48]. Called the interstitium, it's a contiguous, fluid-filled area of the body between the skin and muscles and organs. Lined with collagen bundles, it is analogous to the superficial fascia. There is also a continuity between the interstitium and the lymphatic system. The interstitium's primary function seems to be hydration and cellular transport, potentially opening up whole new frontiers of understanding and treating disease, as well as promoting health and wellness.

REFERENCES

1. Adstrum S. et al. (2017) Defining the fascial system. *J Bodyw Mov Ther.* 21(1):173–177.
2. Lindsay, M. (2008) *Fascia: Clinical Applications for Health and Human Performance.* Clifton Park, NY: Delmar.
3. Vuokko, K. (2002) Intramuscular extracellular matrix: Complex environments of muscle cells. *Exercise Sports Sci Rev.* 30(1):20–25.
4. Lodish, H. et al. (2000) *Molecular Cell Biology,* 4th edn. W. H. Freeman. New York
5. Stecco, C. et al. (2011) Hyaluronan within fascia in the etiology of myofascial pain. *Surg Radiol Anat.* 33(10):891–896.
6. Cretoiu, D. et al. (2016) Telocytes and their extracellular vesicles: Evidence and hypotheses. *Int J Mol Sci.* 17:1322.
7. Langevin, H. (2006) Connective tissue: A body-wide signaling network? *Med Hypotheses.* 66:1074–1077.
8. Oschman, J. (2003) Connective tissue as an energetic and informational continuum. *Struct Integration.* 31(3):5–15.
9. Grinnell, F. (2007) Fibroblast mechanics in three-dimensional collagen matrices (DVD recording). First International Fascia Research Congress, Boston, MA (online). Available: http://www.fasciacongress.org.
10. Kirkwood, J. and Fuller, G. (2009) Liquid crystal collagen: A self-assembled morphology for the orientation of mammalian cells. *ACS Biomatter Sci Eng.* 25:3200–3206.
11. Langevin, H., Stevens-Tuttle, D., Fox, J.R., and Badger, J.G. (2009) Ultrasound evidence of altered lumbar connective tissue structure in human subjects with chronic low back pain. *BMC Musculoskelet Disord.* 10:151.
12. Staubesand, J., Baumbach, K.U.K., and Li, Y. (1997) La structure fine de l'aponévrose jambière. *Phlèbologie.* 50:105–113.
13. Järvinen, T.A. et al. (2002) Organization and distribution of intramuscular connective tissue in normal and immobilized skeletal muscles. An immunohistochemical polarization and scanning electron microscopic study. *J Muscle Res Cell Motil.* 23(3):245–254.
14. Schleip, R. and Müller, D.G. (2013) Training principles for fascial connective tissues: Scientific foundation and suggested practical application. *J Bodyw Mov Ther.* 17(1):103–111.
15. Meltzer, K. et al. (2010) In vitro modeling of repetitive motion injury and myofascial release. *J Bodyw Mov Ther.* 14(2):162–171.
16. Guimberteau, J.-C. (2012) Muscle attitudes (DVD). Endovivo Productions, Pessac, France. Available www.endovivo.com.
17. Passerieux, E. et al. (2006) Structural organization of the perimysium in bovine skeletal muscle: Junctional plates and associated intracellular subdomains. *J Struct Biol.* 154:206–216.
18. van der Wal, J. (2009) The architecture of the connective tissue in the musculoskeletal system: An often overlooked functional parameter as to proprioception in the locomotor apparatus. *Int J Ther Massage Bodywork.* 2(4):9–23.
19. Huijing, P.A. (2009) Epimuscular myofascial force transmission: A historical review and implications for new research. International Society of Biomechanics Muybridge Award Lecture, Taipei, 2007. *J Biomech.* 42(1):9–21.
20. Myers, T. (1997) The "anatomy trains". *J Bodyw Mov Ther.* 1(2):91–101.
21. Myers, T.W. (2013) *Anatomy Trains: Myofascial Meridians for Manual and Movement Therapists,* 3rd edn. Edinburgh: Elsevier.
22. Myers, T. and Lesondak, D. (2010) Anatomy trains revealed; dissecting the myofascial meridians (DVD release). Singing Cowboy Productions, Pittsburgh, PA.
23. Wilke, J., Krause, F., Vogt, L. and Banzer, W. (2016) What is evidence-based about myofascial chains: A systematic review. *Arch Phys Med Rehabil.* 97(3):454–461.
24. Levin, S.M. (1981) The icosahedron as a biologic support system. *Proceedings of the 34th Annual Conference on Engineering in Medicine and Biology,* Houston, Texas, Volume 23, p. 404.
25. Levin, S.M. (2010) Biotensegrity and dynamic anatomy. Lecture (DVD). S.M. Levin, McLean, VA.
26. Kassolik, K. et al. (2013) Comparison of massage based on the tensegrity principle and classic massage in treating chronic shoulder pain. *J Manipulative Physiol Ther.* 36(7):418–427.
27. Ingber, D.E. (1998) The architecture of life. *Sci Am.* 278(1):48–57.
28. Ingber, D.E. (2003) Tensegrity I. Cell structure and hierarchical systems biology. *J Cell Sci.* 116(Pt 7):1157–1173.

29. Ingber, D.E. (2003) Tensegrity II. How structural networks influence cellular information processing networks. *J Cell Sci.* 116(pt 8):1397–1408.

30. Crane, J.D. et al. (2012) Massage therapy attenuates inflammatory signaling after exercise-induced muscle damage. *Sci Transl Med.* 4:119ra13.

31. Banes, A.J. (2012) Mechanical loading & fascial changes: Tendon focus. Plenary lecture, Third International Fascia Research Congress (Conference Proceedings DVD), Vancouver, BC.

32. van den Berg, W.B. (1998) Joint inflammation and cartilage destruction may occur uncoupled. *Springer Semin Immunopathol.* 20:149–164.

33. Boyear, N., Galey, I., and Bernard, B.A. (1998) Effect of vitamin C and its derivatives on collagen synthesis and cross-linking by normal human fibroblasts. *Int J Cosmet Sci.* 20(3):151–158.

34. Kris-Etherton, P.M. et al. (2000) Polyunsaturated fatty acids in the food chain in the United States. *Am J Clin Nutr.* 71:179S–188S.

35. Melanson, S. F. et al. (2005) Measurement of organochlorines in commercial over-the-counter fish oil preparations: Implications for dietary and therapeutic recommendations for omega-3 fatty acids and a review of the literature. *Arch Pathol Lab Med.* 129(1):74–77.

36. Sander, K. and Sanders-Gendreau, K. (2007) The college student and the anti-inflammatory diet. *Explore* 3:410–412.

37. Craig, W. (1999) Health-promoting properties of common herbs. *Am J Clin Nutr.* 70 (Suppl):491S–499S.

38. Aggarwal, B. et al. (2009) Molecular targets of nutraceuticals derived from dietary spices: Potential role in suppression of inflammation and tumorigenesis. *Exp Biol Med.* 234:825–849.

39. Beauchamp, G.K. et al. (2005) Ibuprofen-like activity in extra-virgin olive oil. *Nature.* 437:45–46.

40. Chrysohoou, C. et al. (2004) Adherence to the Mediterranean diet attenuates inflammation and coagulation process in healthy adults: The ATTICA study. *J Am Coll Cardiol.* 44:152–158.

41. Adcocks, C., Colin, P., and Buttle, D. (2002) Catechins from green tea (*Camellia sinesis*) inhibit bovine and human cartilage proteoglycan and Type II collagen degradation. *Vitro J Nutr.* 132:341–346.

42. Stecco, A. et al. (2014) Ultrasonography in myofascial neck pain: Randomized clinical trial for diagnosis and follow-up. *Surg Radiol Anat.* 36:243–253.

43. Langevin, H. et al. (2001) Mechanical signaling through connective tissue: A mechanism for the therapeutic effect of acupuncture. *FASEB.* J15:2275–2282.

44. Langevin, H. et al. (2011) Fibroblast cytoskeletal remodeling contributes to connective tissue tension. *J Cell Physiol.* 226:1166–1175.

45. Langevin, H. and Yandow, J.A. (2002) Relationship of acupuncture points and meridians to connective tissue planes. *Anat Rec.* 269:257–265.

46. Lee, A.S. et al. (2010) Comparison of trunk proprioception between patients with low back pain and healthy controls. *Arch Phys Med Rehabil.* 91(9):1327–1331.

47. Moseley, L. (2008) Tactile discrimination, but not tactile stimulation alone, reduces chronic limb pain. *Pain.* 137:600–608.

48. Benias, P.C. et al. (2018) Structure and distribution of an unrecognized interstitium in human tissues. *Sci Rep.* 8(1):4947.

22 Metabolic Approaches to the Treatment of Back Pain

Carrie Diulus, MD and Patrick Hanaway, MD

INTRODUCTION

Back pain is the most common cause of disability worldwide [1]. Back pain is among the orthopedic conditions that occur when biomechanical forces exceed the patient's metabolic wherewithal to withstand the forces, heal, and manage pain signaling. The aim of this chapter is to help healthcare providers deepen and broaden their awareness of treatable metabolic antecedents of back pain. The chapter uses the functional medicine framework to ascertain and organize patient-specific findings and implement individualized treatment strategies.

LIMITATIONS OF THE PREVAILING MODEL OF PRIMARY CARE MANAGEMENT

Back pain accounts for greater than 10% of visits to primary care physicians within the United States [2]. Despite its common nature, back pain is significantly lacking quality treatment within our healthcare system. In fact, as defined by Porter's Value Equation, the current state of treatment for spine care is classified as poor value with inconsistent outcomes, low patient satisfaction, and high costs [3].

The current practice nationwide demonstrates increased use of advanced imaging, increased use of narcotic prescriptions, and increased referrals to spine surgeons compared to the evidence-based recommendations [4]. Why is that? Outcomes research suggests that the factors driving this trend include the pressures associated with rating pain as a vital sign, improving patient satisfaction measures, and practicing defensive medicine to decrease litigation risk.

Little emphasis gets placed on exercise and movement when it comes to low back pain. The driver for this is often related to the perception that activity increases pain. Physical therapists can at times be culpable in creating this belief by not individualizing the treatment plan or responding to the patient.

Another barrier is the framework by which spine specialists understand back pain. It is reductionistic and in this way doesn't facilitate dialogue with primary care colleagues. In low back pain, we typically divide the spine into a three column structure: anterior, middle, and posterior columns. The anterior column contains the anterior paraspinal muscles, predominately the psoas in the lower back, the vertebral bodies, and the discs. The middle column is considered to contain the neurologic elements, being the spinal cord or the rootlets of the low spine and cauda equina. The posterior column includes the facet joints, the posterior longitudinal ligament, and the posterior paraspinal musculature, including the multifidus and the quadratus lumborum. Low back pain may also arise from the sacroiliac joint, coccyx, and spinopelvic ligamentous structures as well as the piriformis muscle and gluteal myotendinous structures. Each of these areas, in a reductionistic model, has its own associated pathology and inflammatory factors.

Primary care and specialists alike are faced with managing a condition which lacks objective quantification – pain. There is not a diagnostic imaging test that "shows" the pain generator. MRIs and other advanced imaging tests show structural and inflammatory changes that *may or may not be related* to a patient's symptom complex, and even when an imaging study demonstrates what is considered pathology these findings may not be at all associated with the patient's symptoms. Studies have demonstrated that as many as 90% or more of asymptomatic individuals have significant degenerative findings on MRI of the lumbar spine [5, 6]. Even when imaging study findings are associated with a patient's pain, there are often contributing factors that influence a patient's ability to have meaningful resolution of their symptoms. In many ways, the treatment of back pain is as frustrating for the provider as it is for the patient. A sense of helplessness is often felt by the provider in positively impacting the patient's pain, particularly if they focus exclusively on a structural cause and treatment approach to pain. Patients often have confounding socioeconomic issues related to substance use/abuse and employment.

THE FUNCTIONAL MEDICINE MODEL

Functional Medicine is the clinical application of systems biology. Functional Medicine sees health and illness along a continuum that changes over time. Functional Medicine improves patient health by helping clinicians to identify and reverse dysfunction in nutrition, metabolism, and behavior.

> **Definition**: Functional Medicine is a systems biology-based model that empowers patients and practitioners to work together to achieve the highest expression of health by addressing the underlying causes of disease. Functional Medicine utilizes a unique operating system and personalized therapeutic interventions to support individuals in achieving optimal wellness.

Each patient presents a unique set of environmental and lifestyle influences on function, including antecedent genetic vulnerabilities. Lifestyle choices and environmental exposures push us toward (or away from) disease by turning on and off certain genes. We evaluate these triggers and mediators of disease by considering the lifestyle choices (movement, relationships, stress, sleep, and nutrition), as well as external influences (toxins, antigens, and infections). Functional Medicine uses scientific rigor, clinical knowledge, and innovative tools to help identify underlying drivers (both triggers and mediators) of chronic disease, allowing us to reverse these clinical imbalances.

The Institute for Functional Medicine (www.ifm.org) has created innovative ways of representing the patient's signs, symptoms, and common pathways of disease. A timeline of triggers and mediators of dys*function* (symptoms and diseases) is then evaluated through the lens of the seven core clinical imbalances – assimilation, defense and repair, energy production, biotransformation, communication, transport, and structural integrity.

The principal tools for working with patients in this way include therapeutic nutritional interventions, movement, modifying stress responses, and identifying underlying sources of inflammation.

APPLYING FUNCTIONAL MEDICINE TO BACK PAIN

ANTECEDENTS

- Genetic predisposition – Single-nucleotide polymorphisms (SNPs)
  Spine providers have long been aware of genetic predisposition to degenerative changes in the spine and resultant axial back pain. Family history is an important part of the clinical evaluation for patients with back pain. Recent research has identified SNPs and other genetic factors associated with spinal degeneration, including: rs1337185 and rs1676486 in COL1A1 and rs162509 in ADAMTS5. COL1A1 is a structural gene expressed in the intervertebral disc and encodes the alpha-1 chain of type XI collagen. ADAMTS-4 and ADAMTS-5 are degradative genes in the metalloprotease family. COL1A1 SP1 (a collagen I SNP), COL9a3 Trp2 and Trp3 (a collagen IX SNP), and VDR TaqI (a vitamin D receptor

SNP) correlated with lumbar disc degeneration that is proportional to the number of mutations [7–14]. The science around the genetic factors is in its infancy – family history is an important consideration for risk. Genomic SNPs may highlight predisposition to pain, as well as response to standard therapeutic agents, including nonsteroidal anti-inflammatory drugs (NSAIDs) and opioids.

- PreNatal/EpiGenetics – Changes in gene expression or cellular phenotype caused by mechanisms other than DNA sequence. This process has been implicated in inflammation, immune dysregulation, auto-immune diseases, and cancer; though it appears to have global health implications. The primary epigenetic mechanisms are via DNA methylation and histone modification.
  - CpG islands (normally methylated) – hyper-methylation and hypo-methylation varies across different tissues and different regions of DNA, via many different DNA methyl transferases (DNMT). Methylation occurs primarily in the CpG islands, which are proximate to transcription initiation sequences, thus turning on and turning off gene expression.
    - Nutritional factors (B-vitamins, magnesium, omega-3 fats, and antioxidants) affect the production of S-Adenosyl methionine (SAMe) – an essential methyl donor. Methyl-TetraHydroFolate Reductase (MTHFR) genetic variants can affect folate availability to produce SAMe.
    - Environmental factors that affect methylation include Bisphenol A (BPA) and other organotoxins.
  - Histones – over 100 types of post-translational modifications, often acting through deacetylation to modify gene expression.
    - Polyphenols and flavonoids inhibit pro-inflammatory gene expression by downregulating pro-inflammatory cytokines such as NF-κB and "silencing" these genes via histone deacetylation so the DNA condenses and does not allow gene expression.

TRIGGERS/MEDIATORS

- Movement:
  - *Chronic sitting*: It is often felt that manual labor jobs are the most prominent occupational related cause of lower back pain. However, prolonged sitting is a substantial risk factor. An office worker may sit for the majority of their workday. Sitting has been shown to be a risk factor [15–17]. The mechanism for this has not been completely elucidated but it is proposed to be related to increased intradiscal pressure and weakening of the paraspinal musculature as well as alignment-related increased pressures on the facet joints [18]. The metabolic impact of prolonged sitting as it relates to systemic handling of glucose also plays a role.
  - *Poor biomechanics*: There are many factors that impact the biomechanics of the spine. Core strength is important for sound spinal biomechanics. These are the deep spinal muscles, not the superficially observed abdominal "six-pack." Interestingly, a patient can be very lean and have visibly defined abdominal musculature but demonstrate poor spinal muscular stability. Bracing of the back, a practice that was once thought to be protective of the spine, actually leads to weakness of the spinopelvic musculature. In addition, even those who are athletically trained may have substantial strength in the dorsal and ventral muscular planes but weakness in the lateral planes. Athletes and physical therapists often perform strength training in a neutral spine position. However, activities of life often require strength outside of those neutral spine positions (for example, a fireman pulling a morbidly obese patient out of a small bathroom after falling on a wet floor). Paired with overly tight or overly loose tendon and ligamentous structures, these imbalanced forces lead to injury.

- *Connective tissue characteristics*: Flexibility, both hyper- and hypomobility are factors in low back pain [19]. Most clinicians and patients seem to be aware of the impact of tight pelvic, quadriceps, and hamstring myotendinous structures on back pain related conditions. This is related to the pelvic and spinal alignment as well as the ability to generate force without injury through an arc of motion. Hypermobility as a factor is often overlooked and can be exacerbated when treatment focuses on increasing flexibility. Patients with limited mobility benefit from a stretching protocol. Patients who are able to touch or palm the floor with the motion should also be evaluated for other joint hypermobility.
- Relationships/ Employment:
  - *Occupation-related physical and emotional factors*: Independent of other stresses, occupational related stress and job dissatisfaction are independent risk factors for both acute and chronic back pain and should be considered in the evaluation [20].
- Stress:
  - *Psychosocial stressors*: Chronic and acute psychologic stress are linked with numerous pain syndromes. These can be focal such as migraine and back pain or more systemic such as symptom complexes that fall under the category of the diagnosis of fibromyalgia. The specific mechanisms of these associations have not yet been elucidated; however, stress plays a significant role in altering both hormones and neurotransmitters. Chronically elevated cortisol or chronic insufficiency of cortisol impacts the ability to heal an acute injury, resulting in an inflammatory cascade.
  - *Trauma/Acute injury*: Orthopedic injuries are clear causes of acute low back pain. Spinal fracture, even when healed, can change the biomechanical stresses seen within the different spinal columns and segments and this can lead to prolonged pain or remote degenerative changes. Muscle-related injury and the resulting intramuscular scarring are also factors that can contribute to axial back pain and altered spinal biomechanics. Injury, however, does not have to be as dramatic as a fracture. Improper or repetitive lifting places abnormal stresses across spinal elements and can lead to injury. Sometimes this is a muscle-related injury; however, it can also involve the facet joints and the annulus of the intervertebral disc. Annular tears are associated with inflammatory markers and are associated with an increased incidence of back pain and degeneration. Patients will often not remember the moment the "trauma" occurred or report that the pain didn't start for several days after the traumatic event. The mechanism of this delay is felt to be related to an inflammatory threshold. Patients will then report substantial muscle spasm which is intensely painful and can be debilitating. It is this muscle spasm that often causes patients to seek acute care. Under optimal conditions, acute spine-related injury goes through the acute inflammatory process, which leads to tissue healing and resolution of inflammation. There are, however, factors that can lead to impaired healing and prolonged inflammation, which can result in chronic low back pain.
  - *Hormonal factors*: Estrogen seems to play a significant role in disc degeneration. Looking at age-matched controls, young men have higher rates of radiographically identified disc degeneration than pre-menopausal women [21–25]. Post-menopausal women, however, have a higher rate of developing severe degenerative disc changes than age-matched men. There is also a higher incidence of degenerative spondylolisthesis in women who have undergone oophorectomy compared with age-matched women with functioning ovaries [26, 27]. In addition to axial back pain from spine-related disorders, women are more frequently impacted by sacroiliac joint dysfunction in the absence of a history of trauma or instrumented lumbar fusion.
- Sleep:
  - *Poor sleep*: We live in a society that is chronically sleep deprived and, in fact, sleep deprivation is often lauded as a virtue. Sleep deprivation is recognized to increase

inflammation and to increase insulin resistance! [28] Cortisol levels, growth factors, and sex-related hormones are important in healing musculoskeletal injuries. When sleep is not adequate it plays a significant role in prolonging a patient's pain [29, 30]. All patients presenting to a healthcare provider should be asked about their sleep. This includes patients undergoing spinal surgery, as insomnia has been shown to be a risk factor for both poor surgical outcome and what is classified as failed back surgery syndrome. Additionally, sleep apnea plays a significant and increasingly important role in sleep deprivation. Any patient reporting a sense of tiredness after sleeping, or whose spouse reports significant snoring, should be evaluated for sleep apnea.

- Heavy metals and OrganoToxins are environmental influences that can drive inflammation and oxidative stress. In particular, heavy metal toxicity from lead will lead to bone fragility and increased risk of degeneration [31]. Heavy metal toxins are assessed via whole blood to determine current exposure and with the use of DMSA-challenge to assess "total body burden" of heavy metals.
- *Tobacco use*: Tobacco use and smoking are both independent risk factors for back pain as well as for poor surgical outcomes from spinal surgery [32–34]. Patients are very aware of the risks associated with smoking related to the cardiorespiratory system, but often are completely unaware of the role it plays in their low back pain. There are several proposed mechanisms for this as it relates to the intervertebral disc health. In order for an intervertebral disc to remain healthy, the cells within the extracellular matrix must remain nourished and old extracellular matrix needs to be removed and replaced. A full discussion of the mechanisms around how smoking and nicotine impacts the health of the intervertebral disc is beyond the scope of this chapter, but resulting vasoconstriction and carboxy-hemoglobin production interfere with both oxygen and nutrient transport [35, 36]. As such, smoking and nicotine are both triggers for spinal degeneration as well as mediators.
- *Medications*: When looking at a patient with back pain from a comprehensive standpoint, medication use and side effects must also be taken into consideration. An increasing number of patients are being referred for spinal evaluation for low back and leg pain which upon careful evaluation is related to statin use. Statin-related myalgias have been reported to be as low as 1%–2% and as high as 10% in clinical practice [37, 38]. Patients are frequently unaware of this side effect. A drug holiday can usually be safely considered in effected patients, there will be improvement in symptoms within a week or two. In higher-risk patients, consultation with the patient's cardiologist is recommended prior to the drug holiday.
- *Antigens*: Across mucosal barriers, there are numerous ingested and inhaled antigens that generate short-term and long-term inflammatory processes. While allergens create an immediate hypersensitivity response, there are numerous other antigens that will stimulate the innate and the adaptive immune systems, creating chronic inflammation. Seventy-five percent of the immune system is located at the gastrointestinal lining – the interface between self and non-self. These antigens may also cause food sensitivities (non-celiac gluten sensitivity being most common) or food intolerances (e.g. lactose intolerance), as well as non-specific stimulation of the immune system. In addition, we are learning about the effect of food antigens on the gut microbiome. For example, an increased population of gram (−) bacteria in the small intestine will increase lipopolysaccharides (LPS) and induce inflammation via TLR4 and NF-kB.
- *Infections*: Classic infection is not a specific driver of low back pain. Rather, immune alteration due to repeated infection and/or being immunocompromised will alter immune status of the individual. Occult infections, including tick-borne illness, can have an effect on pain perception. Evaluation should be considered if history is applicable and the back pain is of a chronic, intractable, neurologic nature.

- MacroNutrient Status (Proteins, Fats, Carbs)
  - SAD ;-(= Standard American Diet
  - Diet/Insulin resistance/Diabetes

Diet plays a substantial role in low back pain through multifactorial elements. Diet provides the necessary building blocks for maintaining hormonal integrity and for healing tissues. Diet, in and of itself, can be pro-inflammatory. While the pro-inflammatory nature may not be the proximate cause of back pain, it can potentiate an inflammatory response to an injury. Elevated hsCRP is indicative of systemic inflammation and is associated with an increased incidence of low back pain [39]. Diet also impacts a patient's metabolic state and body habitus. Fat mass and fat distribution are independent risk factors for low back pain [40]. This arises from both biomechanical and systemic hormonal and metabolic factors. There is a greater appreciation that adipose tissue is a metabolically active organ rather than being viewed as a passive result of increased calorie consumption. Low levels of both leptin and monocyte chemoattractant protein-1 (MCP-1) are independently associated with back pain [41]. Excess fat and weight loss via bariatric surgery is often recommended for patients prior to spinal surgery, to improve surgical outcomes, because both diabetes and morbid obesity are independent risks factors for poor surgical outcomes and complications. Referring a patient for bariatric surgery for this purpose has been shown to decrease axial back pain prior to surgical intervention; however, it also leads to a reduction of bone mineral density and potentially impacts the ability to get a patients spine to fuse [42].

Diabetes is a risk factor for musculoskeletal-related pain. This is often overlooked as a factor in tendinopathies, such as iliotibial band syndrome and low back pain. As with other diabetic-related complications, musculoskeletal complications are related to deposition of advanced glycation end products (AGEs), which increase the brittleness of tissues [43]. Diabetes is associated with degeneration of the intervertebral disc.

Interleukin-1 beta (IL-1β) is a pro-inflammatory cytokine that has been shown to be involved in the patho-biochemistry of intervertebral disc degeneration [44, 45]. The secretion and activation of IL-1β is the result of the NLRP3-inflammasome activation. Accumulation of AGEs in intervertebral disc, in particular nucleus pulposus tissue, is an activator of the NLRP3-inflammasome [46].

Dietary fats are also known to play a role in inflammatory pathways. With the industrialization of our food supply, the ingestion of omega-3 fatty acids has decreased and we have seen a substantial increase in omega-6 fatty acid consumption. The increase in omega-6 is strongly related to the increased utilization of processed vegetable oils. Omega-3 and omega-6 compete for some of the same enzymes, with omega-3 resulting in an anti-inflammatory cascade and omega-6 resulting in a pro-inflammatory cascade. High omega-6 to omega-3 ratio is associated with increased inflammation and chronic pain. Patients with a high omega-6 to omega-3 ratio have been shown to have a higher degree of knee pain [47–49].

Briefly, the omega-6 to omega-3 ratio is a composite measure. While it can arise from a dietary excess of omega-6 alone it is usually accompanied by intake of processed *trans* fats, which impair the processing of omega-6 fats. High glucose and deficient B vitamins and zinc further impair the enzymes that process dietary fats, causing elevated triglycerides and a backlog of unprocessed dietary fats. Patients with unfavorable omega-6 to omega-3 ratios have the constellation of metabolic findings, not only high levels of lower order omega-6 fats. In fact, they tend to have a deficiency in the higher order omega-6 fats, which have anti-inflammatory properties.

- MicroNutrient Status (Minerals, Vitamins, Phytonutrients)

  Malnutrition, either in the form of protein-calorie deficit or micronutrient deficit, impacts the ability of the body to heal. A detailed discussion of each individual nutrient is beyond the scope of this chapter, but there are several that play a critical role. Ensuring adequate intake of essential amino acids is important for effective tissue healing. Vitamin C is an important factor for collagen synthesis and repair. Vitamin A also plays a notable role in skin and tissue healing. Vitamin D deficiency has been shown to be an independent risk factor for chronic low back pain as well as other pain related syndromes. As many as 82% of patients with chronic low back pain have been shown to have low vitamin D [50].

The Functional Medicine Matrix provides an operating system to evaluate imbalance and disease from a systems medicine perspective. Rather than focusing on symptoms, consideration of functional imbalances can be used to determine optimal leverage points for treatment. Symptoms and diseases express themselves through the following clinical imbalances:

ASSIMILATION

- Body lacking building blocks to heal, secondary to inability to digest/ assimilate nutrients. It is essential to evaluate altered gut function.
  DIG is a pneumonic.
- D=Digestive function
  - *Gastric acidity*: Hypochlorhydria is common when sympathetic overdrive is occurring. Evaluate with Heidelberg pH capsule.
  - *Pancreatic function*: Decreased vagal tone and villous atrophy will both decrease pancreatic excretion of digestive enzymes (proteases, lipases, amylases). Evaluate with fecal pancreatic elastase.
- I=Intestinal permeability
  - Double-sugar Lactulose Mannitol test is "gold standard"
  - Stool and serum markers of Zonulin Occludins protein are emerging
- G=Gut microbiome
  - Measure diversity of organisms present with 16s RNA probes and (emerging) metagenomic sequencing. Microbiome diversity reflects diversity in macronutrient intake and is improved by a rainbow spectrum (ROYGBIV) of fruits and vegetables.
  - Measure stool culture as an expression of growth – this primarily evaluates aerobic bacteria, but gives an indication of dysbiosis
  - Metabolic markers, such as short-chain fatty acids (SCFAs) butyrate, acetate, and propionate give an indication of functional status of the gut microbiome.
  - Note that many different combinations of organisms can create healthy gut function.

DEFENSE AND REPAIR

- Injury healing
  - A full discussion of the injury healing process is beyond the scope of this chapter. There is, however, a need to recognize that abnormalities in the pathways for inflammation, collagen deposition, and bone formation can negatively impact the body's ability to heal an acute injury, leading to chronic dysfunction, inflammation, and structural abnormality.
- Chronic inflammation
  - Osteoclastic activity is generated from chronic inflammation, regardless of its cause. Thus, chronic inflammation will affect bone density as well as bone remodeling in areas of structural stress, increasing pain, dysfunction, and structural abnormalities.

- Type 1 vs Type 3 collagen deposition
  - Typically, tendons and ligaments are primarily Type 1 collagen with small amounts of other collagens and a tissue-specific matrix. In the typical healing process, the body heals an injury in tendons and ligaments with Type 3 collagen. Under electron microscope, Type 1 collagen has long orderly fibrils with regularly spaced cross-links. Type 3 collagen has shorter fibrils and initially it is in a disorganized pattern. Over time, with the forces that are seen across the tissue, the Type 3 collagen will become more linearly oriented and cross-bridging occurs. There are many factors that can impact this, weight-bearing and mechanical stresses being two. Ultimately, the tissue dynamics of a healed tendon or ligament are not the same as the original uninjured structure, based on the different qualities of the collagen. Type 1 collagen is also the predominant collagen of the annulus fibrosus of the intervertebral disc. The intervertebral disc has a high collagen/low proteoglycan ratio. The Type 1 collagen fibrils within the annulus are obliquely orient and provide tensile strength. With injury and aging, the annulus fibrosus loses structural integrity. This may or may not be associated with an associated inflammatory reaction.
- Loss of Type 2 collagen and matrix water content
  - The nucleus pulposus is predominately collagen Type 2, 88% water and proteoglycan. This tissue is a low collagen/high proteoglycan ratio. This makeup gives the disc its compressive properties. With disc aging, there is a loss of water content and conversion to fibrocartilage. This conversion alters the compressive properties of the disc, which in turns changes the forces seen at the vertebral body endplates and across the facet joints, both of which can lead to inflammation.

ENERGY PRODUCTION/MITOCHONDRIAL FUNCTION

- Sarcopenia of aging
  - Muscle weakness places increased stresses across both anterior and posterior elements of the spinal column, which can lead to inflammatory-mediated pain within joint and ligamentous structures as well as within the muscles themselves. Sarcopenia of aging is multifactorial but contributes to significant weakness of the core stabilizing musculature. It has been shown to be associated with degenerative scoliosis and lumbar stenosis in women [51]. Sarcopenia impacts both truncal muscles and appendicular skeletal muscles. This impacts posterior pelvic tilt and, as such, changes the forces seen by the spinal elements and also places patients at increased risk for falls as well as activity-related muscle injury.
- Mitochondrial dysfunction
  - After the brain, the musculoskeletal system is the largest consumer of adenosine triphosphate (ATP) in the body. Alterations in mitochondrial function manifest as pain, weakness, and muscle loss. Mitochondrial function is influenced by oxidative stress, nutritional deficiencies (including CoQ-10), inflammation, infection, and environmental toxin exposure, as discussed previously.
- Chronic muscle contractility (spasm)
  - Muscular contractility dysfunction can be a factor in low back pain, both acutely and chronically. Patients with spasm as a primary component of their pain can describe the pain as "locking up" or that they are unable to walk or sometimes move. The natural response is to limit motion. It is fairly well accepted that limiting motion in these circumstances is counterproductive and encouraging movement and utilization of modalities and medications to assist in this provide benefit.

BIOTRANSFORMATION AND ELIMINATION (SEE TRIGGERS/MEDIATORS)

- Evaluate toxic environmental exposures
  - Heavy metals
  - OrganoToxins
  - Tobacco/Nicotine
- Optimize biotransformation pathways
  - Eliminate constipation
  - Optimize the gut microbiome
  - Provide hepatic support
  - Promote phase 1 (CYP p450) support
  - Stimulate the parallel phase 2 detoxification pathways, including methylation – increase cruciferous vegetables

TRANSPORTATION/COMMUNICATION

- Insulin resistance and diabetes
  - Advanced glycosylated end-product (AGE) accumulation
- Hormonal Imbalances
  - Chronic cortisol issues
  - Testosterone deficiency
  - Estrogen/Progesterone/Relaxin
- Unstable nerve membranes
  - Essential fatty acid imbalance (especially docosahexaenoic acid (DHA))
  - Neurotransmitter abnormality

STRUCTURAL INTEGRITY

- Sarcopenia of aging
- Muscular strength imbalances
  - Strength to stretch imbalances
- Biomechanical changes secondary to structural alignment alterations related to congenital factors and healed injury or arthritic changes
  - Congenital factors
  - Chronic inflammation
  - Healed injury and/or arthritic changes
  - Fatty replacement of multifidus and QL muscles
  - Tendon and ligament composition

THERAPIES

Traditionally, the treatments for back pain include anti-inflammatory medications, muscle relaxants, opioids, and physical therapy. In certain patients, interventional treatments such as dry needling, trigger point injections, medial branch and dorsal rami radiofrequency ablation, and even surgery can be a necessary component of a treatment strategy. Additionally, there is variable efficacy for what are often considered alternative treatments, including acupuncture, spinal manipulation massage therapy, and energy work. These treatments, when included in a robust strategy for a particular patient, do not exclude approaching a patient from a systematic perspective and, in fact, combining traditional treatments with modification of lifestyle factors can be synergistic. This approach can be more satisfying for both the patient and the healthcare provider.

MECHANISMS FOR REDUCING INFLAMMATION

Although the primary pharmaceutical treatment for musculoskeletal pain are NSAIDs, there is mounting evidence that the medications, although with some clear benefits, negatively impact the gut integrity through multiple mechanisms and increase the risk of stroke and heart attack. In many patients, NSAIDs are appropriate and can be a very useful tool in a combined approach. Non-pharmaceutical agents are also potentially useful for decreasing inflammation.

Omega-3 Oils

Omega-3 and omega-6 play an important role in modulating inflammatory pathways and the body needs both but the ratio is important [52]. Marine-based omega-3s have been shown to decrease inflammatory markers such as C-reactive protein (CRP), IL-6, and tumor necrosis factor alpha (TNF-a) [53]. High doses, upwards of 15,000 mg per day, have been shown to have a positive impact on traumatic brain and spinal cord injuries [54]. When combined with curcumin (the most potent bioactive substance found in the turmeric root) in mice with spinal cord injuries simulating cervical stenosis, the combination was found to preserve ambulatory balance and brain-derived neurotrophic factor (BDNF) levels [55]. It is frequently believed that fish oil supplementation increases the risk of bleeding; however, in a recent study in children, it failed to show an increased risk of procedure-related, bleeding even with the use of high dose IV fish oil [56].

Curcumin

Curcumin, as mentioned previously, is found in turmeric root and gives the root its vibrant orange color. It has been found to decrease inflammation by inhibiting the mediators of inflammation, including cytokines, chemokines, adhesion molecules, and Cox-2 [57–59] A randomized double-blind placebo-controlled study in patients with mild–moderate knee arthritis showed symptomatic improvement taking 500 mg of curcuminoids per day [60]. Other studies have shown significant improvement in pain and stiffness, with improved joint function [61, 62]. It may have a positive impact on rheumatoid arthritis. [63, 64] It should be used cautiously in patients taking warfarin as it can potentiate the effects.

Bromelain

Bromelain is derived from both the stem and the pineapple fruit. In Europe, it is approved for both oral and topical use. In the US, however, it is not FDA approved and is classified as a supplement. The mechanism of action is through the kallikrein–kinin pathway-lowering plasmakinin (brady-kinin) at inflammatory sites and lowers prostaglandin E2. Via the arachidonic acid (AA) pathway, it increases platelet-derived cyclic adenosine monophosphate (cAMP). It has immunomodulatory effects on T cells by inhibiting T cell signal transduction. It was shown at a dosage of 90 mg in long bone fractures to significantly reduce pain and swelling and accelerate healing compared to treatment with standard NSAIDs [65].

Alpha-Lipoic Acid

Alpha-lipoic acid (ALA) is an antioxidant that helps turn glucose into energy. It is fat- and water-soluble, unlike other antioxidants; and it is able to pass through the blood–brain barrier. ALA has been used to treat neuropathic pain, with a significant reduction in total symptom scores with 600 mg per day [66–69]. Long-term usage can lower B1 (thiamine) in some patients and supplementation to overcome this may be necessary.

B Vitamins

Neuropathies associated with deficiencies in B1, B6, and B12 are very real and often missed, particularly if a spine provider is focused on an anatomic cause for a patients symptoms. The risk of B12 deficiency is 65% higher in patients who have been on proton pump inhibitors (PPIs) for greater than two years [70]. Supplementation with a B-complex can seem relatively straightforward; however, depending on the population, approximately 28% of individuals will have difficulty processing standard B vitamin supplements because of a mutation in MTHFR. This enzyme is the rate-limiting step in the methylation process. It catalyzes the conversion of 5,10-methylenetetrahydrofolate to 5-methyltetrahydrofolate, a co-substrate for homocysteine. MTHFR variants can be identified in laboratory testing. Homocysteine levels can be measured to screen. Patients with impaired methylation can have signs of nutritional deficiencies. Eating folate-rich leafy green vegetables is recommended and if supplementation is used it should be with methyl-folate and methyl-cobalamin. A great resource is Dr. Kara Fitzgerald's eBook *Methylation Diet and Lifestyle* [71].

Diet

An elimination diet followed by a food challenge has been shown to be very helpful when attempting to uncover problem foods. Food re-challenge is typically performed after 21–28 days of "elimination" (immunoglobulin G (IgG) antigenic half-life = 23 days). IgG blood tests can support the diagnosis of food sensitivities, but there is no compelling data to prove that these tests are as efficacious as the elimination diet and challenge in identifying problem foods.

There are many types of elimination diets, ranging from very restrictive (eating only one food a day or just a few foods each day) to less restrictive (eliminating only one food or food group for a period of time). Our preferred method is a modified version of an elimination diet – avoiding common allergenic and sensitizing foods while encouraging a wide variety of foods that are less likely to cause reaction.

The Modified Elimination Diet, developed by IFM, can be a useful way to begin to identify problem foods, particularly when there is no suggestion of what foods may be connected to your chronic complaints. This dietary approach includes the elimination of gluten and dairy foods, along with pork and beef, corn, eggs, soy, peanuts, shellfish, coffee, tea, alcohol, processed grains, and refined sugars. Some practitioners may prefer the simpler elimination of only gluten or dairy foods if those particular foods are suspicious.

In addition to an elimination diet, which can potentially reduce inflammation, there are several therapeutic strategies specifically related to diet. In patients with significant insulin resistance (carbohydrate intolerance), a low carbohydrate diet can help to decrease systemic blood sugar. The body has minimum requirements for essential amino acids and essential fats, but physiologic mechanisms are in place such that there is no essential requirement for carbohydrates metabolically. That said, both soluble and insoluble fiber are carbohydrates and play an important role in maintaining a healthy gut microbiome. Additionally, constipation in and of itself, as well as gastrointestinal motility disorders, can play a role in chronic low back pain.

Low-carbohydrate diets can also be therapeutic for modulating a patient's insulin sensitivity. Normalization of blood sugar alone helps to decrease systemic inflammation. It also helps to decrease the formation of AGEs. Very-low-carbohydrate ketogenic diets potentially have anti-inflammatory benefits independent of lowered blood sugar and lower AGE production. Ketogenic diets are typically low in carbohydrates, moderate in protein, and higher in fats. The body will preferentially utilize carbohydrates as an energy source, but in the absence of carbohydrates the body can switch to metabolizing fats. When the body is metabolizing fats, either during a fasting state or in ketosis, there are three primary ketone bodies that are produced, beta-hydroxybutyrate (BHOB), acetone, and acetoacetate. A ketogenic diet can be therapeutic in that BHOB suppresses inflammation via AMPK activation, inhibiting IL-1β secretion from neutrophils and NLRP3 activation. In animal models, BHOB has been shown to relieve pain hypersensitivity in mice with spinal cord injuries and lower sensitivity to thermal pain in rats. Further studies in humans specifically related to the anti-inflammatory effects are indicated; however, given the impact on blood sugar and AGE production, a low carbohydrate diet can be a consideration for patients with metabolic syndrome and persistent back pain.

Protein intake is important to focus on as well. The protein source need not be animal-based, but a full complement of amino acids and the digestion and absorption of those amino acids are important to maintain and build muscle. Individual protein needs can vary considerably, from 0.4 g per pound in order to maintain muscle mass up to 1.0 grams per pound in certain individuals for potentially promoting fat loss through an increase in satiation and an increase in thermogenesis. Individuals over 65 also benefit from higher levels of protein in their diets. In patients who are substantially insulin resistant, protein intake may need to be limited, at least initially. The liver increases blood sugar from glycogen stores in response to protein intake and this can cause an elevation in blood sugar despite a relatively low carbohydrate intake. Protein cycling can also be of benefit in some patients, and is beyond the scope of this chapter, but during a protein-restricted "fast" mTOR action is modulated and, as seen with the use of metformin, blood sugar decreases and cell aging is potentially slowed. Interestingly, it has been demonstrated that in a pain management setting, patients on medications such as metformin have lower pain scores than those who are not [72, 73]. Chronic suppression of mTOR, however, is not a desired state from a longevity or healing perspective and, although the data is still in its infancy, there may be some benefit to utilizing dietary strategies to cycle mTOR off and on in order to promote cell autophagy while reducing sarcopenia of aging.

Sleep

It is rare to find a patient in a spine clinic with a primary complaint of back pain that sleeps well. Improving a patient's sleep primarily by focusing on sleep strategies and secondarily by reducing pain are both important. Poor sleep leads to increased cortisol levels which leads to an increase in blood sugar and subsequent elevation of AGE formation as well as having an impact on healing. Additionally, it is necessary to pass through the normal stages of sleep in adequate amounts to have needed levels of testosterone, growth factor, and other hormones that are also important in the healing process. While many of the prescription medications that are used for sleep give the perception of improved sleep, they may have a negative impact on sleep cycles, preventing sleep from playing its role in healing. Sleep hygiene is an important first strategy for improving a patients sleep (see Table 22.1).

Supplementation can be helpful in patients achieving improved sleep. The goal is not to use chemical substances to induce sleep but, rather, to augment natural systems to facilitate normal hormonal and molecular functioning.

Supplementation to improve sleep [74]:

- Magnesium
  - Supplementation of magnesium appears to improve subjective measures of insomnia, such as ISI score, sleep efficiency, sleep time and sleep onset latency, early morning awakening and, likewise, insomnia objective measures such as concentration of serum renin, melatonin, and serum cortisol, in elderly people [75].
- Vitamin D3
  - Required for making melatonin
- Melatonin
  - We advise the use of the lowest possible dose of immediate-release formulation melatonin to best mimic the normal physiological circadian rhythm of melatonin [76, 77].
- L-Tryptophan
  - Precursor to serotonin (via metabolite 5-HTP)
  - Prescription drug in Europe
  - Increases both melatonin and serotonin
  - Multiple trials with conflicting results but generally positive
- Valerian
  - Sedative effect
  - Generally recognized as safe (GRAS)

- gamma-Aminobutyric acid (GABA)
  - Doesn't cross the blood–brain barrier
  - Phenyl-GABA
    - Phenyl-GABA acts as GABA mimetic, mostly at GABA-β and to some extent GABA–α receptors
    - Stimulates dopamine receptors
    - Generally considered safe
- Phenibut (beta-phenyl-GABA) [78]
  - Neuropsychotropic drug
  - Acts as a GABA mimetic, primarily at GABA-β
  - Internationally used for pre and post-operative medication
  - Sold as a supplement in the US (not FDA approved)
  - Similar in structure to baclofen, pictured in Figure 22.1, phenibut does not have the pain-relieving properties of baclofen. Baclofen at 10–20 mg at bedtime can be an effective muscle relaxant and impact sleep in a positive way.

EXERCISE AND MOVEMENT

Patients with spine-related pain often need a different approach than those with other musculoskeletal complaints. Exercise and movement, however, can be both preventative and therapeutic. As discussed above, chronic inactivity, repetitive occupation movements, and chronic sitting play a role in lower back pain. The simple act of encouraging a patient to stand frequently and walk throughout the day can be helpful for both musculoskeletal and systemic health. Sarcopenia of aging and weak muscles from inactivity and disuse also play a significant role. Often, strengthening protocols focus on the anterior–posterior plane, which is important for spinal stability; however, there is often too little attention given to strengthening in the lateral planes. This leads to weakness of the pelvic stabilizing muscles, which leaves the spine more susceptible to injury. Additionally, physical therapy protocols most often focus on strengthening with a neutral spine. The importance of this is not to be diminished, but life and the musculoskeletal stresses of life rarely happen with a neutral spine. Encouraging exercise therapists to work to strengthen a patient in simulated real-life situations can be very helpful in preventing re-injury.

Patients are often able to find relief of back pain with less "clinical" physical movements, utilizing the practices of Pilates and yoga. Movements are illustrated in Figure 22.2. They are called Cat/Cow(a sequence), Plank, Warrior 3 to Balancing Half Moon to Standing, and Reclined spinal twist.

Both Pilates and yoga focus on breath-work in addition to the strengthening and stretch movements. This breath-work can have a profound impact on stress reduction, tolerance of pain, while

---

TABLE 22.1

Strategies for Restoring Sleep During Back Pain

- Blacken room or use a sleep mask
- Minimize nighttime distractions, pets, noise, etc.
- Reduce the room's ambient temperature
- Quit using electronics in bed
- Make a HARD bed time – and stick to it!
- Get up at the same time every day (even weekends).
- Use stress-reducing strategies, particularly prior to bed
- Exercise daily
- Decrease blue light three hours before bed
- Consider sleep enhancing supplements
- Perform sleep study, if snoring

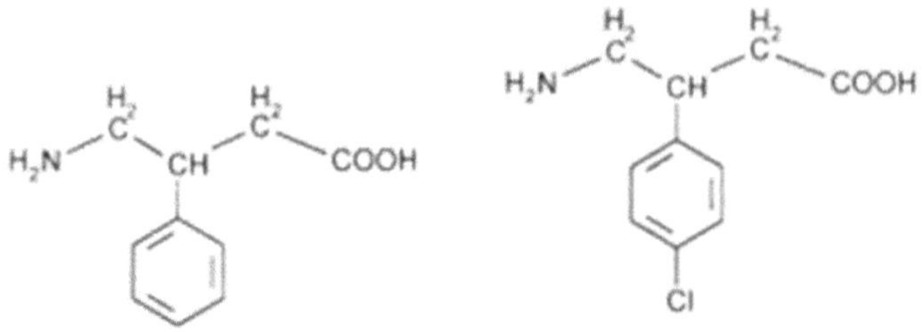

Phenibut   Baclofen

FIGURE 22.1 Baclofen and phenibut are medications similar in structure. Both can favorably impact sleep and baclofen is also effective as a muscle relaxant.

also increasing oxygen and nutrient delivery to the musculoskeletal system. The movements themselves facilitate increased blood flow. Moving through these positions with a "Vinyasa" flow style can also strengthen the smaller stabilizing muscles which are often overlooked but play a crucial role in daily movement. Alignment of the entire musculoskeletal symptom is important with regard to back pain, starting from the way the foot impacts the ground and transmits force through the knee, hip, and pelvis to the spine. The posture of the upper spine is also not to be overlooked in addressing low back pain. Patients who present in a chronic kyphotic state of their cervical and thoracic spine are transmitting forces to the lumbar spine that can have negative implications. Without addressing the entire biodynamic chain, back pain is often recurrent. While the specifics of different yoga methods and positions are beyond the scope of this chapter, there are a few that produce a particularly high yield with many patients. It is important to emphasize that transitioning from one position to the next in the sequences is as powerful as the positions themselves. Focusing on the breath during the practice increases oxygenation but can also decrease the anxiety that often accompanies back pain. "Ujjayi" breathing is a technique in which there is a slight closure of the back of the throat that provides resistance to airflow on both the inhalation and the exhalation as well as an audible sound. Slowly inhaling and exhaling through the nose while listening to the sound of the breath can increase the therapeutic benefit of these movements.

On the other side of the spectrum, there is the subset of patients who over-exercise. Over-exercise itself increases the risk of injury. It also increases systemic inflammation, increases oxidative stress, increases cortisol, and can lead to poor sleep. These can all be factors when addressing someone with chronic low back pain. Helping these patients understand the need to exercise less can be as challenging as getting other patient populations to understand the importance of moving more. It is often helpful to fill up the time that the "over-exerciser" would spend exercising with stress-relieving strategies that are very active and require attention and engagement. Heart rate variability training can be especially helpful in this patient population, providing biofeedback for stress reduction while at the same time being a goal-oriented pursuit.

REFERRING PATIENTS FOR SURGICAL EVALUATION

Fortunately, the natural history for the majority of patients with back pain is favorable. Patients can be reassured that improvement is likely. When initially assessing the patient with back pain, "Red Flag" symptoms (Table 22.2) should prompt x-ray evaluation and perhaps MRI earlier in the process. In the absence of red flag symptoms, imaging is generally unnecessary in the initial time period.

If a patient fails to improve within 6–12 weeks or develops red flag symptoms, X-rays (weight-bearing lumbar AP/lateral and flexion/extension laterals to assess for structural instability) can be obtained and advanced imaging such as an MRI may also be indicated. It is helpful for patients to

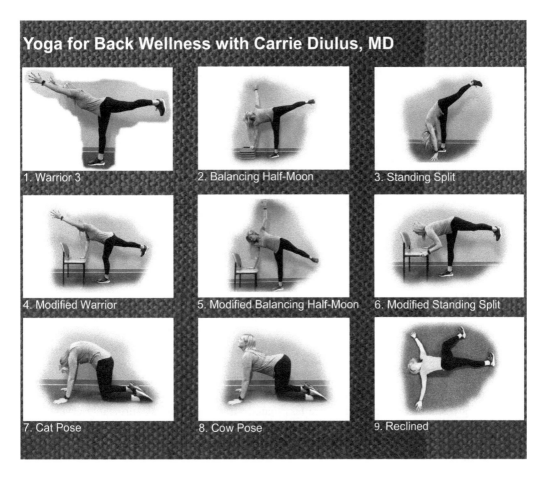

Yoga for Back Wellness with Carrie Diulus, MD

1. Warrior 3
2. Balancing Half-Moon
3. Standing Split
4. Modified Warrior
5. Modified Balancing Half-Moon
6. Modified Standing Split
7. Cat Pose
8. Cow Pose
9. Reclined

FIGURE 22.2 Progress starting with 1–3. Figures D, E, and F are the modified versions with less range of motion and using a chair or other stable object. Focus on slow deep breathing and even "Ujjayi" breathing as detailed in the text. Start with two slow breaths and progress to ten or more. Transition slowly between the three postures. Repeat on the other side. (1) Warrior 3 Focus on keeping the pelvis level to the ground. You can hold out the opposite arm to the leg that is extended or both arms. This helps to stabilize the deep posterior core spinal muscles. (2) Balancing Half Moon (can use a yoga block or balance the lower hand in the air). Turn the pelvis so that it is open with one hip on top of the other. One arm is down to stabilize on a block or suspend in the air. The elevated foot should be flexed as if pressing against a wall. This helps to stabilize the adductors on the lower leg and the obliques and abductors on the upward side and elevated leg. (3) Standing Split. Bending forward with both arms toward the ground, keep the hip of the elevated leg turned slightly out to feel a stretch in the psoas there and in the hamstring on the down leg. Strength should be felt within the gluteal muscles. (4) Modified Warrior 3, (5) Modified Balancing Half Moon, (6) Modified Standing Split. Keep the same principles listed previously but utilize a chair for stability and do not worry about limited range of motion. Both stretching and strengthening can still be felt, and focus should be on breath within the poses and moving through. (7) Cat pose: On all fours, round the neck and the back as high as possible focusing on breathing as described previously. (8) Cow Pose: Drop the lower back and look up to the sky again, breathing as described previously. Can cycle through Cat/Cow poses several times. (9) Reclined twist: Laying on the floor with both arms out-stretched. Outstretch one leg and bend the other leg up toward the chest and then allow it to roll to the opposite side. Turn the head away from the bent leg. Repeat on the other side. Figure is reproduced with permission from C. Diulus, LLC.

TABLE 22.2

**Red Flag Indicators for Diagnostic Imaging
Studies in the Work-up of Back Pain**

**Clinical Indicators for Imaging Studies in the Evaluation
of Chronic Back Pain**

- History of malignancy
- Inability to find a comfortable position
- Pain at night
- Unexplained fever
- Significant spinal trauma
- Bowel or bladder dysfunction
- Gait or balance disturbance
- Progressive weakness
- Known osteoporosis

---

have an MRI before presenting for surgical evaluation. There is a growing trend, however, for insurance providers to create barriers for primary care providers ordering spine MRIs. The rationale for this is that an MRI, given the expense, is seen as a "pre-interventional test," to be ordered by a specialist for consideration and planning of an interventional procedure. There is a growing field of *medical* spine providers, mostly trained in physical medicine and rehabilitation. The majority of these specialists are also trained to perform interventional, although not surgical, treatments. The outcomes for surgical treatment for axial back pain, particularly in the sub-acute stage, in the absence of gross structural instability, are less than desirable. In general, surgical intervention for most axial back pain is not indicated. There is a growing trend for large healthcare systems and even some insurance providers to require a patient see a medical spine provider prior to being referred to a spine surgeon.

CONCLUSION

This chapter has focused on a Functional Medicine approach to back pain. Within this approach, the primary driver of change occurs by identifying macro-nutrient, micro-nutrient, and food sensitivity requirements, providing the basis for personalized therapeutic dietary and nutritional interventions. The Functional Medicine operating system can be applied across myriad diseases. We have focused here on the specific components to consider in patients with back pain, as we have done successfully in our clinical practices. Also presented, from both a surgeon's perspective and a family practitioner's perspective, are the indications for imaging studies and surgical referral.

REFERENCES

1. Cross M et al. The global burden of rheumatoid arthritis: Estimates from the global burden of disease 2010 study. *Ann Rheum Dis.* 2014; 73(7): 1316–1322.
2. Mafi JN, McCarthy EP, Davis RB, Landon BE. Worsening trends in the management and treatment of back pain. *JAMA Intern Med.* 2013; 173(17): 1573–1581.
3. Porter ME. What is value in health care? *N Engl J Med.* 2010; 363(26): 2477–2481.
4. Zheng P, Kao MC, Karayannis NV, Smuck M. Stagnant physical therapy referral rates alongside rising opioid prescription rates in patients with low back pain in the United States 1997–2010. *Spine (Phila Pa 1976.* 2017; 42(9): 670–674.
5. Borenstein DG, O'Mara JW, Jr, Boden SD, Lauerman WC, Jacobson A, Platenberg C, Schellinger D, Wiesel SW. The value of magnetic resonance imaging of the lumbar spine to predict low-back pain in asymptomatic subjects: A seven-year follow-up study. *J Bone Joint Surg Am.* 2001; 83-A(9): 1306–1311.

6. Rajeswaran G, Turner M, Gissane C, Healy JC. MRI findings in the lumbar spines of asymptomatic elite junior tennis players. *Skeletal Radiol*. 2014; 43(7): 925–932.
7. Videman T, Saarela J, Kaprio J, Näkki A, Levälahti E, Gill K, Peltonen L, Battié MC. Associations of 25 structural, degradative, and inflammatory candidate genes with lumbar disc desiccation, bulging, and height narrowing. *Arthritis Rheum*. 2009; 60(2): 470–481.
8. Jiang H, Yang Q, Jiang J, Zhan X, Xiao Z. Association between COL11A1 (rs1337185) and ADAMTS5 (rs162509) gene polymorphisms and lumbar spine pathologies in Chinese Han population: An observational study. *BMJ Open*. 2017; 7(5): e015644.
9. Mio F et al. A functional polymorphism in COL11A1, which encodes the alpha 1 chain of type XI collagen, is associated with susceptibility to lumbar disc herniation. *Am J Hum Genet*. 2007; 81(6): 1271–1277.
10. Pockert AJ, Richardson SM, Le Maitre CL, Lyon M, Deakin JA, Buttle DJ, Freemont AJ, Hoyland JA. Modified expression of the ADAMTS enzymes and tissue inhibitor of metalloproteinases 3 during human intervertebral disc degeneration. *Arthritis Rheum*. 2009; 60(2): 482–491.
11. Stanton H et al. ADAMTS5 is the major aggrecanase in mouse cartilage in vivo and in vitro. *Nature*. 2005; 434(7033): 648–652.
12. Chen S, Huang Y, Zhou ZJ, Hu ZJ, Wang JY, Xu WB, Fang XQ, Fan SW. Upregulation of tumor necrosis factor α and ADAMTS-5, but not ADAMTS-4, in human intervertebral cartilage endplate with modic changes. *Spine (Phila Pa 1976)*. 2014; 39(14): 817–825.
13. Liu S. et al. Association between ADAMTS-4 gene polymorphism and lumbar disc degeneration in Chinese Han population. *J Orthop Res*. 2016; 34(5): 860–864.
14. Toktaş ZO, Ekşi MŞ, Yılmaz B, Demir MK, Özgen S, Kılıç T, Konya D. Association of collagen I, IX and vitamin D receptor gene polymorphisms with radiological severity of intervertebral disc degeneration in Southern European Ancestor. *Eur Spine J*. 2015; 24(11): 2432–2441.
15. Andersen LL, Mortensen OS, Hansen JV, Burr H. A prospective cohort study on severe pain as a risk factor for long term sickness absence in blue- and white-collar workers. *Occup Environ Med*. 2011; 68(8): 590–592.
16. Janwantanakul P, Pensri P, Jiamjarasrangsri V, Sinsongsook T. Prevelence of self-reported musculoskeletal symptoms among office workers. *Occup Med (Lond)*. 2008; 58(6): 436–438.
17. Gupta N, Christiansen CS, Hallman DM, Korshoj M, Carneiro IG, Holtermann A. Is objectively measured sitting time associated with low back pain? A cross-sectional investigation in the NOMAD study. *PLoS One*. 2015; 10(3): e0121159.
18. Nachemson AL. Disc pressure measurements. *Spine (Phila Pa 1976)*. 1981; 6(1): 93–97.
19. Stanitski DF, Nadjarian R, Stanitski CL, Bawle E, Tsipouras P. Orthopaedic manifestations of Ehlers–Danlos syndrome. *Clin Orthop Relat Res*. 2000; 376: 213–221.
20. Hoogendoorn WE, van Poppel MN, Bongers PM, Koes BW, Bouter LM. Systematic review of psychosocial factors at work and private life as risk factors for back pain. *Spine (Phila Pa 1976)*. 2000; 25(16): 2114–2125.
21. Gambacciani M, Pepe A, Cappagli B, Palmieri E, Genazzani AR. The relative contributions of menopause and aging to postmenopausal reduction in intervertebral disk height. *Climacteric*. 2007; 10(4): 298–305.
22. Baron YM, Brincat MP, Galea R, Calleja N. Intervertebral disc height in treated and untreated overweight post-menopausal women. *Hum Reprod*. 2005; 20(12): 3566–3570.
23. Lou C, Chen HL, Feng XZ, Xiang GH, Zhu SP, Tian NF, Jin YL, Fang MQ, Wang C, Xu HZ. Menopause is associated with lumbar disc degeneration: A review of 4230 intervertebral discs. *Climacteric*. 2014; 17(6): 700–704.
24. Lou C et al., Association between menopause and lumbar disc degeneration: An MRI study of 1,566 women and 1,382 men. *Menopause*. 2017; 24(10): 1–9.
25. Nadaud MC, McClure S, Weiner BK. Do facet joint capsular ligaments contain estrogen receptors? Application to pathogenesis of degenerative spondylolisthesis. *AmJ Orthop*. 2001; 30: 753–754.
26. Imada K, Matsui H, Tsuji H. Oophorectomy predisposes to degenerative spondylolisthesis. *J Bone Joint Surg Br*. 1995; 77(1): 126–130.
27. Cholewicki J et al., Degenerative spondylolisthesis is related to multiparity and hysterectomies in older women. *Spine (Phila Pa 1976)*. 2017; 42(21): 1643–1647.
28. Mark RO, Krueger JM. Sleep and immunity: A growing field with clinical impact. *Brain Behav Immun*. 2015; 47: 1–3.
29. Yun SY, Kim DH, Do HY, Kim SH. Clinical insomnia and associated factors in failed back surgery syndrome: A retrospective cross-sectional study. *Int J Med Sci*. 2017; 14(6): 536–542.

30. Finan PH, Goodin BR, Smith MT. The association of sleep and pain: An update and a path forward. *J Pain*. 2013; 14(12): 1539–1552.

31. Patrick L. Toxic metals and anti-oxidants: The role of antioxidants in arsenic and cadmium toxicity. *Altern Med Rev*. 2003; 8(2): 106–128.

32. Elmasry S. Asfour S, Vaccari J, Travascio F. Effects of tobacco smoking on the degeneration of the intervertebral disc: A finite element study. *PloS ONE*. 2015; 10(8).

33. Akmal M, Kesani A, Anand B, Singh A, Wiseman M, Goodship A. Effects of nicotine on spinal disc cells: A cellular mechanism for disc degeneration. *Spine*. 2004; 29: 568–575.

34. Jackson KL, 2nd, Devine JG. The effects of smoking and smoking cessation on spine surgery: A systematic review of the literature. *Global Spine J*. 2016; 6(7): 695–701.

35. Vo N et al. Differential effects of nicotine and tobacco smoke condensate on human annulus fibrosus cell metabolism. *J Orthopaedic Res*. 2011; 29: 1585–1591.

36. Homer HA, Urban JP. Volvo award winner in basic science studies: Effects of nutrient supply on the viability of cells from the nucleus pulposus of the intervertebral disc. *Spine*. 2001; 26: 2543–2549.

37. Nichols GA, Koro CE. Does statin therapy initiation increase the risk for myopathy? An observational study of 32,225 diabetic and nondiabetic patients. *Clin Ther*. 2007; 357: 1761–1770.

38. Shun-Shin MJ, Francis DP. Is this muscle pain caused by my statin? *BMJ*. 2017; 357.

39. Briggs MS, Givens DL, Schmitt LC, Taylor CA. Relations of C-reactive protein and obesity to the prevalence and the odds of reporting low back pain. *Arch Phys Med Rehabil*. 2013; 94(4): 745–752.

40. Hussain SM, Urquhart DM, Wang Y, Shaw JE, Magliano DJ, Wluka AE, Cicuttini FM. Fat mass and fat distribution are associated with low back pain intensity and disability: Results from a cohort study. *Arthritis Res Ther*. 2017; 19(1): 26.

41. Lippi G, Dagostino C, Buonocore R, Aloe R, Bonaguri C, Fanelli G, Allegri M. The serum concentrations of leptin and MCP-1 independently predict low back pain duration. *Clin Chem Lab Med*. 2017; 55(9): 1368–1374.

42. Epstein NE. Bariatric bypasses contribute to loss of bone mineral density but reduce axial back pain in morbidly obese patients considering spine surgery. *Surg Neurol Int*. 2017; 8:13.

43. Wagner DR, Reiser KM, Lotz JC. Glycation increases human annulus fibrosus stiffness in both experimental measurements and theoretical predictions. *J Biomech*. 2006; 39(6): 1021–1029.

44. Phillips KL, Cullen K, Chiverton N, Michael AL, Cole AA, Breakwell LM, Haddock G, Bunning RA, Cross AK, Le Maitre CL. Potential roles of cytokines and chemokines in human intervertebral disc degeneration: Interleukin-1 is a master regulator of catabolic processes. *Osteoarthritis Cartilage*. 2015; 23(7): 1165–1177.

45. Gilbert HT, Hoyland JA, Freemont AJ, Millward-Sadler SJ. The involvement of interleukin-1 and interleukin-4 in the response of human annulus fibrosus cells to cyclic tensile strain: An altered mechanotransduction pathway with degeneration. *Arthritis Res Ther*. 2011; 13(1): 8.

46. Song Y et al., Advanced glycation end products regulate anabolic and catabolic activities via NLRP3-inflammasome activation in human nucleus pulposus cells. *J Cell Mol Med*. 2017; 21(7): 1373–1387

47. Sibille KT, King C, et al. Omega-6: Omega-3 PUFA Ratio, Pain, Functioning, and Distress in Adults With Knee Pain. *Clin J. Pain*. 2018; 34(2): 182–189.

48. Crupi R, Marino A, Cuzzocrea S. n-3 fatty acids: Role in neurogenesis and neuroplasticity. *Curr Med Chem*. 2013; 20(24): 2953–2963.

49. Tokuyama S, Nakamoto K. Unsaturated fatty acids and pain. *Biol Pharm Bull*. 2011; 34(8): 1174–1178.

50. Ghai B, Bansal D, Kanukula R, Gudala K, Sachdeva N, Dhatt SS, Kumar V. Vitamin D supplementation in patients with chronic low back pain: An open label, single arm clinical trial. *Pain Physician*. 2017; 20(1): 99–105.

51. Eguchi Y et al., Association between sarcopenia and degenerative lumbar scoliosis in older women. *Scoliosis Spinal Disord*. 2017; 12: 9.

52. Robinson LE, Mazurak VC. n-3 Polyunsaturated fatty acids: Relationship to inflammation in health adults and adults exhibiting features of metabolic syndrome. *Lipids*. 2013; 48(4): 319–332.

53. Li K, Huang T, Zheng J, Wu K, Li D. Effect of marine-derived n-3 polyunsaturated fatty acids on C-reactive protein, interleukin 6 and tumor necrosis factor α: A meta-analysis. *PLOS ONE*. 2014; 9(2): 88–103.

54. Lei E, Vacy K, Boon WC. Fatty acids and their therapeutic potential in neurological disorders. *Neurochem Int*. 2016; 95: 75–84.

55. Holly LT, Blaskiewicz D, Wu A, Feng C, Ying Z, Gomez-Pinilla F. Dietary therapy to promote neuroprotection in chronic spinal cord injury. *J Neurosurg Spine*. 2012; 17(2): 134–140.

56. Nandivada P et al. Risk of post-procedural bleeding in children on intravenous fish oil. *Am J Surg.* 2016; 214(4): 733–737.

57. Goel A, Aggarwal BB. Curcumin, the golden spice from Indian saffron, is a chemosensitizer and radio-sensitizer for tumors and chemoprotector and radio protector for normal organs. *Nutr Cancer.* 2010; 62(7): 919–930.

58. Goel A, et al. Specific inhibition of cyclooxygenase-2 (COX-2) expression by dietary curcumin in HT-29 human colon cancer cells. *Cancer Lett.* 2001; 172(2): 111–118.

59. Goel A, et al. Curcumin as 'Cure-cumin': From kitchen to clinic. *Biochem Pharmacol.* 2008b; 75(4): 787–809.

60. Reuter S, et al. Epigenetic changes induced by curcumin and other natural compounds. *Genes Nutr.* 2011; 6(2): 93–108.

61. Panahi Y, et al. Curcuminoid treatment of knee osteoarthritis: A randomized double blind placebo-controlled trial. *Phytother Res.* 2014; 28(11): 1625–1631.

62. Belcaro G. et al., Efficacy and safety of Meriva®, a curcuin-phosphatidylcholine complex, during extended administration in osteoarthritis patients. *Alternative Med Rev; J Clin Therapuetics.* 2010; 15(4): 337–344.

63. Park C et al., Curcumin induces apoptosis and inhibits prostaglandin E(2) production in synovial fibro-blasts of patients with rheumatoid arthritis. *Int J Mol Med* 2007; 20(3): 365–372.

64. Chandran B et al. A randomized pilot study to assess the efficacy and safety of curcumin in patients with active rheumatoid arthritis. *Phytother Res.* 2012; 26 (11): 1719–1725.

65. Kamenicek V, et al., Systemic enzyme therapy in the treatment and prevention of post-traumatic and post-operative swelling. *Acta Chir Orthop Traumatol Cech.* 2001; 68: 45–49.

66. Bartkoski S, Day M. Alpha-lipoic acid for treatment of diabetic peripheral neuropathy. *Am Fam Physician.* 2016; 93(9): 786.

67. Jiang DQ, Li MX, Ma YJ, Wang Y, Wang Y. Efficacy and safety of prostaglandin E1 plus lipoic acid combination therapy versus monotherapy for patients with diabetic peripheral neuropathy. *J Clin Neurosci.* 2016; 27: 8–16.

68. Papanas N, Ziegler D. Efficacy of α-lipoic acid in diabetic neuropathy. *Expert Opin Pharmacother.* 2014; 15(18): 2721–2731.

69. Mijnhout GS, Alkhalaf A, Kleefstra N, Bilo HJ. Alpha lipoic acid: A new treatment for neuropathic pain in patients with diabetes? *Neth J Med.* 2010; 68 (4): 158–162.

70. Lam JR, Schneider JL, Zhao W, et al. Acid inhibitor use and vitamin B12 deficiency. *JAMA.* 2013; 310(22): 2435–2442,

71. Fitzgerald K., Methylation Diet and Lifestyle. 2016. Available at: https://www.drkarafitzgerald.com/our-clinic/ebook/

72. Taylor A, Westveld AH, Szkudlinska M, Guruguri P, Annabi E, Patwardhan A, Price TJ, Yassine HN. The use of metformin is associated with decreased lumbar radiculopathy pain. *J Pain Res.* 2013; 6: 755–763.

73. Taylor A, Westveld AH, Szkudlinska M, Guruguri P, Annabi E, Patwardhan A, Price TJ, Yassine HN. The use of metformin is associated with decreased lumbar radiculopathy pain. *J Pain Res.* 2013; 6: 755–763.

74. Yurcheshen M, Seehuus M, Pigeon W. Updates on Nutraceutical Sleep Therapeutics and Investigational Research. *Evidence-based Complementary and Alternative Medicine: eCAM.* 2015;105256. doi:10.1155/2015/105256.

75. Abbasi B et al. The effect of magnesium supplementation on primary insomnia elderly: A double-blind placebo-controlled clinical trial. *J Res Med Sci.* 2012; 17(12): 1161–1169.

76. Leonardo-Mendonca RC, et al. The benefit of four weeks of melatonin treatment on circadian patterns in resistance trained athletes. *Chronobiol Int* 2015; 32(8): 1125–1134.

77. Vural EM. Optimal dosages for melatonin supplementation therapy in older adults: A systematic review of current literature. *Drugs Aging.* 2014; 31(6): 441–451.

78. Lapin I. Phenibut. (Beta-Phenyl-GABA): A tranquilizer and nootropic drug. *CNS Drug Rev.* 2001; 7(4): 471–481.

23 Optimizing Metabolism to Treat Fractures and Prevent Nonunion

Jacob Wilson, MD, Scott Boden, MD,
Kenneth Cintron, MD, MBA and Mara Schenker, MD

INTRODUCTION

Fractures are a commonly encountered patient problem and, depending on the patient and the fracture characteristics, are associated with significant morbidity and in some cases mortality. In the United States alone, it is estimated that 6 million people will incur a fractured bone annually, and of those, nearly 5% (300,000) will develop delayed union or nonunion. Given this prevalence, fracture healing not surprisingly, has received significant interest. Nutrition has been shown to play a significant role in this endeavor. Additionally, the role that nutrition plays in the prevention and treatment of nonunion has now been recognized and has begun to receive attention. In this chapter, we will discuss the role that nutrition and nutrient supplementation plays in the treatment of fractures and the prevention of nonunion.

NORMAL FRACTURE HEALING

Bone is unique in that it retains its ability to heal and repair itself to produce mature bone with the restoration of pre-injury mechanical properties and strength. The process of replacing this bone, however, is complex.

The type of healing that bone undergoes relies primarily on the type of stability applied to the fracture site by orthopedic practitioners. In the setting of anatomic restoration with absolute stability (usually involving compression through the fracture site and rigid internal fixation), where very little shear stress is seen at the abutted cortical surfaces, bone will undergo primary bone healing. This process is reliant on units termed cutting cones. A cutting cone is a unit that is led by osteoclastic reabsorption of bone, followed by osteoblastic layering, which leads to osteoid deposition and bone formation. Put another way, bone resorptive cells cross the fracture to establish a new Haversian system that allows for the establishment of new blood vessels across the fracture site. These blood vessels, then, can deliver mesenchymal stem cells, which differentiate to become osteoprogenitor cells and allow for the direct repair of lamellar bone across the fracture. Again, to achieve this type of healing, rigid fixation and an adequate blood supply at the fracture site are necessary, making primary bone healing rare outside of the setting of Western medicine.[1,2]

In the setting of relative stability, where some movement at the fracture site is allowed, bone will repair by secondary bone healing, that is, there will be a cartilage intermediate. Secondary bone healing has five distinct stages: inflammation, angiogenesis and cartilage formation, cartilage calcification, cartilage removal and replacement with bone, and chronic bone remodeling.[1,3]

The initial hematoma and inflammation at the fracture site are critical. The hematoma—resulting from the disruption of blood vessels, periosteum, and surrounding soft tissue—carries with it important cytokines, growth factors, and signaling molecules that initiate and regulate the complex signaling cascade that drives initial periosteal and endosteal callus formation and repair.[4] These molecules, in conjunction with low oxygen tension at the fracture site, trigger angiogenesis and the next stage of bony reconstitution. The cascade then continues through the aforementioned stages with callus formation, the calcification of callus, conversion to woven bone, and ultimately remodeling of woven bone to lamellar bone.[1,5] For the process of callus and bone mineralization to proceed normally, calcium and vitamin D availability is critical.

The process of fracture healing is complex and requires perfect synchronization of a multitude of factors. Disruption of any of these factors at any point in this process can lead to two entities, known as delayed union and nonunion, which will be discussed going forward.

DELAYED FRACTURE HEALING

While nonunions are relatively uncommon and 90%–95% of fractures heal without incident, they do account for a significant source of patient and physician morbidity and stress.[6,7] Nonunions can be life altering and can have a devastating effect on patient quality of life.[8,9]

A nonunion may be diagnosed when fracture healing has ceased and there is no chance of bony union without further intervention.[10,11] It is worth noting that no consensus definition of nonunion has been agreed upon. Regulatory groups including the United States Food and Drug Administration (FDA) have attempted a temporal definition—a nonunion being defined as diagnosed at a minimum of 9 months, with 3 months of no visible progression of healing.[11] This, however, represents an over-simplification as certain patient factors and comorbidities can contribute to a delay in union; therefore, nonunion must be diagnosed with the specific fracture and patient factors in mind. Clinically, nonunions are marked by continued pain and pathologic motion at the fracture site. Radiographically, there will be lack of bridging bone on all four cortices,[12] persistence of lucency at the fracture site, and sometimes sclerosis on either side of the fracture. Nuclear scans, such as technetium scintigraphy, have also been shown to have reasonable sensitivity and specificity for detecting nonunions and are useful adjuncts.[13]

There are multiple types of nonunions: hypertrophic, oligotrophic, atrophic, septic, and synovial pseudoarthrosis (see Figures 23.1 through 23.3).[14] Diagnosis of the specific type of nonunion is based primarily on radiographic findings. Laboratory findings can also be helpful in the setting of septic nonunion where inflammatory markers (namely C-reactive protein and erythrocyte sedimentation rate) will be elevated.

Nonunions may occur for multiple reasons and are largely attributable to two issues: (1) biomechanics (inappropriate stability for fracture pattern) and (2) biology (vascular, infection, host factors).[15] In clinical practice, host factors are usually present as systemic medical conditions including diabetes, obesity, vascular disease, endocrinopathies, alcohol abuse, cigarette smoking/nicotine, medication adverse effects, malnutrition, and vitamin deficiencies.[10,16]

The surgical management of nonunions is an extensive topic that is beyond the scope of this chapter. Therefore, the remainder of the chapter will focus on modifiable metabolic factors for the prevention of nonunion, as intervention in this realm supplies an opportunity for the prevention of nonunion and enhanced fracture healing in otherwise compromised patients.[17]

METABOLIC FACTORS IN NONUNIONS: A SYSTEMATIC APPROACH

Likely owing to the low incidence of nonunion, there is a paucity of literature examining the effects of nutrition, vitamins, and endocrine disease on the incidence of nonunion in humans. An article in the *Journal of Orthopedic Trauma* in 2007 by Brinker et al., however, suggests that in certain patients endocrinopathies can play a critical role in the development of nonunion and, when corrected, can lead to union without further intervention.[6] In this study, 683 patients presented with nonunion over a 7 year period. Of these patients, 37 met one of the following inclusion criteria: (1) a nonunion that was unexplained and occurred despite lack of technical error on the index

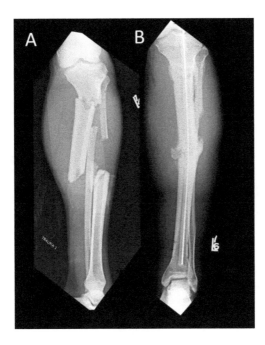

FIGURE 23.1 Radiographic appearance of a septic nonunion. (a) Patient sustained a type IIIA open, segmental tibial shaft fracture that was initially treated with an intramedullary nail. The patient subsequently began draining from his traumatic wound and he presented with elevated inflammatory markers. (b) The patient then underwent irrigation and debridement, removal of hardware and placement of antibiotic rod. He was treated with long-term IV antibiotics, but continued draining from his initial traumatic wound. This radiograph is over 1 year out from his initial injury demonstrating a septic nonunion at his midshaft tibia fracture.

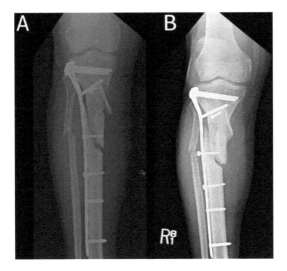

FIGURE 23.2 Radiographic appearance of an oligotrophic/atrophic nonunion. (a) Immediate post-operative films after plate and screw fixation of a comminuted proximal one-third tibial shaft fracture with intra-articular extension. (b) Follow-up imaging at 1 year post-operatively demonstrating little or no callus or bony formation at the distal aspect of the fracture.

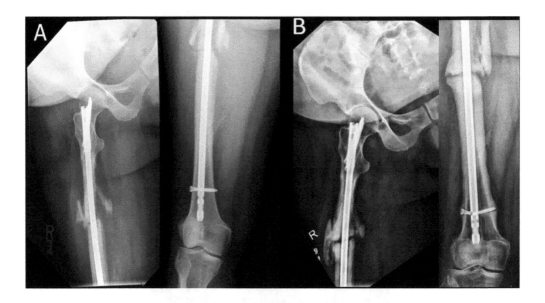

FIGURE 23.3 Radiographic appearance of a hypertrochic nonunion. (a) Anteroposterior (AP) and lateral radiographs, immediately post-operatively from an intramedullary nail of a femoral shaft fracture. (b) AP and lateral films of the same fracture 18 months post-operatively demonstrating the persistence of a lucent line at the fracture site and the classic "elephant hoof" appearance of a hypertrophic nonunion. Also seen is breakage of the distal interlocking screw with auto-dynamization of the fracture site.

operation; (2) a history of multiple low-energy fractures of which at least one did not go on to union; or (3) the nonunion of a nondisplaced pubic ramus or sacral alar fracture (26, 8, and 3 patients, respectively). Once identified as meeting the inclusion criteria, each of the 37 patients (46 fractures in total) was referred to an endocrinologist for evaluation.

The patient cohort included in the study presented at an average of 22 months post-initial injury and had already undergone an average of 2.4 operations prior to presentation. Interestingly, the nonunion sites were diverse in anatomic location and nonunion types. Oligotrophic nonunion was the most common (23 fractures) nonunion subtype, followed by atrophic (12 fractures). Infected nonunion and hypertrophic nonunion were also represented, albeit to a lesser extent (seven and four fractures, respectively). The seven patients with previously diagnosed infected nonunion had no clinical, laboratory, or radiographic signs or symptoms of active infection at the time of endocrinology referral.

Of those referred to endocrinology, 84% were diagnosed with a new metabolic or endocrine abnormality. While power was lacking, the presence of an endocrine abnormality was not significantly different between different nonunion subtypes. Not surprisingly, given the role they play in bone metabolism, vitamin D deficiency and abnormal 24-hour urine calcium were the two most common findings in 68% and 35% of endocrinology-referred patients, respectively. Other identified abnormalities included abnormal thyroid parameters (elevated/depressed thyroid-stimulating hormone [TSH], T3, T4; 24%), reproductive hormone abnormalities (22%), elevated alkaline phosphatase (16%), with others being less common. Of note, those patients who were identified as having vitamin D insufficiency (20–30 ng/mL) or deficiency (<20 ng/mL) were treated with 500 mg calcium with vitamin D 800 IU three times daily.

Impressively, 30 of the 31 patients with identified abnormalities later achieved union at an average of 9.6 months once appropriately medically treated. In addition, after medical therapy was added in accordance with test results, eight patients healed their fracture without further surgical intervention. Given the results of this study, the authors' conclusion that select patients with nonunion should be referred to an endocrinologist seems well justified. Despite this, only 7% of orthopedic surgeons report sending such patients to endocrinologists.[18]

METABOLIC BONE DISEASE

Ultimately, one in three women and one in five men over the age of 50 will have a fracture in their lifetime.[19–22] A fracture in the elderly population is not benign. Hip fractures, in particular, are associated with sobering morbidity and mortality with up to 10%–20% mortality at 1 year post-fracture.[22–26]

Research in osteoporosis and fracture care has focused on the identification of successful secondary preventative techniques. At the forefront of these techniques are nutrition supplementation and medical therapy. These therapies are primarily aimed at reducing fracture rates and also promoting fracture healing. Importantly, patients who are referred for orthopedic or trauma surgery and have previously been prescribed these medications should be assumed to have an accompanying diagnosis of metabolic bone disease.

Medical therapy for fracture prevention is also clinically useful for fracture healing.[27,28] Bisphosphonates (alendronate, risedronate, ibandronate, and zoledronic acid) all have high-quality randomized controlled trial (RCT) proven efficacy in fracture risk reduction. Zoledronic acid, given by intravenous (IV) infusion just once yearly, resulted in a decrease in vertebral fracture by 70%, hip fracture by 41%, and all nonvertebral fracture by 25%.[27,28] While the short-term benefit of bisphosphonates is well established, the long-term benefit (>5 years) seems to be attenuated.[29] Additionally, after being quickly adopted, use has declined steadily since the identification of two significant side effects: osteonecrosis of the jaw and atypical femoral fractures.[30] Hormonal therapy's use, while highly effective in the postmenopausal woman, has all but ceased for fracture prevention after the Women's Health Initiative demonstrated increased risk of breast and other gynecologic cancers with prolonged, high-dose estrogen use. Raloxifene, however, a selective estrogen receptor modulator (SERM) has been approved for the treatment of osteoporosis and decreases the risk of breast cancer concomitantly.

Other therapies—so- called "biologics"—are emerging as potential game changers in fracture prevention and are possibly as powerful for fracture healing. These therapies include denosumab, teriparatide, and the very recently developed romosozumab. Denosumab is a monoclonal antibody to RANK Ligand, and works by decreasing osteoclastic differentiation, thereby decreasing bone resorption. Teriparatide is an anabolic agent (rather than anti-resorptive), which promotes bone formation. Given this mechanism, in addition to in vivo animal data, it has a black box warning for increasing the risk of osteosarcoma. However, this has been reported only once thus far in humans. Lastly, romosozumab is a monoclonal antibody that binds and inactivates sclerostin, a protein that inhibits bone formation. Sclerostin was first discovered in 1999 and the rapid development of a clinically useful biologic in a mere 17 years has bred optimism for the future.[30]

Practitioners must be cognizant of the fact that commonly prescribed medications may alter hormone metabolism and lead to bone resorption and the propensity for delayed fracture healing and avascular necrosis (AVN). In light of this, patient medication lists must be reconciled and appropriate adjustments should be made where clinically appropriate.

VITAMIN D DEFICIENCY

That hypovitaminosis D is related to fracture is clearly not a novel concept. A case-control trial examining 41 male hip fracture patients compared to controls without fracture found that hypovitaminosis D (<50 nmol/L or approximately <20 ng/mL) was the strongest predictor for fracture and was present in 63% of the hip fracture cohort.[31] A meta-analysis, which provides perhaps the highest level of evidence available on the subject, found a hypovitaminosis D prevalence of 73% in elderly fragility fracture patients and, interestingly, 77.5% for younger, nonfragility fracture patients.[32] However, it is worth noting that there is also significant levels of hypovitaminosis D in the nonfracture population and there is some data to suggest that a drop in vitamin D levels may be normal after fracture as a hypothesized consumptive effect during fracture healing.[33]

Despite the fact that compliance remains an issue,[34] supplementation does improve serum vitamin D levels.[32] Several trials have also demonstrated an increase in bone mineral density (BMD) in acute fracture patients with vitamin D and calcium supplementation.[35,36] Another showed increased callus formation when serum calcium was within normal limits, but that supplementation does not improve BMD in these patients.[37] However, there is very little prospective data examining whether supplementation leads to more robust fracture healing or lower nonunion rates. While pilot data, presented at a national meeting, for a randomized control trial suggested that nonunion rates may be lower in vitamin D–supplemented patients (single dose: 100,000 IU),[38] the same group later presented final data that suggested no difference in the nonunion rate.[39]

Studies on vitamin D in fracture healing are underpowered. Sample sizes remain relatively small and supplementation dosing strategies have been highly variable among studies. While there is no data to suggest that vitamin D or calcium supplementation will improve fracture healing or decrease nonunion rates, in the setting of established nonunion, the appropriate medical treatment of endocrinopathies (including vitamin D deficiency) likely has virtue.[6] Until there is definitive research on the subject, patients with fracture should be appropriately advised to adopt the recommendations for the healthy population.

To that end, the United States Preventative Services Task Force (USPSTF) has recommended vitamin D supplementation along with physical therapy in those patients at high risk for falls.[40] This recommendation suggests a dose of 600 IU daily for individuals aged 51–70 years old and 800 IU daily for adults >70 years old or those at risk of fall. (For more information, please reference the USPSTF website at https://www.uspreventiveservicestaskforce.org/.)

MALNUTRITION

Malnutrition commonly affects patients with fracture, especially elderly patients with fragility fractures.[31,41] Not dissimilar to vitamin D deficiency, the definition of malnutrition in the orthopedic literature has been defined multiple ways. A variety of laboratory values (pre-albumin, albumin, total lymphocyte count [TLC]), standardized nutritional assessment scores (chiefly the Mini Nutritional Assessment),[42] and certain anthropometric measures have also been utilized.[43] The most commonly utilized parameters to indicate malnutrition include albumin <3.5g/dL and TLC (white blood cell count multiplied by percent lymphocytes) <1,500cells/mm³. While widely used, TLC has been debated and is not universally accepted as a valid nutritional parameter.[44] Other lab values that have been utilized include low pre-albumin and serum transferrin (<200mg/dL). However, there has been some concern that pre-albumin may be too sensitive a marker to serve as a useful index of nutrition.[43,45] Similarly, while anthropometric measures (namely, body mass index, arm circumference, calf circumference, and triceps skin fold) have proven useful,[45,46] no standardized cutoffs have been established.[43]

Malnutrition has been shown to have many deleterious effects on orthopedic surgery patient morbidity, mortality, and post-operative healing.[43] In the hip fracture population, poor pre-operative nutritional status has been shown to be associated with short- and long-term mortality as well as being predictive of post-operative mobility and living arrangements.[42,47] Additionally, poor nutritional parameters are significantly correlated with increased length of stay and poorer recovery of pre-fracture independence.[47] There is some evidence in this population that nutritional supplementation can ameliorate some of these effects.[48]

Pertaining more closely to this discussion, delayed wound healing and surgical site infection have been associated with poor nutritional parameters, diabetes, and obesity in the trauma, spine, and joint arthroplasty literature.[43,45] While malnutrition may classically be considered in the cachectic patient, it is important to recognize that obesity still represents a malnourished state as obese patients are typically highly deficient in important micronutrients.[49] Given that malnutrition leads to impaired wound healing and increased infection, it is easy to extrapolate that malnutrition could also lead to delayed union or nonunion in fracture patients. This was demonstrated in femoral neck fracture patients, where patients who went on to nonunion or AVN of the femoral head had significantly lower total lymphocyte counts pre-operatively than those patients with non-failed fixation. Additionally, albumin levels were also significantly lower in the nonunion cohort (but not in the AVN group).[50] Importantly, albumin and TLC were independent risk factors for nonunion after controlling for surgeon-dependent factors.[50] No similar studies exist at this time.

Protein malnutrition specifically has also been postulated to be a possible factor in delayed fracture healing.[51,52] Two amino acids, arginine and lysine, are known to stimulate osteoblastic differentiation, proliferation, and activation.[53] A study in rats, which assessed the effect of supplementing malnourished rats with fracture using conditionally essential amino acids (including glutamine, arginine, cysteine, histidine, proline, taurine, and tyrosine), demonstrated that supplementation led to callus formation with increased mineralization and better reconstitution of other nutritional parameters than did a "regular" diet.[54] This report and others suggest there may be benefit to anabolic dietary supplementation.[51,52,54]

A protein-depleted state is a common finding in patients with fracture.[55] Nitric oxide has been shown to be an important regulator in fracture repair and angiogenesis,[56,57] and its sole precursor is arginine, an amino acid. Arginine, citrulline, and ornithine are found in different levels in patients with nonunion versus those with fractures that heal. Interestingly, this varies with nonunion subtype— arginine, and other amino acid levels, are low in atrophic nonunion and elevated in those with hypertrophic nonunion.[58] While not fully elucidated, one reasonable hypothesis is that a lack of certain, necessary, amino acids may contribute to atrophic or oligotrophic nonunion. In addition, hypertrophic nonunion—while previously considered a mechanical condition—may actually have a metabolic contribution.[58] This is a notion that is also supported by the work of Brinker et al.[6] Given these findings, protein supplementation during the healing phase of fracture care could be of some benefit.

In sum, suspected malnutrition is relevant to fracture healing. Surgery, trauma, and hospitalization all increase protein demands. In the hospital setting, suspected malnutrition should prompt referral for dietician consultation and nutritional treatment. Of the various definitions for malnutrition in the US hospital setting, the consensus paper[59] that contains the recommendations from the Academy of Nutrition and Dietetics and the American Society for Parenteral and Enteral Nutrition remains a widely accepted reference standard.

For the purposes of health services analysis, mild to moderate protein calorie malnutrition is a complicating condition and severe malnutrition is a major complicating condition. When malnutrition is present, practitioners are encouraged to document this specifically in patient records. This will facilitate care and help with obtaining the needed resources to best address malnutrition, ideally, ultimately preventing delayed or nonunion.

Diabetes Mellitus

Diabetes has a multifactorial but well-established effect on bone strength and healing, and must be optimally controlled in the setting of fracture to best achieve union. Fracture healing in diabetic patients is often problematic and is delayed by up to 87%.[60] In the foot and ankle literature, diabetic patients have a higher rate of delayed union, nonunion, and pseudoarthrosis after arthrodesis.[60,61] The mechanism behind this delay in healing is multifactorial. Diabetes has a negative impact on both the micro and macrovascular systems, which can lead to decreased blood flow, and subsequently decreased oxygen and nutrient delivery, especially to distal fracture sites. The relative insufficiency of insulin and insulin-like growth factor-1 also results in the loss of an important anabolic protein. Insulin is known to increase osteoblastic proliferation and reduce its apoptosis while osteoclastic activity is reduced by insulin.[60,61] In addition, osteoblastic differentiation is inhibited by hyperglycemia.[62] Lastly, current evidence suggests that thiaziolinediones and other diabetes medications may inhibit osteogenesis.[63,64] Also pertinent to the discussion of nonunion is the fact that diabetic patients and those with poor perioperative glycemic control (even in the absence of diabetes) have a higher rate of surgical site infection.[65] For these reasons, it is of paramount importance to obtain control of diabetes in patients prior to undertaking elective surgery and in the perioperative period of fracture care to have the best chance at achieving bony union.

CIGARETTE SMOKING

Smoking and nicotine intake also have significant negative effects on wound and bone healing. While a history of smoking can also decrease the chance of union, active smokers have a higher rate of nonunion and even when union occurs, it may be delayed by up to 69%.[66–68] Smoking leads to decreased oxygen delivery in multiple ways, thereby decreasing healing potential.[69] Smoke inhalation leads to carbon monoxide binding of hemoglobin, thereby decreasing the oxygen carrying capacity, leading to peripheral tissue hypoxia.[70] Nicotine works at a molecular level by activating the anti-cholinergic anti-inflammatory pathway and is also a potent vasoconstrictor. This, in addition to the aforementioned factors, leads to local tissue hypoxia and ischemia, resulting in impaired tissue healing and repair—increasing the risk for nonunion. It is imperative that patients who smoke make every attempt at cessation, especially in the perioperative and acute fracture healing phases. Nicotine replacement strategies, while obviously better than smoking, are not ideal given the negative effects that nicotine itself has on fracture healing. Given this, medications to treat withdrawal symptoms are preferred and the hospital smoking cessation team (when available) should assist patients with nicotine dependence.

VITAMIN K

While not nearly to the extent of vitamin D, vitamin K has also received some attention with regard to its role in maintaining bone health and prevention of fractures. Vitamin K serves as a co-factor for the enzyme gamma carboxylase, which is responsible for osteocalcin carboxylation. Osteocalcin is a hormone produced by osteoblasts and functions primarily to promote bone formation and mineralization.[71,72] Only a handful of RCTs have examined vitamin K and the risk of fracture.[73–76] Unfortunately, almost all of the trials reporting on fracture rates were conducted in Japan and are of relatively low quality, bringing into question their generalizability.[76]

While small sample sizes and questions regarding quality make generalizable conclusions impossible, multiple small trials have suggested a decreased rate of fracture in vitamin K–supplemented individuals.[73,76] Others showed no difference.[74,75] However, multiple cross-sectional studies have associated a lower concentration of vitamin K1 with increased risk of hip fracture.[72] The data regarding vitamin K and its effect on BMD are conflicting, but trend toward a positive correlation.[72,74] With regard to the clinical application of vitamin K, there is a great need for large RCTs to fully elucidate the potential benefits of supplementation. In the hospital setting, vitamin K optimization should be especially encouraged in alcoholic patients as they are known to have depleted vitamin K stores. A referral to a nutritionist or dietician could be helpful in this endeavor. With regard to the nonalcoholic patient, while it seems reasonable to encourage a diet rich in vitamin K (green leafy vegetables),[76] the current paucity of literature available is not strong enough to make any conclusions or recommendations regarding supplementation.

OBESITY

Obesity has become a health pandemic in the United States.[77] Classical teaching suggests that obesity is protective with regard to fracture and bone health. However, recent evidence has begun to refine this claim.[78] While hip fractures are less common in the obese patient,[79] it seems that other fractures are more common (ankle, leg, humerus, vertebrae).[80] The interplay between obesity and bone health is extraordinarily complex and needs further elucidation. Obesity increases

BMD due to loading; however, due to metabolic disturbances, bone quality at a molecular level can be reduced, negating the theoretical biomechanical benefit of obesity. Additionally, vitamin D is lower and the parathyroid hormone is higher in obese individuals.[81,82] This should be a consideration when choosing at what dose to supplement overweight patients. Obesity, not surprisingly, also decreases mobility and increases fall risk, a known fracture risk.[83] Unfortunately, risk reduction is not as simple as weight loss, and weight loss has actually been demonstrated to increase fracture risk rather than reduce it.[84] It is imperative that clinicians recognize the risk of fracture in obese individuals and supplement and treat medically as indicated in any other patient. Unfortunately, at the current state, medical treatment for fracture prevention occurs less often in obese individuals.[85]

HYPOXIA

Decreased blood flow and compromised vascularity is a known risk factor for delayed or nonunion.[86–88] A sizable portion of this ischemic effect is attributed to not only a lack of nutrient delivery but also the drop in local oxygen tension at the fracture site.

There is scientific proof of concept that oxygen plays an important role in fracture healing.[89,90] In a rat tibia fracture model, rats who were subjected to a hypoxemic environment had delayed healing. While hypoxia did not lead to changes in stem cell differentiation, it did lead to decreased angiogenesis. In straightforward fractures (those without ischemia), hyperoxia also decreased healing relative to normoxia. However, in the setting of ischemia, hyperoxia reversed the effects of ischemia-induced delayed union, an encouraging result.[90]

There has been clinical interest in treating patients with delayed union and nonunion with hyperbaric oxygen therapy. However, a Cochrane review from 2012 failed to locate any evidence for or against its use. There are, however, multiple RCTs in progress.[91] While an extrapolation in patients with sleep apnea (leading to relative hypoxia), it seems a reasonable goal to optimize oxygen delivery in the acute fracture phase so as to avoid the detrimental effects that hypoxia has on fracture healing.

FUSION

In many ways, joint fusion (arthrodesis) is the surgical equivalent of fracture healing. This surgery is therefore prone to many of the same complications that plague fracture healing, making it pertinent to the discussion of preventing nonunion. One joint that is frequently fused is the subtalar joint. A recent study examining the causes of nonunion after subtalar arthrodesis identified the following risk factors as contributing to the formation of a nonunion or pseudoarthrosis: infection, smoking, obesity, diabetes, and alcohol use (OR 4.33, 2.97, 2.93, 1.57, 2.44, respectively). Intriguingly and not surprisingly, the same study found that the accumulation of risk factors led to an increasingly higher risk for nonunion. Specifically, those with three or more risk factors had an odds ratio of 5.5 for the development of nonunion compared to those without any risk factors.[92]

Also, similar to our earlier discussion of fracture nonunion, vitamin D status and other endocrinopathies are important risk factors that predispose to nonunion in arthrodesis patients. A recent case-control study showed that metabolic and endocrine abnormalities are significantly more common in patients who develop nonunion after an attempt at foot and ankle arthrodesis than those who go on to fuse (76% vs. 26% nonunion rate in patients with endocrine abnormality vs. those without, $P < 0.05$).[93] Vitamin D deficiency or insufficiency in particular was associated with an 8.1 times increased risk for nonunion.[93] In light of this information, in the setting of planned, elective arthrodesis, practitioners should correct endocrine abnormalities with medical intervention prior to undertaking operative intervention. Furthermore, every effort should be made to avoid surgical site infection by controlling perioperative glucose and using standard, meticulous sterile technique.

CONCLUSION

Although there is no universal consensus on the specific time frame to make a diagnosis of an established nonunion, there is clear agreement that it represents a very challenging problem to the treating orthopedic surgeon and healthcare system. A fracture or a fusion nonunion could also have devastating unintended consequences for the patient. This fact highlights the importance of avoiding this complication and prevention should start in the perioperative phase of care.

Our recommendation for the fracture or arthrodesis patient is to consider the following:

1. Metabolic and endocrine evaluation coupled with appropriate treatment by an endocrinologist. Balance of the hormonal symphony, including glycemic control, is essential.
2. Evaluation of nutrition status and referral to a nutritionist for optimization when clinically warranted.
3. If indicated, enroll the patient in a smoking cessation program with the use of medications rather than nicotine replacement strategies.
4. For overweight or obese patients with a history of fatigue or sleepiness, a comprehensive sleep assessment is warranted. Obstructive sleep apnea and its musculoskeletal manifestation are further discussed in Chapter 10.
5. For those community-dwelling adults aged 65 or older, 800 IU of vitamin D daily is recommended. This recommendation is for the general population and is for use without the guidance of laboratory testing or consideration of disease conditions. We therefore view this dose and daily frequency of vitamin D as a minimum for any patient at risk of delayed fracture healing.
6. Medications' effects on muscle and bone should be considered, so clinical decision-making can minimize adverse drug effects. In the hospital setting, proton-pump inhibitors are a commonly prescribed class of medications with a known adverse profile. They reduce stomach acid (raise pH), which reduces the absorption of calcium and protein. In turn, this has been shown to impair bone homeostasis in some patients.

While it remains impossible to identify the patient who will develop a fracture nonunion, there are known modifiable risk factors. By incorporating a multidisciplinary approach and utilizing in-hospital resources to address host risk factors, we can enhance the outcomes of our patients in the clinical setting of orthopedic trauma and fracture surgery.

REFERENCES

1. Einhorn TA. The cell and molecular biology of fracture healing. *Clin Orthop Relat Res.* 1998(355 Suppl):S7–S21.
2. McKibbin B. The biology of fracture healing in long bones. *J Bone Joint Surg Br.* 1978;60-B(2):150–162.
3. Watson JT. Fracture repair: Update on mechanism and antagonists. *Orthopaedic Knowledge Online J.* 2016;14(10):1–13.
4. Bolander ME. Regulation of fracture repair by growth factors. *Proc Soc Exp Biol Med.* 1992;200(2):165–170.
5. Giannoudis PV, Einhorn TA, Marsh D. Fracture healing: The diamond concept. *Injury.* 2007;38 Suppl 4:S3–S6.
6. Brinker MR, O'Connor DP, Monla YT, Earthman TP. Metabolic and endocrine abnormalities in patients with nonunions. *J Orthop Trauma.* 2007;21(8):557–570.
7. Lerner RK, Esterhai JL, Jr., Polomono RC, Cheatle MC, Heppenstall RB, Brighton CT. Psychosocial, functional, and quality of life assessment of patients with posttraumatic fracture nonunion, chronic refractory osteomyelitis, and lower extremity amputation. *Arch Phys Med Rehabil.* 1991;72(2):122–126.
8. Schottel PC, O'Connor DP, Brinker MR. Time trade-off as a measure of health-related quality of life: Long bone nonunions have a devastating impact. *J Bone Joint Surg Am.* 2015;97(17):1406–1410.
9. Brinker MR, Hanus BD, Sen M, O'Connor DP. The devastating effects of tibial nonunion on health-related quality of life. *J Bone Joint Surg Am.* 2013;95(24):2170–2176.

10. Brinker MR. Non-unions: Evaluation and treatment. In BD Browner, *JB Jupiter, AM Levine* (eds) *Skeletal Trauma: Basic Science, Management, and Reconstruction*, 2015; Vol. 1, pp. 637–718. Philadelphia, PA: Elsevier Saunders.

11. Cleveland KB. Delayed union and non-union of fractures. In ST Canale, JH Beaty (eds) *Campbell's Operative Orthopaedics*, 2012; Vol. 3, 12th edn, pp. 2981–3016e.2987. Philadelphia, PA: Mosby.

12. Heckman JD, Ryaby JP, McCabe J, Frey JJ, Kilcoyne RF. Acceleration of tibial fracture-healing by non-invasive, low-intensity pulsed ultrasound. *J Bone Joint Surg Am.* 1994;76(1):26–34.

13. Smith MA, Jones EA, Strachan RK, et al. Prediction of fracture healing in the tibia by quantitative radionuclide imaging. *J Bone Joint Surg Br.* 1987;69(3):441–447.

14. Megas P. Classification of non-union. *Injury.* 2005;36 Suppl 4:S30–S37.

15. Egol KA, Bechtel C, Spitzer AB, Rybak L, Walsh M, Davidovitch R. Treatment of long bone nonunions: Factors affecting healing. *Bull NYU Hosp Jt Dis.* 2012;70(4):224–231.

16. Marsh D. Concepts of fracture union, delayed union, and nonunion. *Clin Orthop Relat Res.* 1998(355 Suppl):S22–S30.

17. Schenker MLWN, Lopas L, Hankenson KD, Ahn J. Fracture repair and bone grafting. In L KCannada (ed.) *Orthopaedic Knowledge Update 11*, 2014; pp. 15–25. Rosemont, IL: Academy of Orthopaedic Surgeons.

18. Sprague S, Bhandari M, Devji T, et al. Prescription of vitamin D to fracture patients: A lack of consensus and evidence. *J Orthop Trauma.* 2016;30(2):e64–e69.

19. Melton LJ, 3rd, Atkinson EJ, O'Connor MK, O'Fallon WM, Riggs BL. Bone density and fracture risk in men. *J Bone Miner Res.* 1998;13(12):1915–1923.

20. Melton LJ, 3rd, Chrischilles EA, Cooper C, Lane AW, Riggs BL. Perspective. How many women have osteoporosis? *J Bone Miner Res.* 1992;7(9):1005–1010.

21. Birge SJ, Morrow-Howell N, Proctor EK. Hip fracture. *Clin Geriatr Med.* 1994;10(4):589–609.

22. Cummings SR, Black DM, Rubin SM. Lifetime risks of hip, Colles', or vertebral fracture and coronary heart disease among white postmenopausal women. *Arch Intern Med.* 1989;149(11):2445–2448.

23. Cummings SR, Melton LJ. Epidemiology and outcomes of osteoporotic fractures. *Lancet.* 2002;359(9319):1761–1767.

24. Magaziner J, Hawkes W, Hebel JR, et al. Recovery from hip fracture in eight areas of function. *J Gerontol A Biol Sci Med Sci.* 2000;55(9):M498–M507.

25. Chrischilles EA, Butler CD, Davis CS, Wallace RB. A model of lifetime osteoporosis impact. *Arch Intern Med.* 1991;151(10):2026–2032.

26. Fink HA, Ensrud KE, Nelson DB, et al. Disability after clinical fracture in postmenopausal women with low bone density: The fracture intervention trial (FIT). *Osteoporos Int.* 2003;14(1):69–76.

27. Black DM, Rosen CJ. Clinical practice. Postmenopausal osteoporosis. *N Engl J Med.* 2016;374(3):254–262.

28. Black DM, Delmas PD, Eastell R, et al. Once-yearly zoledronic acid for treatment of postmenopausal osteoporosis. *N Engl J Med.* 2007;356(18):1809–1822.

29. Cheung AM, Papaioannou A, Morin S, Osteoporosis Canada Scientific Advisory Council. Postmenopausal osteoporosis. *N Engl J Med.* 2016;374(21):2096.

30. Rosen CJ, Ingelfinger JR. Building better bones with biologics: A new approach to osteoporosis? *N Engl J Med.* 2016;375(16):1583–1584.

31. Diamond T, Smerdely P, Kormas N, Sekel R, Vu T, Day P. Hip fracture in elderly men: The importance of subclinical vitamin D deficiency and hypogonadism. *Med J Aust.* 1998;169(3):138–141.

32. Sprague S, Petrisor B, Scott T, et al. What is the role of vitamin D supplementation in acute fracture patients? A systematic review and meta-analysis of the prevalence of hypovitaminosis D and supplementation efficacy. *J Orthop Trauma.* 2016;30(2):53–63.

33. Ettehad H, Mirbolook A, Mohammadi F, Mousavi M, Ebrahimi H, Shirangi A. Changes in the serum level of vitamin d during healing of tibial and femoral shaft fractures. *Trauma Mon.* 2014;19(1):e10946.

34. Segal E, Zinman C, Raz B, Ish-Shalom S. Low patient compliance: A major negative factor in achieving vitamin D adequacy in elderly hip fracture patients supplemented with 800IU of vitamin D3 daily. *Arch Gerontol Geriatr.* 2009;49(3):364–367.

35. Doetsch AM, Faber J, Lynnerup N, Watjen I, Bliddal H, Danneskiold-Samsoe B. The effect of calcium and vitamin D3 supplementation on the healing of the proximal humerus fracture: A randomized placebo-controlled study. *Calcif Tissue Int.* 2004;75(3):183–188.

36. Harwood RH, Sahota O, Gaynor K, Masud T, Hosking DJ, Nottingham Neck of Femur Study. A randomised, controlled comparison of different calcium and vitamin D supplementation regimens in elderly women after hip fracture: The Nottingham Neck of Femur (NONOF) Study. *Age Ageing.* 2004;33(1):45–51.

37. Kolb JP, Schilling AF, Bischoff J, et al. Calcium homeostasis influences radiological fracture healing in postmenopausal women. *Arch Orthop Trauma Surg.* 2013;133(2):187–192.

38. Haines NMKL, Seymour R, Karunaker MA. The Effect of Acute High-Dose Vitamin D Supplementation on Fracture Union in Patients with Hypovitminosis D: A Pilot Study. Proceeding of the Orthopaedic Trauma Association Annual Meeting Tampa, FL, 2014.

39. Haines NMKL, Seymour R, Karunaker MA. Healing of Long Bone Fractures in Vitamin D Deficient Patients Treated with High-Dose Vitamin D Supplementation. Poster No. P484.Orlando, FL, 2016.

40. Bischoff-Ferrari HA, Dawson-Hughes B, Willett WC, et al. Effect of vitamin D on falls: A meta-analysis. *JAMA.* 2004;291(16):1999–2006.

41. Drevet S, Bioteau C, Maziere S, et al. Prevalence of protein-energy malnutrition in hospital patients over 75 years of age admitted for hip fracture. *Orthop Traumatol Surg Res.* 2014;100(6):669–674.

42. Helminen H, Luukkaala T, Saarnio J, Nuotio M. Comparison of the mini-nutritional assessment short and long form and serum albumin as prognostic indicators of hip fracture outcomes. *Injury.* 2017;48(4):903–908.

43. Cross MB, Yi PH, Thomas CF, Garcia J, Della Valle CJ. Evaluation of malnutrition in orthopaedic surgery. *J Am Acad Orthop Surg.* 2014;22(3):193–199.

44. Kuzuya M, Kanda S, Koike T, Suzuki Y, Iguchi A. Lack of correlation between total lymphocyte count and nutritional status in the elderly. *Clin Nutr.* 2005;24(3):427–432.

45. Guo JJ, Yang H, Qian H, Huang L, Guo Z, Tang T. The effects of different nutritional measurements on delayed wound healing after hip fracture in the elderly. *J Surg Res.* 2010;159(1):503–508.

46. Jensen JE, Jensen TG, Smith TK, Johnston DA, Dudrick SJ. Nutrition in orthopaedic surgery. *J Bone Joint Surg Am.* 1982;64(9):1263–1272.

47. Koval KJ, Maurer SG, Su ET, Aharonoff GB, Zuckerman JD. The effects of nutritional status on outcome after hip fracture. *J Orthop Trauma.* 1999;13(3):164–169.

48. Avenell A, Smith TO, Curtain JP, Mak JC, Myint PK. Nutritional supplementation for hip fracture aftercare in older people. *Cochrane Database Syst Rev.* 2016;11:CD001880.

49. Via M. The malnutrition of obesity: Micronutrient deficiencies that promote diabetes. *ISRN Endocrinol.* 2012;2012:103472.

50. Bajada S, Smith A, Morgan D. Pre-operative nutritional serum parameters as predictors of failure after internal fixation in undisplaced intracapsular proximal femur fractures. *Injury.* 2015;46(8):1571–1576.

51. Day SM, DeHeer DH. Reversal of the detrimental effects of chronic protein malnutrition on long bone fracture healing. *J Orthop Trauma.* 2001;15(1):47–53.

52. Einhorn TA, Bonnarens F, Burstein AH. The contributions of dietary protein and mineral to the healing of experimental fractures. A biomechanical study. *J Bone Joint Surg Am.* 1986;68(9):1389–1395.

53. Torricelli P, Fini M, Giavaresi G, Giardino R. Human osteopenic bone-derived osteoblasts: Essential amino acids treatment effects. *Artif Cells Blood Substit Immobil Biotechnol.* 2003;31(1):35–46.

54. Hughes MS, Kazmier P, Burd TA, et al. Enhanced fracture and soft-tissue healing by means of anabolic dietary supplementation. *J Bone Joint Surg Am.* 2006;88(11):2386–2394.

55. Patterson BM, Cornell CN, Carbone B, Levine B, Chapman D. Protein depletion and metabolic stress in elderly patients who have a fracture of the hip. *J Bone Joint Surgery Am Volume.* 1992;74(2):251–260.

56. Corbett SA, Hukkanen M, Batten J, McCarthy ID, Polak JM, Hughes SP. Nitric oxide in fracture repair. Differential localisation, expression and activity of nitric oxide synthases. *J Bone Joint Surg Br.* 1999;81(3):531–537.

57. Baldik Y, Diwan AD, Appleyard RC, Fang ZM, Wang Y, Murrell GA. Deletion of iNOS gene impairs mouse fracture healing. *Bone.* 2005;37(1):32–36.

58. Wijnands KA, Brink PR, Weijers PH, Dejong CH, Poeze M. Impaired fracture healing associated with amino acid disturbances. *Am J Clin Nutr.* 2012;95(5):1270–1277.

59. White JV, Guenter P, Jensen G, et al. Consensus statement of the Academy of Nutrition and Dietetics/ American Society for Parenteral and Enteral Nutrition: Characteristics recommended for the identification and documentation of adult malnutrition (undernutrition). *J Acad Nutr Diet.* 2012;112(5):730–738.

60. Retzepi M, Donos N. The effect of diabetes mellitus on osseous healing. *Clin Oral Implants Res.* 2010;21(7):673–681.

61. Jiao H, Xiao E, Graves DT. Diabetes and its effect on bone and fracture healing. *Curr Osteoporos Rep.* 2015;13(5):327–335.

62. Balint E, Szabo P, Marshall CF, Sprague SM. Glucose-induced inhibition of in vitro bone mineralization. *Bone.* 2001;28(1):21–28.

63. Simpson CM, Calori GM, Giannoudis PV. Diabetes and fracture healing: The skeletal effects of diabetic drugs. *Expert Opin Drug Saf.* 2012;11(2):215–220.

64. Simpson C, Jayaramaraju D, Agraharam D, Gudipati S, Shanmuganathan R, Giannoudis PV. The effects of diabetes medications on post-operative long bone fracture healing. *Eur J Orthop Surg Traumatol.* 2015;25(8):1239–1243.

65. Willy C, Rieger H, Stichling M. Prevention of postoperative infections: Risk factors and the current WHO guidelines in musculoskeletal surgery. *Unfallchirurg.* 2017;120(6):472–485.

66. Castillo RC, Bosse MJ, MacKenzie EJ, Patterson BM, Group LS. Impact of smoking on fracture healing and risk of complications in limb-threatening open tibia fractures. *J Orthop Trauma.* 2005;19(3):151–157.

67. Schmitz MA, Finnegan M, Natarajan R, Champine J. Effect of smoking on tibial shaft fracture healing. *Clin Orthop Relat Res.* 1999(365):184–200.

68. Scolaro JA, Schenker ML, Yannascoli S, Baldwin K, Mehta S, Ahn J. Cigarette smoking increases complications following fracture: A systematic review. *J Bone Joint Surgery. Am Volume.* 2014;96(8):674–681.

69. Jensen JA, Goodson WH, Hopf HW, Hunt TK. Cigarette smoking decreases tissue oxygen. *Arch Surg.* 1991;126(9):1131–1134.

70. Copuroglu C, Calori GM, Giannoudis PV. Fracture non-union: Who is at risk? *Injury.* 2013;44(11): 1379–1382.

71. Levinger I, Brennan-Speranza TC, Zulli A, et al. Multifaceted interaction of bone, muscle, lifestyle interventions and metabolic and cardiovascular disease: Role of osteocalcin. *Osteoporos Int.* 2017;28(8):2265–2273.

72. Palermo A, Tuccinardi D, D'Onofrio L, et al. Vitamin K and osteoporosis: Myth or reality? *Metabolism.* 2017;70:57–71.

73. Cheung AM, Tile L, Lee Y, et al. Vitamin K supplementation in postmenopausal women with osteopenia (ECKO trial): A randomized controlled trial. *PLoS Med.* 2008;5(10):e196.

74. Knapen MH, Drummen NE, Smit E, Vermeer C, Theuwissen E. Three-year low-dose menaquinone-7 supplementation helps decrease bone loss in healthy postmenopausal women. *Osteoporos Int.* 2013;24(9):2499–2507.

75. Kasukawa Y, Miyakoshi N, Ebina T, et al. Effects of risedronate alone or combined with vitamin K2 on serum undercarboxylated osteocalcin and osteocalcin levels in postmenopausal osteoporosis. *J Bone Miner Metab.* 2014;32(3):290–297.

76. Cockayne S, Adamson J, Lanham-New S, Shearer MJ, Gilbody S, Torgerson DJ. Vitamin K and the prevention of fractures: Systematic review and meta-analysis of randomized controlled trials. *Arch Intern Med.* 2006;166(12):1256–1261.

77. Flegal KM, Carroll MD, Ogden CL, Curtin LR. Prevalence and trends in obesity among US adults, 1999–2008. *JAMA.* 2010;303(3):235–241.

78. Shapses SA, Pop LC, Wang Y. Obesity is a concern for bone health with aging. *Nutr Res.* 2017;39:1–13.

79. Nielson CM, Srikanth P, Orwoll ES. Obesity and fracture in men and women: An epidemiologic perspective. *J Bone Miner Res.* 2012;27(1):1–10.

80. Premaor MO, Comim FV, Compston JE. Obesity and fractures. *Arq Bras Endocrinol Metabol.* 2014;58(5):470–477.

81. Drincic AT, Armas LA, Van Diest EE, Heaney RP. Volumetric dilution, rather than sequestration best explains the low vitamin D status of obesity. *Obesity (Silver Spring).* 2012;20(7):1444–1448.

82. Ekwaru JP, Zwicker JD, Holick MF, Giovannucci E, Veugelers PJ. The importance of body weight for the dose response relationship of oral vitamin D supplementation and serum 25-hydroxyvitamin D in healthy volunteers. *PLoS One.* 2014;9(11):e111265.

83. Cummings SR, Nevitt MC. Non-skeletal determinants of fractures: The potential importance of the mechanics of falls. Study of Osteoporotic Fractures Research Group. *Osteoporos Int.* 1994;4 Suppl 1:67–70.

84. Meyer HE, Tverdal A, Selmer R. Weight variability, weight change and the incidence of hip fracture: A prospective study of 39,000 middle-aged Norwegians. *Osteoporos Int.* 1998;8(4):373–378.

85. Compston JE, Watts NB, Chapurlat R, et al. Obesity is not protective against fracture in postmenopausal women: GLOW. *Am J Med.* 2011;124(11):1043–1050.

86. Dickson KF, Katzman S, Paiement G. The importance of the blood supply in the healing of tibial fractures. *Contemp Orthop.* 1995;30(6):489–493.

87. Brinker MR, Bailey DE, Jr. Fracture healing in tibia fractures with an associated vascular injury. *J Trauma.* 1997;42(1):11–19.

88. Lu C, Miclau T, Hu D, Marcucio RS. Ischemia leads to delayed union during fracture healing: A mouse model. *J Orthop Res.* 2007;25(1):51–61.

89. Lu C, Rollins M, Hou H, et al. Tibial fracture decreases oxygen levels at the site of injury. *Iowa Orthop J.* 2008;28:14–21.

90. Lu C, Saless N, Wang X, et al. The role of oxygen during fracture healing. *Bone.* 2013;52(1):220–229.
91. Bennett MH, Stanford RE, Turner R. Hyperbaric oxygen therapy for promoting fracture healing and treating fracture non-union. *Cochrane Database Syst Rev.* 2012;11:CD004712.
92. Ziegler P, Friederichs J, Hungerer S. Fusion of the subtalar joint for post-traumatic arthrosis: A study of functional outcomes and non-unions. *Int Orthop.* 2017;41(7):1387–1393.
93. Moore KR, Howell MA, Saltrick KR, Catanzariti AR. Risk factors associated with nonunion after elective foot and ankle reconstruction: A case-control study. *J Foot Ankle Surg.* 2017;56(3):457–462.

24 Treating the Underlying Causes of Synovitis, Degenerative Joint Disease and Osteoarthritis in Primary Care

John C. Cline, MD, BSc

INTRODUCTION

One of the most common conditions that family physicians and other primary care providers face in clinical practice is degenerative joint disease (DJD) or, commonly known as, osteoarthritis (OA) [1]. DJD accounts for one of the greatest causes of disability, loss of productivity, suffering, health decline and social isolation in our society [2]. DJD and OA are the result of synovitis, inflammation of the synovium, which is present often years before cartilage degeneration can be detected by imaging studies.

Western medicine's management of DJD and OA has stagnated. For several decades it has relied on symptom control [3], palliative treatments shown to sometimes accelerate the disease and eventual total joint replacement. The process is often repeated in a patient since OA tends to affect bilateral joints.

This chapter presents emerging treatments for the underlying causes of osteoarthritis. Synovitis' role in the progression of symptoms and structural changes in osteoarthritis provides an important therapeutic focus [4]. Emerging technologies provide new treatment options directed at calming key inflammatory cytokine networks such as IL-1 (interleukin-1). These therapies use the patient's own serum or activated platelets followed by the use of mesenchymal stem cells (derived from autologous adipose tissue or bone marrow) in order to boost anabolic pathways in joints and other tissues. Concurrently, new studies demonstrate that simple approaches utilizing diet, lifestyle and nutrition, calm synovitis progress in all joints and inflammatory processes throughout the body [5]. The emerging technologies and lifestyle approaches are synergistic. Together, they fundamentally shift the primary care approach to OA from management of symptoms to treatment of underlying disease with the potential for cure.

This chapter equips clinicians to translate the cross-specialty research into primary care using a clinical rubric called the Functional Medicine (FM) matrix. This approach helps the clinician to view the patient as a unique individual in terms of antecedents, triggers, mediators, modifiable lifestyle factors, clinical imbalances and so on, with web-like connections and a streamlined approach to therapy. Both emerging technologies and the FM matrix are applied to a clinical case in the primary care setting.

BACKGROUND

Osteoarthritis is a disorder involving movable joints characterized by cell stress and extracellular matrix degradation initiated by micro and macro injury that activates maladaptive repair responses including pro-inflammatory pathways of innate immunity. The disease manifests first as a molecular derangement with abnormal joint tissue metabolism. This is followed by anatomic and/or physiologic derangements characterized by cartilage degradation, bone remodeling, osteophyte formation, joint inflammation and loss of normal joint function. It ultimately culminates in illness [6].

"The synovium is a specialized connective-tissue that lines diarthrodial joints, surrounds tendons and forms the lining of bursae and fat pads. In synovial joints, the synovium seals the synovial cavity and fluid from surrounding tissues. It is responsible for the production and maintenance of synovial fluid volume and composition through the production of lubricin and hyaluronic acid. The synovial fluid aids in chondrocyte nutrition as articular cartilage has no intrinsic vascular or lymphatic supply [7]." In osteoarthritic joints, the histological pattern of the synovial lining is characterized by hyperplasia, sub-lining fibrosis and stromal vascularization [8].

The prevalence of OA of the knee, hip or hand is estimated to be 20%–30% of adults [9] with an estimated lifetime risk of developing knee OA of 40% in men and 47% in women [10]. Risk factors for OA include person-specific factors such as age [11], obesity [12], metabolic syndrome [13], sex, genetics and race/ethnicity as well as joint-specific factors related to abnormal loading of the joints such as history of injury, level of activity, occupation, leg length inequality, strength and joint alignment/flexibility [14]. The main joints affected by OA include the knees, hips, interphalangeal joints, thumb base, first metatarsal-phalangeal joints and spinal facet joints. People who suffer from OA typically develop initial symptoms in middle age with acceleration of symptoms after 50 years of age. Common symptoms include usage-related joint pain, morning- or inactivity-related stiffness and movement restriction, with rest/night pain occurring with severe OA. Common signs of OA include crepitus, joint enlargement, reduced range of motion and joint line tenderness, with muscle weakness, atrophy and joint deformity in severe OA. Joint effusions may or may not be present [15].

DIAGNOSIS

The diagnosis of OA remains clinical and may be made without radiographic or laboratory investigations [16]. OA is also a diagnosis of exclusion and the physician should rule out other forms of arthritis such as rheumatoid arthritis, psoriatic arthritis, septic arthritis, crystal arthropathies which include gout, and so on [17]. Comorbidities often exist, with examples being depression and fibromyalgia [18]. The diagnosis of the severity of OA is therefore based on quality-of-life questionnaires, physical examination and radiography [19]. A commonly used quality-of-life questionnaire is the Western Ontario and McMaster Universities Osteoarthritis Index (WOMAC), with higher scores indicating greater severity of OA [20].

In general, there is poor correlation between symptoms, disability and structural changes. Two large epidemiological studies – the Framingham Osteoarthritis Study [21] and the Osteoarthritis Initiative – demonstrated that hip pain was not present most of the time when there was radiographic evidence of hip OA. Furthermore, many of the participants with painful hips did not have radiographic evidence of hip OA. Therefore, clinicians may miss many elderly people with hip OA by solely relying on radiographic evidence [22].

The presence of synovitis can be detected with the use of ultrasound [23] or MRI (non-contrast enhanced [24] or contrast-enhanced [25]) allowing the visualization of synovial hypertrophy and synovial fluid volume. These changes correlate well with histological findings of inflammation as well as with effusion volume on arthrocentesis [26]. Ultrasound and MRI can detect effusion synovitis up to four years prior to the development of radiological changes associated with osteoarthritis [27].

There is ongoing research attempting to find biomarkers useful in the diagnosis of osteoarthritis [28]. These biomarkers fall into two classes: biomarkers of joint tissue turnover and biomarkers of inflammatory status, which include cytokines, chemokines and cell type markers important in the pathology of OA. At least 70 biomarkers are currently being researched. Unfortunately, there has been little clinical validation of these biomarkers and there remains a large, unmet medical need to identify, test, validate and qualify biomarkers for clinical use [29].

PATHOPHYSIOLOGY

Osteoarthritis results when there is an imbalance between the mechanical forces within a joint and the ability of the articular cartilage to withstand those forces. All the tissues in a joint – cartilage, bone, synovium, ligaments and adipose tissue – are involved in the osteoarthritic process. Once the tolerance of the articular cartilage to mechanical forces is exceeded, inflammatory mediators are released from chondrocytes and the synovium, which may result in the progressive loss of cartilage. Synovial macrophage activation results in the upregulation of NFkB with many cytokines being abundantly expressed and released [30]. The feed-forward, inflammatory cascade of cellular responses to injury results in inflammatory cell infiltration, which leads to erosion and fibrillation of the articular cartilage, fibrosis, subchondral bone sclerosis, synovial hyperplasia and osteophyte formation [31].

An abridged explanation of the inflammatory and reparative responses in osteoarthritis is depicted in Figure 24.1. There are at least 19 cytokine factors as well as growth factors involved in the pathogenesis and repair of joints [32]. The major pro-inflammatory cytokines are IL-1ß, IL-6, IL-15, IL-17, IL-18 and tumor necrosis factor alpha (TNF-α). The collagenase matrix metalloproteinase-13 (MMP-13) is the principal collagen-II-degrading enzyme in articular cartilage. Aggrecanases are the principal aggrecan-degrading enzymes. When these proteinases are activated, the destruction of articular cartilage progresses rapidly. The anti-inflammatory cytokines are IL-4, IL-10 and IL-13.

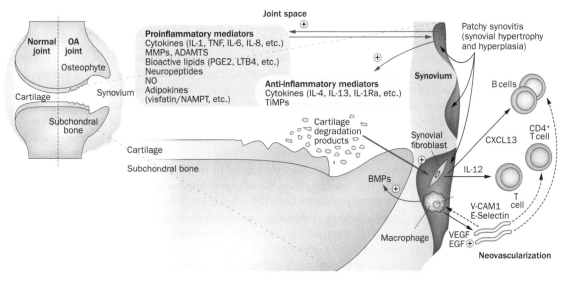

Nature Reviews | Rheumatology

FIGURE 24.1 Involvement of the synovium in OA pathophysiology. Products of cartilage breakdown released into the synovial fluid are phagocytized by synovial cells, amplifying synovial inflammation. In turn, activated synovial cells in the inflamed synovium produce catabolic and pro-inflammatory mediators that leads to excess production of the proteolytic enzymes responsible for cartilage breakdown, creating a positive feedback loop. The inflammatory response is amplified by activated synovial T cells, B cells and infiltrating macrophages. To counteract this inflammatory response, the synovium and cartilage may produce anti-inflammatory cytokines. In addition to these effects on cartilage inflammation and breakdown, the inflamed synovium contributes to the formation of osteophytes via BMPs. *ADAMTS* a disintegrin and metalloproteinase with thrombospondin motifs, *BMP* bone morphogenetic protein, *CXCL13* CXC-chemokine ligand 13, *EGF* endothelial growth factor, *IL* interleukin, *IL-1Ra* IL-1 receptor antagonist, *LTB4* leukotriene B4, *MMP* matrix metalloproteinase, *NAMPT* nicotinamide phosphoribosyl transferase (visfatin), *NO* nitric oxide, *OA* osteoarthritis, *PGE2* prostaglandin E2, *TMP* tissue inhibitor of metalloproteinase, *TNF* tumor necrosis factor, *VCAM-1* vascular cell adhesion molecule 1, *VEGF* vascular endothelial growth factor. (Reproduced with permission from Sellam J, Berenbaum F. The role of synovitis in pathophysiology and clinical symptoms of osteoarthritis. Nat Rev Rheumatol. 2010; 6(11); 625-35. Review. PMID: 20924410.)

The problem arises when the catabolic/inflammatory processes surpass the matrix anabolic/synthetic activities leading to the progressive destruction of the articular cartilage in osteoarthritic joints [33].

IL-1 was the first cytokine discovered in the 1980s [34]. It has long been considered the most potent catabolic cytokine. It coordinates systemic host defense responses to pathogens or various injuries. In the joint, it is released by synovial macrophages [35] as well as by chondrocytes [36]. It results in the downregulation of chondrocyte type II and proteoglycan synthesis. It also stimulates and enhances the release of chondrocyte-mediated cartilage destructive enzymes including matrix metalloproteinases and a disintegrin and metalloproteinase with thrombospondin motifs (ADAMTS), which is a family of peptidases (21). IL-1 has two known isoforms – IL-1α and IL-1β – and both bind to the IL-1R1 (IL-receptor type 1). IL-1α is released intracellularly upon cell death and IL-1β is considered to act as an extracellular cytokine (Figure 24.2.)

Interestingly, cells express a decoy-type, non-signaling IL-1R2 which helps to scavenge excess IL-1. As well, cells that are activated by IL-1 produce and release small amounts of the IL-1 inhibitor – IL-1Ra (receptor antagonist) – which has a downregulating effect on the IL-1 inflammatory cascade [37]. It is understood that high levels of IL-1Ra are needed to effectively balance the impact of IL-1 [38]. There is growing evidence that the introduction of IL-1Ra into joints results in significant downregulation of the inflammatory cascade [39].

CONVENTIONAL NONSURGICAL MANAGEMENT OF OSTEOARTHRITIS

Since OA of the knee is the most common presentation of osteoarthritis in clinical practice, the management will focus on this joint. The factors that influence how OA of the knee is managed are: (1) the presence of comorbidities and (2) the involvement of other joint sites. Thus, four patient groups are identified: patients with knee-only OA and no comorbidities, patients with knee-only OA with comorbidities, patients with multi-joint OA and no comorbidities, and patients with multi-joint OA with comorbidities. Comorbidities include diabetes, hypertension, cardiovascular disease, renal failure, gastrointestinal bleeding, depression or a physical-activity-limiting impairment such as obesity. The consensus-based guidelines were developed by the Osteoarthritis Research Society International (OARSI) and provide the current, evidence-based approach for family physicians and primary care providers in the management of knee OA (Figure 24.3) [40].

Looking carefully at these guidelines, it should be noted that there is no listing of intra-articular injections of hyaluronic acid. This treatment approach remains controversial, with proponents on either side. A recent systematic review concluded that "meta-analysis of only the double-blinded, sham-controlled trials with at least 60 patients did not show clinically important differences of hyaluronic acid treatment over placebo [41]."

The use of intra-articular corticosteroids has been called into question, as demonstrated in a recently published two-year, randomized, placebo-controlled, double-blind trial of intra-articular triamcinolone versus saline for symptomatic knee osteoarthritis [42]. The conclusion: "Among patients with symptomatic knee osteoarthritis, 2 years of intra-articular triamcinolone, compared with intra-articular saline, resulted in significantly greater cartilage volume loss and no significant difference in knee pain. These findings do not support this treatment for patients with symptomatic knee osteoarthritis." The problem with oral anti-inflammatory-type agents is the significant and systemic adverse effects that occur and are routinely observed by family physicians and primary care providers. The ongoing use of oral non-steroidal anti-inflammatory drugs is currently not recommended due to the resultant cardiovascular morbidity and mortality [43, 44]. Based on the current understanding of the pathophysiology of osteoarthritis, none of the recommended OARSI treatments effectively address the upregulated inflammatory cascades and are considered palliative. A potential therapeutic approach may be the use of methotrexate as it is known to have anti-inflammatory effects by suppressing the inflammatory functions of neutrophils, macrophages and monocytes, dendritic cells and lymphocytes through the release

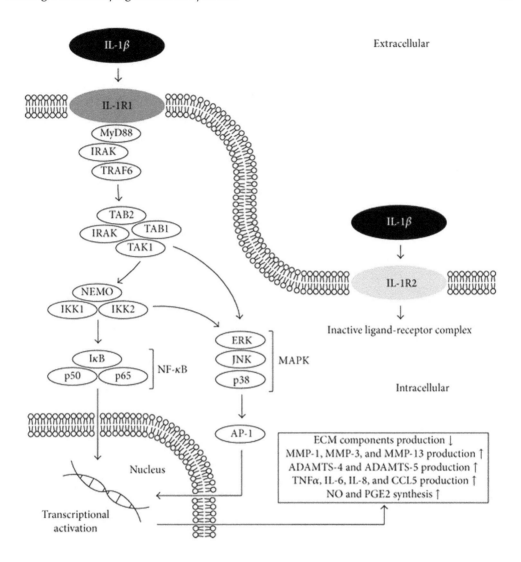

FIGURE 24.2 IL-1β associated intracellular signaling pathways and downstream cellular targets and effects. *IL-1R1* interleukin-1 receptor, type 1; *IL-1R2* interleukin-1 receptor, type 2; *MyD88* myeloid differentiation primary response gene (88); *IRAK* interleukin-1 receptor-associated kinase; *TRAF6* TNF receptor-associated factor 6; *TAK1* also known as mitogen-activated protein kinase kinase kinase 7 (MAP3K7); *TAB1* also known as mitogen-activated protein kinase kinase kinase 7 interacting protein 1 (MAP3K7IP1); *TAB2* also known as mitogen-activated protein kinase kinase kinase 7 interacting protein 2 (MAP3K7IP2); *p50, p65* subunits of proteins forming NF-κB; *IκB* (inhibitor of κB) an endogenous complex of proteins inhibiting the activation of NF-κB; *IKK1,2/NEMO* NF-κB inhibitor kinase 1,2 (IκB kinase 1,2)/NF-κB kinase inhibitor (NF-κB essential modulator); *ERK* extracellular-signal-regulated kinase; *JNK* c-Jun N-terminal kinase; *p38* p38 mitogen-activated protein kinases; *MAPK* mitogen-activated protein kinases; *AP-1* activator protein 1. (Reproduced with permission from Wojdasiewicz et al. 2014. Copyright of Piotr Wojdasiewicz.)

of adenosine. This reduces secretion of inflammatory cytokines including tumor necrosis factor-alpha and interleukin-6. A recently published, small, open-label pilot study of 30 patients with knee osteoarthritis who took methotrexate 15–20 mg/week for six months suggested an analgesic benefit [45]. Finally, these OARSI guidelines make no mention of one of the most important and foundational treatment approaches as taught by Hippocrates including lifestyle approaches such as "Let Food Be Thy Medicine."

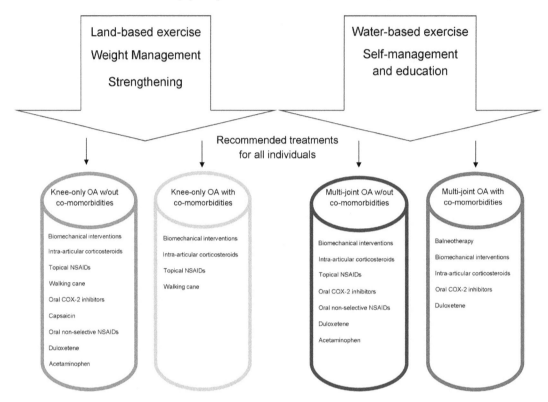

FIGURE 24.3 Osteoarthritis Research Society International guidelines for the non-surgical management of knee osteoarthritis.

FUNCTIONAL MEDICINE

Using a focus on food to modulate the highly complex cascades of the inflammatory orchestra is now a scientifically proven approach to the treatment of OA. The uptake of food interventions in primary care, however, remains poor. A major barrier is the perceived difficulty in incorporating food and other lifestyle approaches into the current models of health care delivery.

Functional Medicine is a personalized, systems-oriented model that empowers patients and practitioners to achieve the highest expression of health by working in collaboration to address the underlying causes of what we call disease [46]. The Institute for Functional Medicine has developed tools to help the clinician think critically about complex health problems. One of these tools – the Functional Medicine Matrix – is a one-page graphic representation of the Functional Medicine approach (Figure 24.4) [47].

The matrix allows clinicians to look carefully at the seven organizing physiological systems (clinical imbalances) in relationship to the: antecedents (factors that predispose the patient to acute or chronic illness), triggers (discrete entities or events that provoke disease or symptoms) and mediators (factors that contribute to the ongoing manifestations of disease). The foundational, personalized lifestyle factors are also reviewed along with the central emotional, mental and spiritual aspects of the individual patient. The FM matrix allows the clinician to think about, and organize, the web-like connections between the various components. Besides being an exceptional tool for critical thinking, the matrix also forces the clinician to think outside of his or her particular area of interest or expertise.

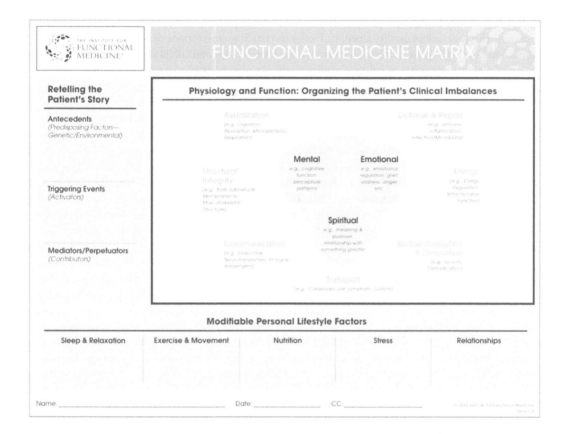

FIGURE 24.4 The Functional Medicine Matrix. (Reproduced with permission from the Institute of Functional Medicine. Copyright of Institute of Functional Medicine.)

LIFESTYLE MODIFICATION

In approaching a chronic disorder like OA it is easy to forget that OA is part of a whole system that may be inflamed or "on fire." There may be a number of antecedent factors that set the patient up to develop osteoarthritis. Examples could be a genetic predisposition, a history of trauma, consuming foods that the patient's system reacts to (such as nightshades, gluten, excess simple sugars, etc.), overuse of antibiotics in childhood resulting in gastrointestinal microbiome alteration, chronic consumption of anti-inflammatory or analgesic medications leading to a breakdown in the integrity of the gastrointestinal lining, certain toxic influences with previous or ongoing exposures to heavy metals or persistent organic pollutants or biotoxins (related to borrelia and coinfections such as bartonella; mycotoxins from fungal overgrowths, chronic dental infections, chronic parasitic illness, etc.) and so on. Triggering events or "tipping points" could include traumatic incidents, repetitive overuse of joints, infections and even toxic emotional events. A common antecedent, trigger and mediator for OA is ongoing obesity, which is an important modifiable factor when it comes to addressing OA [48, 49]. Other mediators of inflammation could include the ongoing consumption of unique foods or beverages that the individual patient is reacting to, a lack of anti-inflammatory foods, herbs and spices in the diet, overuse or misuse of joints, ongoing biotoxin exposure from overgrowths of certain organisms in the microbiome, ongoing exposure to other toxic influences such as heavy metals, chemicals, etc. and so on. When formulating a treatment approach for OA it is important to think in terms of an anti-inflammatory lifestyle.

Thinking through the antecedents, triggers and mediators in each individual patient along with looking carefully at the clinical imbalances seen in the seven physiological systems, the personal lifestyle factors and finally the emotional, mental and spiritual core, will enable the clinician to develop an anti-inflammatory lifestyle program that is unique for each patient. The most common areas affecting osteoarthritis are: lack of quality sleep, lack of or too much exercise, poor diet and nutrition, too much stress and poor coping mechanisms for stress, poor relationships and social support, ongoing dysregulation of mental, emotional or spiritual components, elevated body burdens of toxic metals/chemicals with ongoing exposures to toxicants, ongoing smoldering infections including dental infections and intestinal dysbiosis, obesity with insulin dysregulation and ongoing allergy dysregulation.

One of the most important areas to focus on initially is a careful look at the diet and nutrition as well as the gastrointestinal health of the individual patient. Referring back to the FM matrix, diet and nutrition are at the center of the personalized lifestyle factors. By adjusting this one area, all of the other facets of the matrix are affected through the web-like connections. A simple and profound way to help patients discover which foods or beverages are upregulating the inflammatory cascades is to have them go through the FM Comprehensive Elimination Diet [50]. This is a foundational step towards health recovery that should not be skipped. It is an important tool that allows patients to become their own "medical detectives" and to discover for themselves which foods and/or beverages are triggering and mediating inflammation in general and, specifically, in their joints. This approach takes approximately 4–6 weeks and is a step-by-step, methodical elimination and then reintroduction of various food families. Foods to remove include: corn, dairy, eggs, gluten, simple processed sugars, shellfish, soy, beef, pork, processed meats, coffee, tea, chocolate and nightshades (tomato, white potato, bell peppers, eggplant, goji berries, ashwagandha and tobacco). Foods to include: fruits, healthy oils, lean meats, legumes, nuts, seeds, vegetables and non-gluten grains. One aspect of the FM Comprehensive Elimination Diet is that instead of just giving patients lists of foods, companion recipes are available to make it easier to implement change. This program is given to the patient on the first visit and gives them "homework" to do prior to the second visit which is usually six weeks later. This program helps to engage the patient and, when they discover for themselves the link between consumption of foods/beverages and joint inflammation, they become empowered and are much more likely to eliminate these triggers and mediators on an ongoing basis. Usually, by the second visit, patients observe improvement in their inflammatory symptoms and are then more likely to go on with the other components of the anti-inflammatory lifestyle.

Food and nutrients can also be strategically added to the diet for inflammation-modulating properties. For example, among patients whose food was prepared primarily with processed vegetable oil, extra virgin olive oil was shown to significantly reduce joint edema as well as cartilage destruction by downregulation of pro-inflammatory cytokines such as TNF-α, IL-1β and IL-17 [51]. Piperine from black pepper has a downregulating effect on IL-1β in human osteoarthritis chondrocytes [52]. Piperine also increases the bioavailability of curcumin [53]. *Cordyceps*, a genus of ascomycete fungi, has a similar effect on downregulating IL-1β [54]. It is available in a number of brands such as Cordysen™ or Vitacost® (500 mg capsule daily).

The spice turmeric with its active ingredient curcumin has been used in Ayurvedic medicine for over 4000 years. It is the rhizome of the plant *Curcuma longa* and contains over 20 different active compounds with the most prevalent being the curcuminoids [55]. Curcumin modifies over 80 molecular targets involved in the inflammatory orchestra (Figure 24.5) [56].

A recent randomized controlled trial [57] studied the effects of taking 1 g per day of an oral curcumin formulation (curcumin plus phosphatidylcholine, for better absorption) over eight months. The 50 patients in the treatment group had a >50% decrease in WOMAC score and a threefold increase in treadmill walking distance as compared to the control group. Inflammatory biomarkers such as serum IL-1β, IL-6, soluble CD-40 ligand, soluble VCAM-1 and erythrocyte sedimentation rate (ESR) were significantly decreased in the treatment group. Furthermore, the treatment group experienced decreased gastrointestinal complications, lower limb edema and decreased use of NSAIDS)/analgesics as compared to the control group. Finally, the need for hospital admissions, consultations and laboratory tests were significantly decreased in the treatment group.

Over the years, there has been interest in the use of glucosamine and/or chondroitin as a nutriceutical approach for treating OA. A recent update review concluded that the use of glucosamine/chondroitin has shown inconsistent beneficial effects in large, multi-site placebo-controlled and head-to-head trials [58].

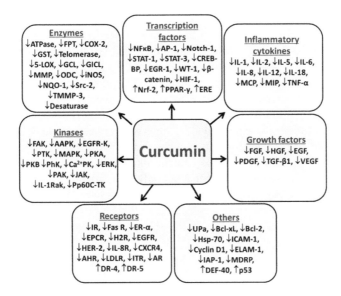

Enzymes
↓ATPase, ↓FPT, ↓COX-2, ↓GST, ↓Telomerase, ↓5-LOX, ↓GCL, ↓GICL, ↓MMP, ↓ODC, ↓iNOS, ↓NQO-1, ↓Src-2, ↓TMMP-3, ↓Desaturase

Transcription factors
↓NFκB, ↓AP-1, ↓Notch-1, ↓STAT-1, ↓STAT-3, ↓CREB-BP, ↓EGR-1, ↓WT-1, ↓β-catenin, ↓HIF-1, ↑Nrf-2, ↑PPAR-γ, ↑ERE

Inflammatory cytokines
↓IL-1, ↓IL-2, ↓IL-5, ↓IL-6, ↓IL-8, ↓IL-12, ↓IL-18, ↓MCP, ↓MIP, ↓TNF-α

Kinases
↓FAK, ↓AAPK, ↓EGFR-K, ↓PTK, ↓MAPK, ↓PKA, ↓PKB ↓PhK, ↓Ca²⁺PK, ↓ERK, ↓PAK, ↓JAK, ↓IL-1Rak, ↓Pp60C-TK

Curcumin

Growth factors
↓FGF, ↓HGF, ↓EGF, ↓PDGF, ↓TGF-β1, ↓VEGF

Receptors
↓IR, ↓Fas R, ↓ER-α, ↓EPCR, ↓H2R, ↓EGFR, ↓HER-2, ↓IL-8R, ↓CXCR4, ↓AHR, ↓LDLR, ↓ITR, ↓AR ↑DR-4, ↑DR-5

Others
↓UPa, ↓Bcl-xL, ↓Bcl-2, ↓Hsp-70, ↓ICAM-1, ↓Cyclin D1, ↓ELAM-1, ↓IAP-1, ↓MDRP, ↑DEF-40, ↑p53

FIGURE 24.5 Molecular targets modulated by curcumin. ↓ downregulated targets; ↑ upregulated targets. (Reproduced with permission from Dr. Muthu K. Shanmugan, National University of Singapore.)

Avocado and soybean oils are often used in the manufacturing of soap. The unsaponifiable fraction of these oils is called avocado/soybean unsaponifiable or ASU.

ASU contains a number of inflammation-modulating phytochemicals such as phytosterols (β-sitosterol, campesterol and stigmasterol), fat-soluble vitamins, triterpene fatty acids and so on, but the active components are unknown. Animal studies, as well as five human clinical trials, have been published showing improvement of OA in the test subjects as compared to the controls [59]. ASU is available as a nutriceutical, for example, Arthrocen® 300 mg once daily.

Boswellia, also known as frankincense, is a group of resins from the *Boswellia serrata* tree. One of these resins, acetyl-keto-beta-boswellic acid inhibits the lipoxygenase pathway and thus decreases inflammation. Nine clinical trials have been published demonstrating some benefit for OA [60]. *Boswellia* can be taken alone or in combination with other plant extracts such as curcumin for synergistic effect in OA.

The author has observed in clinical practice that often a therapeutic oral dose of curcumin capsules can significantly decrease the symptoms of inflammation. If greater efficacy is needed then the combining of various herbal products can be effective. Examples of such products could include: Curcumin Synergy™ Turmeric Supreme Joint by Gaia® Herbs which combines turmeric, *Boswellia*, piperine and other herbs; Inflammatone™ by Designs for Health which combines curcumin, *Boswellia* and other herbs – and so on. Using combination products can also be more cost-effective for the patient.

EMERGING THERAPIES FOR OA

There are now ways to cause tissue to regenerate, increasing the anabolic events within joints. The following are a few of the leading-edge approaches that are now being utilized.

IL-1RA (INTERLEUKIN-1 RECEPTOR ANTAGONIST PROTEIN)

IL-1Ra was first discovered in 1986 and, as previously mentioned, cells such as the chondrocytes which produce and release IL-1β also release small amounts of IL-1Ra. Other cells such as mononuclear cells and macrophages in the blood also produce and release cytokines as well as IL-1Ra [61]. Strategies to inhibit the biological activities of IL-1β have been developed. A recombinant IL-1Ra known as Anakinra has demonstrated the effective blockade of the IL-1 inflammatory cascade. A double-blind, placebo-controlled study ($n = 170$) concluded that it was safe to use in humans but was not associated with improvements in OA symptoms as compared to placebo [62]. Other strategies have been to inject the soluble forms of IL-1 receptors as well as the anti-inflammatory cytokines IL-4, IL-10 and IL-13 with an inhibitory effect on cell synthesis of IL-1. In 1994 it was discovered that if peripheral whole blood is drawn into a syringe containing glass beads coated with $CrSO4$ to initiate monocyte activation, incubated at 37.0°C for 24 hours and then centrifuged, the resulting serum was selectively enriched with the anti-inflammatory cytokines IL-1Ra, IL-4 and IL-10 [63]. Subsequent research has shown that not only is the autologous conditioned serum (ACS) rich in these anti-inflammatory cytokines, but it also contains over 35 other factors including fibroblast growth factor b (FGFb), vascular endothelial growth factor (VEGF), hepatocyte growth factor (HGF), IGF-1, platelet-derived growth factor (PDGF) and transforming growth factor β (TGF β) – as well as a number of the pro-inflammatory cytokines IL-1β and TNF-α [64]. The net effect is anti-inflammatory when the ACS is injected into osteoarthritic joints. This has been demonstrated in animal and human clinical trials with level 1 and 2 scientific evidence – knees [65], hips [66], temporomandibular joint (TMJ) [67]. A recent prospective, observational study demonstrated the therapeutic power of collaboration using ACS and physiotherapy [68]. 118 patients with unilateral knee OA, who were candidates for surgery, were treated with a combination of ACS and physiotherapy. The main endpoints of the study were pain – using the Numeric Rating Scale (NRS) – and functional ability – using the WOMAC global score. Within three months of the ACS/physiotherapy program, there were significant improvements in pain from baseline (-63.0%, $P < 0.001$). These improvements were maintained over 24 months. The mean WOMAC global score was reduced at 24 months compared to baseline (-56.9%, $P < 0.001$). WOMAC subscores for pain (-86.0%, $P < 0.001$) and function (-51.3%, $P < 0.001$) also demonstrated significant improvement in pain from baseline.

PLATELET-RICH PLASMA (PRP)

Platelets are known to contain microvesicles and exosomes which are reservoirs of a multitude of growth factors essential for the regenerative processes in humans. The most relevant growth factors include PDGF, TGF β, FGF, IGF-1, connective tissue growth Factor (CTGF), EGF and HGF [69]. As well, platelet microvesicles also contain a number of microRNAs involved in mesenchymal tissue regeneration, one of which – microRNA-23b – has been hypothesized to be involved in the differentiation of mesenchymal stem cells into chondrocytes [70]. Autologous PRP is defined as a platelet concentration product containing at least 200% of the peripheral blood platelet count [52]. PRP can be obtained in a number of ways including blood filtration and plateletpheresis, centrifugation with "single spinning" method and centrifugation with "double spinning" method. Once obtained, the platelets must be activated with various activators such as thrombin (bovine or autologous) or calcium chloride in the presence of a fibrin matrix. This is then injected into joints, muscles, tendons or ligaments. A recent randomized, prospective study looked at the effectiveness of PRP in the treatment of knee OA [71]. 100 patients with moderate, grade 3, osteoarthritis of the knee were randomized into one of three groups. Group 1 had one injection of PRP, group 2 had two injections of PRP at a two-week interval, and group 3 had three injections of PRP at two-week intervals. Patients were evaluated with Visual Analogue Scores, WOMAC global scores and the Timed Up and Go test at zero, three and six-month intervals. The effectiveness of a single injection of PRP was far less than when two or three injections were given ($P < 0.001$). In all three groups, the improvements in pain, flexibility and function showed a tendency to gradually decrease over time. Unfortunately, because of the lack of standardization of PRP dosing regimens, it is difficult to compare outcomes of studies for the evaluation of clinical effectiveness as the amount and effectiveness of platelet concentration, and thus growth factor content, will vary depending on the various PRP preparation techniques [71].

MESENCHYMAL STEM CELLS (MSCs)

A promising approach to cartilage regeneration in joints is the use of MSCs. MSCs occur in numerous tissues, including bone marrow and adipose tissue [72]. MSCs have the ability to differentiate into bone, cartilage, muscle and adipose tissue [73]. There is a growing scientific literature demonstrating that MSCs can successfully regenerate cartilage in animals and humans [74]. Adipose tissue-derived stem cells (ADSCs) in the form of stromal vascular fraction (SVF) contain stem cells that can differentiate into cartilage, bone, muscle and adipose tissue similar to MSCs [75]. Recent studies have demonstrated that ADSCs can regenerate cartilage in the osteoarthritic knees of human patients [76]. Even more promising is the use of MSCs from bone marrow aspirate concentrate (BMAC) as it is an approved procedure by the United States Food and Drug Administration (FDA). BMAC, besides being a source of MSCs, also contains various growth factors including PDGF, TGF-b as well as bone morphogenetic protein (BMP)-2 and BMP-7 which are known to have both anabolic and anti-inflammatory effects [77]. A recently published review of the BMAC literature [78] concluded that overall the outcomes reported with the use of BMAC for the treatment of early knee osteoarthritis is good to excellent. However, this field is in its infancy and the level of scientific evidence in the studies published varied from grades 2–4. There is a need for large, randomized controlled trials to evaluate the efficacy of BMAC for the treatment of knee pathologies.

CASE STUDY UTILIZING AUTOLOGOUS CONDITIONED SERUM AND THE FUNCTIONAL MEDICINE MATRIX

The following case history was supervised by the author and utilizes the Functional Medicine approach to critical thinking using the principles of the FM matrix. A 64-year-old, married woman presented with a many year history of progressive osteoarthritis affecting both knees (right > left), lower back, neck, and small joints of her hands. She also had one kidney. Over the years, the pain and stiffness in her joints led to an inability to cook and do housework, loss of sleep, fatigue, anxiety and inability to golf, garden and line dance – which she was passionate about. She was careful about her diet and had previously gone through the FM comprehensive elimination diet and she avoided gluten and nightshade foods. Since she had one kidney, she was careful to avoid medications such as NSAIDs and other analgesics. She had tried a number of oral herbal remedies with little improvement. On examination, she appeared tired, moved carefully and walked with a right-sided limp, was unable to flex her fingers more than 50% and demonstrated decreased range of motion in her cervical and lumbar spine regions. Her right knee had a mild–moderate effusion and was warm to touch, with tenderness over the joint lines and lacked full flexion. All standard laboratory work was within normal limits including C-reactive protein (CRP). X-rays showed moderate changes of osteoarthritis in the medial compartment of the right knee as well as many of the proximal interphalangeal (PIP) and distal interphalangeal (DIP) joints in both hands. Her initial WOMAC score was 44/96 or 45%. She met with the family nurse practitioner in my clinic for three, one hour educational sessions reviewing the Functional Medicine anti-inflammatory lifestyle. She was assessed by an excellent physiotherapist for structural and functional problems that she had developed over the years as a result of the OA. She was then coached and supervised on specific flexibility and strengthening exercises by the physiotherapist. She was placed on oral curcumin twice daily with food and began twice-weekly intravenous curcumin treatments over three weeks. A total of five autologous conditioned serum injections to the right knee were given over three weeks and tolerated well. Finally, she was treated twice-weekly with Ondamed® (German electromagnetic, focused field device) over three weeks. Following her third ACS injection, she reported the ability to line dance for two hours with no triggering of inflammation in her knees. The following two days she played 18 holes of golf each day, again without triggering inflammation. She had regained full function of her hands and had no further back and neck pain. Over the subsequent weeks, she noted that she was able to sleep deeply, had increased energy, was able to do housework, cooking and gardening. Importantly, her chronic anxiety also resolved. At the end of the three-week program, her WOMAC score dropped to 11/96 or 11% and one month later the WOMAC score dropped to 6/96 or 6%. At the three-month follow-up, she was clinically doing very well and the WOMAC score dropped to 0/96 and this was maintained at the six, 12- and 18-month follow-ups. As of two years post-treatment, symptoms of osteoarthritis are minimal allowing her to keep engaged in an active lifestyle.

SUMMARY AND CASE DISCUSSION

This case demonstrates the importance of taking a thorough history using the FM matrix to help the clinician think critically about the antecedents, triggers and mediators. Laboratory work should be ordered to rule out serious inflammatory disorders and to look for nutritional insufficiencies. Judicious use of radiological tests should also be done to help rule out serious inflammatory joint disorders. This case also demonstrates the therapeutic power of a multifaceted approach focusing on diet and nutrition and a Functional Medicine anti-inflammatory lifestyle as a means to decrease inflammation. This, combined with leading-edge approaches such as autologous conditioned serum, increases the therapeutic efficacy.

When the patient presents with "arthritis" it is important to distinguish OA from inflammatory-type forms of arthritis such as rheumatoid, psoriatic or ankylosing spondylitis. Once the diagnosis has been made, then the general treatment approach can be based on the OARSI guidelines for the non-surgical management of knee OA (Figure 24.3) in which four categories are reviewed: knee-only OA without or with comorbidities and multi-jointed OA without or with comorbidities. Without forgetting the framework of the OARSI guidelines, an approach using the Functional Medicine model of critical thinking can also be used effectively, as has been discussed and demonstrated in this chapter. The Functional Medicine Matrix (Figure 24.4) becomes the algorithm and is most useful in helping the physician to look critically at the individual patient's key antecedents, triggers and mediators, keeping in mind the timeline of the patient's life.

Then, careful thought is given to the seven core clinical imbalances and the foundational personal lifestyle factors. As one dives into the matrix as it relates to OA, the following key points will be running through one's mind. Did the patient develop OA as a result of: food allergies and/or sensitivities, gastrointestinal dysbiosis, leaky gut or unusual gut microbiota, food additives or excesses, digestive insufficiencies, oxidative stress, mitochondrial dysfunction, toxicant exposures/increased body burden of toxicants, obesity, stress or adrenal fatigue/dysfunction, lack of good quality sleep, hormone imbalances, infections (such as occult dental infections, *Borrelia* and/or coinfections and so on), nutrient deficiencies, prescription drugs (such as statins), genetic predispositions – or combinations of the above? Thinking in terms of the FM matrix forces the physician to think outside of their realm of interest or experience and serves as a good reminder of items that may have been missed in the initial history and physical examination. The lifestyle interventions combined with the emerging therapies can in this way transform osteoarthritis into a treatable, not just a manageable, condition.

REFERENCES

1. Bijlsma JW, Berenbaum F, and Lafeber FP. Osteoarthritis: An update with relevance for clinical practice. *Lancet.* 2011; 377(9783): 2115–2126.
2. Gupta S, Hawker GA, Laporte A, et al. The economic burden of disabling hip and knee osteoarthritis (OA) from the perspective of individuals living with this condition. *Rheumatology (Oxford).* 2005; 44(12): 1531–1537.
3. Yu SP and Hunter DJ. Managing osteoarthritis. *Aust Prescr.* 2015; 38(4): 155–159.
4. Mathiessen A, and Conaghan PG. Synovisit in osteoarthritis: current understanding with therapeutic implications. *Arthritis Res Ther.* 2017; 19(1): 18.
5. Grover AK and Samson SE. Benefits of antioxidant supplements for knee osteoarthritis: Rationale and reality. *Nutr J.* 2016; 15(1): 1–13.

6. Kraus, Blanco, Englund, et al. Call for standardized definitions of osteoarthritis and risk stratifica-
    tion for clinical trials and clinical use. *Osteoarthritis Cartilage*. 2015; 23(8): 1233–1241. doi:10.1016/j.
    joca.2015.03.036. Accessed February 27, 2016.

7. Scanzello CR and Goldring SR. The role of synovitis in osteoarthritis pathogenesis. *Bone*. 2012; 51(2):
    249–257.

8. Prieto-Potin I, Largo R, Roman-Blas JA, et al. Characterization of multinucleated giant cells in
    synovium and subchondral bone in knee osteoarthritis and rheumatoid arthritis. *BMC Musculoskelet
    Disord*. 2015; 16: 226.

9. Murphy L, Schwartz TA, Helmick CG, et al. Lifetime risk of symptomatic knee osteoarthritis. *Arthritis
    Rheum*. 2008; 59: 1207–1213.

10. Oliveria SA, Felson DT, Reed JI, et al. Incidence of symptomatic hand, hip, and knee osteoarthritis
    among patients in a health maintenance organization. *Arthritis Rheum*. 1995; 38: 1134–1141.

11. Loeser, RF. Aging and osteoarthritis. *Curr. Opin. Rheumatol*. 2011; 23(5): 492–496.

12. Wluka, AE, Lombard, CB, and Cicuttini, FM. Tackling obesity in knee osteoarthritis. *Nat. Rev.
    Rheumatol*. 2013; 9(4): 225–235.

13. Zhuo, Q, Yang, W, Chen, J, and Wang, Y. Metabolic syndrome meets osteoarthritis. *Nat. Rev Rheumatol*.
    2012; 8(12): 729–737.

14. Neogi T. OARSI primer: Chapter 1 – epidemiology of OA. *Osteoarthritis Research Society International
    (OARSI)*; 2010 [cited February 27, 2016]; Available from: http://primer.oarsi.org/print/book/export/
    html/2.

15. Dohery M, and Abhishek A. OARSI primer: Chapter 7 – disease diagnosis and clinical presentation.
    Osteoarthritis Research Society International (OARSI); 2011 [cited February 27, 2016]; Available from:
    http://primer.oarsi.org/content/chapter-7-disease-diagnosis-and-clinical-presentation

16. Zhang W, Doherty M, Peat G, et al. EULAR evidence-based recommendations for the diagnosis of knee
    osteoarthritis. *Ann Rheum Dis*. 2010; 69(3): 483–9.

17. Pujalte GG and Albano-Aluquin SA. Differential diagnosis of polyarticular arthritis. *Am Fam Physician*.
    2015; 92(1): 35–41.

18. Sale JE, Gignac M, and Hawker G. The relationship between disease symptoms, life events, coping and
    treatment, and depression among older adults with osteoarthritis. *J Rheumatol*. 2008; 35(2): 335–342.

19. Ashford S and Williard J. Osteoarthritis: A review. *Nurse Pract*. 2014; 39(5): 1–8.

20. Bellamy N, Buchanan WW, Goldsmith CH, et al. Validation study of WOMAC: A health status instru-
    ment for measuring clinically important patient relevant outcomes to antirheumatic drug therapy in
    patients with osteoarthritis of the hip or knee. *J Rheumatol*. 1988; 15(12): 1833–1840.

21. Kim C, Linsenmeyer KD, Vlad SC, et al. Prevalence of radiographic and symptomatic hip osteoarthritis
    in an urban United States community: The Framingham osteoarthritis study. *Arthritis Rheumatol*. 2014;
    66(11): 3013–3017.

22. Kim C, Nevitt MC, Niu J, et al. Association of hip pain with radiographic evidence of hip osteoarthritis:
    Diagnostic test study. *BMJ*. 2015; 351: 1-23. doi:10.1136/bmj.h5983.

23. Sarmanova A, Hall M, Moses J, et al. Synovial changes detected by ultrasound in people with knee osteo-
    arthritis – a meta-analysis of observational studies. *Osteoarthritis Cartilage*. 2016; 24(8): 1376–1383.

24. Neogi T, Guermazi A, Roemer F, et al. Association of joint inflammation with pain sensitization in knee
    osteoarthritis: The Multicenter Osteoarthritis Study. *Arthritis Rheumatol*. 2016; 68(3): 654–661.

25. Guermazi A, Hayashi D, Roemer FW, et al. Synovitis in knee osteoarthritis assessed by contrast-
    enhanced magnetic resonance imaging (MRI) is associated with radiographic tibiofemoral osteoarthritis
    and MRI-detected widespread cartilage damage: The MOST study. *J Rheumatol*. 2014; 41(3): 501–508.

26. De Lange-Brokaar BJ, Ioan-Facsinay A, Yusuf E, et al. Degree of synovitis on MRI by comprehensive
    whole knee semi-quantitative scoring method correlates with histologic and macroscopic features of
    synovial tissue inflammation in knee osteoarthritis. *Osteoarthritis Cartilage*. 2014; 22(10): 1606–1613.

27. Roemer FW, Kwoh CK, Hannon MJ, et al. What comes first? Multitissue involvement leading to radio-
    graphic osteoarthritis: Magnetic resonance imaging-based trajectory analysis over 4 years in the osteo-
    arthritis initiative. *Arthritis Rheumatol*. 2015; 67(8): 2085–2096.

28. Lotz M, Martel-Pelletier J, Christiansen C, et al. Republished: Value of biomarkers in osteoarthritis:
    Current status and perspectives. *Postgrad Med J*. 2014; 90(1061): 171–178.

29. Bay-Jensen AC, Reker D, Kjelgaard-Petersen CF, et al. Osteoarthritis year in review 2015: Soluble bio-
    markers and the BIPED criteria. *Osteoarthritis Cartilage*. 2016; 24(1): 20.

30. van der Kraan PM and van den Berg WB. OARSI primer: Chapter 5 – OA pathogenesis, cell sig-
    nals. *Osteoarthritis Research Society International (OARSI)*; 2011 [cited February 27, 2016]; Available
    from: http://primer.oarsi.org/content/cell-signals

31. Salter DM, Buckwalter JA, Sandell L. OARSI primer: Chapter 4 – pathology of OA. *Osteoarthritis Research Society International (OARSI)* ; 2011 [cited February 27, 2016]; Available from: http://primer.oarsi.org/content/chapter-4-pathology-oa

32. Sellam J and Berenbaum F. The role of synovitis in pathophysiology and clinical symptoms of osteoarthritis. *Nat Rev Rheumatol.* 2010; 6(11): 625–635.

33. Wojdasiewicz P, Poniatowski LA, and Szukiewicz D. The role of inflammatory and anti-inflammatory cytokines in the pathogenesis of osteoarthritis. *Mediators Inflamm.* 2014; 2014: 1–19, 561459. doi:10.1155/2014/561459.

34. Cantarini L, Lopalco G, Cattalini M, et al. Interleukin-1: Ariadne's thread in autoinflammatory and autoimmune disorders. *Isr Med Assoc J.* 2015; 17(2): 93–97.

35. Bondeson J, Blom AB, Wainwright S, et al. The role of synovial macrophages and macrophage-produced mediators in driving inflammatory and destructive responses in osteoarthritis. *Arthritis Rheum.* 2010; 62(3): 647–657.

36. Abramson SB and Attur M. Developments in the scientific understanding of osteoarthritis. *Arthritis Res Ther.* 2009; 11(3)227: 1–9.

37. Dayer JM. Evidence for the biological modulation of IL-1 activity: The role of IL-Ra. *Clin Exp Rheumatol.* 2002; 20(5 Suppl 27): 14–20.

38. Smith DE, Hanna R, Della F, et al. The soluble form of IL-1 receptor accessory protein enhances the ability of soluble type II IL-1 receptor to inhibit IL-1 action. *Immunity.* 2003; 18(1): 87–96.

39. Genemaras AA, Reiner T, Huang CY, et al. Early intervention with interleukin-1 receptor antagonist protein modulates catabolic microRNA and mRNA expression in cartilage after impact injury. *Osteoarthritis Cartilage.* 2015; 23(11): 2046–2044.

40. McAlindon TE, Bannuru RR, Sullivan MC, et al. OARSI guidelines for the non-surgical management of knee osteoarthritis. *Osteoarthritis Cartilage.* 2014; 22(3): 363–388.

41. Jevsevar D, Donnelly P, Brown GA, et al. Viscosupplementation for osteoarthritis of the knee: A systematic review of the evidence. *J Bone Joint Surg Am.* 2015; 97(24): 2047–2060.

42. McAlindon TE, LaValley MP, Harvey WF, et al. Effect of intra-articular triamcinolone vs saline on knee cartilage volume and pain in patients with knee osteoarthritis: A randomized clinical trial. *JAMA.* 2017; 317(19): 1967–1975.

43. Bally M, Dendukuri N, Rich B, et al. Risk of acute myocardial infarction with NSAIDs in real world use: Bayesian meta-analysis of individual patient data. *BMJ.* 2017; 357: 1–13, j1909. doi:10.1136/bmj.j1909.

44. Arfe A, Scotti L, Varas-Lorenzo C, et al. Non-steroidal anti-inflammatory drugs and risk of heart failure in four European countries: Nested case-control study. *BMJ.* 2016; 354: 1–11, i4857. doi:10.1136/BMJ.i4857.

45. Wenham CY, Grainger AJ, Hensor EM, et al. Methotrexate for pain relief in knee osteoarthritis: An open-label study. *Rheumatology (Oxford).* 2013; 52(5): 888–892.

46. Alexander BJ, Ames, BN, Baker SM, et al. 2010. *Textbook of Functional Medicine.* 5. Gig Harbor: The Institute for Functional Medicine.

47. Alexander BJ, Ames, BN, Baker SM, et al. 2010. *Textbook of Functional Medicine.* 691–695. Gig Harbor: The Institute for Functional Medicine.

48. Malfait AM. Osteoarthritis year in review 2015: Biology. *Osteoarthritis Cartilage.* 2016; 24(1): 21–26.

49. Anderson JJ and Felson DT. Factors associated with osteoarthritis of the knee in the first national Health and Nutrition Examination Survey (HANES 1). Evidence for an association with overweight, race, and physical demands of work. *Am J Epidemiol.* 1988; 128(1): 179–189.

50. Institute for Functional Medicine. IFM Elimination Diet – Comprehensive Guide and Food Plan. 2015 [cited February 27, 2016]; Available from: https://www.functionalmedicine.org/page.aspx?uid=37&id=948

51. Rosillo MA, Sanchez-Hidalgo M, Sanchez-Fidalgo S, et al. Dietary extra-virgin olive oil prevents inflammatory response and cartilage matrix degradation in murine collagen-induced arthritis. *Eur J Nutr.* 2016; 55(1): 315–325.

52. Ying X, Chen X, Cheng S, et al. Piperine inhibits IL-1β induced expression of inflammatory mediators in human osteoarthritis chondrocyte. *Int Immunopharmacol.* 2013; 17(2): 293–299.

53. Panahi Y, Alishiri GH, Parvin S, et al. Mitigation of systemic oxidative stress by curcuminoids in osteoarthritis: Results of a randomized controlled trial. *J Diet Suppl.* 2016; 13(2): 209–220.

54. Ying X, Peng L, Chen H, et al. Cordycepin prevented IL-1β induced expression of inflammatory mediators in human osteoarthritis chondrocytes. *Int Orthop.* 2014; 38(7): 1519–1526.

55. Singh G, Kapoor IP, Singh P, et al. Comparative study of chemical composition and antioxidant activity of fresh and dry rhizomes of turmeric (*Curcuma longa linn.*). *Food Chem Toxicol.* 2010; 48(4): 1026–1031.

56. Shanmugam MK, Rane G, Kanchi MM, et al. The multifaceted role of curcumin in cancer prevention and treatment. *Molecules*. 2015; 20(2): 2728–2769.

57. Belcaro G, Cesarone MR, Dugall M, et al. Efficacy and safety of Meriva®, a curcumin-phosphatidyl-choline complex, during extended administration in osteoarthritis patients. *Altern Med Rev*. 2010; 15(4): 337–344.

58. Newberry SJ, Fitzgerald J, SooHoo NF, et al. Treatment of osteoarthritis of the knee: An update review. *Rockville (MD): Agency for Healthcare Research and Quality (US); Comparative Effectiveness Review*. 2017; 190, p. 70.

59. Christiansen BA, Bhatti S, Goudarzi R, et al. Management of osteoarthritis with avocado/soybean unsaponifiables. *Cartilage*. 2015; 6(1): 30–44.

60. Kimmatkar N, Thawani V, Hingorani L, et al. Efficacy and tolerability of boswellia serrata extract in treatment of osteoarthritis of knee – a randomized double blind placebo controlled trial. *Phytomedicine*. 2003; 10(1): 3–7.

61. Frisbie DD. Autologous-conditioned serum: Evidence for use in the knee. *J Knee Surg*. 2015; 28(1): 63–66.

62. Chevalier X, Goupille P, Beaulieu AD, et al. Intraarticular injection of anakinra in osteoarthritis of the knee: A mulitcenter, randomized, double-blind, placebo-controlled study. *Arthritis Rheum*. 2009; 61(3): 344–352.

63. Arend WP and Leung DY. IgG induction of IL-1 receptor antagonist production by human monocytes. *Immunol Rev*. 1994; 139: 71–78.

64. Wehling P, Moser C, Fridbie D, et al. Autologous conditioned serum in the treatment of orthopedic diseases: The orthokine therapy. *BioDrugs*. 2007; 21(5): 323–332.

65. Baltzer AW, Moser C, Jansen SA, et al. Autologous conditioned serum (orthokine) is an effective treatment for knee osteoarthritis. *Osteoarthritis Cartilage*. 2009; 17(2): 152–160.

66. Baltzer AW, Ostapczuk MS, Stosch D, et al. A new treatment for hip osteoarthritis: Clinical evidence for the efficacy of autologous conditioned serum. *Orthop Rev (Pavia)*. 2013; 5(2): 59–64.

67. Alvarez-Camino JC, Vazquez-Delgado E, and Gay-Escoda C. Use of autologous conditioned serum (orthokine) for the treatment of the degenerative osteoarthritis of the temporomandibular joint. Review of the literature. *Med Oral Patol Oral Cir Bucal*. 2013; 18(3): 433–438.

68. Baselga Garcia-Escudero J and Miguel Hernandez Trillos P. Treatment of osteoarthritis of the knee with a combination of autologous conditioned serum and physiotherapy; a two-year observational study. *PLoS One*. 2015; 10(12): 1–10.

69. Marmotti A, Rossi R, Castoldi F, et al. PRP and articular cartilage: A clinical update. *Biomed Res Int*. 2015; 2015: 1–19, 542502. doi:10.1155/2015/542502.

70. Ham O, Song BW, Lee SY, et al. The role of microRNA-23b in the differentiation of MSC into chondrocyte by targeting protein kinase A signaling. *Biomaterials*. 2012; 33(18): 4500–4507.

71. Kavadar G, Demircioglu DT, Celik MY, et al. Effectiveness of platelet-rich plasma in the treatment of moderate knee osteoarthritis: A randomized, prospective study. *J Phys Ther Sci*. 2015; 27(12): 3863–3867.

72. Pak J, Lee JH, Kartolo WA, et al. Cartilage regeneration in human with adipose tissue-derived stem dells: Cerrent status in clinical implications. *Biomed Res Int*. 2016; 2016: 1–12, 4702674. doi:10.1155/2016/4702674.

73. Szilvassy SJ. The biology of hematopoietic stem cells. *Arch Med Res*. 2003; 34(6): 446–460.

74. Centeno CJ, Schultz JR, Cheever M, et al. Safety and complications reporting on the re-implantation of culture-expanded mesenchymal stem cells using autologous platelet lysate technique. *Curr Stem Cell Res Ther*. 2010; 5(1): 81–93.

75. Zuk PA, Zhu M, Ashjian P, et al. Human adipose tissue is a source of multipotent stem cells. *Mol Biol Cell*. 2002; 13(12): 4279–4295.

76. Koh YG, Choi YJ, Kwon SK, et al. Clinical results and second-look arthroscopic findings after treatment with adipose-derived stem cells for knee osteoarthritis. *Knee Surg Sports Traumatol Arthrosc*. 2015; 23(5): 1308–1316.

77. Indrawattana N, Chen G, Tadokoro M, et al. Growth factor combination for chondrogenic induction from human mesenchymal stem cell. *Biochem Biophys Res Commun*. 2004; 320(3): 914–919.

78. Chahla J, Dean CS, Moatshe G, et al. Concentrated bone marrow aspirate for the treatment of chondral injuries and osteoarthritis of the knee: A systematic review of outcomes. *Orthop J Sports Med*. 2016; 4(1): 1–8.

25 Osteoarthritis
Comprehensive Treatment

David Musnick, MD and Richard D. Batson, ND

INTRODUCTION

Physicians in Orthopedic, Physiatry, Sports Medicine, Functional Medicine, Naturopathic Medicine and Primary Care will have a significant number of patient visits in which the patient has complaints of joint dysfunction and pain related to osteoarthritis (OA). The usual approach of prescribing non-steroidal anti-inflammatory drugs (NSAIDS) and pain medications does not adequately address the pathophysiology and can lead to significant side effects. The pathophysiology of OA is complex and should be understood when treating the patient with OA. The clinician should develop a well thought-out treatment plan that addresses not only improvement in pain and function but that also deals with comorbid factors to have more long-term benefits. Pathophysiology, modifiable lifestyle factors, injection therapies, topical therapies modalities, nutritional and other therapies will be discussed.

PATHOPHYSIOLOGY

Osteoarthritis is characterized by progressive loss and degeneration of articular cartilage with resultant joint space narrowing, cysts and osteophyte formation. In addition there can be subchondral bone changes. OA appears to involve changes not only in the articular cartilage but also in all aspects of a joint (bone, capsule, synovium and synovial fluid) (Dieppe, 2011; Martel-Pelletier and Pelletier, 2010; Abramson and Attur, 2009). In the spine, OA is also characterized by disc dehydration, decreased disc space height, facet joint hypertrophy, as well as narrowing of the central canal and neural foramen. OA of the knee may involve the articular cartilage of the patellofemoral joint, proximal tibiofibular joint, as well of the tibia femur joint. OA of the knee commonly involves degeneration and tearing of meniscal cartilage on the medial or lateral meniscus, which increases the risk of degeneration of articular cartilage.

Osteoarthritis is characterized initially by irregularities in and loss of the articular cartilage surface, a thickening of subchondral bone, and formation of marginal osteophytes. Changes include cartilage fibrillation, and focal disintegration within the joint, with the most striking changes usually seen in load-bearing areas of the articular cartilage.

Chondrocytes comprise the entire cellular matrix of the joint. The substrate of the extracellular matrix is comprised of collagen and polysaccharides known as glycosaminoglycans (GAGs). Substantial GAGs in the extracellular matrix include hyaluronic acid, chondroitin-4-sulfate, chondroitin-6-sulfate, dermatan sulfate, and keratan sulfate. The primary roles of the extracellular matrix include absorbing shock, maintaining viscosity, and nourishing chondrocytes. The primary role of the chondrocytes is the ongoing synthesis of matrix components. The chondrocyte also produces enzymes that are involved in the breakdown of components of the matrix. Chondrocytes may be affected by a number of factors, including cytokines, polypeptide growth factors, matrix components and biomechanical stimuli. The health of the joint is dependent on the function and quality of the chondrocyte and the extracellular matrix.

The turnover rate of collagen in the matrix is slow compared to the turnover of proteoglycan which is more rapid (Mow et al., 2005). Trauma or mechanical stress may cause gross damage

419

to chondrocytes and the matrix. Full repair may be possible but often there is inadequate repair. Damaged collagen and proteoglycan taken up by macrophages can stimulate the release of inflammatory cytokines such as IL-1, 6 and TNF-α (Stannus et al., 2010). These cytokines can bind to Chondrocyte receptors and inhibit type II collagen production as well as lead to the production of metalloproteinases (MMP). MMPs act to break down collagen and include MMP-3, MMP-9, MMP-13 and ADAAMTS. IL-1 acts on chondrocytes which can induce NF-κB and activator protein 1 (AP-1), increasing the production of MMP enzymes that break down type II collagen (Wojdasiewicz et al., 2014).

There can be a progressive decrease in collagen and proteoglycans in a joint. There can also be an increase in the rate of apoptosis of chondrocytes in a joint. With a decrease in the collagen and proteoglycan content, fissuring can occur. If there is enough cartilage loss in a surface the subchondral bone can be exposed. More loss is likely in weight-bearing surfaces than in non-weight-bearing surfaces.

There can be a phenotypic switch in certain chondrocytes to a hypertrophic type of chondrocyte. That can produce matrix metalloproteinase (MMP)-13 and type X collagen. As OA progresses, extensive matrix degradation and loss occurs due to the continued production of proteases. Fragments of matrix proteins and pro-inflammatory cytokines can stimulate chondrocytes to produce more proteases and cytokines. As significant matrix damage occurs, chondrocyte cell death progresses, leading to areas of matrix devoid of cells.

OA of a joint can also involve breakdown of the subchondral bone. The receptor activator NF-κB ligand (RANKL) is produced not only by osteoblasts and stromal cells, but also by chondrocytes. Osteoprotegerin (OPG) is produced by osteoblasts and binds to RANKL, thereby preventing RANKL binding to RANK and this decreases and regulates osteoclastogenesis. In OA, various interleukins and cytokines such as IL-1β, IL-6, IL-11, IL-17, and TNF-α lead to increased formation of RANKL and decreased production of OPG, resulting in bone loss. Strategies that increase OPG and decrease RANKL may lead to less bone loss. One such strategy is the use of estrogen in females that are postmenopausal.

OA of a joint may begin due to any number of triggering factors with or without antecedent factors. Antecedent factors may be: trauma and other mechanical factors, systemic or local inflammation, hormone issues, obesity, loss of meniscus in the knee, joint hypermobility and malalignment, etc. The most common triggering factors include trauma, abnormal mechanical force during repetitive motions in sports or walking or an abrupt change in hormones.

Early in the course of OA of a joint there is evidence of enhanced chondrocyte replication, suggestive of attempts at repair. In spite of accelerated metabolism within the chondrocyte, the synthesis of matrix substrates may become insufficient and results in a decreased concentration of sulfur-containing proteoglycans within the extracellular matrix. The failure of chondrocytes to compensate for the proteoglycan loss results in a loss of matrix contents (Loeser et al., 2012).

There are numerous inflammatory mediators in OA. Interleukin-1 (IL-1) is a cytokine implicated in signaling the degradation of cartilage matrix in OA. IL-1 is synthesized by chondrocytes and mononuclear cells lining the synovium and it suppresses the synthesis of type 2 (articular) cartilage and promotes formation of type 1 (fibrous) cartilage. IL-1 induces catabolic enzymes such as stromelysin and collagenase and IL-1 upregulates the production of aggrecanases which cleave proteoglycan. Intra-articular injection of IL-1 induces proteoglycan loss and an IL-1 receptor antagonist slows progression of cartilage loss in animal models of OA (Loeuille et al., 2005). Given the role of IL-1 in promoting cartilage degradation, IL-1 inhibition is a logical treatment target in OA.

In addition to the production of aggrecanases, IL-1 triggers an entire cascade of pro-inflammatory and catabolic cytokines including tumor necrosis factor alpha (TNF-α), IL-6, IL-8, and PGE-2, which act synergistically with IL-1 to perpetuate the pro-inflammatory cascade (Loeuille et al., 2005). TNF-α induces cartilage degeneration by increasing cytokine production and the expression of collagenases and aggrecanases (Baker et al., 2010).

In response to IL-1, chondrocytes secrete neutral metalloproteinases (MMP) and active oxygen species that are directly implicated in the destruction of cartilage matrix. IL-1 is a potent inhibitor of proteoglycan and collagen synthesis (Loeser, 2013). There are other cytokines that may play a role in OA and these include IGF 1, transforming growth factor beta and osteopontin. These cytokines may be primarily anabolic for cartilage.

A number of proteases including metalloproteinases can lead to degeneration of cartilage. These include collagenases, which are a family of enzymes known to cleave helical type 2 cartilage and have activity against type X cartilage. Connective tissue cells produce tissue inhibitors of metalloproteinases (TIMPs). There is likely an imbalance between the level of TIMPs and the metalloproteinases that may lead to a catabolic effect and subsequent cartilage degradation (Brophy et al., 2012).

Osteoarthritic cartilage is characterized by an increase in anabolic and catabolic activity. At first, compensatory mechanisms such as increased synthesis of matrix molecules (collagen, proteoglycans, and hyaluronate) and proliferation of chondrocytes in the deeper layers of the cartilage, are able to maintain the integrity of the articular cartilage, but in the end, loss of chondrocytes and changes in the extracellular matrix predominate and osteoarthritic changes develop.

Most people with moderate to severe OA will have some degree of synovial inflammation or synovial hypertrophy during the course of their OA (Baker et al., 2010). Synovitis may contribute to pain and disease progression, including cartilage destruction and may be mediated by the production of inflammatory factors and proteins referred to as damage-associated molecular patterns (DAMPs), including alarmins (Liu-Bryan and Terkeltaub, 2011). Secondary OA may be seen in joints previously affected by inflammatory arthritis.

Soft-tissue components of the joint, in addition to the cartilage, including ligaments, joint capsule, and, in the knee, the menisci, are commonly affected by OA. These tissues exhibit loss of chondrocyte cells and disruption of their extracellular matrix. The joint capsule may thicken and calcification of the matrix can lead to osteophytes and joint hypertrophy. Studies have shown that torn menisci can be a source of inflammatory mediators in the joint (Brophy et al., 2012). Muscles and nerves are also affected by OA, resulting in weakness and pain (Roos et al., 2011).

Age is the risk factor most strongly correlated with OA and some studies suggest that more than 80% of individuals over the age of 75 are affected. Age-related tissue changes are believed to be due to a decrease in the repair mechanisms of chondrocytes. With age, chondrocytes are unable to maintain synthetic activity, exhibit decreased responsiveness to anabolic growth factors, synthesize smaller and less uniform proteoglycans and fewer functional link proteins.

OA progresses when tissue regeneration cannot keep pace with the rate of cartilage loss. Joint damage may occur when the biomaterial properties of the articular cartilage are inadequate or the load on the joint is excessive. Contributing factors related to the development or progression of OA in a particular joint are: traumatic injury including sprains and contusion, joint malalignment, prolonged myofascial tightness, ligament laxity with joint hypermobility, prolonged muscle recruitment weakness in muscles stabilizing or moving the joint, genetic predisposition, obesity, aging, gender, hormone issues and nutritional factors. Additional insult on the total joint load can come from the extra weight burden associated with obesity and certain physical activities such as high-impact sports. Recent scientific literature suggests that, in addition to the extra weight burden associated with obesity, inflamed adipose tissue and dyslipidemia associated with obesity can contribute to OA.

PATIENT EVALUATION

In order to determine the extent of joint osteoarthritis the clinician should order an X-ray of the joint. One is looking for joint space narrowing, osteophytes, sclerosis of bone. The X-ray should be shown to the patient and a discussion should be held regarding what is OA and what the goals are going to be for that joint or joints. This will aid patient compliance, especially in designing a long-term as well as a short-term treatment program.

In general severe degenerative joint disease (DJD) is associated with significant pain and disability. A patient may have mild to moderate OA of the knee and hip and not be very symptomatic. Patients can progress to becoming symptomatic and having significant dysfunction with progress of OA of the involved joint. OA appears to progress in perimenopause and menopause in women. Given the vulnerability of aging joints to OA it is advisable to include in a yearly physical exam visit, a preventative history and physical examination directed at the knee and hip joints.

In this exam evaluate lower extremity joint mechanics and alignment, looking especially for varus or valgus knee alignment and excessive pronation or supination of the feet. Evaluate and make suggestions on gait and footwear as many people, especially women, have footwear that does not support their feet well, especially against the pronation forces of gait, and this could place abnormal forces on their knees and hips. Evaluate and make suggestions to help patients sit in neutral spine posture to slow or prevent neck and low back OA. Evaluate and treat muscle weakness, muscle tightness and age-related sarcopenia.

Assessing dysfunctional biomechanics of the knee and hip are essential for a complete treatment approach for OA. Osteoarthritis occurs more commonly in a number of areas of the body: the C5-7 areas of the cervical spine, the L4-S1 areas of the lumbar spine, the knees, hips and the IP and DIP joints of the hands, as well as the CMC joint of the thumb. The hips and knees are weight-bearing joints and excessive or abnormal loads can contribute to the development and progression of OA. Dysfunctional mechanics at a joint can create excessive shearing and abnormal forces on articular cartilage contributing to the progression of DJD. Dysfunctional mechanics can result from alignment dysfunction from tight muscles (myofascial factors), loss of cartilage, gait dysfunction, weak muscles, poor posture, lax ligaments and non-supportive footwear. It is important to evaluate a patient that has OA for these factors and to suggest treatment. Biomechanical assessment also forms the basis of exercise recommendations to avoid excessive impact on the affected joints and to maximize the safe exercise in which patients will engage.

BIOMARKERS

Biochemical changes in joint tissues precede those anatomical changes which can be identified via standard radiology. Identifying these biochemical alterations via specific biomarkers is an important endeavor in order to identify and treat individuals at risk, as well as for targeting early interventions which may slow or prevent the gross anatomical expression of OA upon articular degradation, osteophytosis and joint space narrowing (JSN). There remains a potential use of biomarkers in tracking the efficacy of early interventions aimed at mitigating those biochemical changes which precede the gross anatomical development of OA, thereby halting the process of OA progression. At present, this area is entirely investigational, but may hold promise for clinicians interested in addressing OA pathophysiology prior to the gross anatomical development of the disease. The diagnostic and prognostic value of OA biomarkers is currently an area requiring further research in order to delineate which, if any, biomarkers may be clinically reliable with respect to assessment, prevention and treatment of OA.

In a six-year population-based cohort study of middle-aged subjects with chronic knee pain, researchers report several diagnostic associations between serum and urinary biomarkers and progressive osteophytosis. The researchers assessed cartilage degradation by urinary C-telopeptide fragments of type II collagen (uCTx-II), synthesis by serum type II A procollagen N-terminal propeptide (sPIIANP), and articular tissue turnover by cartilage oligomeric matrix protein (sCOMP). COMP and uCTX-II were shown to have positive predictive value for subsequent progressive osteophytosis in multiple knee compartments, while uCTX-II also showed a positive predictive value for progressive joint space narrowing (JSN). The researchers demonstrated that the biomarker utility with regards to its predictive value may be linked to the timing of the stage of osteoarthritis with respect to progressive osteophytosis and JSN. The formation and progression of osteophytes is characteristic of early-stage OA and was correlated with a higher level of sCOMP in years 0–3 of the study, with a 33% higher risk for tibiofemoral osteophyte progression for every unit increase in sCOMP. On the other hand, joint space narrowing (JSN), a later development in the progression of OA, was significantly associated with an increase in CTX-II in years 3–6 of the study. The researchers note that this is the first study to demonstrate a phasic and nonpersistent character of knee OA with periods of progression and stabilization, associated with biochemical differences revealed through the study's biomarkers (sCOMP, uCTX-II) (Kumm et al., 2013).

C-terminal telopeptide of type II collagen (CTX-II) is primarily generated by matrix metalloproteinase activity during cartilage degradation in OA. It is known to show a closer link with progression of articular cartilage degradation in OA patients. Its increased serum, urine or synovial fluid levels, and correlations with articular cartilage degradation were reported in both preclinical and clinical studies (Garnero et al., 2001; Oestergaard et al., 2006). CTX-II is available as an ELISA assay and may be considered as a method of doing a functional assay of an OA intervention for a patient. The goal is to demonstrate a significant reduction in CTX-II within 8–12 weeks of a new intervention.

A clinical exam can also evaluate the following comorbidities.

RISK FACTORS

The development of OA is thought to be a combination of local joint-specific factors which arise in the context of systemic susceptibility to OA (Suri et al., 2012). Local biomechanical factors include weight-bearing effects of obesity, mechanical environment of the joint (knee laxity, proprioception, knee alignment), occupational factors, physical activity and sports participation and muscle weakness. Systemic risk factors for OA include age, sex, ethnicity, obesity (non-weight bearing mediators including dyslipidemia, inflammatory mediators, adipokines), hormonal status, menopause and bone density, nutritional status, and genetics (Felson et al., 2000; Suri et al., 2012).

Sports activities that may increase the risk of OA include high-intensity, acute, direct joint-impact activities such as football and soccer. Repetitive joint impact with torsional (twisting) is also associated with joint degeneration and occurs in the elbows of baseball pitchers and knees of soccer players. Modification of sports-related OA risk factors includes preparticipation evaluation of individual risk factors, inclusion of playing surfaces that decrease joint impact loading, use of equipment including braces, pads, shoes, and training that improves joint dynamic stability.

Comorbidities

The prevalence of comorbidities in patients with OA is very high, with common comorbidities including hypertension, depression, chronic obstructive pulmonary disease, cardiovascular disease, diabetes, metabolic syndrome and epilepsy. Comorbidities must be considered and addressed when treating the OA patient; however, an in-depth discussion of these factors is beyond the scope of this chapter.

Overweight and Obesity

One of the main risk factors for OA is obesity. Historically, the link between obesity and OA was solely attributed to excessive joint loading resulting from increased body weight. Obesity adds to abnormal alignment and loads at weight-bearing joints, especially the knee and hip. Greater body mass index (BMI) in both women and men has been associated with an increased risk of knee OA. In addition, obesity may lead to altered posture (in standing, sitting and sleeping), altered biomechanics of gait, and less physical activity, any or all of which may further contribute to altered joint biomechanics (Jadelis et al., 2001). In addition, to weight-bearing joints being affected, non-weight-bearing joints are also affected in obesity-induced OA, suggesting a more complex etiology than previously recognized. Non-weight-bearing mechanisms contributing to OA include disturbed lipid metabolism, low-grade inflammation and adverse adipokine profiles. (Thijssen et al. 2015) These mechanisms will briefly be discussed in order to better appreciate the important role of addressing obesity with respect to OA prevention and management.

Obesity is characterized by dyslipidemia including high plasma levels of triglycerides (TGs), low levels of HDL cholesterol (HDL-c), increased levels of LDL cholesterol (LDL-c), increased levels of oxidized LDL (Ox-LDL), as well as elevated levels of free fatty acids (FFAs). High serum total cholesterol has been associated with generalized OA (Sturmer et al. 1998). In addition, osteoarthritic chondrocytes have been shown to accumulate lipids and researchers have shown that the amount of intracellular lipid accumulation correlates positively with OA severity (Lippiello et al. 1991).

Previous research has demonstrated reduced serum HDL cholesterol levels in OA patients (Soran et al., 2008). Recent research has shown a significant inverse relationship between HDL cholesterol levels and risk of hand osteoarthritis (Garcia-Gil et al., 2017). Obesity-related dyslipidemia is also characterized by elevated oxidized LDL. Oxidized LDL has been shown to induce joint inflammation and cartilage destruction via activation of the Ox-LDL receptor-1 (LOX-1). Activation of the LOX-1 by oxidized LDL stimulates the release of vascular endothelial growth factor (VEGF), thereby increasing the expression of inflammatory cytokines IL-1β, IL-6 and TNF-α. In addition, Ox-LDL can directly induce matrix metalloproteinases (MMP), leading to further cartilage degradation, while decreasing chondrocyte cell viability and proteoglycan synthesis.

Free fatty acids (FFAs) may also play a role in the pathophysiology of OA in the context of obesity-related dyslipidemia. Obesity-related dyslipidemia is characterized by an impaired inhibition of intracellular lipolysis resulting in increased release of FFAs from adipose tissue, as well as reduced clearance from the blood. (Ishikawa et al., 2012; Mook et al., 2004). FFAs influence the progression of OA by stimulating toll-like receptor 2/4, leading to systemic as well as local synovial lining macrophage activation. Macrophages located in the synovial lining, under the influence of increased FFAs, upregulate the release of TNF-α, thereby inducing local joint inflammation (Thijssen et al., 2015).

Recent research has revealed an additional role of adipokines in the etiology of OA. Obesity is characterized by altered levels of adipokines secreted by the adipose tissue resulting in increased expression of pro-inflammatory mediators in articular cartilage and synovium. The altered adipokine secretory profile includes increased levels of leptin, resistin and visfatin, with decreased levels of adiponectin in both the plasma and synovial fluid. Adipokines may play a direct role in OA pathogenesis with a positive correlation of leptin, resistin and visfatin and cartilage destruction. Conversely, adiponectin has been shown to have a negative correlation with cartilage destruction with lower levels of adiponectin associated with obesity-related OA.

In conclusion, understanding the important role of obesity in the etiology and morbidity of OA calls the clinician to actively target obesity as a primary modifiable risk factor of OA. Furthermore, weight reduction in patients with established OA may directly affect the underlying biochemical milieu unique to obesity, in addition to reducing the load on susceptible weight-bearing joints. Understanding the key role of these biochemical mediators in obesity-related OA moves us beyond the "wear and tear" model of OA and compels the clinician interested in addressing "root-cause" factors, to actively and aggressively pursue weight loss as a primary prevention and intervention in the obese OA population.

HORMONES

The connection between hormonal status and the risk of OA and OA morbidity is a complex area requiring additional research prior to forming definitive conclusions about the role of hormones and hormone replacement in the OA population. There are numerous studies investigating the correlations between endogenous hormones and OA, as well as the use of exogenous hormones in the treatment of OA. A primary area of focus is the sex hormones, including estrogens and testosterone. Other areas of exploration include progesterone, sex hormone binding globulin, DHEA and aromatase.

The largest meta-analysis to date on sex hormones and OA resulted in mixed data regarding the role of endogenous estrogen and testosterone in OA and regarding the use of estrogen and testosterone replacement. The researchers concluded that there is insufficient evidence to form strong conclusions based on the heterogeneity of the studies, while available evidence supports the effects of both endogenous and exogenous estrogen, as well as estrogen receptor polymorphisms on joint health (Tanamas et al., 2011). One MRI study of men with asymptomatic OA showed a positive cross-sectional association between testosterone and tibial cartilage volume in the medial compartment.

Researchers examined the relationship between serum levels of estradiol, progesterone, testosterone and sex hormone binding globulin (SHBG) and symptomatic knee OA at baseline and 24-month follow-up. The researchers reported a positive correlation between cartilage volume and progesterone levels in females, with an inverse association between estradiol, progesterone and testosterone and effusion-synovitis volume. No statistically significant associations were observed for males. The researchers concluded that low serum levels of estradiol, progesterone and testosterone are associated with increased knee effusion-synovitis and possible other OA-related structural changes (Jin et al., 2017).

ESTROGENS AND MENOPAUSE

The role of estrogens in the development and prevention of OA, and as a potential modifiable risk factor for it, is an important area of consideration. OA is more common in women after menopause, with a world-wide estimate of 10% of men and 18% of women aged 60 or over presenting with symptomatic OA.

The pathophysiology of OA and obesity has been reviewed in a previous section with a focus on additional non-weight-bearing factors which contribute to the increased risk and morbidity of OA in the obese population. Both weight-bearing and non-weight-bearing joints are equally affected in obese women, suggesting a systemic etiology which contributes to the onset and progression of OA. The combination of menopause and obesity may further contribute to the risk and progression OA in a compounded manner and should be taken into consideration when evaluating and treating the postmenopausal obese patient.

Estrogen Replacement

Estrogens act as antiresorptives that directly and indirectly reduce osteoclastogenesis and osteoclastic bone resorption. In addition, chondrocytes express estrogen receptors (ER), primarily ER-β, and are responsive to estrogens (Karsdal et al., 2012). Research has demonstrated that cartilage degradation is significantly lower in women using hormone replacement therapy compared with control. In addition, cartilage degradation has been shown to be significantly higher in postmenopausal women compared to age-matched premenopausal women, suggesting that estrogens play a key role in the potential development and progression of OA (Christgau et al., 2004a; Mouritzen et al., 2003).

Additional research has demonstrated a lower risk of radiographic knee and hip OA in women receiving estrogen replacement therapy (Bay-Jensen et al., 2013). A recent analysis of the Women's Health Initiative (WHI) studies showed a 45% reduction in joint surgery for women taking estrogen compared to the control group (Cirillo et al., 2006). The potential role of estrogen replacement therapy in the prevention of OA is an important area of continued exploration. Initial research points to the possibility that menopause and hormonal status may be considered among the modifiable risk factors for OA. While the need for additional scientific research in this area is most certainly warranted, estrogen replacement therapy is currently an FDA-approved medication for the prevention of osteoporosis. Women who are eligible for estrogen replacement may receive additional benefits with respect to the prevention and treatment of OA in this context.

Testosterone

Testosterone levels and bone density have been inversely correlated in a number of studies in both male and female populations. Studies on testosterone, testosterone replacement therapy (TRT) and OA are currently limited in the medical literature. One MRI study showed a positive correlation between testosterone and tibial cartilage in the medial compartment in healthy men; however, longitudinal follow-up showed reversal of these findings (Cicuttini et al., 2003; Hanna et al., 2005). The researchers acknowledged that definitive conclusions regarding an association between cartilage status and testosterone levels could not be made, noting that factors such as increased physical activity in the higher T group leading to accelerated cartilage degradation could have accounted for the reversal of findings on longitudinal examination (Hanna et al., 2005).

Other studies on testosterone replacement therapy (TRT) have shown equivocal results. Limitations of these studies may include insufficient statistical power to detect statistically significant results due to a small sample size, insufficient dosages of testosterone (median values not established via serological measurement during study), and lack of objective radiological measurements (cartilage volume, bone marrow lesions, effusion-synovitis volume, etc.). At this time a connection between low testosterone and risk of OA or OA morbidity has not been clearly established in the medical literature.

Androgens upregulate transforming growth factor beta (TGF-β) and insulin-like growth factors (IGFs) which stimulate bone formation and downregulate IL-6, thereby inhibiting the formation of osteoclasts. In addition, androgens inhibit parathyroid hormone (PTH), thereby limiting bone resorption. In addition, dihydrotestosterone (DHT) has been shown to reduce osteoprotegerin (OPG) levels, which may play a role in the stimulation of osteoclastic activity (Clarke and Kholsa, 2009).

Clinicians experienced with testosterone replacement therapy (TRT) should consider the individual patient and testosterone status when prescribing TRT, especially with respect to OA comorbidities. Low testosterone has been associated with a number of adverse health outcomes including, but not limited to, reduced muscle strength and mass, increased body fat mass and weight gain, dyslipidemia, and decreased bone density (Morgantaler et al., 2015).

Numerous intervention studies have consistently found improvement in cardiovascular risk factors including fat mass, obesity, waist circumference, blood pressure and glycemic control with the use of TRT in males with baseline low testosterone levels (Morgantaler et al., 2015). The role of obesity and dyslipidemia in contributing to OA has been discussed in a previous section. While understanding the direct effects of testosterone on OA requires additional research, treatment and prevention of OA in eligible males with low testosterone may prove beneficial via improvement in adverse lipid profiles and reduction of fat mass.

Hypermobility syndromes: Patients that have ligament laxity in a single joint have a higher risk of developing OA in that joint. Patients that have joint laxity in numerous joints have a higher risk of developing OA in lower and upper extremity joints. This is more common in patients that have the Benign Hypermobile Joint Syndrome (BHJS) as well as Ehler Danlos Syndrome (EDS) (Bridges et al., 1992). Patients should be screened on history and physical exam for evidence of hypermobility. Patients with hypermobility of their hands are at higher risk of thumb OA at the first CMC joint. Patients with ligament laxity in the knee are at higher risk of progression of knee OA. Patients with BHJS or EDS should be given information regarding how to protect each hypermobile joint. They should be seen by a Physical Therapist trained in this disorder. It is also advisable for the patient to be on daily joint support such as glucosamine sulfate. Extra-articular ligament injections (Prolotherapy) may be appropriate to stabilize hypermobile joints to decrease the likelihood of significant OA developing in a particular hypermobile joint.

Hemochromatosis, an iron storage disease, is a comorbid condition as it can predispose to OA, especially of the MCP joints of the hand. Serum ferritin, iron and transferrin saturation should be checked in any patient with widespread OA or OA at an early age to rule out hemochromatosis.

TREATMENT

TARGETS FOR TREATMENT

The primary treatment targets for OA include the reduction of pain, reducing swelling, reducing inflammation and improving function. Addressing comorbid biomechanical issues is important. This includes: joint biomechanical alignment, muscle recruitment, decreasing biomechanical stress on the joint and stabilizing hypermobility. Addressing other comorbidities such as obesity and hormone issues should be part of a long-term plan. Slowing joint degeneration and encouraging regeneration of cartilage are important. Increasing range of motion is an important goal and may involve manual therapies along with interventions mentioned in this chapter. Increasing joint space on an X-ray may be a desired goal but should not be promised as it is difficult to accomplish and may require long periods of time. Increasing joint space should be discussed on a case-by-case basis in regard to the amount of joint space narrowing that exists and the options for treatment that the patient can undergo. Injection therapies such as stem cell injections may have the greatest likelihood of increasing joint space, along with the non-injection therapies mentioned in this chapter.

When treating a patient it is reasonable to pick treatments that address the pathophysiology as well as comorbid factors. It is reasonable to have a short-term plan to reduce symptoms and a longer-term plan to work on comorbidities. Short-term therapies should address joint pathophysiology including but not limited to: decreasing inflammation (especially IL-1, IL 6, IL-17, TNF-α, NF-κB and PGE-2), providing precursor nutrients for chondrocytes and the matrix, inhibiting matrix metalloproteinases and other damaging enzymes.

Nutritional therapies may be especially useful in the treatment of OA because they may provide substrates for cartilage regeneration, decrease inflammation and have demonstrated efficacy in controlling pain and improving function. Nutritional therapies are outlined in Table 25.1.

NSAIDs AND NSAID SIDE EFFECTS

NSAIDS, both OTC and prescription, have been the primary treatment of OA. They appear to be moderately effective for pain control and in improving function. They are often used in doses that are more analgesic than anti-inflammatory. NSAIDs inhibit cyclooxygenase (COX-2) and block prostaglandin synthesis. NSAIDs may also decrease pro-inflammatory cytokines such as interleukin-6 (IL-6) and tumor necrosis factor alpha (TNF-α) in synovial fluid in knee OA (Gallelli et al., 2013).

NSAIDs are, unfortunately, associated with a significant side-effect profile. These side effects include increased risk of cardiovascular events including MI, stomach and duodenal ulcers, aggravation of ulcerative colitis, liver damage, and decreased renal blood flow along with potential decline in renal function.

While NSAIDs are effective in the reduction of pain, the long-term use of NSAIDs is not recommended in OA due to their side-effect profile of these agents. If a practitioner is set on the use of long-term NSAIDs it appears that Naprosyn is less likely to cause cardiovascular side effects compared to Celebrex and ibuprofen. The authors of this chapter would advocate not using long-term OTC or prescription NSAIDS but would advocate using anti-inflammatory supplements as outlined below.

In addition to the inherent side effects of NSAIDs, there is evidence, both in animals with experimental OA and in humans, that administration of NSAIDs may actually accelerate joint destruction (Brandt, 1987a,b). Due to the high incidence of side effects from NSAIDS, clinicians may consider avoiding them or minimize their use when possible and only use on a short-term basis when necessary.

NSAIDs may lead to defects in the mucous lining of the gastric mucosa, small or large intestine. They can lead to damage of the wall of the intestine. The former may be treated with nutritional support to improve the mucous lining. NSAIDs may also lead to an iron deficiency anemia, which

TABLE 25.1

Mechanism of Action by which Nutrients Protect Against Osteoarthritis

Supplement	Mechanism of Action	Dose
Analgesic		
Avocado/soybean unsaponifiable residues (ASU)	Analgesic	
Chondroitin sulfate	Analgesic	
Glucosamine sulfate	Analgesic	
SAMe	Analgesic	
Modulate Inflammation		
Avocado/soybean unsaponifiable residues (ASU)	Modulate inflammation by suppressing IL-1, PGE-2, IL-6, IL-8	300 mg/day
Omega-3 fatty acids	Modulate inflammation by suppressing IL-1, TNF-α, PGE-2, 5-LOX, FLAP, COX-2	3–4 grams per day
SAMe	Modulate inflammation by suppressing IL-1, TNF-α	400 mg 2× a day
Glucoasamine sulfate	Modulate inflammation by suppressing PGE-2	1500 mg one time per day
Devil's claw	Decrease NF-κB	
Lyprinol	Decrease COX-2	900–1200 mg per day
Hyaluronic acid	Binds to TLR-4; increase I IL-10	80–240 mg/day
Hops, THIAA	Decrease NF-κB and TNF-α	
Boswellia	Inhibit LOX and COX	500–600 mg 3× a day
Curcumin	Decrease IL-1B, IL-6, TNF-α, PGE-2, COX-2 and NF-κB	500 mg 2–3× a day
Cartilage Regeneration		
Undenatured type II collagen	Increase type II collagen synthesis	40 mg 2–3× a day
Chondroitin sulfate	Increase proteoglycan synthesis	800 mg 1× per day
Glucosamine sulfate	Increase proteoglycan synthesis; increase chondrocyte matrix gene expression	1500 mg 1× per day
SAMe	Increase proteoglycan synthesis	400 mg 2× a day
Avocado/soybean unsaponifiable residues (ASU)	Increase collagen synthesis; stimulate TGF-β1; stimulate plasminogen activator inhibitor-1 expression	300 mg/day
Vitamin C	Increase collagen and proteoglycan synthesis; stabilization of the mature collagen fibril	250–500 mg 3× a day
Strontium	Increase IGF1	680 mg/day
Decrease Degradation		
Glucosamine sulfate	Decrease collagen degradation	
Omega-3 fatty acids	Decrease degradation by inhibiting ADAMTS-4, MMP-3, MMP-13, aggrecanase	2–4 grams per day
Vitamin C	Decrease degradation by inhibiting aggrecanase	250–500 mg 3× a day
Avocado/soybean unsaponifiable residues (ASU)	Decrease degradation by inhibiting metalloproteinase activity and collagenase synthesis	
Strontium	Increase OPG;	680 mg per day
Curcumin	decrease MMP-1, -3 and -13 and ADAMTS-5; increase OPG	500 mg 2–3 times a day
Tetrahydro-Iso-Alpha-Acids	Decrease MMP-9	300 mg/day 2× a day

Source: Table is reprinted with permission from Taylor and Francis from *Scientific Basis for Musculoskeletal, Bariatric and Sports Nutrition*.

may be treated with supplemental iron. Prolonged NSAID use may increase the permeability of the small intestine and may predispose an individual to food allergies or increased intestinal permeability, which may further aggravate joint pain.

NSAIDS appear safer when administered topically. This is reasonable for the knee, elbow, feet and hands. It is reasonable to use a topical NSAID two times a day over the involved joint for 2–4 weeks to determine if there is clinical benefit and to continue it if there is. When treating knee OA there has been evidence that topical NSAIDS have decreased pain at about the same level as with oral NSAIDs, but are much safer. The NSAIDS diclofenac, ibuprofen, and ketoprofen have been shown to be most efficacious when administered topically (Rannou et al., 2016). They can be applied to areas such as the knee, wrist, hands, feet, elbows where the joints with OA are not too deep.

Narcotic pain -relieving medications are not recommended for OA pain but are still being used. Narcotics can slow intestinal motility and lead to constipation, and may also lead to addiction. These drugs may also lead to pain sensitization and aggravate chronic pain.

Several nutritional supplements have been shown to be as effective as NSAIDs in reducing pain and improving functional limitation in patients with OA without adverse effects common to NSAIDs. These include glucosamine sulfate, Lyprinol and SAMe. A 2004 study demonstrated SAMe (1200 mg/d) was as effective as a commonly prescribed COX-2 inhibitor, but with a slower onset of action and a lower incidence of side effects (Soeken et al., 2002).

TOPICAL AGENTS

Topical NSAIDS have been studied and appear most effective for OA of the knee and hands. There appears to be a role for topical lidocaine in a 4%–5% patch. This role would be to provide some pain relief in patients with chronic pain from OA. Lidocaine does not exhibit an anabolic or anti-inflammatory effect.

INJECTION THERAPIES

There are a number of injection therapies that have shown benefit in OA, especially of the knee. Cortisone injections can have a significant anti-inflammatory effect in patients with moderate to severe OA. Cortisone injections may lead to cartilage degeneration in the long run and should not be the mainstay of treatment. The effects may wear off after about two months.

Platelet-rich plasma (PRP) is thought to provide high concentrations of growth factors, including tissue growth factor and platelet-derived growth factors, which may increase the proliferation of mesenchymal stem cells and increase collagen production and matrix synthesis (Anderson et al., 2005). PRP can reduce inflammation in an OA joint by enhancing the expression of NF-κB inhibitor, and thus reduce NF-κB signaling and dampen its downstream inflammatory cytokine activation (Andia and Maffulli, 2013). PRP when injected in a knee has shown the ability to switch off the inhibition of type II collagen and aggrecan gene expression in IL-1β-activated NF-κB in chondrocytes (van Buul et al., 2011).

A meta-analysis of ten trials assessing the effect of PRP injections in patients with knee OA found a significant difference in pain scores in the PRP-treated groups (Laudy et al, 2015). However, only one of the trials compared PRP injections with placebo.

There have not been any trials examining the structural effects of PRP in OA joints in regard to joint space. There is also a lack of standardization of the preparations of PRP amongst the trials, with varying concentrations of platelet, frozen versus fresh preparations, and the filtration of white cells.

STEM CELL INJECTIONS

Mesenchymal stem cell (MSC) injections of stem cells derived from bone marrow and adipose tissue have been used in severe OA of knees and hips. The procedures can vary widely in regard to what type of stem cell is used, as well as how it is then prepared after harvesting (culture expanded, etc.). There are studies that show efficacy with stem cells injected into knee and other joints (Filardo et al, 2016; Chahla et al., 2016; Burke et al., 2016; Freitag et al., 2016; Centeno et al., 2014). A recent article has outlined some of the adverse effects of stem cell injections (Centeno et al., 2016).

It appears that MSC injections may be efficacious in knee and hip OA that is moderate to severe and in which patients are trying to avoid operative management. It is important for clinicians who do not do this injection to be aware of the research and the different methods available and to refer to centers that they believe are using the safest and most research-based methods for efficacy.

Fibroblast Growth Factor (FGF): A recombinant FGF-18 (sprifermin) has been used in human trials. There is study evidence that FGF-18 may be efficacious for OA. FGF-18 has been shown in animal models of injury-induced OA to have an anabolic effect on cartilage, stimulating proteoglycan synthesis and cartilage matrix formation (Ellman et al., 2008; Moore et al., 2005).

Two phase 1 trials of intra-articular recombinant human FGF-18 for knee OA have demonstrated a statistically significant dose-dependent improvement in tibiofemoral cartilage volume and a reduction in joint space narrowing after 12 months (Mastbergen et al., 2013). An initial proof-of-concept trial with *intra-articular sprifermin* in 180 knee OA patients has shown some promise (Lohmander et al., 2014). There was a statistically significant dose-dependent reduction in loss of total and lateral tibiofemoral cartilage thickness but no change in medial or central tibiofemoral cartilage. There was improvement in WOMAC pain scores in those receiving the highest doses of sprifermin (100 µg). At this time this drug is in phase 2 clinical trials.

Nutritional Therapies Can Reduce Inflammation

Inflammatory mediators are integral in the pathogenesis of OA. Human OA cartilage expresses modulators of inflammation (COX-2, 5-LOX, FLAP, IL-1α, TNF-α) (Curtis et al., 2002) that normal human cartilage does not. Inhibition of inflammatory mediators may slow disease progression and has long been a target for treatment. Table 25.1 summarizes the mechanism by which avocado/soybean unsaponifiable residues, omega-3 fatty acids, SAMe, and glucosamine interfere with the inflammatory cascade. Other agents that can be considered to decrease inflammation are curcumin and Boswellia.

The clinician should consider placing a patient on an anti-inflammatory, low-toxin diet rich in food-based antioxidants as part of a long-term treatment program to reduce inflammatory mediators. The clinician may also want to recommend a trial of a nightshade (potatoes, tomatoes, peppers and eggplant) free diet for 3–4 weeks to see if a patient has pain reduction and to continue it if they do.

Omega-3 Fatty Acids

Osteoarthritic cartilage expresses markers of inflammation that contribute to the dysregulation of chondrocyte function and the progressive degradation of the cartilage matrix. *In vitro*, when human OA cartilage explants are exposed to omega-3 polyunsaturated fatty acids, the molecular modulators of inflammation are inhibited. Curtis et al. cultured human OA articular cartilage with various fatty acids and concluded omega-3 fatty acids, but not other fats, have the capacity to improve late-stage OA chondrocyte function. They found culture for 24 hours with omega-3 fatty acids resulted in a decreased loss of GAGs, reduced collagenase cleavage of type II collagen, a dose-dependent reduction in aggrecanase, and all studied modulators of inflammation (COX-2, 5-LOX, FLAP, IL-1α) and joint destruction (ADAMTS-4, MMP-3, MMP-13) were abrogated or reduced (Curtis et al., 2002).

The concentration and distribution of fatty acids in the diet has long been known to exert influence over the inflammatory cascade.

When treating patients with omega-3 fatty acids it is reasonable to use fish oil products consisting of the triglyceride form of EPA and DHA because it may be better absorbed. It is reasonable to choose products that have been tested for purity and that are extremely low in contaminants of pesticides, mercury and PCBs. It is reasonable to use approximately 2–4 g of high-EPA fish oil per day. In patients with sluggish delta-6-desaturase enzymes the omega-6 equivalent GLA may also need to be taken even though it is omega-6. This would be recommended for patients that are obese as well as for patients that have metabolic syndrome. It is reasonable to use about 240 mg of GLA in most patients on 2–4 g of fish oil. Side effects of fish oil are minimal but caution should be used if a patient is on a medication such as Coumadin because of the platelet effects of fish oil.

Lyprinol is a patented extraction of New Zealand green-lipped mussel powder derived from *Perna canaliculus*. It has been shown to provide significant pain relief and improvement in joint function in 80% of subjects after 8 weeks of treatment without adverse effect. The therapeutic value of Lyprinol has been attributed, in part, to its high concentration of omega-3 fatty acids (Cho et al., 2003).

There have been variable results in efficacy of trials using Lyprinol in patients with OA at the current starting dose of 900–1200 mg per day. It would not be a first-line approach and EPA/DHA capsules or oil should be used first for their anti-inflammatory effect because of extensive research on safety and beneficial effects in joints and non-joint systems. It appears that Lyprinol does not have the same adverse GI side-effect profile as NSAIDS and therefore could be used as a safe anti-inflammatory for patients with OA.

SAMe (S-Adenosyl Methionine)

SAMe is synthesized endogenously from methionine and adenosine triphosphate (ATP). It is a methyl donor to numerous acceptor molecules and plays an essential role in many biochemical reactions involving enzymatic transmethylation. In addition it has proved efficacious in the treatment of OA in regard to treatment of inflammation and cartilage regeneration and its use is primarily limited by quality and cost factors.

SAMe has been shown to inhibit the synthesis and the activity of IL-1 and TNF-α at multiple locations in its signal transduction pathways. SAMe has demonstrated the ability to upregulate the proteoglycan synthesis and proliferation rate of chondrocytes, thereby promoting cartilage formation and repair. SAMe is an alternative to NSAIDs for treatment of joint inflammation and pain caused by trauma and disease states such as OA. It is a proven therapy for OA and has a low side-effect profile. The consensus among several published reviews is that SAMe appears to be of equivalent effectiveness to NSAIDs in reducing pain and improving functional limitations, with fewer side effects. One study suggested SAMe has a slower onset of action than NSAIDs with equivalent results at 4 weeks (Najm et al., 2004).

B12 and folate aid the body in using SAMe, and it may be useful to supplement with these nutrients as well. The amounts in a good multiple would usually be sufficient but one may want to choose methylated forms of folate. SAMe can interact with tramadol as well as serotonergic antidepressants. One should try and use other agents when these drugs are already prescribed or use SAMe with caution and monitor patients for a serotonergic syndrome. There appears to be some efficacy of SAMe in patients with fibromyalgia, therefore it would be a good choice in a patient with OA and fibromyalgia (Jacobsen et al., 1991).

SAMe is efficacious in depression so that its use would be indicated in a patient with OA and comorbid depression. One would then evaluate its efficacy on mood as well as its effect on pain.

Patients should be encouraged to use enteric-coated SAMe. The dosage of SAMe is typically 200–400 mg three times per day for OA and 800 mg per day if one was treating OA and fibromyalgia.

Curcumin

Curcumin has anti-inflammatory effects and can suppress inflammatory mediators such as IL-1Beta, IL-6, IL-8, TNF-α, PGE-2, lipooxygenase and COX-2, as well as inhibiting the activation of nuclear factor kappa-B (NF-κB) (Yeh et al., 2015; Henrotin et al., 2010; Matis and Shakibaei, 2010).

Curcumin may also decrease damaging enzymes such as MMP-1, -3 and -13, as well as aggrecanase ADAMTS-5 (Yeh et al., 2015). It may also upregulate a chondroprotective transcriptional regulator CITED2, in cultured chondrocytes in the absence or presence of IL-1β, and decrease reactive oxygen species (Aggarwal et al., 2013; Henrotin et al., 2010). Curcumin may inhibit RANKL in the joint (Yeh et al., 2015). Curcumin can increase the OPG/RANKL ratio and thus may be protective of subchondral bone (Bharti et al., 2004).

Curcumin may have direct effects on production of type II collagen and glycosaminoglycans. It may inhibit apoptosis of chondrocytes by inhibiting capsase 3 (Henrotin et al., 2009).

Of note is that curcumin has low solubility, poor GI absorption and poor systemic bioavailability (Mirzael et al., 2017). If it is to be used orally for OA it should be taken in a form that increases curcumin absorption including nanoparticle, liposomal, phospholipid complexes and BCM-95 forms. The best studied form of curcumin for OA is the Meriva liposomal form. Doses varied between 200 and 1500 mg per day (Mirzael et al., 2017). It is the authors' protocol to start with this form of curcumin at 500 mg 2× a day and reassess in 4 weeks and increase to 3× a day to see if there is an increase in effect with regard to pain and swelling reduction, and improvement in function. Studies with nanoparticle topical curcumin showed slowing of OA progression in knees in a mouse model (Zhang et al., 2016). It is reasonable to use curcumin in a nanoparticle topical form for joints with OA that are a short distance from the skin.

NUTRITIONAL THERAPIES CAN PROVIDE SUBSTRATES FOR CARTILAGE REPAIR AND REGENERATION

The regeneration of cartilage must be an emphasis of treatment to minimize disease progression. Substantial evidence, *in vitro* and *in vivo*, attests to the ability of nutritional agents to enhance proteoglycan synthesis, increase strength of the collagen network, decrease proteinases that degrade collagen and proteoglycans (aggrecanase), and decrease IL-1 and subsequent pro-inflammatory cytokines that further perpetuate cartilage degradation.

Nourishment of the joint is complicated in that articular cartilage is neither vascularized nor supplied with nerves or lymphatic vessels. The outer third of the knee meniscus has a reasonable blood supply. Chondrocytes receive their nourishment from synovial fluid. The use of nutritional supplements to support joints with osteoarthritic changes makes sense primarily if there is cartilage surface remaining, as opposed to bone-on-bone anatomy. It also makes sense as prevention for other joints in the setting of a joint that has minimal cartilage remaining or in one that has been replaced. Most of the studies regarding nutraceutical support have been done regarding osteoarthritis of the knee, but it is very reasonable to consider its use in other joints with OA.

JOINT SUPPORT SUPPLEMENTS

Glucosamine

"Glucosamine therapy for treating osteoarthritis" was first published in the *Cochrane Database of Systematic Reviews* in the year 2001 and was updated both in 2005 and 2009. The findings from the Cochrane Collaboration provide level 1 evidence in support of the use of the Rotta preparation (stabilized) of glucosamine sulfate in OA. In 2001 publication researchers identified 16 randomized controlled trials (RCTs) providing evidence that glucosamine sulfate is both safe and effective in OA. Most of the trials only evaluated the Rotta preparation of glucosamine sulfate. In 13 RCTs glucosamine was compared to placebo and was found to be superior to placebo in 12 out of 13 studies. Glucosamine was compared to NSAIDs in four RCTs and was found to be superior in two and equivalent in two (Towheed et al., 2001). The 2005 update analyzed 20 RCTs and found that glucosamine favored placebo with a 28% improvement in pain and 21% improvement in function, using the Lequesne index. RCTs using a non-Rotta preparation of glucosamine failed to demonstrate effects beyond placebo (Towheed et al., 2005). In a 2007 editorial by two of the authors, they highlight the importance of ensuring the content and purity of over-the-counter preparations of glucosamine sulfate with respect to safety and efficacy (Towheed and Anastassiades, 2007). The conclusions of the 2009 updated Cochrane Review, which included an additional five RCTs, total 25, found no benefit in pain and WOMAC function in those studies using a non-Rotta preparation, while those using the Rotta preparation showed glucosamine to be superior to placebo. In addition, none of the additional studies included in this review contradicted the original finding of the authors' 2001 publication regarding the superior effect of glucosamine compared to NSAIDs in two studies, and equivalent effects in two others (Towheed et al., 2009).

The vast majority of published clinical research studies have demonstrated that glucosamine is effective for decreasing pain, improving range of motion and improving function. N-acetyl-D-glucosamine is a naturally occurring amino sugar found in all human tissues. It functions as a building block in the synthesis of structural cartilage matrix substrates such as glycoproteins, glycolipids, GAGs, hyaluronate, and proteoglycans and is required to manufacture joint lubricants and protective agents such as mucin and mucus secretions (Matheson and Perry, 2003). Glucosamine sulfate has been found to inhibit NF-κB and PGE-2 and thus can have anti-inflammatory effects (Argo et al., 2003).

Crystalline stabilized GS has been shown to inhibit IL-1β-induced gene expression of matrix degradation factors MMP-3 (stromelysin-1) and ADAMTS-5 (aggrecanase 2), thus having an effect of decreasing enzyme mediated chondrocyte degradation (Chiusaroli et al., 2011). Crystalline stabilized GS was introduced in studies as the "Dona" form. Other companies now have stabilized GS. When prescribing GS it is important to ask a company if their GS is stabilized.

Although glucosamine is not generally found in the human diet, it is made from the exoskeletons of shrimp, crabs, and lobsters for use in medical applications. It is also available in a vegan form that is made from corn. It is important to make sure that the form is the sulfate and not the HCL form and that the product is stabilized. As a supplement, glucosamine is available as glucosamine sulfate, glucosamine hydrochloride, and N-acetyl glucosamine. Thus far, the majority of clinical research demonstrating efficacy in OA has been conducted with the sulfate form. Glucosamine sulfate is the recommended form at this time.

When administered orally, the absorption rate for glucosamine sulfate (GS) in the human GI tract is approximately 87% (Setnikar et al., 1993). In recent years, topical cream containing glucosamine and chondroitin sulfate has shown efficacy in relieving pain in OA of the knee (Cohen et al., 2003). Topical GS (10% and 30%) is reasonable to use for peripheral meniscus tears in patients with reasonable knee function, chondromalacia patella, and OA of the great toe, thumb and fingers. It should be applied 1–2 times per day over the joint line areas.

Glucosamine sulfate has been shown in a number of studies to slow progression of joint space narrowing in the knee. One study compared GSA 1500 mg per day vs. placebo and followed the patients for three years. It demonstrated a mean joint space narrowing of 0.04 mm in the GS group vs 0.19 mm in the placebo group (Pavelka et al., 2002). These results were similar to another three-year study of GS vs. placebo study published in the *Lancet* in 2001 (Reginster et al., 2001). In 2004, a study was published documenting that glucosamine sulfate had the ability to reduce joint space narrowing in postmenopausal women with osteoarthritis of the knee (Bruyere et al., 2004). The mechanism of action is purported to be the increased availability of substrate for proteoglycan synthesis as well as anti-inflammatory actions.

All of the above studies used a single daily dose of GS of 1500 mg. This can be done as three 500 mg capsules or two 750 mg capsules. It is reasonable for the clinician to recommend that their patient use this dose and a dosing method as a minimum dose to achieve structure-modifying effects.

While studies of glucosamine and OA are largely positive, there are a few negative studies that raise several interesting questions about whether or not glucosamine may be more effective in OA subtypes. In a 2004 study, Christgau et al. explored using specific markers of collagen turnover to help classify patients at baseline. Using these markers, they were able to demonstrate that those patients who initially had high cartilage turnover were particularly responsive to glucosamine therapy (Christgau et al., 2004b). Another question remaining for clinical investigation is the generalizability of glucosamine to treating OA of all joints, since the knee has been the most widely studied. The authors have had experience using stabilized GS for all extremity joints and spinal joints with OA and have found efficacy.

The one constant found in all studies reported in the medical literature is that glucosamine appears to be remarkably safe and well tolerated at 1500 mg per day. Side effects are significantly less common with glucosamine than either NSAIDs. Studies have addressed concerns that glucosamine, a sugar, can have adverse effects on levels of plasma glucose and insulin, but further research has found these concerns to be unfounded (Tannis et al., 2004; Scroggie et al., 2003).

Glucosamine is often derived from shellfish and several authors have expressed concern that the supplement may cause allergic reactions in people who are sensitive to shellfish. Glucosamine is derived from the exoskeletons of shellfish but antibodies in individuals allergic to shellfish are targeted at antigens in the meat, not the shell. Thus far, there have been no documented reports of allergic reactions to glucosamine among shellfish-sensitive patients, but it is prudent to recommend the synthetically derived, generally vegan (corn-based) form of the supplement be used in this population (Gray et al., 2004).

Most studies have concluded that patients taking glucosamine do not seem to notice much effect for at least six weeks. Patients need to be educated in regard to the duration of supplementation and how long it may take to notice an effect. In general GS should be taken for about ten weeks after an acute extremity joint injury or sprain of the neck or low back. GS should be taken for a minimum of ten weeks by the patient with moderate to severe OA to determine if there is efficacy.

Chondroitin Sulfate

Chondroitin sulfate (CS), a mucopolysaccharide, is a proteoglycan component that functions in the maintenance of cartilage elasticity, strength, and mass. It may inhibit COX-2 and stimulate the cartilage matrix. In humans, chondroitin sulfate is made from glucosamine sulfate derivatives. Chondroitin sulfate, like glucosamine, is not present in significant amounts in the human diet. It is extracted from either bovine trachea or marine shell sources for use in OA.

The medical literature contains numerous studies, of varying quality, pertaining to the use of chondroitin as a therapy for OA. Many early studies have shown efficacy in relieving pain and improving function whereas some later studies and meta-analyses have not (Reichenbach et al., 2007). Chondroitin studies have often used combinations of chondroitin with glucosamine (often in the HCL form). CS has been shown in many studies to alleviate pain, decrease NSAID use and improve joint mobility. Studies have shown that CS may be able to slow the progression of joint space narrowing with osteoarthritis of the knee Reginster et al., 2003). A study demonstrated reduction in joint space narrowing of 0.1 mm compared to 0.24 mm in the placebo group (Kahan, 2006).

Results of chondroitin supplementation typically take 8–12 weeks to become apparent, as is the case in the glucosamine studies. The recommended dosage is 800–1200 mg per day given in one or two doses.

There is not enough evidence to suggest an additive benefit of chondroitin when glucosamine sulfate is already being used in therapeutic doses, but CS is generally relatively inexpensive and without side effects. Because of this it is recommended that the clinician recommend glucosamine sulfate as a first-line agent and make sure the patient is using glucosamine sulfate because of the research to support that formulation. One could then add 1200 mg per day of CS after a minimum of 12 weeks on GS to see if the patient improved in pain and function. It would also be reasonable to choose a second agent other than CS, based on the recent meta-analysis.

An important controversy in the medical literature as it pertains to the efficacy of chondroitin is whether or not clinically significant amounts are available to the body via oral dosing, given the large size of the molecule. During the past few years, several studies have demonstrated a low oral absorption of chondroitin sulfate and shown absorption estimates across the gut mucosa range from 10 to 70% (Barthe et al., 2004). Low molecular weight CS was developed to improve absorption of CS.

Other than mild gastrointestinal distress, the incidence of adverse effects with chondroitin sulfate is extremely low. Chondroitin is typically extracted from bovine trachea and concern has been expressed about the potential risk of contamination by animals infected with bovine spongiform encephalopathy (BSE, or "mad cow disease"). There are currently no documented cases of such contamination and risk of transmission is thought to be low. Low molecular weight CS is made from shellfish sources. Vegetarian patients should be informed of the bovine or shellfish origin of chondroitin products.

Of interest is that chondroitin sulfate has been shown to have an action as a mast cell stabilizer. There are patients that have worsening pain when they are having concurrent allergies. In this population CS is an excellent supplement to use. There are some studies documenting increased mast cells in osteoarthritic joints that would make a trial of CS worthwhile (de Lange-Brokaar et al., 2016).

Collagen Type II

Undenatured type II collagen (UC-II) is a nutritional supplement which is derived from chicken sternum cartilage. In an RCT of 190 individuals with symptomatic knee OA, UC-II (40 mg) over a 180-day period significantly improved knee joint symptoms in knee OA, as measured by the Western Ontario McMaster Universities Osteoarthritis Index (WOMAC). Secondary outcome measures included the Lequesne Functional Index (LFI), Visual Analog Scale (VAS) and WOMAC subscales. UC-II supplementation resulted in significant improvement in all three WOMAC subscales (Lugo et al., 2016).

Another clinical trial investigated the efficacy of UC-II versus glucosamine and chondroitin (G+C) in knee OA patients. Twenty-five patients were randomized to each intervention group. The patients were treated for 90 days with either UC-II 40 mg once daily or G+C 1500/1200 mg twice daily. Each UC-II capsule contained 20 mg of UC-II standardized to 5 mg of bioactive undenatured type II collagen. The G+C capsules contained glucosamine HCL (USP grade) and chondroitin sulfate (USP grade). Outcome measures included the WOMAC, VAS and LFI. Both treatments reduced WOMAC, VAS and LFI scores with a reduction of 33%/40%/20% (WOMAC/VAS/LFI) by UC-II versus 14%/15.4%/6% (WOMAC/VAS/LFI) by G+C. The authors disclosed that the research was supported by InterHealth Research, a producer of UC-II (Crowley et al., 2009).

Limitations of this study include the use of glucosamine hydrochloride (HCL) instead of glucosamine sulfate, which has been shown to demonstrate increased efficacy when compared to glucosamine HCL, particularly the Rotta preparation. At present, glucosamine sulfate has a more robust body of evidence regarding its efficacy, as previously cited in the Cochrane Systematic Review entitled "Glucosamine therapy for treating osteoarthritis." This study should therefore be interpreted with caution regarding conclusions about the increased efficacy of UC-II over glucosamine. In conclusion, patients with OA may benefit from both UC-II as well as standardized glucosamine sulfate in the form of the Rotta or another stabilized form.

Methylsulfonylmethane (MSM)

MSM is a source of sulfur as well as a methyl donor. In one study MSM and glucosamine sulfate (GS) were used alone and in combination. Both agents were found to be efficacious in OA but the combination of 500 mg of MSM and 500 mg of GS was found to be more efficacious than the use of one of them alone. Also in this study patients reported improvement in symptoms with less lag time than with the individual agents alone (Usha and Naida, 2004). MSM has been shown at doses of 3 g two times per day in a placebo-controlled trial to decrease pain and increase function in activities of daily living (Kim et al., 2006). MSM appears to have a minimal side-effect profile. Although there have only been two studies, MSM appears to show efficacy. Doses of 3000 mg twice a day are recommended if used alone or 500 mg three times a day if used concurrently with GS.

Hyaluronic Acid

Hyaluronic acid (HA) is a main component of the extracellular matrix within the joint. It is a hydrophilic polysaccharide varying in length from 250 to 25,000 disaccharide units. The large size of this molecule and the water it holds give the matrix solution remarkable viscosity, tensile, and shock-absorption properties. HA is present in joints in the cartilage matrix as well as the synovial fluid. In moderate to severe OA the synovium may produce less HA and the synovial fluid may become dysfunctional.

Intra-articular hyaluronans (viscosupplementation) have been used extensively to treat pain and mechanical dysfunction associated with osteoarthritis of the knee. Many controlled clinical studies have demonstrated their efficacy and a low side-effect profile for this indication and application (Kelly et al., 2004; Aggarwal and Sempowski, 2004).

Intra-articular injections of the knee are indicated if the patient has very little cartilage surface and wishes to avoid surgery. They are done one time per week for 3–5 weeks (depending on the viscosupplementation formulation used). An improvement in pain levels and in function appears to have clinical benefit lasting from 6 to 9 months. The treatment often needs to be repeated after 6–9 months. Side effects are minimal and may include swelling. It is of note that this treatment is usually given to patients who have little cartilage and joint space remaining in the tibia femur joint. It can in fact be very beneficial in patients with moderate joint space narrowing with patellofemoral OA.

There appears to be a role for oral hyaluronic acid in the treatment of osteoarthritis of the knee and possibly other joints. One of the mechanisms of action of HA appears to be on the epithelial cells of the intestine. It has been shown to bind to toll-like receptor 4 (TLR-4), which can lead to an increase in an anti-inflammatory cytokine IL-10 and increase the production of suppressor of cytokine signaling 3 (SOCS3), which can lead to the suppression of pro-inflammatory cytokine expression. The binding of HA to TLR-4 also suppresses the expression of pleiotrophin, which can contribute to the suppression of inflammation (Asari et al., 2010).

Doses have varied from 80 to 240 mg per day in various studies. The studies have all been done on knee OA and have been done in animal and human studies. They have shown efficacy in regard to a reduction in knee pain, an improvement in function and some of them have shown a decrease in synovitis. A good review of all of the human studies has been done by Mariko Oe in the *Nutrition Journal* (Oe et al., 2016).

Cetylated Fatty Acids

Cetylated fatty acids (CFAs) have been used in studies both orally and topically. They have been marketed under the name of Celadrin and Cetyl Myristoleate and have minimal side effects. CFAs have been demonstrated in short-term studies to improve range of motion and function of patients with knee OA (Hesslink and Armstrong, 2002) A single short-term study has demonstrated efficacy of topical cetylated fatty acids on wrist and elbow function and endurance during exercise (Kraemer et al., 2004). CFA may be taken orally in a dose of 350 mg or used topically to improve pain and function in OA of the knee, elbow and wrist. It appears to be more useful when used topically 2× a day. It is best used for chondromalacia when applied on either side of the patella. One could extend this use to the thumb at the CMC joint. It should be used 2× a day for at least 8–10 weeks.

Vitamin C/Ascorbic Acid

Ascorbic acid plays a role in the synthesis of joint components, encourages cartilage synthesis *in vitro*, and epidemiologic data suggests dietary intake of ascorbic acid is associated with a reduction of OA progression. Vitamin C is necessary for the synthesis of collagen and GAGs within the joint capsule. In collagen synthesis, ascorbic acid is a cofactor for enzymes essential for stabilization of the mature collagen fibril. The role of vitamin C as a carrier of sulfate groups also makes it a requirement for GAG synthesis (Schwartz and Adamy, 1977).

In vitro, the addition of ascorbic acid to OA cultures results in a decreased level of aggrecanase, the primary enzyme responsible for the degradation of proteoglycan. Vitamin C has been shown to significantly increase the biosynthesis of proteoglycan in both normal and osteoarthritic tissues, suggesting it may be helpful in joint repair (Schwartz and Adamy, 1977).

In the Framingham Osteoarthritis Cohort Study, a moderate intake of vitamin C (120–200 mg/d) was associated with a threefold lower risk of OA progression. The association was strong and highly significant and was consistent between sexes and among individuals with different severities of OA. The higher vitamin C intake also reduced the likelihood of development of knee pain (McAlindon et al., 1996a).

Avocado/Soybean Unsaponifiable Residues (ASU)

ASU is a manufactured product, distributed in France as Piascledine, consisting of one-third avocado oil and two-thirds soybean unsaponifiables (Hauselmann, 2001). Three of four rigorous clinical trials suggest that ASU is an effective symptomatic treatment of OA. A dose of 300 mg ASU per day has demonstrated efficacy in both knee and hip OA but appears to have been studied more extensively for hip OA. Outcome measures have included a reduction in NSAID and analgesic intake, a reduction in pain, and an increase in function. ASU has been shown to have structure-modifying effects in the hip (Lequesne et al., 2002). No serious side effects were reported in any of the published studies.

Based on *in vitro* research, the apparent mechanism of effect of ASU is via the attenuation of inflammatory mediators and the stimulation of anabolic processes within the cartilage. The anti-inflammatory effects of ASU include the inhibition of IL-1 and the inhibition of IL-1-stimulated PGE-2 and pro-inflammatory cytokines IL-6 and IL-8 *in vitro*, and it prevented the deleterious action of IL-1 on synovial cells and on articular chondrocytes of rabbits *in vivo* (Boumediene et al., 1999; Henrotin et al., 1998).

Several *in vitro* studies on cultured chondrocytes have demonstrated these unsaponifiable residues have an inhibitory action on collagenase synthesis, metalloproteinases, pro-inflammatory cytokines IL-6 and IL-8, the inducible form of nitric oxide synthase and PGE-2, all of which decrease inflammation (Spector et al., 1994; Ernst, 2003). The anabolic effects of ASU include the *in vitro* stimulation of collagen synthesis and transforming growth factor beta-1 in articular chondrocyte cultures and the expression of plasminogen activator inhibitor-1 by articular chondrocytes (Boumediene et al., 1999). ASU has also been found in a lab model to promote tissue inhibitors of metalloproteinases and limit MMP-3 production (Henrotin et al., 2003).

Niacinamide/Vitamin B-3

Niacin, or vitamin B-3, occurs in two forms, nicotinic acid (usually referred to as niacin) and nicotinamide (typically referred to as niacinamide). While both forms have many functions in the body and are crucial to cellular energy production as precursors of NAD and NADP, their therapeutic uses differ considerably.

Niacinamide has been in use as a therapy for osteoarthritis since the 1940s, based on preliminary work by Kaufman (Kaufman, 1983). In-office clinical research, reported by Kaufman on 455 patients receiving 1500–4000 mg/d niacinamide compared against untreated age-matched controls suggested an increase in joint range index and subsequent reduction in pain in 4–8 weeks. More recently investigators have examined efficacy and potential mechanism of action of niacinamide in OA more closely. Jonas et al. demonstrated in a 12-week randomized double-blind placebo-controlled trial ($N=72$) that patients who took niacinamide (3000 mg daily) experienced an improvement in the global impact of their osteoarthritis, increased joint flexibility, reduced inflammation, and decreased use of anti-inflammatory medication, compared to controls (Jonas et al., 1996).

While the mechanism of action of niacinamide in OA has yet to be fully elucidated, current theories suggest that niacinamide acts on chondrocytes to decrease cytokine-mediated inhibition of aggrecan and type II collagen synthesis. In addition, reduction in either production or effect of IL-1 on chondrocytes has been suggested as a plausible mechanism (McCarty and Russell, 1999).

Adverse affects have not been widely reported with pharmaceutical-grade niacinamide, although nausea, heartburn, flatulence and diarrhea have been reported. Elevated liver enzymes can occur with niacinamide and for this reason it is advisable to insure niacinamide supplement quality and evaluate baseline liver function tests prior to, and periodically after, niacinamide administration. While large-scale safety, efficacy, and dosing studies are clearly lacking for the general recommendation of niacinamide treatment for osteoarthritis, preliminary research suggests the nutrient has therapeutic value and warrants further investigation.

Strontium

Strontium ranelate is a nutrient that is being used in some European countries for the treatment of postmenopausal osteoporosis. A number of formulations of strontium have been used in the United States for the same purpose (including strontium citrate). Studies have provided a preclinical basis for the use of strontium ranelate in osteoarthritis. In OA and normal chondrocytes that are treated with or without interleukin 1β (IL-1β), strontium ranelate has been shown to stimulate the synthesis of type II collagen and proteoglycan (Henrotin et al., 2001). In a three-year post-hoc analysis of the pool of Spinal Osteoporosis Therapeutic Intervention (SOTI) and Treatment of Peripheral Osteoporosis studies, strontium ranelate was shown to significantly decrease the levels of urinary C-terminal telopeptides of type II collagen (u-CTX-II), a cartilage degradation biomarker, compared with placebo (Alexanderson et al., 2007).

A post-hoc analysis was done of pooled data on 1,105 women with osteoporosis and osteoarthritis of the spine (Bruyere et al., 2008). The data was from the Spinal Osteoporosis Therapeutic Intervention (SOTI) and Treatment Of Peripheral Osteoporosis (TROPOS) trials. In this study one group of women took 2 g of strontium ranelate daily for three years and they were compared to a placebo group. The admission criteria for these studies were women age 50 and older who had been postmenopausal for at least five years and had osteoporosis documented by DEXA scan. The conclusions of the post-hoc study were, "The proportion of patients with worsening overall spinal OA score was reduced by 42% in the strontium ranelate group compared to a placebo group" (Bruyere et al., 2008). There appears to be a symptom- and structure-modifying effect of strontium in the spine. Studies have not looked at other joints. This study appears to indicate a role for strontium in patients that have spinal OA and osteoporosis. Because of the mechanism of action of strontium it is highly likely that it would be efficacious in women with osteoporosis and OA who were perimenopausal and or immediately postmenopausal, as well as for women who were quite far out from the onset of menopause. Strontium ranelate at 2 g per day would be the preferred form and delivers 680 mg of elemental strontium. Strontium citrate could be dosed at the same dose but has not been adequately studied as has the ranelate form. Strontium ranelate appears to have interactions with calcium and vitamin D. There also may be a slight increased risk of venous thrombosis. The clinician should follow vitamin D levels and augment as necessary and consider using strontium in patients with combined osteoporosis and OA of the spine.

Vitamin D

Vitamin D has been used for many years for prevention of rickets and in the treatment of osteoporosis. Recently vitamin D has been recommended for cancer prevention and for reduction in all-cause mortality.

The expression of vitamin D receptors is upregulated in human OA chondrocytes (Tetlow and Woolley, 2001). Vitamin D receptors have been found in muscle. The Framingham Study found a threefold increase in risk of OA progression for patients in the middle and lowest tertiles of serum levels of 25-OH vitamin D. Low serum levels of vitamin D also predicted osteophyte growth and loss of joint space (McAlindon et al., 1996b). It is recommended that clinicians check serum 25-OH vitamin D levels in their patients with OA. It is recommended, based on the physiology and clinical research, that clinicians use supplemental vitamin D3 to increase the serum level of vitamin D to well within the normal range (above 32 ng/ml). Results of a study from Tufts University on the relationship of vitamin D deficiency and symptoms of knee OA were presented in the Fall 2007 meeting of the American College of Rheumatology. Having a low vitamin D level was associated with more knee pain and greater functional limitations. The above information is convincing enough to support serum testing and supplementation of vitamin D in patients with OA.

Selenium

Low selenium levels have been reported as a risk for osteoarthritis (Jordan et al., 2005). The primary organic forms of selenium are the amino acid-based selenocysteine and selenomethionine. Selenium is used in the body in a number of enzyme systems. Selenium can be obtained from dietary sources although the soils are deficient in selenium in many countries. A dose of 100 mcg per day is usually recommended either in dietary or supplement sources.

Devil's Claw (*Harpagophytum procumbens*)

There have been a number of studies assessing the effectiveness of supplementing with devil's claw for low-back pain or for OA. Most of the studies are short-term or lack controls. A study of patients with hip or knee OA using an aqueous extract of devil's claw used 2400 mg of extract daily, corresponding to 50 mg of harpagoside, showed efficacy in pain reduction and improvement in function but was carried out for only 12 weeks (Wegener and Lüpke, 2003). The long-term safety of devil's claw needs more investigation before it can be recommended for long-term use.

Taking devil's claw orally alone or in conjunction with nonsteroidal anti-inflammatory drugs (NSAIDs) seems to help decrease osteoarthritis-related pain.

Hops

There are lipophilic extracts of hops that can be modified to the family of isohumulones. These compounds can reduce inflammation, insulin resistance dyslipidemia and obesity. They have been found to reduce post-prandial endotoxemia and subsequent inflammation. THIAA is a particular isohumulone that has been produced as a supplement and has been found to have actions in regard to osteoarthritis, including the inhibition of NF-κB, attenuation of TNF-α, and MMP-9 expression. This supplement should be considered in a patient that has osteoarthritis with any of the following comorbidities: insulin resistance, obesity and dyslipidemia (Van Cleemput et al., 2009; Bland et al., 2015).

Scutellaria baicalensis

Research has been done in a rat model with a compound comprised of *Acacia* (A), *Scutellaria* (S), and *Morus* (M) extracts and it was found to decrease urinary CTX-II significantly (Yiman et al., 2017). Human trials are not yet available for this herb in regard to OA.

Bone Morphogenic Protein (BMP)

BMP has been shown in a number of animal model studies to decrease certain inflammatory mediators and decrease certain destructive enzymes (aggrecanase, MMP-3, and MMP-13). These studies have used injectable BMP. Some *in vitro* studies have shown BMP-7 has an anabolic effect on cartilage by stimulating synthesis of cartilage matrix components and increasing proteoglycan and collagen synthesis (Flechtenmacher et al., 1996; Chubinskaya and Kuettner, 2003). There are no available studies on the use of oral BNP in humans with OA.

Hydration

It is important to recommend to patients that they remain well hydrated. There is evidence that chronic low-grade dehydration may contribute to OA of the knee and low back. The clinician can recommend a minimum intake of fluid with most of it in the form of filtered water. Water may also

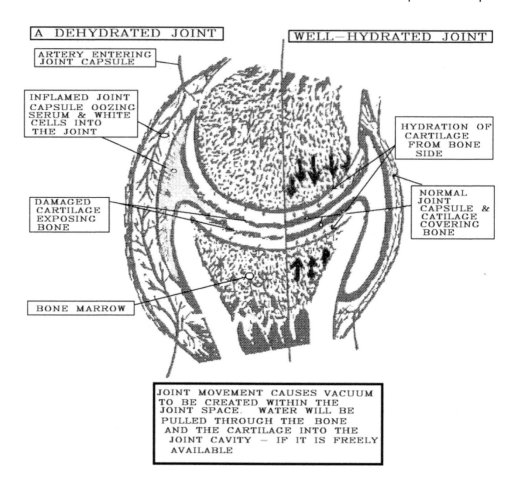

FIGURE 25.1 A well-hydrated joint is contrasted with a dehydrated joint. (Figure is reprinted with permission from Taylor and Francis from *Scientific Basis for Musculoskeletal, Bariatric and Sports Nutrition.*)

be obtained from juices low in sugar and in higher water-content fruits and vegetables. Figure 25.1 demonstrates in visual form some of the effects of dehydration on the joint.

Duration of Joint Support Supplementation

The duration of supplementation depends on the pathology that the clinician is treating. If you are treating an acutely injured joint (knee, hip or spinal joint) it is reasonable to start supplementation immediately upon diagnosis and continue treatment for approximately 12 weeks. It is also reasonable to consider an X-ray of the joint six months after the original injury to make sure that no significant OA changes have occurred. If OA has developed consider the guidelines below. If you are treating a joint with osteoarthritis that has articular cartilage remaining you will need to make a long-term plan for nutritional joint support.

Choice and Timing of Nutritional Support Supplements

The choice of nutritional support for patients with osteoarthritis can be based on a number of factors including the monthly cost of an individual supplement, the efficacy of each nutritional intervention, current clinical studies, and side-effect profiles. It is also related to the pathology and clinical progression of OA in the joint or joints being treated. The clinician should always make recommendations for exercise, posture, stable shoe wear, physical therapy, ligament laxity and manipulative therapies when appropriate to normalize joint mechanics and forces. Although most of the research has been in regard to OA of the knee and hip, one can use the following nutritional approach with OA of any joint including the spine.

Start a patient on an anti-inflammatory diet. At about four weeks into the program you may decide to put the patient on a nightshade-free diet for four weeks. If they have food allergies have them off of those foods. If you suspect food allergies you can put the patient on an allergy-elimination diet or order a food allergy blood test.

The patient with OA should also be started on a balanced and well-formulated multivitamin mineral formula because of the information on selenium, vitamin D and vitamin C. This formula should contain at least 100 µg of selenium, at least 200 mg of vitamin C and at least 1000 IU of vitamin D3. Vitamin D levels should be tested and patients should be supplemented appropriately to bring their level up to at least 40 ng/ml.

Nutritional approaches can block proteases and inflammatory cytokines and also augment sulfur and chondrocyte nutrients and anabolic agents. When starting or adding any supplement for joint support it is important to inform the patient that they should monitor their pain level and functional abilities in a journal, wait at least eight weeks before starting any new supplement, and compare pain and function to just before they started the new product.

Along with a good multiple vitamin, glucosamine sulfate should be a foundation of any short- and long-term treatment plan. Start a patient on stabilized glucosamine sulfate (preferably the vegan corn form) at the 1500 mg one time per day dose for a minimum of ten weeks. A second dose of 1500 mg may be considered depending on the patient's body weight and the number of osteoarthritic joints.

Two to four grams of a triglyceride fish oil can be started with the GS. Because curcumin interrupts the pathogenesis of OA at so many locations it should be used as a foundation treatment in a highly absorbable form like Meriva or BCM-95. Doses of 500 mg 3× a day should be considered. This could also be started in the first phase of treatment. (The authors would advise phasing in every 2–4 days the new supplements in case a patient reacts adversely to one of them.)

In the first 1–2 months of treatment the clinician could consider using Physical Therapy with manual and STEP approaches. The clinician may also consider referring for Frequency Specific Microcurrent or Pulsed Electromagnetic Field treatment although there are no human trials. In the authors' experiences these are the two most effective modalities to decrease pain and inflammation in OA joints and appear to have an excellent side-effect profile.

At about eight weeks the patient should be experiencing reduced pain and improved function.

At approximately ten weeks assess the patient's functional abilities and pain level. At this point the clinician has a number of options on what to add. The clinician could add both oral HA and type II collagen for another 6–8 weeks then reassess. The clinician can consider adding chondroitin sulfate (unless the patient is vegetarian) at the 800–1200 mg dose to see if there is an added benefit in symptoms and function after 8–12 weeks. It would be reasonable to use the low molecular weight form for better absorption. CS would also be especially beneficial in the person with mast cell activation.

Lyprinol could be helpful for moderate pain and inflammation-related symptoms.

SAMe would also be an excellent second-line agent. Because of its cost it may be prohibitory for a lot of people as a long-term supplement. It could be started at a dose of 400 mg 2× a day and kept there if efficacious. This would be an especially good agent if a patient has comorbid depression.

A hops extract formula with THIIA would also be an appropriate second-tier agent. Hops extract would be a good choice if there is insulin resistance, obesity and dyslipidemia.

If there is no significant additive effect after 10 weeks it is not reasonable to continue chondroitin sulfate (unless they come to you already on a CS product and they feel that it is working well for them).

Avocado/soybean unsaponifiable (ASU) residues would be a reasonable second-tier or third-tier agent because of the research regarding its utility in blocking cytokines as well as blocking metalloproteinases. One could use 300 mg of ASU per day. If this agent was too costly or not efficacious. One should monitor liver enzymes if this agent is added.

After 3 months of treatment the clinician should do a thorough reevaluation.

Intra-articular hyaluronic acid should be considered for advanced knee and hip OA. This would be added to nutritional support and if it is efficacious can be repeated approximately every 9 months. It is reasonable to consider it for moderate OA as well as chondromalacia patella. Long-term use of glucosamine, curcumin, chondroitin, SAMe and vitamin D appear safe and patients can be maintained on any combination of these for long periods of time. ASU has not been used long term but it should be safe unless there is an allergy to soy.

Nutritional Support for Sprains and Osteoarthritis Prevention

There is a rationale for the use of joint-support nutrients after traumatic injury that involves meniscus or articular cartilage, including moderate to severe sprains or contusions to a joint. This would include motor vehicle injuries to the facets of the neck, thoracic and lumbar spine, contusions to the patella, ankle, knee meniscus and other extremity sprains. No long-term studies document the prevention of osteoarthritis with joint-support nutrients after traumatic injury but the rationale of nutritionally supporting the cartilage after a sprain injury is very sound. Glucosamine sulfate with or without chondroitin sulfate may be started at the time of the diagnosis and continued for a minimum of eight weeks and preferably for 12 weeks after the sprain. There is a definite preventative indication here with low chance of side effects. In addition to traumatic injuries, there appears to be good clinical response to the use of glucosamine sulfate in problems involving the articular cartilage of the patella in both patellofemoral tracking syndrome and chondromalacia. The clinician can recommend starting joint support nutrients 6–8 weeks before high use of the knee in sports. If the problem and use of the knee are ongoing, then nutritional support should be continuous.

Limit higher-risk activities such as contact sports and sports with a high risk of falling. Limit running in patients with moderate OA of the knee or hip. Encourage cross-training for exercise. Limit work and household-related activities of squatting, kneeling and excessive stair-climbing.

If there is hypermobility of a joint with laxity on stress tests then Prolotherapy should be done to stabilize a joint. If there is moderate cartilage loss and inadequate response to the former treatments then a trial of PRP in the joint could be done perhaps at eight-week intervals for two to three injections. If this is not effective enough, stem cell treatment or joint-replacement surgery could be entertained.

With any approach significant education of the patient should be done so that the patient can be on board with a short- and long-term treatment plan.

CLINICAL SUMMARY

A nutritional approach to osteoarthritis is theoretically justified and has been overwhelmingly validated in laboratory and clinical trials. Whereas conventional therapeutics may offer the most effective short-term pain relief in OA, long-term pain relief, improvement in function and regeneration of the joint is better accomplished with nutritional and other therapies with fewer side effects. Nutritional support when combined with assessment and optimization of biomechanics, strength and balance can offer both immediate and long-term improvements in function and in pain relief of OA. It may also offer a slowing or stopping of joint surface loss.

REFERENCES

Aggarwal, B.B., Gupta, S.C., and Sung B. Curcumin: An orally bioavailable blocker of TNF and other proinflammatory biomarkers. *Br J Pharmacol* 2013; 169: 1672–1692.

Aggarwal, A. and Sempowski, I.P. Hyaluronic acid injections for knee osteoarthritis. Systematic review of the literature. *Can Fam Physician* 2004; 50: 249–256.

Alexanderson, P., Karsdal, M., Qvist, P., Reginster, J.Y., and Christiansen, C. Strontium ranelate reduces the urinary level of cartilage degradation biomarker CTX-II in postmenopausal women. *Bone* 2007; 40: 218–222.

Andia, I. and Maffulli, N. Platelet-rich plasma for managing pain and inflammation in osteoarthritis. *Nat Rev Rheumatol* 2013; 9: 721.

Argo, R., Alvarez-Soria, M.A., Diez-Ortego, I. et al. Glucosamine inhibits IL-1beta-induced NFkappaB activation in human osteoarthritic chondrocytes. *Osteoarthritis Cartilage* 2003; 11: 290–298.

Asari, A., Kanemitsu, T., and Kurihara, H. Oral administration of high molecular weight hyaluronan (900kDa) controls immune system via Toll-like receptor 4 in the intestinal epithelium. *J Biol Chem* 2010; 285: 24751–24758.

Baker, K., Grainger, A., Niu, J., et al. Relation of synovitis to knee pain using contrast-enhanced MRIs. *Ann Rheum Dis* 2010; 69: 1779.

Barthe, L. et al. In vitro intestinal degradation and absorption of chondroitin sulfate, a glycosaminoglycan drug. *Arzneimittelforschung* 2004; 54(5): 286–292.

Bay-Jensen, A.C., Slagboom, E., Chen-An, P., Alexandersen, P., Qvist, P., Christiansen, C., Meulenbelt, I., and Karsdal, M.A. Role of hormones in cartilage and joint metabolism: Understanding an unhealthy metabolic phenotype in osteoarthritis. *Menopause* 2013; 20(5): 578–586. doi:10.1097/GME.0b013e3182745993.

Bharti, A.C., Takada, Y., and Aggarwal, B.B. Curcumin (diferuloylmethane) inhibits receptor activator of NF-kappa B ligand-induced NF-kappa B activation in osteoclast precursors and suppresses osteoclastogenesis. *J Immunol* 2004; 172: 5940–5947.

Bland, J., Minich, D., Lerman, R., Darland, G., Lamb, J., Trip, M., and Grayson, N. Isohumulones from hops (*Humulus lupulus*) and their potential role in medical nutrition therapy *Pharma Nutrition* 2015; 3(2): 46–52.

Brandt, K.D., Effects of nonsteroidal anti-inflammatory drugs on chondrocyte metabolism in vitro and in vivo. *Am J Med* 1987a; 83(5A): 29–34.

Brandt, K.D. Nonsteroidal antiinflammatory drugs and articular cartilage. *J Rheumatol* 1987b; 14: 132–133.

Bridges, A.J., Smith, E., and Reid, J. Joint hypermobility in adults referred to rheumatology clinics. *J Soann Rheum Dis* 1992; 51(6): 793–796.

Brophy, R.H., Rai, M.F., Zhang, Z., Torgomyan, A., and Sandell, L.J. Molecular analysis of age and sex-related gene expression in meniscal tears with and without a concomitant anterior cruciate ligament tear. *J Bone Joint Surg Am* 2012; 94:385.

Bruyere, O., Pavelka K., Rovati L.C., Deroisy R., Olejarova M., Gatterova J., Giacovelli G., and Reginster J.Y. Glucosamine sulfate reduces osteoarthritis progression in postmenopausal women with knee osteoarthritis: Evidence from two 3-year studies. *Menopause* 2004; 11(2): 138–143.

Bruyere, O., Delferriere, D., Roux, C., Wark, J.D., Spector, T., Devogelaer, J.P., Reginster, J.Y. Effects of strontium ranelate on spinal osteoarthritis progression. *Ann Rheum Dis* 2008; 67: 335–339.

Burke, J., Hunter, M., Kolhe, R., Isales, C., Hamrick, M., and Fulzele, S. Therapeutic potential of mesenchymal stem cell based therapy for osteoarthritis. *Clin Transl Med* 2016; 5(1): 27.

Centeno, C., Pitts, J., Al-Sayegh, H., and Freeman, M. Efficacy of autologous bone marrow concentrate for knee osteoarthritis with and without adipose graft. *BioMed Res Int* 2014; 2014: 370621–370629.

Centeno, C., Al-Sayegh, H., Freeman, M.D., Smith, J., and Murrell, W. A multi-center analysis of adverse events among two thousand, three hundred and seventy two adult patients undergoing adult autologous stem cell therapy for orthopaedic conditions. *Int Orthopaedics* 2016; 40(8): 1755–1765.

Chahla, J., Dean, C.S., Moatshe, G., Pascual-garrido, C., Serra-Cruz, R., and Laprade, R.F. Concentrated bone marrow aspirate for the treatment of chondral injuries and osteoarthritis of the knee: A systematic review of outcomes. *Orthop J Sports Med* 2016; 4(1): 2325967115625481.

Chiusaroli, R. et al., Experimental pharmacology of glucosamine sulfate. *Int J Rheumatol* 2011; 2011: 939265. doi:10.1155/2011/939265.

Cho, S.H. et al., Clinical efficacy and safety of Lyprinol, a patented extract from New Zealand green-lipped mussel (Perna Canaliculus) in patients with osteoarthritis of the hip and knee: A multicenter 2-month clinical trial. *Allerg Immunol (Paris)* 2003; 35(6): 212–216.

Christgau, S. et al., Osteoarthritic patients with high cartilage turnover show increased responsiveness to the cartilage protecting effects of glucosamine sulphate. *Clin Exp Rheumatol* 2004a; 22(1): 36–42.

Christgau, S. et al., Suppression of elevated cartilage turnover in postmenopausal women and in ovariectomized rats by estrogen and a selective estrogen-receptor modulator (SERM). *Menopause* 2004b; 11: 508–518.

Chubinskaya, S. and Kuettner, K.E. Regulation of osteogenic proteins by chondrocytes. *Int J Biochem Cell Biol* 2003; 35: 1323–1340.

Cicuttini, F.M. et al., Factors affecting knee cartilage volume in healthy men. *Rheumatology* 2003; 42: 258–262.

Cirillo, D.J., Wallace, R.B., Wu, L., and Yood, R.A. Effect of hormone therapy on risk of hip and knee joint replacement in the Women's Health Initiative. *Arthritis Rheum* 2006; 54: 3194–3204.

Clarke, B.L. and Khosla, S. Androgens and bone. *Steroids* 2009; 74(3): 296–305.

Cohen, M., et al., A randomized, double blind, placebo controlled trial of a topical cream containing glucos-amine sulfate, chondroitin sulfate, and camphor for osteoarthritis of the knee. *J Rheumatol* 2003; 30(3): 523–528.

Crowley, D.C., Lau, F.C., Sharma, P., Evans, M., Guthrie, N., Bagchi, M., Bagchi, D., Dey, D.K., and Raychaudhuri, S.P. Safety and efficacy of undenatured type II collagen in thetreatment of osteoarthritis of the knee: A clinical trial. *Int J Med Sci.* 2009; 6(6): 312–321.

Curtis, C.L. et al., Pathologic indicators of degradation and inflammation in human osteoarthritic cartilage are abrogated by exposure to n-3 fatty acids. *Arthritis Rheum* 2002; 46(6): 1544–1553.

de Lange-Brokaar, B.J. et al., Characterization of synovial mast cells in knee osteoarthritis: Association with clinical parameters. *Osteoarthritis Cartilage* 2016; 24(4): 664–671. doi:10.1016/j.joca.2015.11.011.

Ellman, M.B., An, H.S., Muddasani, P., and Im, H.J. Biological impact of the fibroblast growth factor family on articular cartilage and intervertebral disc homeostasis. *Gene* 2008; 420: 82.

Ernst, E., Avocado-soybean unsaponifiables (ASU) for osteoarthritis – a systematic review. *Clin Rheumatol* 2003; 22(4–5): 285–288.

Filardo, G., Perdisa, F., Roffi, A., Marcacci, M., and Kon, E. Stem cells in articular cartilage regeneration. *J Orthop Surg Res* 2016; 11: 42.

Flechtenmacher, J., Huch, K., Thonar, E.J., Mollenhauer, J.A., Davies, S.R., Schmid, T.M., and Kuettner, K.E. Recombinant human osteogenic protein 1 is a potent stimulator of the synthesis of cartilage proteogly-cans and collagens by human articular chondrocytes. *Arthritis Rheum* 1996; 39: 1896–1904.

Freitag, J. et al., Mesenchymal stem cell therapy in the treatment of osteoarthritis: Reparative pathways, safety and efficacy – a review. *BMC Musculoskelet Disord* 2016; 17: 230.

Gallelli, L. et al., The effects of nonsteroidal anti-inflammatory drugs on clinical outcomes, synovial fluid cytokine concentration and signal transduction pathways in knee osteoarthritis. A randomized open label trial. *Osteoarthritis Cartilage* 2013; 21(9): 1400–1408.

Garcia-Gil, M., Reyes, C., Ramos, R., Sanchez-Santos, M.T., Prieto-Alhambra, D., Spector, T.D., Hart, D.J., and Arden, N.K. Serum lipid levels and risk of hand osteoarthritis: The Chingford prospective cohort study. *Sci Rep.* 2017; 7(1): 3147. doi:10.1038/s41598-017-03317-4.

Garnero, P., Piperno, M., Gineyts, E., Christgau, S., Delmas, P.D., and Vignon, E. Cross sectional evalu-ation of biochemical markers of bone, cartilage, and synovial tissue metabolism in patients with knee osteoarthritis: Relations with disease activity and joint damage. *Ann Rheum Dis* 2001; 60(6): 619–626.

Gray, H.C., Hutcheson, P.S., and Slavin, R.G., Is glucosamine safe in patients with seafood allergy? *J Allergy Clin Immunol* 2004; 114(2): 459–460.

Hanna, F. et al., Factors influencing longitudinal change in knee cartilage volume measured from magnetic resonance imaging in healthy men. *Ann Rheum Dis* 2005; 64(7): 1038–1042.

Hauselmann, H.J. Nutripharmaceuticals for osteoarthritis. *Best Pract Res Clin Rheumatol* 2001; 15(4): 595–607.

Henrotin, Y.E. et al., Effects of three avocado/soybean unsaponifiable mixtures on metalloproteinases, cyto-kines and prostaglandin E2 production by human articular chondrocytes. *Clin Rheumatol* 1998; 17(1): 31–39.

Henrotin, Y.E. et al., Avocado/soybean unsaponifiables increase aggrecan synthesis and reduce catabolic and proinflammatory mediator production by human osteoarthritic chondrocytes. *J Rheumatol* 2003; 30: 1825–1834.

Henrotin Y. et al., Biological actions of curcumin on articular chondrocytes. *Osteoarthritis Cartilage* 2010; 18(2):141–149. doi:10.1016/j.joca.2009.10.002.

Henrotin, Y. et al., Strontium ranelate increases cartilage matrix formation. *J Bone Miner Res* 2001; 16: 299–308.

Hesslink, R. Jr, Armstrong, D., Nagendran, M.V., Sreevatsan, S., and Barathur, R. Cetylated fatty acids improve knee function in patients with osteoarthritis. *J Rheumatol.* 2002; 29(8): 1708–1712.

Ishikawa M et al., Lectin-like oxidized low-density lipoprotein receptor 1 signal is a potent biomarker and therapeutic target for human rheumatoid arthritis. *Arthritis Rheum* 2012; 64: 102434.

Jacobsen, S., Danneskiold-Samsoe, B., and Andersen, R.B. Oral S-adenosylmethionine in primary fibromyal-gia. Double-blind clinical evaluation. *Scand J Rheumatol* 1991; 20: 294–302.

Jadelis, K. et al., Strength, balance, and the modifying effects of obesity and knee pain: results from the Observational Arthritis Study in Seniors (OASIS). *J Am Geriatr Soc* 2001; 49(7): 884–891.

Jonas, W.B., Rapoza, C.P., and Blair, W.F., The effect of niacinamide on osteoarthritis: A pilot study. *Inflamm Res* 1996; 45(7): 330–334.

Jordan, J.M. et al., Low selenium levels are associated with increased risk for osteoarthritis of the knee. *American College of Rheumatology Annual Meeting.* San Diego November 12–17, 2005. Abstract 1189.

Jin, X., Wang, B.H., Wang, X., Antony, B., Zhu, Z., Han, W, and Ding, C. Associations between endogenous sex hormones and MRI structural changes in patients with symptomatic knee osteoarthritis. *Osteoarthritis Cartilage* 2017; 25(7): 1100–1106.

Kahan, A. STOPP (Study on Osteoarthritis Progression Prevention): a new two-year trial with chondroitin 4&6 sulfate (CS). 2006. Available at: www.ibsa-ch.com/eular_2006_amsterdam_vignon-2.pdf.

Karsdal, M.A., Bay-Jensen, A.C., Henriksen, K., and Christiansen, C. The pathogenesis of osteoarthritis involves bone, cartilage and synovial inflammation: May estrogen be a magic bullet? *Menopause Int.* 2012; 18(4): 139–146. doi:10.1258/mi.2012.012025.

Kaufman, W., Niacinamide: A most neglected vitamin. *J Int Acad Prev Med* 1983 (Winter): p. 5–25.

Kelly, M.A., P.R. Kurzweil, and R.W. Moskowitz, Intra-articular hyaluronans in knee osteoarthritis: Rationale and practical considerations. *Am J Orthop* 2004; 33(2 Suppl): 15–22.

Kim, L.S., Axelrod, L.J., Howard, P., Buratovich, N., Waters R.F. Efficacy of methylsulfonylmethane (MSM) in osteoarthritis pain of the knee: A pilot clinical trial. *Osteoarthritis Cartilage* 2006; 14: 286–294.

Kraemer, W.J., Ratamess, N.A., Anderson, J.M., Maresh, C.M., Tiberio, D.P., Joyce, M.E., and Hesslink, R, Jr. Effect of a cetylated fatty acid topical cream on functional mobility and quality of life of patients with osteoarthritis. *J Rheumatol* 2004; 31(4): 767–774.

Kumm, J., Tamm, A., Lintrop, M., and Tamm, A. The prevalence and progression of radiographic knee osteoarthritis over 6 years in a population-based cohort of middle-aged subjects. *Rheumatol Int* 2012; 32(11): 3545–3450.

Kumm, J., Tamm, A., Lintrop, M., and Tamm, A. The value of cartilage biomarkers in progressive knee osteoarthritis: Cross-sectional and 6-year follow-up study in middle-aged subjects. *Rheumatol Int* 2013; 33(4): 903–911.

Laudy, A.B., Bakker, E.W., Rekers, M., and Moen, M.H. Efficacy of platelet-rich plasma injections in osteoarthritis of the knee: A systematic review and meta-analysis. *Br J Sports Med* 2015; 49: 657.

Lequesne, M. et al., Structural effect of avocado/soybean unsaponifiables on joint space loss in osteoarthritis of the hip. *Arthritis Rheum* 2002; 47(1): 50–58.

Lippiello L, Walsh T, and Fienhold M. The association of lipid abnormalities with tissue pathology in human osteoarthritic articular cartilage. *Metabolism* 1991; 40: 5716.

Loeser, R.F. Aging processes and the development of osteoarthritis. *Curr Opin Rheumatol* 2013; 25: 108.

Lohmander, L.S. et al., Intra-articular sprifermin (recombinant human fibroblast growth factor 18) in knee osteoarthritis: a randomized, double-blind, placebo-controlled trial. *Arthritis Rheumatol* 2014; 66: 1820.

Lugo, J.P., Saiyed, Z.M., and Lane, NE. Efficacy and tolerability of an undenatured type II collagen supplement in modulating knee osteoarthritis symptoms: A multicenter randomized, double-blind, placebo-controlled study. *Nutr J* 2016; 15: 14.

Mastbergen, S.C., Saris, D.B., and Lafeber, F.P. Functional articular cartilage repair: Here, near, or is the best approach not yet clear? *Nat Rev Rheumatol* 2013; 9: 277.

Matheson, A.J. and Perry, C.M. Glucosamine: A review of its use in the management of osteoarthritis. *Drugs Aging* 2003; 20(14): 1041–1060.

Matis, U. and Shakibaei M. Curcumin mediated suppression of nuclear factor-kB promotes chondrogenic differentiation of mesenchymal stem cells in a high-density co-culture microenvironment. *Arthritis Res Ther* 2010; 12: R127.

McAlindon, T.E. et al., Do antioxidant micronutrients protect against the development and progression of knee osteoarthritis? *Arthritis Rheum* 1996a; 39(4): 648–656.

McAlindon, T.E. et al., Relation of dietary intake and serum levels of vitamin D to progression of osteoarthritis of the knee among participants in the Framingham Study. *Ann Intern Med* 1996b; 125: 353–359.

McCarty, M.F. and Russell, A.L., Niacinamide therapy for osteoarthritis – does it inhibit nitric oxide synthase induction by interleukin 1 in chondrocytes? *Med Hypotheses* 1999; 53(4): 350–360.

Mirzael, H. et al., Phytosomal curcumin: A review of pharmacokinetic, experimental and clinical studies. *Biomed. Pharmacotherapy* 2017; 85: 102–112.

Mook S., Halkes C.C., Bilecen S., and Cabezas M.C. In vivo regulation of plasma free fatty acids in insulin resistance. *Metabolism* 2004; 53: 1197201.

Moore, E.E. et al., Fibroblast growth factor-18 stimulates chondrogenesis and cartilage repair in a rat model of injury-induced osteoarthritis. *Osteoarthritis Cartilage* 2005; 13: 623.

Morgentaler, A., Miner, M.M., Caliber, M, Guay, A.T., Khera, M., and Traish, A.M. Testosterone therapy and cardiovascular risk: Advances and controversies. *Mayo Clin Proc* 2015; 90(2): 224–251.

Mouritzen, U., Christgau, S., Lehmann, H.J., Tanko, L.B., and Christiansen, C. Cartilage turnover assessed with a newly developed assay measuring collagen type II degradation products: Influence of age, sex, menopause, hormone replacement therapy, and body mass index. *Ann Rheum Dis* 2003; 62: 332–336.

Najm, W.I. et al., S-adenosyl methionine (SAMe) versus celecoxib for the treatment of osteoarthritis symptoms: A double-blind cross-over trial. [ISRCTN36233495]. *BMC Musculoskelet Disord* 2004; 5(1): 6.

Mow, V.C., Gu, Y.W., and Chen, H.F. Structure and function of articular carilage and meniscus. In Mow V.C. and Huiskers R. eds, *Basic Orthopaedic Biomechanics and Mechano-Biology*, 3rd edn, 2005, Philadelphia: Lippincot Williams & Wilkins, 181–258.

Oe, M., Tashiro, T., Yoshida, H., Nishiyama, H., Masuda, Y., Maruyama, K., Koikeda, T., Maruya, R., and Fukui, N. Oral hyaluronan relieves knee pain: A review. *Nutr J.* 2016; 15: 11. doi:10.1186/s12937-016-0128-2. Review.

Oestergaard, S. et al., The utility of measuring C-terminal telopeptides of collagen type II (CTX-II) in serum and synovial fluid samples for estimation of articular cartilage status in experimental models of destructive joint diseases, *Osteoarthritis Cartilage* 2006; 14 (7): 670–679.

Pavelka, K. et al., Glucosamine sulfate use and delay of progression of knee osteoarthritis: A 3-year, randomized, placebo-controlled, double-blind study. *Arch Intern Med* 2002; 162: 2113–2123.

Rannou, F., Pelletier, J.P., and Martel-Pelletier, J. Efficacy and safety of topical NSAIDs in the management of osteoarthritis: Evidence from real-life setting trials and surveys. *Semin Arthritis Rheum* 2016; 45(4 Suppl): S18–S21. doi:10.1016/j.semarthrit.2015.11.007.

Reginster, J.Y. et al., Long-term effects of glucosamine sulfate on osteoarthritis progression: A randomized, placebo-controlled trial. *Lancet* 2001; 357: 251–256.

Reginster, J.Y. et al., Naturocetic (glucosamine and chondroitin sulfate) compounds as structure-modifying drugs in the treatment of osteoarthritis. *Curr Opin Rheumatol* 2003; 15(5): 651–655.

Reichenbach, S. et al., Meta-analysis: Chondroitin for osteoarthritis of the knee or hip. *Ann Intern Med* 2007; 146: 580–590.

Roos, E.M., Herzog, W., Block, J.A., and Bennell, K.L. Muscle weakness, afferent sensory dysfunction and exercise in knee osteoarthritis. *Nat Rev Rheumatol* 2011; 7: 57.

Schwartz, E.R. and Adamy, L. Effect of ascorbic acid on arylsulfatase activities and sulfated proteoglycan metabolism in chondrocyte cultures. *J Clin Invest* 1977; 60(1): 96–106.

Scroggie, D.A., Albright, A., and Harris, M.D., The effect of glucosamine-chondroitin supplementation on glycosylated hemoglobin levels in patients with type 2 diabetes mellitus: A placebo-controlled, double-blinded, randomized clinical trial. *Arch Intern Med* 2003; 163(13): 1587–1590.

Setnikar, I. et al., Pharmacokinetics of glucosamine in man. *Arzneimittelforschung* 1993; 43(10): 1109–1113.

Sharif, M., Kirwan, J.R., Elson, C.J., Granell, R., and Clarke, S. Suggestion of nonlinear or phasic progression of knee osteoarthritis based on measurements of serum cartilage oligomeric matrix protein levels over five years. *Arthritis Rheum*. 2004; 50(8): 2479–2488.

Soeken, K.L. et al., Safety and efficacy of S-adenosylmethionine (SAMe) for osteoarthritis. *J Fam Pract* 2002; 51(5): 425–430.

Soran N et al., Assessment of paraoxonase activities in patients with knee osteoarthritis. *Redox Rep* 2008; 13: 1948.

Spector, T.D., Hart, D.J., and Doyle, D.V. Incidence and progression of osteoarthritis in women with unilateral knee disease in the general population: The effect of obesity. *Ann Rheum Dis* 1994; 53: 565.

Stannus, O., Jones, G., Cicuttini, F., Prameswaran, V., Quinn, S., Burgess, J., and Ding, C. Circulating levels of IL-6 and TNF-alpha are associated with knee radiographic osteoarthritis and knee cartilage loss in older adults, *Osteoarthritis Cartilage* 2010; 18(11): 1441–1447.

Sturmer T. et al., Serum cholesterol and osteoarthritis. The baseline examination of the Ulm Osteoarthritis Study. *J Rheumatol* 1998; 25: 182732.

Suri, P., Morgenroth, D.C., and Hunter, D.J. Epidemiology of osteoarthritis and associated comorbidities. *PM&R* 2012; 4(5): S10–S19.

Tanamas, S.K., Wijethilake, P., Wluka, A.E., Davies-Tuck, M.L., Urquhart, D.M., Wang, Y., and Cicuttini, F.M. Sex hormones and structural changes in osteoarthritis: A systematic review. *Maturitas* 2011; 69(2): 141–156. doi:10.1016/j.maturitas.2011.03.019.Epub.

Tannis, A.J., Barban, J., and Conquer, J.A. Effect of glucosamine supplementation on fasting and non-fasting plasma glucose and serum insulin concentrations in healthy individuals. *Osteoarthritis Cartilage* 2004; 12(6): 506–511.

Tetlow, L.C. and Woolley, D.E. Expression of vitamin D receptors and matrix metalloproteinases in osteoarthritic cartilage and human articular chondrocytes in vitro. *Osteoarthritis Cartilage* 2001; 9: 423–431.

Thijssen E., van Caam, A., and van der Kraan P.M. Obesity and osteoarthritis, more than just wear and tear: Pivotal roles for inflamed adipose tissue and dyslipidaemia in obesity-induced osteoarthritis. *Rheumatology (Oxford)* 2015; 54(4): 588–600.

Towheed, T.E., Anastassiades, T.P., Shea, B., Houpt, J., Welch, V., and Hochberg, M.C. Glucosamine therapy for treating osteoarthritis. *Cochrane Database Syst Rev* 2001; 1: CD002946.

Towheed, T.E. and Anastassiades, T. Glucosamine therapy for osteoarthritis: An update. *J Rheumatol* 2007; 34(9): 1787–1790.

Towheed, T.E., Maxwell, L., Anastassiades, T.P., Shea, B., Houpt, J., Robinson, V., Hochberg, M.C., and Wells. G. Glucosamine therapy for treating osteoarthritis. *Cochrane Database Syst Rev* 2005; 18(2): CD002946.

Usha, P.R. and Naidu, M.U.R. Randomised, double-blind, parallel, placebo-controlled study of oral glucosamine, methylsulfonylmethane and their combinations. *Clin Drug Invest* 2004; 24: 353–363.

van Buul, GM. et al., Platelet-rich plasma releasate inhibits inflammatory processes in osteoarthritic chondrocytes. *Am J Sports Med* 2011; 39: 2362.

Van Cleemput, M., Cattoor, K., De Bosscher, K., Haegeman, G., De Keukeleire, D., Heyerick, A., Hops (*Humulus lupulus*)-derived bitter acids as multipotent bioactive compounds. *J Nat Prod* 2009; 72(6): 1220–1230.

Wegener, T. and Lüpke N.P., Treatment of patients with arthrosis of hip or knee with an aqueous extract of devil's claw. *Phytother Res.* 2003; 17(10): 1165–1172.

Wojdasiewicz, P., Poniatowski, Ł.A., and Szukiewicz, D. The role of inflammatory and anti-inflammatory cytokines in the pathogenesis of osteoarthritis. *Mediators Inflamm* 2014; 2014: 2014561459.

Yeh, C.C. et al., Evaluation of the protective effects of curcuminoid (curcumin and bisdemethoxycurcumin)-loaded liposomes against bone turnover in a cell-based model of osteoarthritis. *Drug Des Devel Ther* 2015; 9: 2285–2300.

Yimam, M. et al., Cartilage protection and analgesic activity of a botanical composition comprised of *Morus alba*, *Scutellaria baicalensis*, and *Acacia catechu*. *Evidence-Based Complementary Alternative Med* 2017; 2017: 10.

Zhang, Z. et al., Curcumin slows osteoarthritis progression and relieves osteoarthritis-associated pain symptoms in a post-traumatic osteoarthritis mouse model. *Arthritis Res Ther* 2016; 18: 128.

26 Integrative Approaches to Autoimmune Arthritis

George E. Muñoz, MD

INTRODUCTION

This chapter addresses the management of steroids and secondary steroid effects on orthopedic treatment interventions. It does so in light of emerging research on the gastrointestinal mucosa as a key regulator of autoimmune arthritis. The chapter applies the research to clinical rheumatology and concludes with a case study.

CORTICOSTEROIDS

Corticosteroids are key regulators of whole-body homeostasis. The effects of corticosteroids are widespread, including profound alterations in carbohydrate, protein, and lipid metabolism, and the modulation of electrolyte and water balance. Corticosteroids affect all the major systems of the body, including the cardiovascular, musculoskeletal, nervous, and immune systems [1]. The purpose of this section is to review some pertinent effects of corticosteroids relevant to the integrative orthopedic approach presently and not simply rehash all too well-known effects and complications of chronic and supra-physiologic dosing of corticosteroids. One focal point of emphasis is to update the GI mucosal effects secondary to steroids that alter immunity, the microbiome, and secondary signaling pathways. Ulcerogenic and gastritis and gastric ulcers have been well delineated and will not be covered. The concept that steroids alter the microbiome through transmissible mechanisms via commensal bacteria in susceptible hosts has been clearly verified in animal mouse models. Knockout mice injected with commensals previously treated with corticosteroids, possessed an anti-inflammatory effect on IL-10 knockout mice without further steroid exposure to the test subjects. Conclusion—immunity can be shaped by direct transmission of commensal bacteria and possesses anti-inflammatory effects in mouse models. Fecal transplants in humans are now fully underway and this concept is clinically operative. Understanding that steroids have numerous immune effects that include the GI mucosa and their secondary microbiome change which in turn exerts other immunologic signaling pathways is the newest model to focus upon the clinical implications for both beneficial therapeutics and iatrogenic effects [2]. Clinically, monitoring the microbiome for diversity, adequate commensals, and the suppression of potential pathogens makes sense to maintain not only health and nutrition but optimal immune functions that include adequate defenses against secondary infection.

Another area of update is the use of sustained release prednisone that is dosed nightly instead of the classic morning dosing we are accustomed to with regular prednisone. Not only are inflammatory cytokine levels highest at night during sleep, but secondary complications of all forms of apnea further augment the inflammatory burden. TNF and IL-6 both begin to rise at night during sleep and peak about 4–6 hours after REM sleep is initiated. This dangerous pattern could account for why emergency rooms encounter acute myocardial infarctions first thing in the morning around 5–7 a.m. These 2 cytokines when elevated shift the inflammatory effect into a later and longer time frame of the morning and create a sustained pattern of clinical inflammation in rheumatoid arthritis (RA) patients particularly. Furthermore, targeting steroid use to direct anti-inflammatory effect during this chronobiology and the circadian pharmacokinetic phenomenon has been explored and is now presently being utilized in clinical practice as a therapeutic option in RA patients and others with inflammatory systemic rheumatic disorders [3, 4]. Ultimately, the bio-engineering of new forms of slower and controlled delayed release steroids for nightly or p.m. dosing have added an option for clinicians when facing patients more recalcitrant to steroid taper as well as an opportunity for improvement in quality of life and morning stiffness in RA patients by targeting nighttime cytokine elevations [5]. This innovation in 4 hour delayed delivery has provided a new therapeutic option worth noting for the practicing orthopedist.

INFECTION

The incidence of infection with corticosteroid use is obviously a critical subject and minimizing the risk of utmost importance to all clinicians irrespective of specialty. The same applies to orthopedics. Dosing and infectious complications seem to go hand in hand in a fairly linear and predictable fashion based on the literature and well-established norms. Maintaining the dose of chronic steroids (4–6 weeks or longer) under a top physiologic range of 5–7.5 mg prednisone is desirable to mitigate risk. As steroid dose is increased, infection, hospitalizations, and other secondary complications increase including diabetes, cataracts, skin thinning (and its important immune barrier function) are all compromised. Other studies cite <10 mg and total 700 mg prednisone exposure as cutoffs for infectious complications [6].

The use of high-dose steroids has been shown to be associated with increased morbidity and mortality in patients with SLE, RA, and other autoimmune conditions [7].

Low-dose methylprednisilone was effective in controlling SLE flares and associated with fewer serious infections than traditional high-dose methylprednisilone [8].

GRAFT AND PROSTHETIC FAILURE IN AUTOIMMUNE PATIENTS

In more recent studies, the risk of infection in the general population was analyzed. Risk stratification was noted as follows: The main factors distinctly associated with infection after total knee arthroplasty (TKA) were BMI (BMI >30: OR = 2.53, 95% CI 1.25, 5.13; BMI >40: OR = 4.00, 95% CI 1.23, 12.98), diabetes mellitus (OR = 3.72, 95% CI 2.30, 6.01), hypertension (OR = 2.53, 95% CI 1.07, 5.99), steroid therapy (OR = 2.04, 95 % CI 1.11, 3.74), and RA (OR = 1.83; 95% CI 1.42, 2.36). So, while RA has its own inherent risk, the associations of BMI, diabetes, and hypertension further complicate the picture. Adequate preparation of the individual surgical candidate for fat/BMI reduction, lowering of BP to optimal levels, and glycemic control can all be achieved through a healthy nutritional program incorporating anti-inflammatory with low glycemic index nutritional patterns. Hence, lifestyle, nutrition, and a total person approach makes sense to optimize outcomes. An interdisciplinary approach in the preop phase, which may be 3–6 months of preparation or more if needed, makes sense to reduce risk and improve surgical outcomes with goals to reduce patient BMI to <40 range in normal height range individuals [9]. Whether calorie restriction, elimination of processed carbohydrates, low impact cardiovascular exercise (swimming, recumbent stationary bike), or nutrition counseling and weekly or bi-weekly follow up and patient contact and engagement are useful if not essential to encourage and improve patient compliance and goal attainment. Technology has aided significantly in this regard and secure texting applications exist for such purposes, especially in lifestyle and weight loss arenas. Consideration of a multi-disciplinary team approach makes sense and is a recommendation for successful implementation as well as coordination with the primary physician and relevant engaged subspecialist (cardiology, endocrinology for type 2 DM, rheumatology) if part of the health care team.

IMPLANTS AND STEROIDS

The issues of implants, infection, and their failures follow similar patterns, as has been discussed with respect to total joint replacements in RA and SLE patients in the literature.

The literature, unfortunately, compares many heterogeneous types of populations with varying doses of steroids and patients with many other comorbidities which often makes it difficult to extrapolate the effects of only the steroid dose for specific patient types. This is especially true in retrospective data sets and meta-analysis, which therefore lend themselves towards type 2 errors statistically. What can be said, however, is that again, the higher the dose of steroids and the longer the patient has been on them, the more the risk. Identifying several factors may be highly relevant in selecting or de-selecting patients for interventions. These include Vitamin D deficiency and insufficiency. Deficiency defined as serum levels less than 30 ng/ml and insufficiency as 30–40 ng/ml. Optimal levels depending upon who is speaking, as there is no global consensus, will range between 45 and 65 ng/ml. Epidemiologic data in 2010 in the USA describes that for 60,000 TKAs the "most common causes of revision TKA were infection (25.2%) and implant loosening (16.1%)" [10]. My contention is that loosening is either primary prosthetic failure or primarily bone failure to hold the prosthetic device/implant in place for the required biomechanical loads. While there may be many causes of these failures, the lack of adequate bone matrix is potentially remedial to a point and should be targeted by optimization of the Vitamin D level and supplementation with high-quality absorbable calcium (such as microcrystalline hydroxyapatite, magnesium as glycinate or malate, phosphorous, and Vitamin K2 to enhance bone calcification and not extra-articular bone deposits in soft tissue or the vascular tree.) The amount of Vitamin D required will depend on the serum levels of the patient and their pre-treatment level, GI absorption, and body size as well as their genomics with respect to vitamin D receptor binding affinities and ranges between 2,000 and 10,000 IU daily are not uncommon to attain the required goal. Monitoring of Vitamin D levels by the orthopedist, rheumatologist, internist, or primary care physician needs to occur to optimize levels as discussed. Implanting patients with prosthetics of any type and not correcting Vitamin D levels predisposes to potential bone, graft, or prosthetic loosening. Loosening accounts for 16% of infections in this large retrospective analysis. Careful preoperative planning and patient selection helps reduce this risk, in theory, and makes sense as good medicine given current knowledge of insufficiency spontaneous fractures, osteoporosis, athletics, and the like in Vitamin D deficient individuals.

HEALTH TEAM INTERVENTIONS AND PREOP CONSIDERATIONS

Patient goals to reach healthier body composition for general health, decreasing other comorbidities associated with obesity including hypertension, cardiovascular disorders, and type 2 DM are the tip of the ice berg as to *why* optimizing body composition is important for the orthopedic and arthritis patient. For the operative candidate patient, this is even more essential and more of a time line priority. A professional team approach makes sense with a nutritionist or dietician, physical therapist, medical physician and orthopedist specialist, and when possible a psychosocial care specialist/ health coach to achieve optimal preoperative condition. This team approach enhances the patient journey and compliance and improves value by raising expectations and discovering potential hindrances and blocks as to *how* an individual patient will execute lifestyle changes and weight loss and have enough resources preop and postop to comply with what is asked. Patients with chronic illnesses like RA, SLE, chronic OA, and pain, often have anxiety and depression as well which can further impact their care negatively. These individuals have higher risk, more complications, use more emergency resources, and in the RA population have a higher mortality. For these reasons, quick psychosocial and pain and depression screening are an important aspect of the whole person care approach to identify higher risk individuals before surgery is contemplated. Doing so allows the health care team to prepare, correct, educate, and support the patient's needs and enhance their journey and improve rendered care value. This is part of improving the value proposition, a current mandate of The Patient Protection and Affordable Care Act.

DIET AND NUTRITIONAL INTERVENTIONS

Dietary and nutritional interventions have become an important aspect of patient care in all specialties. The current rise in obesity as a global epidemic will increase health care costs, morbidity and premature mortality across a wide patient population if changes are not reversed. The current fast food diet in the United States, dubiously termed the standard American diet or known by its acronym the SAD diet, is high in sugar, processed carbohydrates, and unhealthy types of fats (trans). This dietary pattern is highly pro-inflammatory and as such increases systemic inflammation. This situation can further increase inflammatory cytokines including TNF Alpha, Interleukin 6, and other pro-inflammatory signaling molecules. Their effect on an individual increases pain, inflammation, and dysfunction of endothelial functions leading to the earliest hypertension cardiovascular physiologic defect. Left unchecked, metabolic syndrome, insulin resistance, elevated lipids and inflammatory markers (CRP), and blood vessel markers for inflammation (Lp-PLA2, MPO) all increase. The net effect here is that left unchecked, this silent inflammation is the main health threat resulting in blood vessel inflammation with enhanced risk of stroke, heart attack, and sudden death. For the arthritis patient, this cascade generally means more pain from inflammatory arthritis such is the case in RA but it is also a factor for the osteoarthritis patient. For the orthopedic surgeon, caring for patients with inflammation increases the risk of complications from a cardiovascular standpoint and will possibly cause more pain, potentially resulting in poorer postop results due to pain and more inflammation at healing sites. Therefore, addressing diet preoperatively is beneficial from this standpoint and also has additional benefits in avoidance of or reduction in chronic meds for hypertension and cardiovascular disease and Type 2 Diabetes, which may have untoward metabolic side effects. Once again there is no single dietary plan that is best for everyone but an anti-inflammatory diet (such as the Mediterranean diet) has been found to be effective, appropriately balanced for the general population, and recommended for wider use as a viable option [11, 12]. While other nutritional dietary patterns exist, and may be more appealing to individual patients, such as the Paleo diet, where eliminating grains, dairy, nutritional products of industry and sticking to an ancestral hunter-gatherer dietary pattern of "eating what you can catch, fish, or gather" including legumes, nuts, seeds, fish, fowl, and occasional meats is the general theme [13]. In contrast, the more restrictive carbohydrate, South Beach diet, changes metabolism from carbohydrate sugar-based energy to relying on healthy fats and lean protein resulting in fat loss, body composition benefits, and significant weight loss if adhered to diligently and coupled with lifestyle changes. For the Mediterranean diet, ample scientific references abound including reduction in cardiovascular markers and inflammatory markers [14]. Since chronic disease is driven by inflammation, the balance of macronutrients and omega-6 and omega-3 fatty acids in an anti-inflammatory Mediterranean diet can alter the expression of inflammatory genes. In particular, the balance of the protein to the glycemic load of a meal can alter the generation of insulin and glucagon further influences how the balance of omega-6 and omega-3 fatty acids affect eicosanoid formation and other inflammatory mediators to amplify or downregulate. One pathway to overcome silent inflammation requires an anti-inflammatory diet with omega-3s and polyphenols abundant in veggies and fruits and other anti-oxidant rich super foods. The most important aspect of such an anti-inflammatory diet is the stabilization of insulin and reduction in intake of omega-6 fatty acids. The ultimate treatment lies in reestablishing hormonal and genetic balance to generate satiety instead of constant hunger. Anti-inflammatory nutrition, balanced macronutrient ratios of carbohydrate: healthy fats: lean protein in a ratio of 40:30:30 in conjunction with caloric restriction, should be considered as a form of gene-silencing lifestyle approach that deals with silent inflammation. In addition to this foundation, supplemental omega-3 fatty acids at the level of 2–3 g of eicosapentaenoic acid (EPA) and docosahexaenoic acid (DHA) per day is recommended to optimize the omega-3 to omega-6 fatty acid ratios in vivo and measurable by commercial labs today. Additionally, the Mediterranean diet has been established as an effective intervention for cardiovascular primary prevention as cited in 2013 in the *NEJM* by Ramon Estruch, MD, PhD and colleagues [11]. They state that "The traditional" Mediterranean diet is characterized by a high intake of olive oil, fruit, nuts, vegetables, and cereals; a moderate intake of fish and poultry; a low intake of dairy products, red meat, processed meats, and sweets; and wine in moderation, consumed with meals. In observational cohort studies and a secondary prevention trial (the Lyon Diet Heart Study), increasing adherence to the Mediterranean diet has been consistently beneficial with respect to cardiovascular risk. A systematic review ranked the Mediterranean diet as the most likely dietary model to provide protection against coronary heart disease [14]. Small clinical trials have uncovered plausible biologic mechanisms to explain the salutary effects of this food pattern. In a particular randomized study, a 30% reduction per 1000 at-risk patients was found by following the Mediterranean diet. Therefore, the same type of risk reduction can be expected for the obese inflamed orthopedic joint replacement candidate being evaluated by the academic or hospital-based musculoskeletal interdisciplinary care team or the solo joint reconstruction specialist in a community practice. Irrespective of the clinical setting, engaging and resourcing a care team model makes sense and in this instance the data for clinical benefit is well established. Whatever nutrition plan or diet is chosen, encouragement to make a lifestyle decision rather than a temporary diet should be the preferred mindset to invoke long-term benefit, compliance, and better surgical and health outcomes all around. A diet rich in colorful, non-starchy vegetables that contributes adequate amounts of polyphenols to help not only to inhibit nuclear factor (NF)-κB (primary molecular target of inflammation) but also activate AMP kinase is desirable. Understanding the impact of an anti-inflammatory diet on silent inflammation can elevate the diet from simply a source of calories to being on the cutting edge of gene-silencing technology [15]. Portion control coupled with calorie restriction and this type of high quality nutrient-dense, low glycemic index eating along with adequate hydration (6–10, 8oz glasses of water), elimination of soda and juices containing high fructose corn syrup (HFCS) content are all recommended changes to be made for a healthy lifestyle change. In the end, sugar is sugar, and, if excessive, its biologic effect is generally deleterious or causes insulin spikes. Artificial sweeteners should be added to our list for elimination, as a group they abnormally reset the taste and brain receptors to abnormal levels of desirable sweetness in foods, thereby creating a drive to consume even more sugar or food despite caloric needs. This is another area to address in aiding patients with both weight loss, fat loss, and satiety concerns along with adequate fiber intake, optimally achieved with 3–4 servings of fruits and vegetables per day [16]. (https://www.cdc.gov/nccdphp/dnpa/nutrition/pdf/rtp_practitioner_10_07.pdf). Resources for physicians and patients also exist at: (https://www.cdc.gov/healthyweight/healthy_eating/index.html) [17].

Unfortunately, even healthy eating may not eliminate or ensure that micronutrient vitamin and mineral deficiencies do not exist. For individuals with inflammation, adequate Vitamin D3 to maintain optimal range levels between 30 and 50 ng/ml is recommended by experts in the field including AACE [18] although no global consensus exists. The IOM recommendation for Vitamin D [19] for adults is 800 IU daily which is profoundly inadequate for active RA and SLE patients who have active systemic inflammation. The AACE recommendations for optimal levels and my 25-year experience with inflammatory patients as a whole point to the higher recommended level of 50 ng/ml as a more desirable treatment goal. Patients with obesity, type 2 DM, chronic gout, chronic pain, elevated CRP for any reason, or vascular inflammatory markers and endothelial markers of dysfunction all require higher levels of Vitamin D intake due to upregulation of inflammatory cytokines and signaling. Vitamin D has a beneficial effect on gene silencing and effects on both innate and adaptive immunity have been well established, including enhanced phagocytosis and chemotaxis in innate immunity and for adaptive immunity, expression of the nuclear VDR with inhibition of pro-inflammatory TH1 responses including gamma interferon, TNF Alpha and direct interleukin suppression consistent with T-regulatory cell function responses [20]. The IOM recommendations are solely for bone health and of marginal benefit to the population of rheumatic patients. For this reason, Vitamin D3 should be dosed according to the patient individual needs and may vary from 1,000 IU daily up to 10,000 IU daily and in rare instances higher. Experts in Vitamin D have recommended the concept "go low and slow approach" with lower daily divided doses rather than single high-level dosing. Additionally, the Endocrine Society recommended a much, much higher minimum blood level of Vitamin D. The society's clinical practice guideline was developed by experts in the field assigned to a Vitamin D Task Force, and they concluded: "Based on all the evidence, at a minimum, we recommend Vitamin D levels of 30 ng/mL, and because of the vagaries of some of the assays, to guarantee sufficiency, we recommend between 40 and 60 ng/mL for both children and adults." [21] In any case, only blood monitoring will ensure that safe and adequate levels of Vitamin D3 are maintained (optimal range 40–60 ng/ml) in addition to metabolic bone parameters including calcium, phosphorous, and magnesium and in osteopenia or osteoporotic patients, bone turnover markers (serum CTX or urinary NTX) are also monitored. Furthermore, 1,000–1,500 mg of elemental calcium, 250–500 mg of magnesium and phosphorous combination along with adequate Vitamin D (1,000–10,000 IU daily) is supportive of bone, cartilage, muscle, and nervous system functions. From a GI perspective, the mucosa is also benefited by all of the above minerals and Vitamin D along with Vitamin A as water-soluble beta carotene 10,000 IU daily with mixed carotenoids. Vitamin A is essential for barrier function epithelial skin, respiratory, GU and GI function [22].

In the orthopedic candidate, this is crucial to reduce potential portals of entry for infection and improving innate immunity function. We have focused on the obese and overweight patient, but patients with chronic diarrhea for any reason and very low BMI would definitely benefit from both Vitamin D and Vitamin A supplementation for all of the above reasons. L-glutamine and anti-inflammatory botanicals such as curcumin (1,000–2,000 mg twice daily) and Boswelia Serrata (100–250 mg twice daily) are other important supplements and nutraceuticals worth mentioning. All of these benefit the GI tract and by inference support a healthy microbiome which plays a role in immunity, ability to fight infection and ongoing inflammation, or silencing of pro-inflammatory cascades. In so doing, normal physiologic and metabolic functions are supported and if we help the microbiome, it, in turn, helps maintain health and improve recovery. Hence probiotics should be administered with routine antibiotic use to maintain beneficial commensal bacterial diversity and numbers. Both are needed. Which probiotic to recommend remains controversial and without uniform opinion as the data and studies are thus far insufficient for specific recommendations. High quality probiotics containing *Lactobacillus* and *Bifidobacterium* species make good clinical sense. VSL#3 has some reported outcome data in treating mild to moderately severe ulcerative colitis but in too small numbers to make generalized recommendations for all-comers and varied clinical scenarios [23]. Stool transplants have been utilized clinically in cases of severe microbiome disturbances including managing refractory *Clostridium difficile* superinfection, especially in a hospital setting. This technology is in its infancy and seems a bit too extreme for the average situation and preventative measures. Further research and data in this arena are pending and clearly will have a role in select situations. As a general recommendation for patients it makes sense that besides healthy eating, the use of a probiotic along with prebiotic foods (fermented foods such as sauerkraut, pickled ginger, pickles, and others) makes good clinical sense to recommend to patients to support the microbiome. Stress reduction techniques including mindfulness are recommended along with breathing techniques and exercise as part of a comprehensive stress reduction program. It has been shown that these activities have a positive impact on the immune system, help reduce inflammation, and help to reduce chronic pain. Furthermore, using mind–body exercises such as guided imagery as part of a preoperative and postoperative care has been established as beneficial in mainstream medicine including academic centers for cancer treatments. The same may be applied to orthopedics, healing, and utilizing the mind–body connection to enhance patient experience.

MANAGEMENT OF DMARDS AND BIOLOGICS IN ORTHOPEDICS

DMARD management in general medicine is an area of need in terms of clarification and simplification holding true for the practicing orthopedist. The medical pharmacologic management of the rheumatology patient is becoming more and more complex, however, some guiding principles will clarify the relevant points to be focused upon. For ease of use, we will use the lenses of the preoperative, intraoperative, and postoperative time periods as the pertinent natural reference points to base our discussion of these class of meds. Also, certain DMARDS are much less or hardly used depending on training or prescribing habits of the rheumatologist and the frequency of the rheumatic disease being treated. An example of this would be D-penicillamine, a drug much less utilized now than 15–25 years ago when it was used for both RA and scleroderma or progressive systemic sclerosis (PSS). Current treatment paradigms no longer utilize D-penicillamine use for RA since so many other DMARD and biologic agents including newer small molecule oral biologics exist or are on the pipeline. The main DMARDs and immunosuppressive drugs currently in use commonly for RA are hydroxychloroquine (Plaquenil), methotrexate (oral or injectable), sulfasalazine (Azulfidine), azathioprine (Imuran), and leflunomide (Arava). DMARDs used more rarely include cyclophosphamide (Cytoxan) and cyclosporin (Sandimmune, Neoral, Gengraf) [24]. The complexity of medical decision-making for the entire musculoskeletal health care team in coordinating total hip arthroplasty (THA) and TKA in both stable and active disease rheumatic patients has been murky, complex, and nonuniform. The proposed 2017 American College of Rheumatology Guideline in its final phase of development streamlines this array of medication management in the RA, PsA (psoriatic arthritis), SLE, AS (ankylosing spondylitis), and JIA (juvenile inflammatory arthritis) patients [25].

Please refer to the guideline document above for specifics on each drug and diagnosis but, for general discussion, understanding the pharmacokinetics and half-life of each drug dictates when to schedule elective surgery. Based on this pharmacology, 4 important points are worth mentioning as per the proposed ACR guidelines:

1. Patients with rheumatic diseases undergoing THA and TKA are at increased risk for periprosthetic joint infection.
2. Appropriate management of antirheumatic medication in the perioperative period may provide an important opportunity to mitigate risk.
3. Nonbiologic disease-modifying antirheumatic drugs may be continued throughout the perioperative period in patients with rheumatic diseases who are undergoing elective THA and TKA.
4. Biologic medications should be withheld as close to 1 dosing cycle as scheduling permits prior to elective THA and TKA and restarted after evidence of wound healing, typically 14 days, for all patients with rheumatic diseases.

The recommendations are focused on THA and TKA and not on fractures or spinal surgery or foot and ankle procedures. Questions as to NSAID, corticosteroid management, and methotrexate use in these latter settings still need to be clarified. For this, the orthopedic surgeon, rheumatologist PCP, and the health care team must individualize and coordinate care to establish the best individual decision making. For THA and TKA, however, we now have more specific recommendations that may serve as a background with which to help base future decision making. "Withhold all current biologic agents prior to surgery in patients undergoing elective THA or TKA, and plan the surgery at the end of the dosing cycle for that specific medication" as per the guideline proposal and follow the specific drug recommendation for each drug as listed in Table 26.1.

Specific examples include adalimumab which is dosed every 2 weeks and therefore elective orthopedic surgery for THA and TKA should be booked during week 2–3 *after the last dose*. For

TABLE 26.1

ACR Proposed 2017 Guidelines for Perioperative Management of Antirheumatic Meds

DMARDs: *continue* these Medications through surgery	Dosing Interval	Continue/Withhold
Methotrexate	Weekly	Continue
Sulfasalazine	Once or twice daily	Continue
Hydroxychloroquine	Once or twice daily	Continue
Leflunomide (Arava)	Daily	Continue
Doxycycline	Daily	Continue
Biologic agents: *stop* these medications prior to surgery and schedule surgery at the end of the dosing cycle. *resume* medications at minimum 14 days after surgery in the absence of wound healing problems, surgical site infection, or systemic infection	**Dosing Interval**	**Schedule Surgery (relative to last biologic agent dose administered) during**
Adalimumab (Humira)	Weekly or every 2 weeks	Week 2 or 3
Etanercept (Enbrel)	Weekly or twice weekly	Week 2
Golimumab (Simponi)	Every 4 weeks (SQ) or every 8 weeks (IV)	Week 5 and 9
Infliximab (Remicade)	Every 4,6, or 8 weeks	Week 5, 7, or 9
Abatacept (Orencia)	Monthly (IV) or weekly (SQ)	Week 5 and 2
Certolizumab (Cimzia)	Every 2 or 4 weeks	Week 3 or 5
Rituximab (Rituxan)	2 doses 2 weeks apart every 4–6 months	Month 7
Tocilizumab (Actemra)	Every week (SQ) or every 4 weeks (IV)	Week 2 and 5
Anakinra (Kineret)	Daily	Day 2
Secukinumab (Cosentyx)	Every 4 weeks	Week 5
Ustekinumab (Stelara)	Every 12 weeks	Week 13
Belimumab (Benlysta)	Every 4 weeks	Week 5
Tofacitinib (Xeljanz): STOP this medication 7 days prior to surgery	Daily or twice daily	7 days after last dose
Severe SLE-specific medications: *continue* these medications in the perioperative period	**Dosing Interval**	**Continue/Withhold**
Mycophenolate mofetil	Twice daily	Continue
Azathioprine	Daily or twice daily	Continue
Cyclosporinc	Twice daily	Continue
Tacrolimus	Twice daily (IV and PO)	Continue
Not severe SLE: *discontinue* these medications 1 week prior to surgery	**Dosing Interval**	**Continue/Withhold**
Mycophenolate mofetil	Twice daily	Withhold
Azathioprine	Daily or twice daily	Withhold
Cyclosporins	Twice daily	Withhold
Tacrolimus	Twice daily (IV and PO)	Withhold

etanercept (Enbrel), a weekly-dosed TNF biologic self-injectable, schedule surgery during week 2 according to the guideline. For medications with much longer half-lives with variable dosing regimens such as infliximab (Remicade), the recommendation for surgery schedule mirrors this variability in dosing but recommends the surgery 1 week *after the last dose*. For example, dosing infliximab every 4 weeks leads to a surgery scheduled during week 5 after the last dose; for every 5 weeks, schedule surgery during week 6; for every 8 weeks dosing, surgery should be scheduled during week 9 after the last dose of infliximab. For general DMARDS such as methotrexate, Plaquenil, sulfasalazine, and leflunomide, the drugs may be continued through the operative period without discontinuation.

The guideline also discusses specific situations for patients with SLE who are stable or *not* severe. For these SLE patients, withhold the current dose of mycophenolate mofetil, azathioprine, cyclosporine, or tacrolimus 1 week prior to surgery in all patients undergoing THA or TKA. However, for severe SLE continue the current dose of methotrexate, mycophenolate mofetil, azathioprine, cyclosporine, or tacrolimus through the surgical period in all patients undergoing THA or TKA.

MANAGEMENT OF CORTICOSTEROIDS INTRAOPERATIVELY

This has been an area of further debate, confusion, and some degree of clinical inconsistency in management of the rheumatic patient. In general, the weight gained by corticosteroid use is sometimes lost, but the body composition at the lower weight is almost always changed. The set-up for sarcopenia is as daunting as the obesity. Having mentioned this fact, the management of corticosteroids by the orthopedist as per the guideline proposal are to be handled in the following manner:

> "For RA, SpA including AS and PsA, or SLE: Continue the current daily dose of glucocorticoids in patients who are receiving glucocorticoids for their rheumatic condition and undergoing THA or TKA, rather than administering perioperative supra-physiologic glucocorticoid doses (so-called "stress dosing"). The literature review found information on hemodynamic instability in a systematic literature review on patients with rheumatic diseases whose mean prednisone (or equivalent) dose was < or =16 mg/day. The CDC considers the cut-off for immunosuppression at 20 mg of prednisone/day for at least 2 weeks, and observational studies demonstrate an increase in arthroplasty infection risk with long-term steroid use >15 mg/day. Optimization for THA and TKA should include carefully tapering the glucocorticoid dose prior to surgery to <20 mg/day, when possible." This recommendation does not refer to JIA patients receiving glucocorticoids who may have been treated with glucocorticoids during childhood developmental stages, or to patients receiving glucocorticoids to treat primary adrenal insufficiency or primary hypothalamic disease. Low-quality RCT evidence (rated down for indirectness due to varying glucocorticoid doses, heterogeneity of surgical procedures, and imprecision due to small numbers) and evidence from observational trials summarized in a systematic review suggested that there was no significant hemodynamic difference between those patients given their current daily glucocorticoid dose compared to those receiving "stress-dose steroids" [26].

IMMUNOTHERAPY AND CHECKPOINT THERAPY

Immune checkpoint therapy, which targets regulatory pathways in T cells to enhance antitumor immune responses, has led to important clinical advances and provided a new weapon against cancer. This therapy has elicited durable clinical responses and, in a fraction of patients, long-term remissions where patients exhibit no clinical signs of cancer for many years [27]. The associated complications of this very promising approach to cancer therapies have been reviewed and include neurologic and dermatologic, including some life threatening such as Sweet's syndrome, Stevens-Johnson syndrome, immune endocrinopathies, and sometimes death [28]. These complications will be seen in increasing numbers as this technology continues to expand and both orthopedic surgeons and rheumatologists need to become familiar with this broad variety of secondary disorders that are sometimes life threatening, appearing in about 15% of a nearly n = 500 patient cohort treated with PD-1 blockade [29]. Digital or extremity amputations may be needed in situations of superinfection or vascular compromise as a direct result of this form of therapy. Skeletal physicians will be called upon as the numbers of patients rises utilizing checkpoint immune therapies in oncology.

THE MICRBIOME IN RHEUMATOLOGY-ORTHOPEDICS

The explosion of science, technology (17S RNA PCR and gene analysis GWAS) and immune system interactions, and revolutionary probes has led to a massive amount of data regarding the microbiome commensals inhabiting the human body and their symbiotic effect on health, metabolism, infection, and cancer. The Human Microbiome Project has been one of the main platforms for this revolutionary science. Understanding the relationships of these beneficial bacterial species and their role in immune trafficking and secondary metabolism has become a priority in rheumatology. Various inflammatory types of arthritis, specifically RA and the spondyloarthropathy are being studied extensively in this regard. Approximately 18 months ago, Shur and his group published a breakout paper on this topic delivering specific correlations between rheumatic disease (RA, PsA, AS, Reiters), microbiome imbalance, and specific bacterial imbalance detected along with a corresponding cytokine signature. This coordination of science tracking the microbiome alterations within disease specificity and ascribing the secondary immune response may lead to a therapeutic needed to approach these inflammatory conditions from another perspective. This concept is not new. Functional medicine, other non-primary immunologists, gastroenterologists, and mainstream medicine players have promoted microbiome interventions for quite a while before the science was developed as it is now. The gap between the clinical observations and the research science is now closing [30]. It is now recognized that more than 100 trillion cells inhabiting our human bodies are rather prokaryotic in nature. At any given time, we carry 3–6 pounds of bacteria that contain roughly 3 million protein-coding genes [31].

While a diverse number and type of probiotics exist in the marketplace for our consumer patients, the data is missing for this degree of specificity to be aligned with specific conditions that are generally marketed. This does not mean they are of no benefit, but it does mean that the consumer and physician, are not 100% clear on best probiotic choice, for specific conditions including routine maintenance, preop, postop, etc. The general literature on probiotics has included very few good studies to clarify the aforementioned questions. One probiotic for which there is some literature is VSL#3 that contains ample numbers of colonies and was found effective in an IBD population but in small numbers. Research on wider disease entities utilizing advanced probes and genomic typing is needed to answer the many questions regarding probiotic use, their indication, efficacy, types and bacterial commensal variety, and specificity required in various clinical settings. Studies on the use of probiotics at present have been too small in number to make general recommendations in RA and spondyloarthropathy are not yet possible [32]. Also, it has been confusing to make specific probiotic recommendations to all comers as the science has been unclear as is the case of *Lactobacillus* in 2 animal model examples, hence more study and clarification is required. Implementation of therapy with single-strain live organisms leading to a modification of the host microbiome composition that does not depend on fecal microbial transplantation is an area of investigation. Several animal studies have demonstrated successful treatment of autoimmune manifestations with this methodology, including amelioration of IBD by either *Bacteroides fragilis* [33] or a cocktail of *Clostridia* [34] through induction of colonic Treg cells. This is in contrast to the pro-colitogenic and pro-arthritogenic effects of *Bacteroides* in HLA–B27–transgenic rats and the detrimental role of *Lactobacillus* in adjuvant-induced arthritis in some rat models contrasted with a beneficial effect of *Lactobacillus* strains in other studies. Still, the evidence that probiotics have therapeutic value in RA is scarce. Most studies conducted so far are rather small and usually show modest or no effect [30]. This notwithstanding, the orthopedic surgeon or musculoskeletal health care team can recommend some general principals to their patients. These include consuming a healthy diet as has already been discussed such as a plant-based, high fiber, low refined sugar, moderate protein, low glycemic index, and containing healthy fats such as omega-3 from nuts, seeds, oily fish, avocado, and omega-3 olive oil. Additionally, consuming prebiotic foods supports the microbiome and should be part of the nutritional pattern.

Fermented foods were previously mentioned and they support the commensal balance and are also very important. These include sauerkraut, keifer, yoghurt, and pickled foods such as ginger, herring, and pickles. If antibiotics are prescribed, concurrent prescription of probiotics makes good clinical sense both preoperatively and postoperatively to help mitigate superinfection and reduce the incidence of GI side effects, *Clostridium difficile*, and other antibiotic related GI effects. In severe situations, the orthopedist may require a more formal or aggressive approach to treat or manage GI superinfection in their postoperative patient. The use of stool transplant as an adjunctive therapy is in clinical use as a tool to address and leverage the microbiome-immune interactions in clinical setting refractory to conventional medical therapies as well as to treat IBD. Antibiotic resistant *Clostridium difficile* can be approached through microbiome manipulation and stool transplantation with good results [35].

ORTHOPEDIC-RHEUMATOLOGY COLLABORATION

The patient journey and the patient-centric care model calls for an integrated approach from the relevant health care team for improvement in the patient's experience and better clinical results coupled with increased value and a goal of cost reduction. This is an ACA mandate known as the "triple aim" cited within its legislative health care law of the Patient Protection and Affordable Care Act [36].

That being said, the push–pull that can or has occurred between orthopedics and rheumatology must focus on this unified patient-centric care model. It addresses all aspects of the patient in their journey from diagnosis, to preoperative stages, intraoperative and postoperative care, and convalescence and rehabilitation. The crossover of the orthopedic patient's care to other health care providers, including rheumatology, primary care, or needed subspecialists, plays a role in this journey. However, the entire health care team and anyone who "touches" the patient physically, verbally, or by influence or perception can affect the journey in either a beneficial or detrimental fashion. This, therefore, creates the opportunity to impact patient care through experience. Identification of care barriers is another important aspect of this global approach. Validated research tools now exist to assess patient risk and compliance to potentially very expensive treatments such as joint reconstruction and the specialized postoperative care and rehabilitation required for best outcomes. Patient depression, anxiety, and social situation with work, school, family, or their core life situations may impact compliance or ability to comply with treatment programs. A lack of understanding by any of the health care team providers may increase the risk of failure or non-compliance in certain regards. Identifying these patients proactively through validated care instruments, as has been researched and done by Reiss and others in the IBD space and is now being applied to rheumatology, makes sense for all chronic care subspecialists including orthopedics and joint reconstruction or surgical intervention settings [37].

Finally, interdisciplinary rounds, networking, conferences, and social interactions are all recommended to bolster relationships and discussion relevant to improving and streamlining care and identifying mutual areas of interest for research. In the end, we all want the same thing which is to do right by our patients and create life-enhancing benefits through our craft and professions. *How* we get there may be specialty specific but the *why* should be considered and unified through patient-centric care and the focus on their journey through our realms of specialty care [38].

CONCLUDING CASE STUDY

History of present illness: Mary B is a 59-year-old woman with relatively new onset RA of 8 months duration referred by her PCP and rheumatologist for integrative orthopedic management and evaluation for right knee TKR. She has gone to physical therapy for the right knee pain and OA for 4 months with minimal improvement and had a longstanding history of pain in that joint following a ski injury 15 years prior. The rheumatologist is treating her with various DMARDS including methotrexate 25 mg weekly by injection, Plaquenil 200 mg twice daily, and Remicade 10 mg/kg every 8 weeks and tapering doses of corticosteroids of 5 mg every other day which she required about 3 months ago for a flare prior to her Remicade dose escalation from 5 mg/kg per infusion. She also uses over-the-counter anti-inflammatory meds and Tylenol, and Tramadol for more significant pain. She has trouble sleeping at night due to pain graded at 5–8/10. Mary stand at 5'6". She weighs 195lbs (BHI 31.5). Her waist circumference is 38 inches (BP 138/88).

General Exam: Normal other than increased abdominal visceral fat. Joint and Orthopedic Exam is normal except for her right knee. She has medial and lateral joint line tenderness of the right knee with pain on range of motion and decreased flexion to 90 degrees. Her gait is antalgic due to the right knee and she uses a cane in the left hand for the past 6 months. The right knee demonstrates medial instability, slight warmth, no significant effusion, and no popliteal masses noted. Drawer sign is negative. Both hips and the contralateral knee are normal. Her ankle and foot exam are WNL.

X-rays: confirm bicompartmental advanced degenerative changes of the right knee with near bone-on-bone findings, small osteophytes of the medial tibial plateau, and erosion of the lateral tibial plateau consistent with healed RA erosion.

Diagnostic Ultrasound: confirms a negative power doppler of the right knee, synovial proliferation, intact MCL, LCL, and both medial and lateral meniscus protrusions and degeneration.

Labs: confirm fasting blood sugar 110 mg/dl with HgBA1C 6.5%/ Fasting insulin elevated 40/ RF positive-60 units/ CCP POSITIVE >250 units/ Chemistry: otherwise normal. Liver Profile: normal. Triglycerides elevated 150 mg/dl (normal 60 mg/dl) Vitamin D 3 – 20 ng/ml. CBC reveals normal WBC 6000 with normal differential. HgB 11, Hct 33% with MCV 100 and normal platelets.

What preoperative advice and or *lifestyle* measures would be advisable in Mary's case, based on the clinical history, physical findings, and laboratory results for the following specific areas?

1. BMI
2. Hyperglycemia and insulin resistance, metabolic syndrome
3. Vitamin and/or nutritional deficiencies
4. Referrals
5. Specific dietary plans to consider

When Mary returns 5 months later, she reports diligence in her nutrition and low impact exercise on a stationary bike and swimming. She has lost 27 pounds since the last visit and you coordinate an operative surgical date. Based on her current DMARDS, biologic meds

1. *How would you coordinate her surgical intervention (TKR) relative to the Remicade, Methotrexate and Plaquenil DMARD therapies?*
2. You learn that Mary is off steroids and are quite pleased. *How do you manage and plan for corticosteroid recent use in the perioperative and operative day?*

CASE ANSWERS: LIFESTYLE

1. BMI: while there is no singular perfect diet or nutritional plan for everyone, the *anti-inflammatory Mediterranean diet* meets many individual patients needs for both weight loss and improvement in inflammatory mechanisms as well as being effective in hypertension, type 2 DM, and cardiovascular prevention. Combining some degree of processed carbohydrate restriction and low impact exercise if possible would be the best scenario.

2. Hyperglycemia and insulin resistance, and metabolic syndrome: can all be addressed through a carbohydrate-restrictive plant-based diet.

3. Vitamin D: correcting Vitamin D deficiency is an important aspect of integrative rheumatology and orthopedic care. Doing so preoperatively is even more important to ensure optimal bone healing, metabolism, and improved immune function overall. Dosing Vitamin D3 tailored to individual patient needs, weight requirements, and their response as measured by serial blood monitoring is the recommended best practice. Optimal serum levels of 40–60 ng/ml are desirable and achievable with various regimens outlined within the chapter. Pharmacologic dosing of 50,000 units weekly for 1–3 months followed by oral daily dosing of 2,000 to up to 10,000 units daily single dose or split 2–3 (*bid* or *tid*) daily are possible treatment routes. Using lower doses and slowly correcting deficiency utilizing multiple dosing regimens is recommended by some experts as noted in the chapter. In all instances, serum determinations of D, calcium magnesium, phosphorous, and PTH and urinary calcium if a history of stone formation is elicited are all recommended. Coordination of this care with an integrative rheumatologist or PCP is advised for this type of detailed care.

4. *Omega-3, EPA/DHA, probiotics, B12 Vitamins, L-5-methyltetrahydrofolate, curcumin,* and *boswelia* are all recommended to be considered for use in this RA patient with OA, chronic pain, and metabolic syndrome.

COORDINATION OF DMARDS AND BIOLOGICS

Based on the proposed ACR Guidelines the following is recommended:

1. Remicade—infusions every 8 weeks. Book surgery week 9
2. Methotrexate oral or injectable—continue through surgery
3. Plaquenil—continue through surgery
4. Corticosteroids—this patient was on low-dose alternate day prednisone 5 mg every other day. She was tapered off steroids since her last visit with you. General medical clearance and rheumatology clearance preoperatively are done. The patient exhibits no sign of adrenal insufficiency and has normal BP. No intraoperative corticosteroids are indicated as per the guideline proposal. Note, however, that individual patients may require more in-depth evaluation, cortisol determinations, endocrine evaluations for further adrenal cortical and pituitary axis evaluations. Proposed guidelines are not to supplant good clinical decision-making in individual situations or patient needs but rather be used as general guides only.

REFERENCES

1. McKay, L.I. et al., Physlogic and Pharmacologic effects of Croticosteroids, https://www.ncbi.nlm.nih.gov/books/NBK13780/.
2. Huang EY, et al., Using corticosteroids to reshape the gut microbiome: Implications for inflammatory bowel diseases. *Inflamm Bowel Dis*, 2015; 21(5): 963–972.
3. Buttgereit F, et al., Targeting pathophysiological rhythms: Prednisone chronotherapy shows sustained efficacy in rheumatoid arthritis. *Ann Rheum Dis*, 2010; 69(7): 1275–1280.
4. Buttgereit F, et al., Efficacy of modified-release versus standard prednisone to reduce the duration of morning stiffness of the joints in rheumatoid arthritis, (CAPRA-1); a double-blind, randomized controlled trial. *Lancet*, 2010; 371(9608): 205–214.
5. Cutolo M, Seriolo B, Craviotto C, Pizzorni C, and Sulli A, Circadian rhythms in RA. *Ann Rheum Dis*, 2003; 62: 593–596.
6. Stuck, A, et al., Risk of infectious complications in patients taking glucocorticosteroids. *Rev Infect Dis*, 1989; 11: 954–963.

7. Fan PT, Yu DT, Clements PJ, Fowlston S, Eisman J, and Bluestone R, Effect of corticosteroids on the human immune response: Comparison of one and three daily 1 gm intravenous pulses of methylprednisolone. *J Lab Clin Med*, 1978; 91: 625–634.

8. Wallace DJ, et al., Systemic lupus erythematosus—survival patterns. Experience with 609 patients. *JAMA*, 1981; 245: 934–938.

9. Chen J, et al., Risk factors for deep infection after total knee arthroplasty: a meta-analysis. *Arch Orthop Trauma Surg*, 2013; 133(5): 675–687.

10. Bozic KJ, et al., The Epidemiology of Revision Total Knee Arthroplasty in the United States. *Clini Orthop Related Res*, 2010; 468 (1): 45–51.

11. Estruch N, et al., Primary prevention of cardiovascular disease with a editerranean diet. *N Engl J Med*, 2013; 368: 1279–1290.

12. Castro-Quezada I, et al., The Mediterranean diet and nutritional adequacy: A review. *Nutrients*, 2014; 6(1): 231–248.

13. Manheimer EW, et al., Paleolithic nutrition for metabolic syndrome: Systematic review and meta-analysis. *Am J Clin Nutr*, 2015; 102(4): 922–932.

14. Casas R, et al., Anti-inflammatory effects of the mediterranean diet in the early and late stages of atheroma plaque development, *Med Inflammation*, 2017; 2017: 12.

15. Sears B, Anti-inflammatory Diets. *J Am Coll Nutr*, 2015; 34 Suppl 1: 14–21.

16. Centers for Disease Control and Prevention. Can eating fruit and vegetables help people to manage their weight? 2012. www.cdc.gov/nccdphp/dnpa/nutrition/pdf/rtp_practitioner_10_07.pdf

17. Centers for Disease Control and Prevention. Healthy Eating for a Healthy Weight. 2016.www.cdc.gov/healthyweight/healthy_eating/index.html

18. The American Association of Clinical Endocrinologists. The long awaited institute of medicine report on "dietary reference intakes for calcium and vitamin d" was released november 30th and is available. 2018. https://www.aace.com/article/106.

19. National Academy of Sciences. Dietary Reference Intakes for Calcium and Vitamin D. 2010. www.nationalacademies.org/hmd/Reports/2010/Dietary-Reference-Intakes-for-Calcium-and-Vitamin-D.aspx

20. Prietl B, et al., Vitamin D and immune function. *Nutrients*, 2013; 5(7): 2502–2521.

21. Holick MF, et al., Evaluation, treatment, and prevention of vitamin D deficiency: an Endocrine Society clinical practice guideline. *J Clin Endocrinol Metab*, 2011; 96(7): 1911–1930.

22. Villamor E, et al., Effects of vitamin A supplementation on immune responses and correlation with clinical outcomes. *Clin Microbiol Rev*, 2005; 18(3): 446–464.

23. Sood A, et al., Probiotic preparation, VSL#3 induces remission in patients with mild-to-moderately active ulcerative colitis. *Clin Gastroenterol Hepatol*, 2009; 7(11):1202–1209.

24. American College of Rheumatology. Treatments. 2018. www.rheumatology.org/I-Am-A/Patient-Caregiver/Treatments

25. American College of Rheumatology. Perioperative. 2017. www.rheumatology.org/Practice-Quality/Clinical-Support/Clinical-Practice-Guidelines/Perioperative

26. Somayaji R, Barnabe C, and Martin L, Risk factors for infection following total joint arthroplasty in rheumatoid arthritis. *Open Rheumatol J*, 2013; 7: 119–124.

27. Sharma P and Allison, JP, The future of immune checkpoint therapy. *Science*, 2015; 348(6230): 56–61.

28. Calabrese L and Velcheti V, Checkpoint immunotherapy: good for cancer therapy, bad for rheumatic diseases. *Ann Rheum Dis*, 2017; 76(1): 1–3.

29. Zimmer L, et al., Neurological, respiratory, musculoskeletal, cardiac and ocular side-effects of anti-PD-1 therapy. *Eur J Cancer*, 2016; 60: 210–225.

30. Sher J, et al., Review: Microbiome in inflammatory arthritis and human rheumatic disease. *Arthritis Rheumatol*, 2016; 68(1), 35–45.

31. Peterson J, et al., The NIH human microbiome project. *Genome Res*, 2009; 19 : 2317–2323.

32. Alipour B, et al., Effects of Lactobacillus casei supplementation on disease activity and inflammatory cytokines in rheumatoid arthritis patients: A randomized double-blind clinical trial. *Int J Rheum Dis,* 2014; 17: 519–27.

33. Mazmanian SK, Round JL, and Kasper DL, A microbial symbiosis factor prevents intestinal inflammatory disease. *Nature,* 2008; 453:620–625.

34. Atarashi K, et al., Induction of colonic regulatory T cells by indigenous Clostridium species. *Science* 2011; 331: 337 role="italic">–341.

35. Van Nood E, et al., Duodenal infusion of donor feces for recurrent Clostridium difficile. *N Engl J Med*, 2013; 368:407–415.

36. Institute for Healthcare Improvement. IHI triple aim initiative. http://www.ihi.org/offerings/Initiatives/TripleAim/Pages/default.aspx. Accessed March 26, 2016.
37. Reiss M and Sandborn WJ, The role of psychosocial care in adapting to health care reform. *Clin Gastroenterol Hepatol,* 2015; 13(13): 2219–2224.
38. American College of Rheumatology. Managing Your Rheumatic Disease. 2016. www.rheumatology.org/I-Am-A/Patient-Caregiver/Diseases-Conditions/Living-Well-with-Rheumatic-Disease/Managing-Your-Rheumatic-Disease. Accessed March 23, 2016.

Index

5-HT, *see* 5-hydroxytryptamine (5-HT)
8-oxoguanine/8-ohdg, 51–54

A

Acidifying foods, 152
ACS, *see* autologous conditioned serum (ACS)
ADH, *see* antidiuretic hormone (ADH)
Allergenic foods, 152–153
Angiotensin converting enzyme inhibitors, 243
Antipsychotic drug therapies, 218
    5-hydroxytryptamine (5-HT), 218
Autoimmune Arthritis
    corticosteroids, 449
    diet and nutritional interventions, 452–454
    graft and prosthetic failure, 450
    health team interventions and preop considerations, 451–52
    immunotherapy and checkpoint therapy, 457
    implants and steroids, 451
    infection, 450
    management of corticosteroids intraoperatively, 457
    management of DMARDS and biologics, 455–457
    micrbiome in rheumatology-orthopedics, 458–459
    orthopedic-rheumatology collaboration, 459
Autologous blood-derived products, 67–68
    platelet-rich plasma (PRP), 67

B

Biotensegrity
    overview, 93–94
    perspective, 94–108
        bones float and fascia communicates, 99–100
        clinical application, 101–104, 106–108
        diagnostics, 100–101
        interventions, 105
        misframing of anatomy, 95–97
        prolotherapy, 105–106
        tensegrity, 97–99
BMD, *see* bone mineral density (BMD)
BMU, *see* bone remodeling units (BMU)
bone densitometry testing (DXA), 272
bone mineral density (BMD)
    in determination of peak bone mass, 266–267
    due to inflammatory bowel disease, 267
    help in nutrition and bone health, 284–286
    in orthogenomics, 28
    in osteoporosis, 254–257
    in treatment of drug-related sarcopenia, 249–253
    linked with diuretics, 220
    linked with genome-wide association studies, 28
    linked with thyroid replacement drugs, 219

C

Canine tendinopathy, 76–77
CDKN1A, *see* cyclin-dependent kinase inhibitor 1A (CDKN1A)

Celiac disease, 150, 271, 272
Chromophores, 113–116
    green and blue-light, 115–116
    light/heat gated ion channels, 115
    mitochondria, 114
CIRS, *see* chronic inflammatory response syndromes (CIRS)
CK, *see* creatine kinase (CK)
CKD2, *see* cyclin-dependent kinase 2 (CKD2)
clinical diagnosis for sarcopenic obesity, 224–227
    metabolic, 224–225
        decreased dihydroepiandrosterone (DHEA), 225
        decreased sex hormone binding globulin (SHBG), 225
CNV, *see* copy number variation (CNV)
CoQ10, *see* Coenzyme Q10

D

DHA, *see* docosahexaenoic acid (DHA)
DHEA, *see* dehydroepiandrostedione (DHEA)
Diuretics, 220, 243
Drug-related muscular pain
    alteration in metabolism of vitamin D, 220
    antipsychotic drug therapies, 218
        5-hydroxytryptamine (5-HT), 218
    cholesterol-lowering agents, 217–218
    Coenzyme Q10 (CoQ10), 215–216
    corticosteroid, 217
    diuretics, 220
    hormone-dependent cancers, 219
    influenza vaccination, 221
    management of drug-induced musculoskeletal disorders, 221
    mechanisms to induce myopathies, 215–217
    non-steroidal anti-inflammatory drugs (NSAIDS), 218–219
    overview, 215
        creatine kinase (CK), 215
        rhabdomyolysis, 215
        upper limit of normal (ULN), 215
    quinolone antibiotics, 218
    synthetic PTH- forteo, 220
    thyroid replacement drugs, 219
Drug-related sarcopenia
    allopurinol in management of gout, 244
    angiotensin converting enzyme inhibitors, 243
    corticosteroids, 244–245
    diagnosis, 239–240
    diuretics, 243
    epidemiology, 239
    formoterol in the management of asthma, 244
    HMG-CoA reductase inhibitors, 244
    pathophysiology, 240–241
        fatigue-resistant fibers, 240
        insulin like growth factor-1 (IGF-1), 241
    proton pump inhibitors, 245
    psychotropic medications, 245
    risk factors, 241–242

cyclin-dependent kinase 2 (CKD2), 242
cyclin-dependent kinase inhibitor 1A (CDKN1A), 242
dehydroepiandrostedione (DHEA), 242
myogenic differentiation antigen 1 (MYOD1), 242
parathyroid hormone (PTH), 242
retinoblastoma (RB1), 242
vitamin D receptor (VDR), 242
selection of oral antidiabetic drugs, 243–244
treatment, 245–248
DXA, *see* bone densitometry testing (DXA)

E

Emulsifiers, 142–143
EPA, *see* eicosapentanaeoic acid (EPA)

F

Fascial syndromes and musculoskeletal pain
anatomy, 359–360
biotensegrity, 360–361
components, 357–358
extracellular matrix (ECM), 357
low back pain (LBP), 358
diagnosis, 362–363
metabolic pathways, 361–362
therapies, 363
manual, 363
movement, 363
stretch, 363
treatment plans, 365–366
Fatigue-resistant fibers, 240
Formoterol, 244
β2-adrenoceptor-selective agonist, 244
Fractures and Prevent Nonunion healing
normal, 389
delayed, 390
systematic approach
metabolic bone disease, 393
vitamin D deficiency, 393–394
malnutrition, 394–395
diabetes mellitus, 395–396
effect of cigarette smoking, 396
vitamin K, 396
obesity, 396–397
hypoxia, 397
fusion, 397
Functional medicine cure for back pain
antecedents, 370–371
genetic predisposition, 370–371
prenatal and epigenetics, 371
assimilation, 375
biotransformation and elimination, *see* triggers
and mediators
defense and repair, 375–376
energy production and mitochondrial function, 376
structural integrity, 377
transportation/communication, 377
triggers and mediators
micronutrient status, 375
movement, 371–372
relationships and employment, 372
sleep, 372–373
stress, 372
toxins, 373

G

GALT, *see* gut-associated lymphoid tissue (GALT)
GCF, *see* gingival crevicular fluid (GCF)
Gene mutation and gene polymorphisms differences,
21–22
Hemophilia and Cystic Fibrosis, 21
Tay Sachs Syndrome, 21
Gluten-sensitive enteropathy, *see* Celiac disease
Glycosylated hemoglobin/ hemoglobin a1c/hgb a1c/hba1c,
41–44
GWAS, *see* genome-wide association studies (GWAS)

H

HCY, *see* homocysteine (HCY)
Heel pain therapy management
advanced concepts, 354
advanced imagining of plantar aponeurosis, 353–354
case study, 351
functional podiatry approach, 354–355
metabolic considerations, 351–353
pathoanatomical features of plantar fascia, 349–351
Hormone-dependent cancers, 219
HSCRP, *see* high sensitivity c-reactive protein (HSCRP)

I

IAOMT, *see* International Academy of Oral Medicine and
Toxicology (IAOMT)
IBD, *see* Inflammatory bowel disease (IBD)
IMT, *see* Initial military training (IMT)
Inflammatory bowel disease (IBD), 142, 267, 271
Initial military training (IMT), 283
IGF-1, *see* insulin like growth factor-1 (IGF-1)
Inflammatory responses to environmental exposures
beta endorphins and pain, 177–178
biotoxin pathway, 165–169
proopiomelanocortin (POMC), 168
relative risk, 165
vascular endothelial growth factor (VEGF), 169
vasoactive intestinal polypeptide (VIP), 169
chronic inflammatory response syndromes (CIRS),
162–164
cytokines and OA, 172–173
enthesium, 176–177
herniated nucleus pulposus and innate immune
effectors, 170–171
nucleus pulposus cells (NP), 171
platelet derived growth factors (PDGF), 170
microRNA and OA, 173–174
osteoarthritis and VIP, 172
overview, 159–162
pain regulators, 164, 178–179
SP, VIP and CGRP, 178–179
symptoms, 164–165
antidiuretic hormone (ADH), 165
TGF beta-1 and OA, 173
TGF beta-1, smad 2, smad-3, fibrosis and scars, 177
TGF beta-1, tendon injury and repair, 174–176
transcriptomics, 169–170
copy number variation (CNV), 170
Post Lyme Syndrome, 170
transient receptor potential receptors (TRPV1), 179
Influenza vaccination, 221

Irradiation, 150–151
   cold pasteurization, 151
   radura, 151

J

Joint support supplements
   avocado and soybean unsaponifiable residues (ASU), 437
   cetylated fatty acids, 436
   chondroitin sulfate, 434–435
   collagen type II, 435
   devil's claw (*Harpagophytum procumbens*), 439
   glucosamine, 442–444
   hops, 439
   hyaluronic acid, 436
   methylsulfonylmethane (MSM), 435
   niacinamide/vitamin B-3, 437–438
   Scutellaria baicalensis, 439
   strontium, 438
   vitamin C and ascorbic acid, 436–437
   vitamin D, 438–439

M

Mechanisms to induce myopathies, 215–217
Mechanisms for reducing inflammation
   B vitamins, 378–379
   diet, 394
   exercise and movement, 396
   sleep, 379–380
   use of alpha-lipoic acid, 378
   use of bromelain, 378
   use of curcumin, 378
   use of omega-3 oils, 378
Mesenchymal stem cells, 70–73
   adipose-derived MSCs (AdMSCs), 70
   adipose-derived stromal vascular fraction (AdSVF), 70
   bone marrow-derived MSCs (BMSCs), 70
   cytokine licensed, 70
   total nucleated cell count (TNCC), 70
Metabolic interventions for sarcopenic obesity
   clinical case and diagnosis, 224–227, 233–234
      functional, 225–227
      metabolic, 224–225
      ratio of muscle to fat, 227
      structural, 224
   overview, 223–224
      basal metabolic rate (BMR), 223
      body mass index (BMI), 223
   therapies, 227–233
      exercise, 222–223
      protein, 228–229
      protein quality, 229–230
      Time of Protein Intake, 230–232
      weight loss, 232
Microarray studies, 24
Mitochondrial medicine, 13–14
MMA, *see* maxillomandibular advancement (MMA)
MSC, *see* mesenchymal stem cells (MSC)
Muscle injury therapies
   clinical evaluation, 319–321
      classification, 319–320
      predisposing factors, *see* Predisposing factors of muscle injury

phases of muscle recovery, 321–332
   treatment modalities, 322–332
      physical, 322
MYOD1, *see* myogenic differentiation antigen 1 (MYOD1)

N

Nanoparticles, 151–152
Nanotechnology, 12–13
NAS, *see* noncaloric artificial sweeteners (NAS)
NP, *see* nucleus pulposus cells (NP)
NSAIDS, *see* non-steroidal anti-inflammatory drugs (NSAIDS)

O

Omega 3 test, 51
   docosahexaenoic acid (DHA), 51
   eicosapentanaeoic acid (EPA), 51
Osteoporesis
   metabolic syndromes, 263
   pathophysiology, identification, 264–272
      by decreased mineral availability, 266–267
      by decreased osteoblast activity, 268–269
      by impaired protein metabolism, 270–271
      by increased osteoclast activity, 268–269
      by peak bone mass determination, 266–267
      by systemic inflammation, 271
      by uncertain etiologies, 271–272
   patient evaluation, 272–274
      by imaging studies, 272–273
      by laboratory diagnosis, 272
      by physical exam, 272
      by use of biomarkers, 274
   physiology, identification, 272–275
      through bone-building nutrients, 265–266
      of bone morphogenetic proteins (BMP) 2 and 4, 264
      by intervention trials, 264
      by osteoclastic activity, 263
   treatment, 274–276
      through caffeine intake, 274
      through calcium intake, 274
      through fiber intake, 274
      through isoflavones intake, 276
      through nutritional supplements, 275–276
      through vitamin C intake, 274
Oral antidiabetic drugs, 243–244
   sodium glucose co-transport inhibitors (SGLT2), 244
Orthobiologics, 3
   platelet-rich plasma (PRP), 3–7
      clinical applications, 5–7
      limitations, 7
      preparation, 4–5
      working process, 3–4
Orthobiologics clinical tips, 11
Orthogenomics, 14–15
   Single nucleotide polymorphisms (SNP), 14
Orthogenomics, genome-directed therapies
   candidate gene studies and molecular mechanism, 23–24
   co-morbidities, 27–28
   construction of clinician's genomic tool box, 24–31, 30–31
      monogenic, 25–27
      polygenic, 27

gene mutation and gene polymorphisms differences, 21–22
  Hemophilia and Cystic Fibrosis, 21
  Tay Sachs Syndrome, 21
genome-wide association studies (GWAS), 24, 28–29
  receptor activator of nuclear factor-kappa B ligand (RANKL), 30
identification of gene polymorphisms linked to osteoarthritis or osteoporosis, 22–23
microarray studies, 24
osteoarthritis, 22–23
  DIO2, 23
  GDF5, 23
  SMAD3, 23
osteoporosis, 28
overview, 21
pharmacogenomics, 32–33
  osteoarthritis, 32–33
  osteoporosis, 33
OSA, *see* obstructive sleep apnea (OSA)
OSAS, *see* obstructive sleep apnea syndrome (OSAS)
Osteoarthritis, 22–23
  comprehensive treatment
    pathophysiology, 434
    patient evaluation, 436, *see* Patient evaluation for Osteoarthritis treatment
  DIO2, 23
  GDF5, 23
  SMAD3, 23

P

Pain regulators, 178–179
  SP, VIP and CGRP, 178–179
Parenteral nutrition (PN), 271, 299
Patient evaluation for osteoarthritis treatment
  biomarkers, 422–423
  bone morp hogenic protein, 439
  comorbidities and, 423
  estrogens and menopause, 425
    estrogen replacement, 425
    testosterone, 426
  hormones and, 424–425
  overweight and obesity, 423–424
  risk factors, 423
  treatment
    curcumin, 431–432
    injection therapies, 429
    joint support supplements, *see* Joint support supplements
    NSAID s and NSAID side effects, 427–429
    nutritional therapies, 430
    omega-3 fatty acids, 430–431
    SAM e (S-adenosyl methionine), 431
    stem cell injections, 429–430
    targets, 427
    topical agents, 429
PBC, *see* Primary biliary cirrhosis (PBC)
PBM, *see* Peak bone mass (PBM)
Peak bone mass (PBM), 264
Perioperative metabolic therapies
  application in regenerative medicine, 308
  epidemiology, 293–294
  guidelines for recovery, 294–295

optimization by metabolic agents
  amino acids, 301–305
  antioxidants, 305–306
  hormones, 305
  minerals, 306
  probiotics, 308
  vitamins, 306–307
pharmacology, 295
preoperative patient evaluation
  nutrition-specific laboratory evaluation, 296–297
  physical exam, 295–296
risks involved, 295–297
treatment recommendations
  diet, 297–299
  pain control, 299–301
PDGF, *see* platelet derived growth factors (PDGF)
Periodontal disease
  epidemiology, 185–186
  overview, 185
    pregnancy gingivitis, 185
  pathophysiology, 186
    gingival crevicular fluid (GCF), 186
    heavy metal mercury, 186–187
    reactive oxygen species (ROS), 186
  patient evaluation, 187–188
    International Academy of Oral Medicine and Toxicology (IAOMT), 187
  prevention, 188–189
  treatment, 189
Physical methods for muscle injury treatment
  acupuncture, 325–326
  cryotherapy and heat, 322
  deep heat: ultrasound, 323
  exercise, 326–327
  extracorporeal shock wave therapy (ESWT), 324
  high galvanic electrical stimulation (HVPGS), 323
  massage, 325
  micro-electric nerve stimulation (MENS), 324
  nutritional interventions, 327–329
  orthobiologics
    stem cells, 329–330
    platelet-rich plasma, 330
    musculotendinous junction case study, 330–332
  photobiomodulation (PBMT), 324–325
  superficial heat, 322–323
  transcutaneous electrical nerve stimulation (TENS), 323
Platelet-rich plasma (PRP), 3–7
  clinical applications, 5–7
    ACL reconstruction, 7
    osteoarthritis, 5–6
    rotator cuff injuries, 6
    tendinopathies, 5
  preparation, 4–5
  working process, 3–4
  α-granules, 3
PN, *see* Parenteral nutrition (PN)
"Porous bone," *see* Osteoporesis
POFD, *see* pharyngorofacial disorders (POFD)
POMC, *see* proopiomelanocortin (POMC)
Post Lyme Syndrome, 170
Potobiomodulation therapy
  chromophores, 113–116
    green and blue-light, 115–116

light/heat gated ion channels, 115
    mitochondria, 114
effects on inflammation, 121–124
    autoimmune diseases and T-cells, 123–124
    macrophage phenotype, 123
    NF-kBin normal cells, 121
    reduces levels of pro-inflammatory cytokines, 122
metabolic effects, 116–120
    effects on stem cells, 121
    oxidative stress, 116–119
    synergy with exercise, 119–120
    systemic effects, 121
orthopedics, 128–131
    arthritis, 128–129
    bones, 130
    elbow, 130
    lower back pain, 129
    muscles, 129–130
    shoulder, 130–131
    tendonitis, 129
overview, 113
pain, 127–128
    central, 128
    local inflammatory, 127
    local neuropathic, 128
traumatic brain injury, 124–127
Predictive biomarkers in personalized laboratory
            diagnoses
    8-oxoguanine/8-ohdg, 51–54
    glycosylated hemoglobin/ hemoglobin a1c/hgb a1c/
            hba1c, 41–44
    high sensitivity c-reactive protein (HSCRP), 44–45
        reactive oxygen species (ROS), 44
    homocysteine (HCY), 45–47
    immune tolerance cell cultures lymphocyte response
            assay (LRA), 47–49
    omega 3 test, 51
        docosahexaenoic acid (DHA), 51
        eicosapentanaeoic acid (EPA), 51
    overview, 39
    selection criteria, 40–41
        usual test results *vs.* predictive goal value
            results, 41
    urine pH, 49–50
    vitamin d, 50–51
Predisposing factors of muscle injury
    extrinsic, 320
    hormone balance, 321
    intrinsic, 320
Pregnancy gingivitis, 185
Primary biliary cirrhosis (PBC), 267, 271
Proton pump inhibitors, 245
PRP, *see* platelet-rich plasma (PRP)
PTH, *see* parathyroid hormone (PTH)

Q

Quinolone antibiotics, 218

R

RB1, *see* retinoblastoma
RDA, *see* recommended dietary allowance (RDA)
recommended dietary allowance (RDA) 295

Reduction in orthopedic conditions through
            teledontic treatment
    correcting pharyngorofacial disorders, 204–210
        maxillomandibular advancement (MMA), 208
        surgically assisted mandibular expansion
            (SAME), 208
    metabolic disturbances, 195–204
        clinical considerations, 203–204
        degeneration, 195–197
        musculoskeletal pain, 199–203
        obstructive sleep apnea (OSA), 197–199
    overview, 193
        obstructive sleep apnea (OSA), 193
        obstructive sleep apnea syndrome (OSAS), 193
        pharyngorofacial disorders (POFD), 193
        temporomandibular joint (TMJ), 193
    POFD and biomechanics of musculoskeletal pain,
            193–195
Regenerative immunology, 12–13
    total joint arthroplasties (TJA), 12
Regenerative orthopedics enabled by cross-cutting
            technologies
    orthobiologics, 3
        platelet-rich plasma (PRP), 3–7
    overview, 3
    stem cells, 7–10
        cellular therapy for tissue repair, 8–10
Rhabdomyolysis, 219
ROS, *see* reactive oxygen species (ROS)

S

Safeguard musculoskeletal structures
    acidifying foods, 152
    allergenic foods, 152–153
    clinical costs of food technology, 153–156
        artificial intelligence, 156
        charting the newly connected data points, 153
        collaboration, 156
        food as medical treatment, 155–156
        food as prescribed, 155
        group clinic visits, 156
    emulsifiers, 142–143
    food colorings, 145–146
    GMO enables glyphosates, 150
        genetically modified organisms (GMOs), 150
        Salmonella, 150
    interesterification of fats, 143–145
    irradiation, 150–151
        cold pasteurization, 151
        Radura, 151
    nanoparticles, 151–152
    overview, 141–142
    sweeteners, 146–148
        noncaloric artificial sweeteners (NAS), 147
    ultra-pasteurization and emerging dairy technologies,
            148–150
        gut-associated lymphoid tissue (GALT), 149
        Lactobacilli, 149
        ultra-heat treatment (UHT), 148
SAME, *see* surgically assisted mandibular
            expansion (SAME)
Sex hormones and their impact on sarcopenia and
            osteoporosis

osteoporosis, 254–257
    bone remodeling units (BMU), 255
overview, 251
sarcopenia, 251–254
    Akt, 254
    c-Jun HN2-terminal kinase, 254
    myostatin, 254
    Notch, 254
Stem cells, 7–10
    cellular therapy for tissue repair, 8–10
        bone regeneration, 9
        cartilage regeneration, 9–10
        contraindications, 10
        tendon regeneration, 8–9
    types, 7–8
Stress fracture risk in military personnel
    nutrition and bone health determination
        by calcium and vitamin D, 284–285
        by iron content, 284–285
    pathophysiology and epidemiology, 283–284
    patient evaluation, 288
    prevention by nutritional interventions
        using iron, 286–287
        using calcium and vitamin D, 287–288
Sweeteners, 146–148
    noncaloric artificial sweeteners (NAS), 147

T

Tendinopathy
    clinical presentation and diagnosis, 339–340
    comorbidities, 341–342
    pathology and etiologies, 340–341
    treatment
        frequency specific microcurrent, 343
        injection therapies, 344–345
        low-level laser therapy (photobiomodulation),
            343–344
        physical therapy, 343
        topical treatments, 344
TGF beta-1 and OA, 173
Therapies for sarcopenic obesity, 227–232
    exercise, 232–233
        progressive resistance training (PRT), 233
    protein, 228–229
        acceptable macronutrient distribution range
            (AMDR), 228
        dietary reference intakes (DRI), 228
        estimated average requirement (EAR), 228
        recommended dietary allowance (RDA), 228
    protein quality, 229–232
        essential amino acids (EAA), 229
TMJ, *see* temporomandibular joint (TMJ)
Treatment of back pain
    functional medicine model, 370
        application, 370–377, *see also* Functional medicine
            cure for back pain
    primary care management model, 369–370
    surgical evaluation, 382–384

therapies for
    reducing Inflammation, 378, *see also* Mechanisms
        for reducing inflammation
Treatment for synovitis, degenerative joint disease and
        osteoarthritis
    background, 403–404
    diagnosis, 404
    pathophysiology, 405–406
    conventional nonsurgical management, 406–408
    functional medicine application, 408–409
    lifestyle modification, 409–411
    emerging therapies
        IL-1Ra (interl eukin-1 receptor antagonist protein),
            411–412
        platelet rich plasma (PRP), 412
        mesenchymal stem cells (MSCs), 412
        case study, 413
TRPV1, *see* transient receptor potential receptors (TRPV1)

U

UHT, *see* ultra-heat treatment (UHT)
ULN, *see* upper limit of normal (ULN)
Ultra-pasteurization and emerging dairy technologies,
        148–150
    gut-associated lymphoid tissue (GALT), 149
    Lactobacilli, 149
    ultra-heat treatment (UHT), 148

V

VDR, *see* vitamin D receptor (VDR)
VEGF, *see* vascular endothelial growth factor (VEGF)
Veterinary medicine advances in regenerative orthopedics
    comparative orthopedics, 61–65
        osteoarthritis, 61–64
        tendinopathy, 64–65
    regenerative therapies in veterinary orthopedics,
            77–78
        autologous *vs.* allogeneic use, 78
        stem cell tissue source, 77–78
    overview, 59–61
    regenerative therapies on dogs and horses for
            osteoarthritis, 67–73
        autologous blood-derived products, 67–68
        autologous conditioned serum (ACS), 68
        mesenchymal stem cells (MSC), 70–73
        platelet-rich plasma for osteoarthritis, 69–70
    regenerative therapies on dogs and horses for
            tendinopathy, 73–78
        canine tendinopathy, 76–77
        platelet-rich plasma, 76
        stem cell s for treatment of equine tendinopathy,
            73–75
    species as models for human orthopedic disease,
            65–67
        osteoarthritis, 65–67
        tendinopathy, 67
VIP, *see* vasoactive intestinal polypeptide (VIP)

T - #0881 - 101024 - C488 - 254/178/22 - PB - 9781032094854 - Gloss Lamination